LIFESTYLE MEDICINE
AN INCREDIBLE JOURNEY

LIFESTYLE MEDICINE
AN INCREDIBLE JOURNEY

ANTHONY ARMSTRONG

ISBNs
Paperback: 978-1-80541-343-1
eBook: 978-1-80541-342-4

Disclaimer

This book provides a wide range of health information, but it should not be taken as direct medical advice. It is not intended to be a substitute for the advice of physicians or suitably qualified practitioners and nutritionists when considering prescribed medications, nutritional therapies and other treatments. Neither the publisher nor the author accepts liability for readers who choose to self-prescribe.

All supplements should be kept out of the reach of infants and children.

Preface

Future generations will at some point look back in disbelief at what is unfolding before our very eyes. Despite all the medical advances of the last 100 years, more people than ever before are falling ill with life-taking and life-destroying degenerative, chronic and autoimmune diseases. These can only be classed as epidemics and the increases are so staggering they are almost unbelievable. Below are the UK figures:

- In 1960 1 in 100 11-year-old children were obese. In 2019 the figure was 1 in 5 (a 20-fold increase or 2,000%). In 2022 the figure is now 1 in 4.
- Around 200,000 people had type 2 diabetes 60 years ago. Today the figure is over 4 million and by 2035 it will be 6 million (a 30-fold increase or 3,000%).
- In 1970 1 in 10,000 children were autistic. Today the figure is around 1 in 35 (a 280-fold increase or 28,000%). The numbers continue to increase exponentially every single year.
- Cancer used to affect 1 in 4 people. Today, half of the entire population will develop cancer at some point in their life.
- Half of all children now have at least one chronic disease.
- The number of strokes is projected to increase by a further 60% over the next 20 years.

These are not isolated examples. The number of people suffering from most other diseases are also escalating alarmingly. These range from food allergies, IBS, asthma, infertility, psoriasis, and ADHD to mental illness, Crohn's disease, type 1 diabetes, and Alzheimer's and Parkinson's disease. In addition, the age at which many of them start to develop is also falling every year. Type 2 diabetes, for example, used to affect only people over 60 years of age but today, children as young as eight are developing the disease. The sad fact is very few people know anything about these disease epidemics or that many of the diseases barely existed 60 years ago. But these epidemics are a global human tragedy of immense proportions, and it is happening despite hundreds of years of modern medical research and the trillions of dollars that medicine spends globally each year.

Why are these epidemics occurring? Why are no official organisations exposing them? Why are medicine, governments, regulators and charities not demanding that research be carried out to uncover the reasons? Why are the press and media not alerting the public? The NHS and other health services simply cannot keep up with these incredible increases in disease and cannot treat people effectively. The truth is all this was happening well before the Covid pandemic started, although it has, of course, made things worse. Is there a universal reaction to this medical disaster? Apparently, most people simply believe we just need more doctors, nurses, hospitals and ambulances. But is this a real solution? The truth is simple. The only solution to disease epidemics is to discover their true causes so that prevention becomes the key priority. The problem is medicine simply does not know the causes of nearly all of them and so can do little or nothing to prevent them. When a disease develops, medicine simply starts to use drugs to help minimise symptoms or slow down the rate of decline in health. Cures are only rarely achieved.

However, here is the most amazing fact of all. Most of these chronic life-destroying diseases really can be prevented by simple lifestyle changes. Even when a disease has already developed, lifestyle changes can usually provide better outcomes than drugs and, in many cases, cure or remission is also possible. Of course, there are also infectious diseases like colds, influenza, pneumonia and COVID-19 that cannot be prevented, but even for these diseases, lifestyle changes can radically improve the human immune system and help the body overcome them quickly and with minimal symptoms. This is one of the greatest stories in the history of mankind, but the fact that medicine does not promote lifestyle solutions is also one of the greatest tragedies. If you find all this impossible to believe, the evidence you will see will surprise and shock you. It is a story I have tried to explain to friends and relatives for over ten years. The problem is the entire world has been led to believe over many decades that – with a few exceptions (like smoking and lung cancer) – most diseases are just a normal part of ageing, down to chance or caused by faulty genes, and medicine and the drugs they use are quite simply the only option people have after these "inevitable" diseases develop.

Whenever I tried to explain to friends about the miraculous benefits of lifestyle medicine and how it can prevent or treat disease, it was clear they did not believe any of it could be true because, if it was, their doctor would be telling them about it. Eventually, I realised it was impossible to explain the complex and shocking reasons why medicine continues to ignore effective lifestyle solutions, even in a 30-minute conversation. That is why, five years ago, I wrote a 200-page fact-filled prequel to this book and gave it to a dozen friends to gauge their reaction. Most of these people were "devout disciples" of conventional medicine, so it was very encouraging to receive positive responses and even suggestions on what to do next, like trying to get the book published. Of course, there are some things they still find difficult to believe, but overall the hard evidence clearly struck a chord that caused most of them to rethink some of their original beliefs. They are using several lifestyle changes they would once have ignored or dismissed out of hand and are continuing to do so.

It took 18 months to write the prequel and a further three and a half years to write this book. So, why have I devoted so much of my life to this project? As you will see later, lifestyle medicine has transformed my health and my life. The fact so few people know what is possible must be one of the greatest tragedies in the entire history of the world. My aim is simply to help spread the message that the lifestyle you lead can completely transform both your health and life expectancy and provide people with the evidence to help get them motivated to take control of their own health. Here are just two tantalising examples that will help set the scene on what lifestyle changes can achieve.

A small but increasing number of conventionally trained doctors are using lifestyle techniques with incredible success – the sort of success that medicine can only dream of achieving. For example, medicine has maintained for decades that type 2 diabetes is a disease that cannot be cured. They also know that, even with the best drugs available, patients will still experience a slow inevitable decline which can lead to heart disease, amputations, blindness, kidney disease and liver damage. But this conventional medical dogma is wrong because thousands of doctors across the world are reversing the disease in hundreds of thousands of patients just by changing their diet. One UK surgery alone, which adopted a simple dietary protocol, is saving well over £50,000 each year on diabetes drugs, curing many of its diabetic patients and transforming their health. The NHS spends 10% of its entire budget on treating diabetes, so imagine how many billions of pounds could be saved and how many lives transformed if this protocol was adopted around the country and indeed worldwide. Amazingly, this is not happening, and you will also discover the terrible reasons why.

An increasing number of studies are also revealing incredible variations in life expectancy of over 20 years within geographical regions and social strata of society. These show that not only is a significantly increased life expectancy possible for virtually anyone who knows the "secrets", but that most of the major life-taking and life-destroying diseases like heart disease, cancer and Alzheimer's can be prevented or at least deferred until much later in life. This means not just extra years, but extra years blessed with good vibrant health.

Around 25 years ago, a friend suggested I should read a book about lifestyle medicine that led to a transformation in my health. I believe this book can help do the same for anyone who reads it, because a significantly longer, happier and healthier life is possible for most people.

I hope you take the "incredible journey".

Anthony Armstrong

Contents

Introduction

Around 25 years ago, I was diagnosed with very high cholesterol. A friend suggested that I should read a book called *The 8 Week Cholesterol Cure* and, after eight weeks, doing nothing more than changing my diet and taking a few supplements, the level came down from 7.3 to 5.2. I remember feeling a sense of achievement, but only later did I fully understand how remarkable this outcome was. A typical statin drug at that time reduced cholesterol by about 20% whereas by diet alone I had achieved a 30% reduction. I would possibly have needed two different drugs to achieve the same result and, of course, all drugs have potential side effects whereas changing diet has none.

It was clear just how powerful natural solutions to health could be and this led me on a life-long quest to learn everything I could. I have read nearly 100 books and thousands of articles, papers and studies. Every year I discover new ways to improve my health and I am significantly healthier now than I was 30 years ago which, according to conventional medicine, is almost "impossible". I will be forever grateful to the friend who recommended the book, for not only did it ultimately lead to a transformation in my health, but it also changed my life immeasurably. I want to share with anyone who is interested what I have learnt, so they too can experience the incredible power of lifestyle medicine. The benefits are far reaching. From simply having more energy and love of life, to slashing your risk of most serious diseases and significantly increasing not just your life expectancy, but your healthy life expectancy.

There is, of course, one fundamental problem. Most people reply, "Surely what you say cannot be true. If it was, then my doctor would be telling me about it." So, there are two key questions. Why does your doctor know almost nothing about natural solutions that could transform your health? Why does he or she only use drugs? These are questions I will answer in evidence-based detail. Of necessity, it is a long, deeply disturbing, but ultimately rewarding journey. You will learn about the toxic relationship between the drug industry and medicine. How "Big Pharma" controls charities and patient groups and, in fact, how it has gained almost total control over the entire health agenda. But you will also learn how natural solutions to health can achieve far better outcomes. These are just some of the unbelievable true facts that will surprise and shock you:

- Prescription drugs are the third leading cause of death after heart disease and cancer.
- Fraudulent medical research involving beta blocker drugs caused the deaths of 800,000 people in Europe. Incredibly, this story was subject to almost universal censorship. The researcher responsible was never tried or convicted of any crime. You will discover how it all happened.
- Most of the big killer diseases can be prevented by lifestyle changes. In fact, just one single lifestyle intervention could simultaneously reduce the numbers of people having heart attacks, strokes, diabetes, dementia, Alzheimer's, many types of cancer, depression and premature death by an average of 30%. Absolutely impossible you must be thinking. But before you dismiss this claim out of hand, let me give you the immediate proof. Who says so? Medicine itself. The NHS provides these figures and says, "This is no snake oil. If it were a pill, it would be one of the most cost-effective drugs ever invented." The shocking thing is not that this is all true, but that virtually no one knows anything about it. You will have to wait to find out what it is, and exactly why it has been "suppressed".

- Thalidomide was not just a tragic accident. You will be saddened and appalled by what you read. But you will be even more shocked to learn that since the thalidomide scandal in the 1960s there have been three more drugs that have caused serious deformity or severe learning difficulties in as many as 1 million children.
- The American Heart Association has unequivocally stated that 80% of heart attacks are preventable.
- The American opioid crisis is a drug-induced medical scandal that has so far caused the deaths of 500,000 people. But it has also created incalculable drug addiction and destroyed the lives of many millions. But this is no longer just an "American problem". It is spreading to many European countries and other parts of the world.

The main purpose of this book is to show that simply improving your lifestyle is the best way to stay healthy, live longer and avoid most diseases. To do this logically and with proof, however, I also need to provide a complete overview of all the other key aspects of health, disease and the human body, as well as all the organisations, industries and key individuals involved, plus the main conventional medical treatments. I also need to explore in detail the real reasons why doctors know almost nothing about lifestyle medicine. What you will learn is deeply disturbing. It will shock you to the very core. You will not want to believe it because it will challenge everything you thought you knew about medicine, health and humanity. But please read with an open mind and remember that most of the evidence I give is factual and a matter of public record. I have included all the essential key facts. However, for some aspects, more detailed information is needed and, where necessary, I give recommendations for further reading.

Part 1

Conventional Medicine Versus Lifestyle Medicine

What are the main differences?

Let us start our journey by looking at the main differences between conventional and lifestyle medicine.

Conventional medicine

Apart from a few exceptions, such as vaccination and maternity services, medicine is all about treating sick people. Its two weapons of choice are drugs and surgery. This is how it has worked for around 100 years. People get sick, go to their doctor and hope the treatments they prescribe will help to alleviate their symptoms to bearable levels. Complete cures do not occur very often.

This simple paragraph sums up medicine's overriding approach to treating chronic diseases like cancer, strokes, dementia and diabetes that fill up our hospitals and surgeries. Prevention in the true sense of the word is not seriously on the medical agenda. The ultimate proof of this is the fact that only 1% of all medical research throughout the world is aimed at finding out how to prevent disease. The other 99% is spent on finding drugs and surgical techniques that alleviate symptoms and slow down disease progression. The NHS really should be called the NIS – the National Illness Service.

If you look at any medical textbook and the NHS website, you will see the cause of virtually every disease is listed as unknown, which is not surprising given the derisory amount of research that takes place. But if, as a profession, you do not know the causes of disease, can you really be sure there isn't something that would provide much better results than the drugs and treatments you currently use? Surely if you knew the real causes of disease you could, in many cases, simply prevent it from happening in the first place or provide a real lasting cure. Medicine's absolute priority should be to find the real causes of every disease, but this is not happening. We will come back to this issue many times as we look at different diseases, as well as exploring the shocking reasons for this unscientific approach. Here are just two examples of how you can make huge, devastating mistakes when you do not know the real causes of disease.

Up until around 1950 doctors recommended that patients who had anxiety problems should smoke cigarettes to reduce the symptoms. This may sound impossible to believe now, but medicine had no idea then that tobacco was the main cause of lung cancer or that it increased the risk of heart attacks by at least 100%. It is impossible to know how many people around the world died prematurely from these diseases because of this medical advice, but over the decades it must have been hundreds of thousands and more likely millions.

Stomach ulcers used to affect around 10% of the population of western countries. There were no cures, and they were a major cause of death and suffering. Then around 1990 it was discovered that the main cause was a bacterium. Given that antibiotics were available from around 1950 and that they cured most ulcers in a matter of days, over the next 40 years, millions and probably tens of millions of people died or suffered unnecessarily. All because the true cause of the disease was unknown.

Even today the causes of virtually every disease are still unknown. This really does mean that, around the world, millions of lives are still being lost or destroyed each year, and in Parts 4 and 5 you will see several serious and current examples of this. It is true that tens of billions of dollars are spent on medical research each year, but this is simply to develop drugs that minimise the symptoms of disease. Medicine claims that everything it does is based on science, but if it adopted real science, its absolute priority would be to understand the true causes of every disease and not just treat the symptoms with drugs that have minimal benefits. Only then can you help prevent diseases or develop the best treatments for those that still occur.

Mankind has made incredible progress in understanding every part of the vital science in physics and chemistry. Without this, modern society would not have been able to reap the benefits of technical innovations we often take for granted, like electric lighting, the world wide web and modern transport systems. By comparison, medicine's understanding of the key scientific part of why diseases develop is almost non-existent. Medicine should be embarrassed it has allowed this lack of crucial knowledge to prevail for 100 years, and unless something amazing occurs, it is likely to continue for another 100 years. If a patient ever went to a doctor and asked how they could prevent a disease from happening, the doctor really would be non plussed and probably embarrassed.

Even though medicine knows so little about the causes of disease, it seemingly believes the human body is a frail thing riddled with things like faulty genes and other imperfections and that developing many diseases is, for many people, just a matter of chance and an inevitable part of ageing. Anyone who is healthy now can expect to become unhealthy soon, and the older we become, the more inevitable this is. Medicine claims only drugs and medical procedures can help to slow down this "inevitable" deterioration. These sorts of claims are unscientific and in fact incorrect.

The drugs medicine uses generally disrupt one or more of the body's biological processes. By doing so they may provide temporary relief from some symptoms, but they are actually working against the body's natural processes and functioning. Trillions of finely balanced and interlinked biological processes occur naturally within the body every second. Disrupting one or two of these by using a drug causes a cascade of other unwelcome and often dangerous reactions. This is why drugs cause so many side effects and deaths.

Medicine's modus operandi has spawned huge global industries that include pharmaceuticals, medical equipment, diagnostic testing and medical research. Annual global GDP (the value of everything produced in the world each year) is around $90 trillion. Medicine and the industries that supply it account for about $9 trillion. In other words, around 10% of the world's total GDP is spent on treating sick people. The pharmaceutical industry alone accounts for over $1 trillion. These figures do not include social care costs for the sick and disabled. This medical industrial complex, which controls 10% of global GDP, is, as we will discover, an immensely powerful group. *It* controls governments – not the other way around.

Lifestyle medicine

Lifestyle medicine has one overriding aim which is to prevent people from becoming ill. You can see immediately that this is the ultimate threat to medicine and the powerful industries that supply it, because they rely almost completely on a never-ending stream of sick people.

The human body is the most complex and miraculous thing in the universe and lifestyle medicine's main priority is to understand why diseases occur so they can be treated or prevented in the best ways possible. It simply does not believe that things like biological and genetic imperfections and even ageing automatically lead to disease. Quite simply, disease occurs when the body's natural, finely balanced and interlinked processes, like cell regeneration, detoxification processes and immune function, are compromised by inappropriate environmental and lifestyle factors.

Human evolution has occurred over millions of years and the profound complexity of the body at a cellular level is mind-boggling. Countless operations occur naturally and simultaneously each second, with multiple level feedback layers adding to the complexity. Lifestyle medicine works with nature rather than against it. It looks at the whole body and its entire environment and seeks simply to keep this most remarkable organism in balance and functioning as it has evolved to do. As you will see later, people who live healthy lifestyles with healthy diets really do live much longer and have far less sickness and disease. Of course, there are some things the human body and its natural defence, regeneration and healing mechanisms cannot do. Serious accident victims need modern medical interventions. Type 1 diabetics need insulin. Nevertheless, the human body has the innate ability to prevent or recover from many diseases and infections provided it has the environment and nutrients that allow it to operate optimally. It would indeed be a damning indictment of evolution if this wasn't the case!

To end this section, here is one simple example of how medicine and lifestyle medicine treat the same condition which illustrates the gulf in ideas and treatments. Acid reflux occurs when stomach acid gets through the pyloric valve at the base of the oesophagus. It then moves up the oesophagus causing a burning sensation, heartburn and other unpleasant effects. Stomach acid contains several compounds but the key one is hydrochloric acid, but where does this come from? Quite simply, it is produced by the body. Why does the human body literally manufacture its own hydrochloric acid? Primarily because it is needed as an initial stage in breaking down food so it can be properly digested and absorbed. But it also acts as a potent barrier to dangerous bacteria, viruses and other pathogens and helps to kill them before they can enter the stomach.

Medicine's main weapons for treating acid reflux are antacid drugs and proton pump inhibitor (PPI) drugs. These neutralise much of the stomach acid and can also prevent its formation. For many people, the drugs do indeed provide some short-term relief, but they don't prevent the problem from continually reoccurring. Also, there are some unpleasant side effects, like bloating and indigestion, as well as much more serious ones. For PPI drugs, for example, there is strong evidence that long-term use can, quite shockingly, cause a 50% increase in the risk of developing Alzheimer's, a 20–50% increase in kidney disease and up to a 20% increase in heart attacks. A 2018 study also showed an increased risk of stomach cancer of up to 800% for those taking the drugs for several years. They also increase the risk of pneumonia and other infectious diseases as well as leading to nutrient deficiencies because of poor food digestion which can lead to bone fractures and many other conditions. PPI drugs are also difficult to stop taking because the symptoms of reflux can then return with a vengeance.

Lifestyle medicine takes a completely different approach. The body produces stomach acid for essential reasons, so the priority is not to destroy it. Adopting the key lifestyle factors that are examined in detail in Part 4 really will significantly help to prevent acid reflux from ever starting. They can also reduce its effects and even cure it. However, there are some very specific factors like digestive enzymes, gut bacteria and certain foods that play a crucial role, and for anyone who wants to learn more and wants to avoid taking the very dangerous PPI drugs, I would recommend the book *Improve Your Digestion* written by Patrick Holford.

In summary, lifestyle medicine works with nature rather than against it. It can prevent many diseases from occurring or reoccurring and there are no side effects. Drugs, however, work against the body's natural processes. They do not cure the problem and just minimise symptoms, meaning they often have to be taken indefinitely and they come with a host of side effects, many of them serious and even life-threatening. These are the dominant themes you will see detailed evidence for throughout the book.

What are the strengths and weaknesses of medicine and lifestyle medicine?

Conventional medicine

Modern accident and emergency treatments are remarkable. It is without doubt a true jewel in the crown of medicine. Millions of lives are saved each year around the world because of it. However, whilst accidents and war and violence are, to a large part, unpreventable, many of the other cases that end up in A&E departments, such as heart attacks, are preventable. So, it is true that someone who suffers a heart attack and reaches hospital alive has a much greater chance of surviving thanks to modern medical techniques, but would it not be better to prevent the heart attack in the first place?

Antibiotics deserve the name "wonder drugs". They have saved millions of lives. They used to cure 100% of infected patients, something no other drug has ever come remotely close to replicating. However, largely due to their overuse and abuse, the golden age of antibiotics really is in decline and around 700,000 patients now die each year because of their failures. Some experts predict this will increase to 10 million by 2050. In addition, research also now shows they have previously unknown side effects and are a major cause of many modern diseases. Evidence on this will be given throughout the book which is truly concerning.

Insulin is another truly life-saving "drug". Although to be strictly accurate it is not a drug, but a natural substance produced by the body to regulate blood sugar. Those people who are born with type 1 diabetes cannot produce insulin. Historically, these people had very short lives until a way was developed to enable insulin to be produced in a form that could be injected. Now type 1 diabetics can lead close to a normal life provided they also adhere to sensible diets and blood sugar monitoring.

Anaesthetics are a further example of life-saving medicines. Without modern anaesthetics, most complex surgery would be impossible.

Hip replacement operations permit people to regain mobility that would otherwise have consigned them to a life of increasing disability. But again, preventing arthritis would still be a better solution and, for most people, this really is possible provided a healthy lifestyle is started from a young age.

However, as we start to move from these incredible medical success stories, a different picture starts to emerge.

Almost 50% of people who have cancer eventually die from it. Cancer survival rates have improved only marginally over the last few decades despite countless claims of "breakthroughs" and despite the truly enormous sums of money being spent on it each year – over $100 billion. Meanwhile, the number of people diagnosed with cancer continues to increase year on year and even children are seeing frightening increases.

Heart attacks are still the leading cause of death despite the countless number of drugs used to try to prevent it.

Other diseases fare much worse. There are no effective treatments for Alzheimer's, dementia, Parkinson's, multiple sclerosis, ulcerative colitis, motor neurone disease, autism, neuropathy and many other such conditions.

Type 2 diabetes is raging out of control. Sixty years ago, the number of cases in the UK was around 200,000, now it is 4 million and is projected to reach 6 million by 2035. The NHS spends around £14 billion each year, around 10% of its entire budget, on treating type

2 diabetes and yet, despite all the drugs that are prescribed, most people do not have control of their blood sugar levels. This triples the risk of heart disease, it is the leading cause of blindness in working aged people, the single greatest cause of kidney failure and leads to serious liver problems and nerve damage that can necessitate amputations. Around 9,000 people each year have limbs amputated. All this means that type 2 diabetics have, on average, a ten-year lower life expectancy.

Mental illness is fast becoming an epidemic to rival type 2 diabetes. Antidepressant and antipsychotic drugs provide very limited benefits and come with incredibly dangerous side effects, such as an increased risk of suicide, heart disease, obesity and diabetes. In addition, they are incredibly addictive. They are not solving the problem and yet they are medicine's first line of treatment.

Knee operations are risky. In fact, studies have shown that some people undergoing knee operations have worse outcomes than those who decide not to have them. Some people do, of course, benefit but many suffer complications that worsen their long-term situation.

"Doctor, I feel tired all the time." In medical circles this condition even has its own acronym, TATT. It is the most common reason for an appointment, and most doctors confess to a feeling of dread when they hear these seven words because they have no answer or treatments to offer. Indeed, at medical school, doctors are taught first to eliminate any serious medical causes of tiredness, such as cancer, but once this has been done, they learn it is "all in the mind". If the patient is unlucky, he or she may even be offered an antidepressant which, of course, will bring its own set of side effects. Can millions of people just be hypochondriacs or malingerers as medicine believes or are doctors just looking in the wrong place for a solution? Lifestyle medicine, on the other hand, really does have many of the answers.

If you do not like sad, tragic stories then brace yourself. Ricketts and scurvy were Victorian diseases that had long been consigned to the history books. But recently they have been making a comeback. In 2014 around 4,500 people in the UK were diagnosed with rickets and many hundreds with scurvy. The causes of these diseases are so well known – lack of vitamin D for rickets and lack of vitamin C for scurvy – that even most of the public know about it let alone every medical processional in the world. That medicine has allowed, and continues to allow, these dreaded diseases to re-emerge is difficult to believe, especially when cheap and safe vitamin supplements would prevent both diseases with 100% effectiveness. We will discover the scandalous reason for this situation later.

Did you know 1 in 5 men die before the age of 65. I was shocked when I read this statistic. It's still hard to believe.

These, of course, are just snapshots, and I could have highlighted many more examples, but they show that, despite the brilliant successes in some parts of medicine, there are serious and deadly shortcomings in many other areas.

Lifestyle medicine

Lifestyle medicine excels at the prevention of disease. Of course, the adoption of the same lifestyle principles also helps people who have already developed diseases and, in most cases, produces better outcomes than drugs.

There is strong evidence that lifestyle is a key factor in the development of most chronic diseases. Even medicine tacitly agrees that diet and exercise, as well as many other lifestyle factors, play a significant role in many diseases, but for reasons we will explore in detail later, this tacit understanding is about as far as medicine goes. You will not find doctors pushing lifestyle solutions with any real enthusiasm or purpose. But the following are realistic estimates of the level of prevention that could be achieved by lifestyle changes for some of the most common diseases:

- heart attacks and stroke – 90% plus (even the World Health Organization and the American Heart Association put the figure at over 80%)
- type 2 diabetes – 90% plus
- TATT – 90% plus
- IBS – 90% plus
- Alzheimer's and dementia – 80% plus
- cancer – 50–90%

When we examine lifestyle medicine in detail later, I will give copious evidence to help substantiate these "seemingly impossible claims". But here are just four brief examples of what is to follow.

As outlined, just one single lifestyle intervention that almost everyone could do can simultaneously prevent around 30%, on average, of all these diseases – statistic courtesy of the NHS. So, there is already definitive proof for about a third of these claims. You will find out what it is in Part 4.

Consider the progression of type 2 diabetes. Sixty years ago, there were around 200,000 cases but by 2035 it will be 6 million. There simply cannot be any explanation for a 30-fold increase in such a disease other than from environmental and lifestyle factors, and even medicine really does accept that type 2 diabetes is caused by an inappropriate lifestyle. This means that once the causes are understood, it must be possible to prevent it and even reverse it. Period. The simple fact is, for type 2 diabetes, the causes are well understood by those who advocate lifestyle medicine, and the ultimate proof is it has been reversed successfully in over 100,000 patients in the UK alone.

For Alzheimer's, there is considerable evidence that B vitamins alone can significantly slow down the progression of the disease. There is even a clinical trial to prove it. But there is a dark and deeply disturbing side to this story that will be explained in Part 5.

Three impeccable randomised clinical trials have shown that a daily intake of nuts, fish oil or extra virgin olive oil can cut the risk of heart disease by 30%.

Of course, lifestyle medicine cannot do everything. Serious accidents require modern medical interventions and when people do have a heart attack, medicine can often keep them alive in ways lifestyle medicine cannot. So, in a logical, truly scientific and sane world, medicine and lifestyle medicine would co-exist and concentrate on what they do best. Millions of cases of serious diseases would be prevented by lifestyle changes and the half empty hospitals and surgeries would then be able to provide the most immaculate and speedy treatments for those who still need them. The never-ending NHS crises and waiting time scandals would be a thing of the past. Of course, this is not happening nor is it likely to happen any time soon. Why? Medicine's universal answer is that there is "insufficient proof" that lifestyle intervention works and because of this they are largely ignored.

But medical proof is elusive.

Proving something works medically and that it is safe is not as easy as you may think. It is hugely complex, costly and challenging. So complex, in fact, that probably half of what you are going to read is given over to addressing this divisive and difficult issue. The main reason for this is that the human body is an almost infinitely complex organism. In addition, the thousands of variables like foods, emotions, vitamins, minerals, chemicals, sleep and physical activity that affect how it works are difficult and sometimes almost impossible to separate. Indeed, it can be so difficult that leading medical experts can often disagree on what causes a disease and what works to treat it even when they are all looking at the same basic information. Let me give you just a few examples.

Medical experts simply cannot agree on what the optimum diet for promoting health should be. Some experts maintain that a low fat, high carbohydrate diet is best while others advocate the exact opposite: a low carbohydrate, high fat diet, or indeed an almost endless range of other permutations. These differences have led to serious conflicts, the dismissal of medical personnel and even legal trials. This deadlock has persisted for decades and will almost certainly continue for many more.

The original trials on HRT drugs showed they caused a 5% risk of developing breast cancer. A re-evaluation of exactly the same data has recently revealed that the risk is actually twice as high as originally predicted. How can the same data be interpreted with a 100% difference in outcomes? Can this really be called science? How many women would have decided not to take HRT drugs over many decades if they had known the latest data about their increased risk, and how many have died because of it?

Imagine a hypothetical trial where a group of people who eat virtually no vegetables agrees to go on a diet that increases their intake to 50% and they stop eating the highly processed ready-made meals that make up half of their existing diet. After a year, the results show that, compared to a similar group who carries on eating the original processed diet, the vegetable group has significantly lower rates of heart disease and cancer. Does that prove that vegetables help to prevent these two diseases? The answer is no. Highly processed ready-made foods contain lots of chemicals and the improvement in disease risk could simply be because they have stopped eating these "potentially dangerous" foods. How can you decide whether it is the benefits of vegetables or the removal of the dangers of processed foods that have caused the improvement in health? In this trial, you cannot. (Please do not be put off eating vegetables because of this hypothetical example. As you will see later, the truth is that both facts are correct. Vegetables significantly decrease the risk of developing serious diseases and highly processed foods increase the risk.) This hypothetical trial is the simplest one involving food you can imagine. There are just two variables and yet it is impossible to determine what caused the improvement in health. Imagine how much more difficult it would be if you compared two completely different diets, each with many dozens of different foods.

Drugs are approved using scientifically based clinical trials. They are meant to provide the ultimate proof that a drug works and that it is safe. But 20% of all the drugs that have ever been used by doctors have either subsequently been taken off the market or given the ultimate black box warning because they are killing people or causing serious diseases, like cancer and heart attacks. Millions of people have died because the trial process, which is supposed to detect serious drug side effects, has failed. And yet, these clinical trials are supposed to be *the* "gold standard" of medical proof.

Statins are the most prescribed drugs of all time with total sales recently reaching $1 trillion. You might imagine that the evidence behind these drugs must, therefore, be irrefutable. But even though the official medical position advocates their use, behind the scenes there is what can only be described as open warfare within medicine regarding statins.

The British Medical Journal (BMJ) is one of the top three most respected medical journals in the world. In 2016 it published a study claiming that around 20% of people who took statins suffered from significant side effects. Professor Sir Rory Collins, who is Britain's top statin expert, demanded they retract the study saying it was incorrect. The BMJ refused.

In 2017 medical guidelines were changed so that people over 55 with a low risk of heart attack should be given statins. This effectively doubled the number of people who should take statins overnight from 6 million to 12 million. The Royal College of GPs objected to this needless change which was based just on age.

In 2018 a group of highly respected researchers issued a paper highlighting how new medical research on statins had been blatantly manipulated to make them look more effective and safer than they are.

The queen's former doctor, many other prominent medical experts and the authors of over 30 books have questioned the safety and efficacy of statins.

Medicine's claim that everything it does is based on rigorous science is not true, otherwise these contradictions would never happen. The copious hard evidence to back this up will be explored in detail in Part 3. Medicine's claim that lifestyle medicine has insufficient proof to support it is also not correct and Part 4 will provide clear evidence that most diseases are, in large part, preventable.

Part 2

Essential Background Information

Some background information is necessary to fully understand all the evidence that will be presented. This includes sections on the placebo effect, clinical trials, drug patent law, the pharmaceutical business model and drug regulation. If all this sounds too boring, please do not be tempted to skip this section as it is essential reading. It also contains fascinating insights that I guarantee will surprise and shock you.

Placebo effects

The placebo is one of the most powerful treatments ever discovered. If a doctor gives a patient who is depressed or in pain a "sugar pill", they will report a significant improvement in symptoms even though there cannot be any clinical effect. For depression, the patient will experience, on average, a 20% improvement in symptoms with a placebo and 25% with an antidepressant. The drug produces just an extra 5% real benefit over the placebo, but, as we will see later, there is a final twist that I guarantee will shock you even more. The placebo effect works for many conditions in varying degrees, but it does not work for everything. For example, someone with a serious infectious disease can be cured with antibiotics but not a placebo. The placebo effect, however, can be so great that it must be considered when assessing whether, and by how much, drugs really work. The clinical trial was developed for this exact purpose as we will see in the next section.

How does the placebo work? It was originally thought that because the patient expects a doctor to improve their symptoms with, say, a drug, when given a placebo (which they think is a drug) they experience a positive outlook which leads to lower perceived symptoms and also because this positive mood triggers the release of chemicals within the body, such as natural painkillers and mood enhancers, which further benefit the symptoms. There are, however, other factors involved. Several trials have been carried out where the patients have been told they were being given a placebo that would provide no clinical effect. The patients, however, still reported improved symptoms. In one trial, when the doctors said the trial was to end and the placebo withdrawn, the patients protested because they felt so much better and wanted to keep taking the dummy pills. In a further trial, patients were split into two groups. In one group the doctor was told to have no interaction with the patient. He did not look up when the patient entered the room, wrote a prescription, pushed it across the desk and told the patient to return in two weeks. In the other group the doctor greeted the patient by name, with a smile and maintained eye contact throughout. He empathised and said he was sure the treatment would help and he looked forward to seeing them in two weeks. Even though both sets of patients were given the same placebo and both reported an improvement in symptoms, the second group had better outcomes.

So, the placebo works on several levels. Patients expect an improvement and, psychologically, they perceive one. The psychologically positive thoughts trigger the release of natural chemicals that further improve symptoms. A positive empathetic relationship between doctor and patient further magnifies the effect. There are other effects at work, but these examples are sufficient for this simple brief examination. What the placebo clearly shows is that it has a significant effect on the mind and an individual's health. But the mind alone (without any placebos) can also exert a significant effect on our health or ill health as we will see in Part 4.

The randomised clinical trial

Medicine claims the randomised clinical trial is the ultimate proof that a drug or any other treatment works. So, what exactly does a clinical trial entail? In the examples below we are considering drugs, but the logic still applies to other treatments, like acupuncture and vitamin therapy, that can be prescribed by nutritionists.

As we have seen, the placebo effect can be so great we could never be sure a drug works because of a genuine clinical effect or simply due to the placebo effect without some method that separates the two. The clinical trial does this by measuring the drug's outcomes directly against a placebo. Only if the drug performs better than the placebo can it be said to have a genuine clinical effect. The randomised clinical trial or, to give it its full title – the randomised, double blind, placebo-controlled trial – works as follows.

People are recruited to take part in the trial and split into two groups. Around half of them receive the drug and the other half, the placebo. This is the placebo-controlled part of the trial. Randomised means that the people in each group are chosen entirely at random – by drawing names out of a hat, for example. This stops unscrupulous researchers or drug companies from rigging the trial by placing, for example, all the patients who they judge most likely to benefit from the drug in that half of the trial. During the trial, the patients are assessed and monitored by doctors. Double blind means that neither the patient nor the doctor knows who is taking the drug or the placebo. This stops any bias in interpreting the results. The only person who knows is the one who "drew the names out of the hat" and they also supply the identical packets containing identical-looking capsules that are either placebo or drug.

So, in theory, the clinical trial excludes any possible bias, fraud or manipulation. So, what could possibly happen to undermine this "jewel in the crown of modern medicine"? Well, actually, just about every type of fraud and manipulation you can think of occurs regularly and some that you could never imagine. We will explore this in detail in Part 3. There are several other things we need to understand about clinical trials. They are fiendishly complex and typically the data and analysis from a large trial covers around 100,000 pages, with some requiring 300,000 pages. It would take someone many months to read and fully absorb all this data. The clinical trial report also covers thousands of pages of data which include complex statistical tables. The money involved is huge, with a single trial costing hundreds of millions of dollars. To gain approval for most new drugs the company has been required to submit two clinical trials to the drug regulators. There are three stages in the clinical trial process.

Stage I involves animal testing and then giving the drug to a small number of human "guinea pigs" for the very first time. This is potentially a dangerous moment, so the dosage is extremely low, and the patients are carefully monitored. Nevertheless, there have been around 1,000 cases of serious harm and death over the years from this initial part of the trials.

Stage II occurs after it has been established that people are not going to be harmed or killed immediately. It involves testing various people with different doses to try to establish the optimum levels.

Stage III is the actual clinical trial.

There is a stage IV trial which is carried out after the drug has been approved and is already being used and prescribed. Its stated purpose is to assess how the drug is performing in the "real world". The important point is it is nowhere near as rigorous as the original stage III clinical trial. There are, for example, no placebo comparisons, no randomisation and no double blinding. The costs are low and the timescales generally just a few weeks. As we will see later, the pharmaceutical industry uses them mainly for drug promotion, even though they have little or no clinical validity.

Another term you will often hear about is meta-analysis. This is simply a pooled analysis of several individual clinical trials on the same drug. If this pooled analysis shows positive results, it is considered an even better level of overall proof than a single or even two clinical trials.

Epidemiological studies

An epidemiological study monitors groups of people to try to establish cause and effect relationships between risk factors for disease, such as smoking, alcohol, exercise and diet. The study period can be very long, and the numbers of people can be in the thousands. The Framingham Heart Study and the Nurse's Health Study in America are well-known examples. The people involved complete regular detailed questionnaires about their lifestyle, such as how much they drink and smoke, comprehensive breakdowns of diet and exercise, drugs taken, and health issues and outcomes. This type of study can give valuable insights into the relationship between lifestyle and health, although scientists claim they cannot provide definitive proof of cause and effect. Nevertheless, the analysis of well-conducted studies, especially if backed up by other studies, can provide evidence that is hard to dismiss. For example, every study that has analysed the effects of smoking shows smokers consistently live shorter lives than non-smokers. It is true a few smokers live to 100, but equally some die in their thirties. On average, however, heavy smokers can expect to live 15 years less than non-smokers and moderate smokers seven to ten years less. Some ten years before their death, they also start to experience significant health problems, such as heart and respiratory problems. What these studies also show is that those people who live the healthiest lifestyle also live longer and have less illness than those with the unhealthiest lifestyle. So, someone who eats plenty of vegetables and fruit, exercises and has a fulfilling social life will live longer than "couch potatoes" who gorge on Coca Cola and McDonalds and whose interests revolve around TV and video games.

As we will see later, much medical research is open to bias, manipulation and fraud and it is important to look at who funded the trial or study before deciding whether to believe its findings. If Coca Cola sponsored a study that showed its sugar laden drink was not responsible for weight gain, then quite rightly you would be deeply suspicious. In fact, Coca Cola did fund such a study – costing over $1 million – and it backfired badly when it was exposed in the Times newspaper. The study claimed it was a lack of adequate exercise that caused weight gain and obesity and not sugary drinks. This caused anger amongst many health experts, and Coca Cola's science and health officer later resigned over the affair. The true reality is sugary cola drinks contribute to around 180,000 deaths a year through diabetes, heart disease and cancer according to a study from Tufts University. Coca Cola's shoddy research is the same as that employed by the tobacco industry to try to protect cigarette sales. It shows to what depths some researchers will sink in their quest for money, and how they are willing to ignore the serious health problems their research will perpetuate. The Coca Cola example is blatant and easily discredited, but fraud and bias in research is common and not always so easy to expose.

Another example is a study in the journal Advances in Nutrition that claimed refined grains have no impact on health and the main culprits are red and processed meats. Unsurprisingly, the study was funded by the Wheat Foods Council and the Grain Foods Foundation. We will see later that refined grains are indeed one of the major causes of diseases like diabetes and obesity.

Drug patent law

When a pharmaceutical company develops a chemical compound they believe could have a therapeutic effect, they can apply for a patent that is enforceable worldwide and is valid for 20 years. At the end of 20 years the patent expires, and any company can then make the drug. Generic drug manufacturers exist for this sole purpose. As we will see in the next section, the cost of producing most drugs is usually small, so when there is free competition the price typically falls by about 90%. It usually takes seven years to develop and test the drug through the various trial phases. This leaves the company around 13 years during which time they can sell the drug at any price they choose to maximise their profit. Drugs are tested for one specific outcome – to lower blood pressure, for example – and are approved only for that condition. It is illegal for drug companies to promote the use of a drug for any other reason because by definition there is no proof that it would work. Nevertheless, as we will see later, promoting such "off-label prescribing" is one of the most prolific frauds the pharmaceutical industry commits. A drug patent is the most valuable thing a pharmaceutical company possesses. Without it, their business literally would not exist. The law does not theoretically allow anyone to patent a natural substance, such as a vitamin, so anyone can make them and therefore the price for vitamins is very low in comparison to drugs.

The pharmaceutical business model

The business model of the pharmaceutical industry is like no other industrial sector. Drugs that can be produced for less than a few tens of dollars for a year's supply can sell for tens of thousands of dollars. Not all drugs have this type of mark up, of course, but the fact that when a drug comes off patent, the company can still make a profit, even though its price falls by around 90%, says it all.

In 2009 a detailed analysis was carried out on the most widely prescribed drugs at that time comparing ingredient costs and selling prices. Here are the figures for just three randomly selected drugs and are for 100 tablets of each. The costs are all US dollars. Mark ups like this are normal.

Drug	Ingredients	Selling Price	Mark Up
Celebrex (painkiller)	0.60	130.27	21,722%
Lipitor (statin)	5.80	272.37	4,690%
Prozac (antidepressant)	0.11	247.47	224,973%

When a drug does come "off patent", the loss of revenue can seriously damage the company's profitability and, therefore, its share price. It is, therefore, a financial imperative to replace the off-patent drug with a new drug for the same condition so the high price can be maintained or, ideally, even improved upon. This is why you will see, for example, new classes of drugs unleashed on the public every 15 or 20 years. Not because they are clinically better or safer, not because the new drugs are actually needed, but simply because of financial necessity. If new drugs are not found and approved, the very existence of the company is at risk. It is that serious.

The pharmaceutical industry would tell you that drug development costs are huge and drug prices simply reflect these enormous costs. To get approval for a drug, the company must submit two stage III clinical trials to the regulator. The pharmaceutical industry claims that to bring a single drug to market costs an average of $2.4 billion. Independent experts say this cost has been grossly exaggerated to try to justify obscenely high drug prices and that a more realistic figure is $100 million. But even $100 million is still a huge sum of money. Whatever the true figure is, the only people who can fund such incredible sums are the pharmaceutical industry itself, other global corporations and governments. This business model means the pharmaceutical industry remains the most profitable industry bar none, seriously outpacing all others including oil, banking and mining.

Blockbuster drugs

Producing blockbuster drugs is the goal of every pharmaceutical company. It is the name given to a drug that achieves annual sales of over $1 billion.

Drug regulation

Each major country has a drug regulator. Their mandate is to protect the public by assessing new drugs and granting licences only if they meet certain conditions for effectiveness and safety, and to take action if unexpected side effects occur at a later stage. This includes taking the drug off the market or requiring special disclosures to doctors such as black box warnings that spell out clearly the life-threatening side effects. Doctors would normally only use such drugs in patients who already had life-threatening conditions and where it was judged the benefits might outweigh the risks.

The US has the Federal Drug Agency (FDA) which has been in existence for over 100 years. Most smaller countries cannot afford to assess all the drugs coming onto the market nor do they have the resources to look at all the reported side effects. So, what usually happens is they will often "rubber stamp" the decisions of the FDA. The FDA is, therefore, on a global scale, the pre-eminent drug regulator and any shortcomings in the US would also affect many other people in many other countries. As we will see later, the shortcomings at the FDA, and indeed in drug regulation generally, are deeply disturbing. The EU has the European Medicines Agency (EMA). Whilst the EMA is gaining traction it has only been in existence since 1995. The UK has the Medicines and Health Regulatory Authority (MHRA).

Big Pharma, Big Food, Big Agriculture, Big Data, Big Tobacco, Big Chemical and Big Finance

These are the names used to describe major global cartels which are controlled by a relatively small number of giant companies that exert dominant control over their particular sector. For example, just ten major food producers control around 70% of American and European processed food supply. Just three global agriculture companies control 60% of seed, fertiliser, herbicide and pesticide supplies across the world. These companies have immense influence and if governments offend them too much or bring in strict laws against them, they risk losing thousands of jobs because the companies can threaten to move their businesses to other countries that are prepared to have laxer laws just to gain jobs and the prestige of having a global business in their country.

All these companies are governed by one simple thing: money. Many of the products of these companies are responsible in part for much of the sickness and disease escalating around the globe. They are so powerful. however, that they are usually able to fight off demands for unsafe products to be banned from sale or at least to do so for many years.

There will be many examples of this throughout the book, but I will explore one classic case now.

In the late 1940s doctors and researchers started to understand that cigarette smoking was a major cause of lung cancer and studies were carried out to demonstrate this link. This, of course, represented a major threat for Big Tobacco. The tobacco companies fought back by saying the evidence was inconclusive and they hired a number of scientists who were also prepared to challenge this evidence. The infamous Hazleton Laboratories, for example, carried out studies that "proved" that second-hand smoke is not harmful to human health which no doubt provided a significant boost to their profits. This "muddying of the water" had the desired effect because it delayed government action to bring in legislation relating to the dangers of smoking for many years. Even when the evidence against smoking continued to mount to an unchallengeable level, the industry's response was always the same – they denied any such link. Nevertheless, nearly two decades later, and despite their best efforts, legislation was eventually passed requiring cigarette packets to carry warning notices about the cancer link. Further legislation continued to be passed and tightened over subsequent years, like banning tobacco advertising and indoor smoking. What is equally shocking is that many politicians also sided, at least initially, with the industry, probably to protect jobs and possibly because in the US they also received significant funding from the tobacco companies. Even now, Big Tobacco still officially refuses to acknowledge that smoking causes lung cancer.

Of course, companies should have a right to challenge laws they feel are unjust and that threaten their business because governments can, of course, sometimes "get it wrong". But the shocking twist in this story is that the tobacco industry actually knew cigarettes caused cancer and knew they were addictive almost from the beginning, even when they were strenuously denying such links. How do we know? Because there were leaked internal company documents. In other words, they were blatantly lying. But what is perhaps even more shocking is that independent scientists and research organisations were also willing to manipulate the science to get the results Big Tobacco wanted. Is it possible they were unaware of the truth? Or is the truth simply that they were being paid huge sums of money to help keep cigarettes on the market for as long as possible? It seems almost inconceivable that they didn't know, and this means that both they and the companies were prepared to allow cigarettes to continue to kill millions of people each year in return for what must have been huge sums of money and huge profits. However, the evidence against the industry continued to mount and more people began to understand the devastating human cost of smoking (including the fact it also significantly increased the number of heart attacks) as well as the huge economic cost. Eventually, in 1998, the tobacco industry agreed to pay a $246 billion settlement to the US government (paid over many years) to help offset the huge medical costs caused by smoking-related diseases. When Big Tobacco agreed this settlement, however, they simply increased cigarette prices, so, in effect, the public ended up paying the fine. They knew they could get away with this because of the addictive nature of cigarettes – a fact they had also denied for decades. Then, to increase their profits even further, they started huge advertising campaigns to promote cigarette smoking in developing countries. These countries are now seeing rising epidemics of lung cancer, heart attacks and early deaths. There isn't much more I can say about this devastatingly evil industry.

You may think the tobacco scandal must surely be a rare type of event, but sadly, this is not the case, as you will see in the numerous examples relating to Big Ag, Big Pharma and Big Food yet to be explored.

PART 3

Medicine and the Drug Industry – The Truth You Won't Want to Believe

Why does your doctor know virtually nothing about lifestyle solutions to health? It is a complex story that will take over 60 pages to explain. It will ultimately shock you to the core. The title of the first section alone will probably make you angry because you will not want to believe it. But please look at the indisputable evidence before you make a final judgement.

Medicine – a hierarchical profession dominated by dogma, reputation and ego

Resisting new ideas is, in varying degrees, a natural human trait. Virtually every profession, every organisation, every expert and most individuals do so when new ideas are proposed which contradict their own beliefs, even though the new ideas are often subsequently shown to be correct. In 1615 Galileo Galilei worked out that the earth revolves around the sun. However, the orthodox view that the sun revolved around the earth was sacrosanct and those in power made it clear that, unless he repudiated his theory, he would be executed. He had no choice but to recant even though he knew he was right. In 1905 Albert Einstein developed his theory of relativity, but the scientific status quo was so firmly entrenched that it took another 14 years before it finally started to gain official acceptance. These two examples simply involved science and established dogma. The retention of reputations and ego almost certainly played a part in why it took so long to accept these incredible new facts. There is, however, another factor which can also play a vital part in resisting new ideas and that is money. This will be covered in extensive detail shortly, but in this section, I will concentrate simply on how medicine resists new ideas.

If every example throughout history, where a new idea was initially ridiculed and dismissed, but eventually proven to be correct was written down, it would probably fill dozens of books. Medicine really has played a part in all of this, but what you will find shocking and almost impossible to believe is the extent to which it occurs within this most trusted of professions. Given that medicine is inextricably linked to human life, there is also an even more frightening outcome which is it often leads to serious and even deadly outcomes for patients on a scale that makes it even more unbelievable. The facts are simple. Medicine's rigid hierarchical structure resists change to an alarming degree, and new ideas and medical breakthroughs can take decades before they gain traction and start to help patients. Here are six quotes that illustrate the depth of the problem:

- "It takes 50 years to get a wrong idea out of medicine. And 100 years to get a right one into medicine." John Hughlings Jackson
- "All truth passes through three stages. First, it is ridiculed. Second, it is violently opposed. Third, it is accepted as being self-evident." Arthur Schopenhauer

- "Truth never triumphs – its opponents just die out. Science advances one funeral at a time." Max Plank
- "The scientific establishment is permeated with opinions which pass for valid scientific inductions and with contradictions which are disregarded because it is too painful to face the prospect of revisions of the theory which would be required to reconcile the contradictory observations with the dominant theory." Carl Lindegren
- "Paradigm shifts in science often take 20 to 40 years to become established after a period of resistance." Thomas Kuhn
- "Let's be clear: the work of science has nothing whatsoever to do with consensus. Consensus is the business of politics. Science, on the contrary, requires only one investigator who happens to be right, which means that he or she has results that are verifiable by reference to the real world. In science, consensus is irrelevant. What is relevant is reproducible results. The greatest scientists in history are great precisely because they broke with the consensus." Michael Crichton, MD, bestselling author

These quotes expose one of the most devastating problems in science and medicine and they play a crucial role in helping to expose the truth. Here are seven "deadly" examples which illustrate this deeply disturbing problem. They encompass distant history to the present day.

Scurvy

The basic history of scurvy is well documented. When early merchant ships embarked on long journeys across the oceans, the lack of fresh foods meant vitamin C was virtually non-existent, and scurvy was the inevitable result. Of course, the exact cause was only known centuries later when vitamin C was discovered. The death toll was horrific, and many ships lost more than half of their crew. When they reached the new continents, they took on board new supplies, including fruits and vegetables, and even most of those already suffering from scurvy recovered. The British Navy also suffered from scurvy and many lives were being lost. Then, in 1753, James Lind, who was a naval surgeon, carried out an early version of a clinical trial which showed that citrus fruit could cure scurvy. But it was 42 years later in 1795 that the naval hierarchy started giving their crew lemon juice because of the further efforts of another Scottish physician, Sir Gilbert Blane. Scurvy then disappeared almost entirely, but not before an estimated 130,000 naval seamen had died of this horrific and preventable disease. It is impossible to know exactly what was going on in the minds of all those involved and why it took so many years, but it is quite likely that the idea that such a terrible disease could be treated and prevented just by eating fruit was almost impossible to believe.

Puerperal fever

Puerperal fever was one of the most tragic and most avoidable diseases in the history of medicine. It is the name given to a deadly infection that affected many mothers just after they had given birth. The cause was an infection introduced by the contaminated hands of doctors and unsterilised medical instruments. The consequences were unbearable pain, pelvic abscesses, sepsis, high fever and agonising death. Wherever male obstetricians took over from female midwives, puerperal fever followed. It was a disease caused by doctor arrogance.

One of the earliest records of this disease is from 1746 in a Paris hospital where more than 50% of mothers who gave birth died. However, the most detailed account of the problem came from Dr Ignaz Semmelweis of Austria in the 1850s. He noted that mothers who were assisted by doctors had more than three times the rate of death than those helped by midwives. He suspected a contagious agent. One of the main problems was that doctors often went from touching infected corpses in the cadaver dissection lab to the maternity ward and delivered babies without any form of washing or disinfectant.

Dr Semmelweis directed the doctors at his hospital to use a chlorinated lime solution on their hands prior to touching the mother. When this procedure was adopted, the mortality rate went from a high of 32% to almost zero. Dr Semmelweis held several other senior staff positions and wherever his hygiene methods were followed, mortality rates dropped. Dr Breisky of Prague also adopted good hygiene methods and reported in 1882 that he had helped 1,100 women deliver in succession without a single death. Dr Semmelweis, Dr Breisky and Dr Oliver Wendell Holmes of the USA were the most prominent advocates of hand washing and they all desperately tried to convince other doctors and hospitals to do the same.

Dr Semmelweis published all his work, but most of his contemporaries ignored such outrageous and offensive "nonsense". Doctors were insulted at the suggestion that their hands were dirty and were unwilling to admit culpability in the injury and deaths of so many patients. The medical community expelled him from their profession. His former colleagues also tricked him into visiting a mental institution in 1865 and then committed him against his will. He died mysteriously two weeks later.

A decade later, Louis Pasteur's germ theory and Joseph Lister's work on hospital sanitisation provided further proof for Semmelweis' work. Despite all this evidence, the medical profession took many more decades to fully embrace these new ideas and even up to around 1940 women were still dying from puerperal fever. It was only after the invention of the antibiotic Prontosil that puerperal fever deaths finally dropped to almost zero. But the records of Dr Semmelweis and Dr Breisky proved that doctors could have stopped most of the puerperal fever deaths from as early as the 1850s if only they had washed their hands and instruments.

Considering that one-fifth of the population at that time consisted of women of child-bearing age, and that a 30% maternal mortality rate was common, the impact on society was enormous. It would be impossible to calculate accurately the number of women killed in the westernised world by puerperal fever in the 90-year period up to 1940, but it is unlikely to be less than 50 million. As well as this horrific death toll, there were millions of motherless children relegated to die or live a life of malnutrition and disease, often forced to work in mines, factories and sweat shops. It is important that we never forget the history of puerperal fever because the massive loss of maternal life also devastated the family unit and society as a whole, as well as savagely reducing overall life expectancy. But I'll hazard a guess that you have never even heard of puerperal fever.

Radical mastectomy

In the 1890s, William Halstead developed a radical mastectomy procedure for women with breast cancer. It involved not just removal of the breasts, but underlying chest muscles and lymph nodes. It soon became established as the standard breast cancer treatment. In the 1940s, however, some senior surgeons, like Sir Geoffrey Keynes, questioned the surgery but their ideas were dismissed or just ignored. Several other studies raised similar concerns over the next few decades, but again they also were effectively ignored. Then in 1980 a randomised clinical trial was carried out that compared radical mastectomy with a conservative breast-saving surgery. The researchers were amazed to find there was no difference in the death rates. But radical mastectomy was still so engrained within medicine that virtually no one would believe the results. The researchers then carried out two more trials in the 1990s, and finally, everyone had to agree this type of radical mastectomy did not achieve better results than simple surgery. Since then, radical mastectomy has only been used on rare occasions. The real tragedy is that during its use it caused many severe long-term side effects, including chronic pain and restricted arm movements. Up to the year 2000, around 500,000 women in the US alone had undergone this devastating and unnecessary surgery. When you saw John Hughlings Jackson's quote that it takes 50 years to get a bad idea out of medicine you probably thought this was silly, but even though some doctors challenged its use, medical dogma persisted, and it took 80 years to get rid of the devastating treatment of radical mastectomy.

Bed rest for heart attacks

In 1912 Dr James Herrick was the first physician to fully describe a myocardial infarction (heart attack) which made it a landmark paper in medical research. In the paper, he stated "the importance of absolute rest in bed for several days". Having just described this "new disease", how could he be so sure this was the right thing to do? Well, the logic was seductive. After a heart attack, the heart muscle is damaged and, therefore, it must be protected from further damage by complete inactivity – surely this was simple common sense. What then happened was that a few days rapidly became a standard six weeks. Medical dogma then exacerbated the problem further by declaring that if a patient was allowed to move during this period it amounted to medical malpractice. A prominent physician from the 1930s said, "The patient is to be guarded by day and night nursing and helped in any way to avoid voluntary movement or effort." This practice went unchallenged for over 50 years.

How did it end? It all ended abruptly in the mid-1960s never to be mentioned again. In preparation for the Apollo moon mission, young volunteers were asked to remain immobile in bed to mimic the lack of exercise the astronauts would encounter in space and to see what effect it would have. Several weeks later, their heart function had deteriorated so alarmingly that the trial had to be stopped. The penny dropped, and bed rest after a heart attack was gone forever to be replaced by...? You probably know the answer: exercise.

What were the consequences of bed rest? For those people who reached hospital alive after a heart attack, the mortality rate was 30%, while the rate today is 8%. Of course, the treatments available today save more lives, but enforced bed rest accounted for around half of the difference. A researcher has estimated the global death toll from enforced bed rest at well over 10 million. All this happened because medicine's hierarchical and ego driven structure resists change to an alarming degree. This time it took over 50 years to get rid of this devastating medical treatment.

Stomach ulcers

Medicine had decided as early as the nineteenth century that stomach ulcers were caused mainly by stress. Drastic operations were performed in severe cases to remove part of the stomach. For everyone else there were no effective treatments. Around 10% of the adult population suffered from ulcers at some point in their life. Many died from internal bleeding and many more suffered almost unbearable pain. Then in the 1970s it was discovered that antacids, like Zantac and Tagamet, could help reduce the symptoms by lowering stomach acid which irritated the ulcers. At that time antacids were so widely used they were making $3 billion profit each year (this is equivalent to $30 billion today after taking inflation into account). Whilst these drugs helped to reduce the pain, they did not stop it and patients were still suffering appallingly.

Nothing much would have changed but for two physicians and researchers – Barry Marshall and Robin Warren who were based at the Royal Perth Hospital in Australia. When they carried out biopsies on ulcer patients, they discovered there was a common denominator, a bacterium known as Helicobacter pylori, and because of this it should be possible to cure the condition with antibiotics. They presented the data in a paper at a meeting of the Royal Australian College of Physicians in 1981 and were met with total scepticism. To gastroenterologists, the concept of a germ causing ulcers was like saying the earth was flat. But there may also have been other considerations. This discovery threatened not just a "$30 billion drug market" but the entire field of endoscopy. Every gastroenterologist would treat around 25 patients each week and because it could not be cured the patients just kept coming back. Did commercial and career interests affect their judgement? We will never know, but it would perhaps be naive to assume it played no part at all.

Over the next few years, the physicians carried out more research and tried without success to get anyone interested. In desperation, Barry Marshall did the only thing he could think of. He needed to prove a causal relationship between the bacterium and ulcers on a human volunteer, but it would be unethical to use anyone but himself. So, he drank a solution containing a culture of H. pylori bacteria. Within a few days, he was severely ill. He underwent endoscopy which disclosed the development of severe inflammation, the precursor to actual ulcers. He then took antibiotics which soon cleared up the inflammation and underwent a second endoscopy to prove the treatment's effectiveness. All this was written up and presented in a paper published in the Medical Journal of Australia in 1985. If he had assumed his suffering and the proof it yielded would this time sway minds, he was to be disappointed yet again. The paper was met with the same total disregard. Once medical dogma is entrenched, it stays entrenched. Barry Marshall then spent time working in the US and managed to get stories printed in some popular newspapers and periodicals with titles such as "Guinea-pig doctor experiments on himself and cures ulcers". Slowly, the idea gained traction. Other doctors started to try antibiotics and by the mid-1990s, even the FDA was publicising the data, and medicine finally came on board. The use of antibiotics soon became a standard treatment for ulcers.

It is impossible to predict how many people died and suffered unnecessarily between this discovery in 1981 and medicine's reluctant acceptance 15 years later, but it must surely have been many millions and more likely tens of millions. Eventually, the work of Barry Marshall and Robin Warren and their enormous contribution to medicine was recognised when, in 2005, they were awarded the Nobel Prize for medicine. The medical journals and senior medical experts who refused to recognise and even consider their work were left red-faced. But perhaps we should not feel too sorry for them given the immense suffering and death toll their arrogance, ego and dogma had caused.

How many researchers would just have "given up" when faced with such ridicule and hostility? How many similar medical breakthroughs are thwarted by dismissive medical dogma even today? You will see more examples in Parts 4 and 5.

The scandal of beta blocker drugs used during surgery

This scandal is so important it will be covered in much more detail later, but I will outline one important part now which is particularly relevant to this section. In 2009 a medical guideline involving the use of beta blocker drugs to protect the heart during surgery was endorsed by a committee of leading experts of the European Society of Cardiology. This guideline was implemented across the entire EU. At the time it was implemented, many other researchers could see the claims made for the drugs were too good to be true because there were also other trials that showed the drugs did not work and some in fact showed they caused harm. But because these researchers and doctors were further down the hierarchical ladder, this evidence and these concerns were ignored by the leading experts.

Five years later, it was discovered that the drugs had in fact caused the deaths of around 800,000 EU citizens. Medical dogma and the extreme, unchallengeable hierarchical nature of medicine were some of the major causes of this scandal, much like the senior gastroenterologists in the 1980s who ignored the evidence about the real cause of stomach ulcers for 15 years which resulted in millions of cases of death and unnecessary suffering.

Type 2 diabetes

Medicine has consistently maintained that once someone develops type 2 diabetes, it cannot be cured. But the fact is some doctors and other lifestyle practitioners had been reversing the disease for many decades. This is just one more example of how medical dogma perpetuates human suffering. Type 2 diabetes increases the risk of heart attacks by 300% and causes thousands of amputations and liver diseases each year as well as reducing life expectancy. In the last 60 years there have probably been at least 8 million people in the UK who have developed diabetes. The total number of deaths and serious outcomes this has caused is again impossible to calculate accurately, but it is certainly in the hundreds of thousands. We will see later that the NHS has recently approved a dietary method for reversing type 2 diabetes. So, there is now tacit acceptance that a simple lifestyle change can indeed reverse the disease for many people. This is yet another example vindicating John Hughlings Jackson's "impossible to believe" claim that "it takes 50 years to get a wrong idea out of medicine".

Chronic fatigue syndrome

Chronic fatigue syndrome (CFS) is not to be confused with "tired all the time". Most people who experience TATT manage to live some sort of normal life even though they experience lethargy and tiredness. Chronic fatigue syndrome, on the other hand, is so severe the lives of most sufferers are effectively destroyed. CFS affects about 250,000 people in the UK, 10% of them children. It is a horrible condition and many patients become bedridden for years. There are around 60 symptoms linked to the disorder, including severe movement pain, constant exhaustion and being very sensitive to sound, light, heat and cold. The disability benefits and costs for the NHS and other public services run into billions of pounds each year.

Many years ago, medicine concluded that chronic fatigue syndrome is not an actual medical condition, and that it is all in the patient's mind. They believe patients mistakenly think they cannot exercise and move and this is the main underlying cause of the condition. A clinical trial was conducted in 2011 called PACE to provide definitive proof for this theory. This used cognitive behaviour therapy (CBT) and graded exercise therapy (GET) as treatments. The main conclusion of the trial was that 22% of the patients taking the therapy recovered compared to just 7% in the non-therapy group. The trial protocols had been approved by the Research Ethics Committee, and the results peer reviewed by the Medical Research Council. This is just about as high an endorsement as any medical research could ever achieve, so the results were indisputable. This led the National Institute for Health and Care Excellence to endorse the use of CBT and GET as the standard medical treatment for chronic fatigue syndrome throughout the UK.

This standard treatment involves using psychologists to implement CBT and get patients to exercise a little bit more each day with graded exercise therapy. The problem is many patients felt, and still feel, angry that they were being blamed for inflicting these distressing symptoms upon themselves. They maintain that it does not work and, in some cases, makes the condition worse. Medicine, on the other hand, claims patients resist the treatment because they do not want to be stigmatised as being mentally ill.

When pharmaceutical companies carry out clinical trials, they are allowed to keep the trial data completely secret, other than submitting it to the regulators. But when research is funded by the government, like the PACE trial, the data and results are meant to be freely available to anyone. Disturbed by what had happened and still doubting the results, a group of patients made repeated freedom of information requests to get access to the raw trial data. They repeatedly came up against a brick wall from Queen Mary's University who held all the trial data. The university in fact then spent £200,000 on legal fees in a desperate attempt to challenge the freedom of information requests. Why would a university spend such an enormous sum of money in trying to block a legal right of access to such data? Did it try to prevent access because it realised that any subsequent analysis could prove very damaging to the researchers and all the elite bodies who had approved and positively reviewed the PACE trial? In the end, a tribunal forced the university to release the data in 2016.

A team of leading academics were then able to re-analyse the data and found that the claimed benefits did not reflect what the results had shown, and the treatments were virtually worthless. After a year those receiving the treatment, for example, could walk just 30 metres more than those in the control group. The academics discovered that the original researchers had changed their "definition" of recovery to a much more lenient version. For example, a patient entering the trial under the original rules could show worse symptoms in two out of the four criteria and still be classed as recovered in the new version. They pointed out that the scientific principles governing clinical trials state that once the protocols for the trial have been established, they must not be altered. This is designed to stop any subsequent manipulation of the results which is what seemingly occurred in the PACE trial. There were several other disturbing findings, but I will outline just one of them. Most of the people with CFS are so ill they receive government benefits. If the PACE treatment really worked, the cost of benefits would be expected to fall. Instead, for those taking the treatment, the numbers receiving benefits increased overall.

Faced with this serious challenge, the authors of the PACE trial simply ignored the reanalysis and declared CBT and GET did work for some people. They did not address the serious issues raised. There was also virtually no interest from any other medical body, individual doctors or psychologists. This meant there could be no resolution of this serious issue and so the stalemate continued. Since 2016 there have been two other papers published, one by the PACE authors, and a response by the academic critics. The PACE authors tried to justify changing the definition of recovery with the following logic. They said they preferred their modified definition because it was more consistent with their own clinical experience and it generated results more in line with previous studies. The academics responded that the purpose of a clinical trial is to find out the truth. It is not to confirm what you expect to find, but to discover if your expectations are correct. They added sternly, "It is not appropriate to loosen the definition of recovery because things did not go as expected."

While all this was happening, the House of Commons in January 2019 held a debate on the controversial issues surrounding the PACE trial and the current medical treatments. Carol Monaghan MP reported what she had been told by patient groups about their experience of PACE type treatments: "Many who were able to walk when they embarked on a course of graded exercise dropped out of the treatment in wheelchairs or bedbound. Furthermore, patients were pressurised to describe improvements that they did not feel. As the trial progressed and the results did not meet the authors expectations, they simply lowered the threshold to define improvement. In some cases, those whose condition had deteriorated were classed as recovered. That is simply not good science."

At the end of the debate, the House of Commons supported the proposal that the use of this standard medical treatment should be suspended. Some very high-profile academics and researchers have recently added their weight behind a change to the current treatments. Hilda Bastian, a veteran public health researcher in the UK, Germany and America, said, "I think the balance should, and ultimately will, tip towards the consumer movement." A very diplomatic way of saying that the current treatment should be stopped. Jonathan Edwards, emeritus professor of connective tissue medicine at University College London, said, "For most patients now, the real issue has become that the treatment just doesn't work. That's what a careful reading of the PACE trial indicates."

However, despite all this powerful evidence and the high profiles of those calling for action, the situation still currently remains unchanged. Patients are being given treatments that do not work in any meaningful way and medicine is still laying the blame on the patients themselves without any real understanding of what might be causing the condition. While all this is happening, the lives of a quarter of a million people continue to be effectively destroyed. This is leading to open hostility between patients and their doctors.

Ten years ago, medicine decided it knew the cause of chronic fatigue syndrome. Research was conducted and then seemingly "adjusted" to "prove" this idea was correct. Now it will not listen to the damning evidence that it was wrong. This is another tragic example of how medicine's rigid hierarchical structure, dominated by dogma, ego and the preservation of reputations, resists change to an alarming degree. Only when this changes will new research be carried out on CFS to try to find its real causes, and only then will it be possible to finally help the quarter of a million patients with this devastating condition. CFS patients will be praying that John Hughlings Jackson is wrong on this occasion and that it will not take another 50 years to get this bad idea out of medicine. Chronic fatigue syndrome epitomises a major and devastating problem within modern medicine that very few people know anything about. The PACE trial was originally given one of the highest endorsements any medical research can ever achieve. Will all the experts, researchers, doctors and psychologists involved ever be prepared to admit they were wrong? It is all very sad and very frightening.

To summarise this section so far, once a particular medical idea takes hold it is difficult to change it even when wrong, because it simply becomes a consensus view that is universally adopted and too many reputations and egos are then at stake. The simple fact, however, is that medicine really has only evolved and improved because the greatest scientists in history have had the courage to challenge it. The world owes all of them the greatest debt of gratitude because without their heroic efforts, much of medicine really would still be in the dark old days. As you will see now, however, many of them have paid a great personal price for the way they put science and truth above everything else.

Challenges to the medical status quo

So, what happens to scientists and doctors who challenge conventional medical beliefs? The answer to this question explains in part why so many medical catastrophes keep occurring. Medicine really does need to be challenged and, in a sane world, it would welcome this to help ensure that what it does really works and to reduce the huge loss of human lives when it gets things wrong. But the reality is that, even today, the medical profession rarely tolerates any challenges to its beliefs. Instead, dogma, reputation and ego still seem to reign supreme, despite medicine's indisputable history of mistakes. Many of the challenges, however, also involve drugs, so the pharmaceutical industry protecting its profits is also a key player in silencing and discrediting those involved.

The process of dealing with those who speak out against conventional medical beliefs follows several well-worn paths which have been used for many decades. Those involved are initially ridiculed for their ideas. Researchers may then trawl through their past life and career to try to find any embarrassing or controversial situations they might have been involved in. If they do find anything it will be blown out of proportion and used to discredit their reputations. Researchers will also examine their research data to try to find anything, however small, that is debatable. They then exaggerate and misrepresent it. At that point they attack the authors and demand their paper(s) be retracted. Pharmaceutical companies also have specially trained employees whose purpose is to attack scientists and academics who speak out against any drug. Official company papers which have been seized during the many legal cases brought against drug companies show lists of such doctors and researchers with words like "neutralise" or "discredit" placed against each name. All this is accompanied by curtailing their medical influence which will include not receiving invites to medical conferences, not receiving any additional funding, being excluded from meetings, censoring their ability to communicate information, and not getting any future research papers published. If everything else fails, there is a final option of revoking their medical licences. This all-out attack usually works, and many reputable scientists, doctors and academics have seen their careers and reputations severely diminished and even destroyed for speaking out, even though they have eventually been proven right. Here are just a few examples of the many hundreds of such attacks.

John Yudkin was a high-profile nutritional physiologist who set up the nutrition department in Queen Elizabeth College at the University of London. In the 1970s Yudkin was emphatically making the case that sugar was the main culprit for the huge rise in diseases like heart attacks. But medicine's elite had already decided that fat was the main cause, so they would not allow any of his ideas to gain traction. He was subjected to all the established attacks like ridiculing his evidence, never being invited to conferences (even the ones he had organised were cancelled), and all the new papers he submitted were never published. His own college even refused to let him use the research facilities he had created once he retired. He died in 1995 a forgotten and discredited scientist. And yet today, medicine now accepts that sugar plays a significant role in many diseases which has led governments to introduce things like sugar taxes. If his ideas had been examined objectively at that time and sugar had been given the ranking it deserves as one of the most dangerous foods ever – probably on a par with smoking – then in the intervening 40 years, many cases of serious diseases and early deaths really could have been prevented.

In the 1940s, Dr Alice Stewart was the youngest fellow ever elected to the Royal College of Physicians. She started to investigate the increasing levels of childhood cancers at that time and found strong evidence that they were caused by the practice of giving X-rays to pregnant women. The results of her work were published in the Lancet in 1957. British and US medical establishments, government regulators and the nuclear industry were outraged by this evidence which represented a major threat. They launched a brutal attack on Dr Stewart. She never received another research grant in England. It took 25 years before medical establishments finally accepted her research and stopped the practice of giving X-rays to expectant mothers. It is impossible to calculate how many children developed unnecessary cancers and how many died from them over the quarter of a century that this tragic treatment continued to be given.

Herbert Needleman of the University of Pittsburgh published a study in 1979 in the New England Journal of Medicine which revealed the effect of lead on the brain. It showed that children with high lead levels in their body had significantly poorer scores in intelligence tests, speech processing, and auditory and attention measurements. The main source came from the fumes of leaded petrol and both the oil and lead industries coordinated a vicious attack against Needleman since his work threatened the viability of their businesses. They used scientific and medical consultants as well as public relations firms to destroy his research and credibility and pressurised the Environment Protection Agency and other organisations to launch investigations against him. All this ruined Needleman's academic career even though it was all eventually confirmed to be true and leaded petrol was subsequently phased out and finally banned from use years later. Once again it is impossible to calculate the huge numbers of children who suffered unnecessarily.

We have seen how the two Australian researchers Barry Marshall and Robin Warren found the true cause of stomach ulcers – a bacterium that could easily be cured by antibiotics. Probably because they were junior researchers and not considered a real threat, their work was simply dismissed, ignored and treated with disdain. Had they been high-profile scientists like John Yudkin and Dr Stewart, they would almost certainly have been viciously attacked in the same way and their research papers probably retracted. It is lucky for mankind they were not prevented from continuing to try to promote their ideas, and that they had the courage to continue to do so despite facing total ridicule and dismissal, otherwise, by now, tens of millions more people would have died from ulcers or suffered from unbearable pain.

UK cardiologist Dr Aseem Malhotra and Harvard Medical School's Dr John Abramson analysed several studies which showed that, overall, side effects affected 18–20 % of statin users. The paper was published in the British Medical Journal. They were attacked by the pro-statin lobby with calls for the paper to be immediately retracted. So far, the BMJ is heroically holding firm and refusing the retraction because it clearly believes the conclusions of the paper are correct. So, this attack is still ongoing.

Professor Tim Noakes is a very eminent scientist with over 550 peer-reviewed publications and two lifetime achievement awards. He believes firmly in the concept of evidence-based medicine. For years he had followed the conventional low fat medical guidelines with his patients until he started to look at the evidence in detail and realised it was not supported by any science. He is now an advocate of LCHF diets (low carb, high fat). But when he made a low carb recommendation to a mother and her daughter in 2014, he was hauled before the Health Professional Council of South Africa for not following the conventional low fat guidelines. He refused to change his position and a legal high-profile court case was brought against him that lasted three years. The judges finally acquitted him in 2017 because of the incredible evidence he provided, The Health Professional Council's "evidence" of the benefits of a low fat diet consisted of just one meta-analysis and even this was subject to a devastating critique by Noakes and his star witness – UK nutritionist Dr Zoe Harcombe. Noakes, on the other hand, produced the following overwhelming evidence for the LCHF diet: 47 clinical trials, 11 meta-analyses and 28 intervention trials. The evidence included a European study which showed a raised intake of saturated fats was linked to lower rates of cardiovascular disease.

Sadly, but perhaps not unexpectedly, the medical establishment was not prepared to accept such an embarrassing judgement and they immediately appealed. The new appeal case lasted another year but thankfully, in 2018, he was again acquitted on all counts. The Health Professional Council tried for four years to simply protect their reputations and to destroy Professor Noakes for challenging them, even though the low fat diet they advocate has no scientific evidence, while the low carb diet used by Professor Noakes has overwhelming wide-ranging evidence. Having lost the legal case, you really should have expected them to change their diet recommendations, but they haven't. They still officially recommend the low fat diet and South Africa, sadly and unsurprisingly, has one of the highest rates of obesity in Africa.

Dr Gary Fettke, an Australian surgeon, was also an advocate of low carb diets. He recommended them to a number of his patients who had type 2 diabetes. Most of them then saw their diabetes reverse. But despite this success, Dr Fettke was subsequently banned from giving nutritional advice to his patients or speaking about low carb diets for the rest of his medical career with no ability to appeal this ruling. He was then subject to over four years of bullying and harassment, but all this failed to silence him. Then, unexpectedly, in 2018 the Australian Health Practitioner Regulation Authority dropped all charges against him. They even sent a letter of apology and confirmed that no harm had come to his patients and said there was no significant risk from the low carb, high fat diet he recommended. Could this decision have been influenced by the South African legal case? It is impossible to say with any certainty, but whatever the reason, this seemed like another significant win for those advocating low carb diets. However, the reality is much more sanguine. Every single health authority and government throughout the entire world simply, and almost unbelievably, continues to officially promote the low fat diet they approved nearly 40 years ago with all the devastating health outcomes it produces, and this will be explored in much more detail in Parts 4 and 5.

In 2007 Dr Irene Frachon at the Brest hospital in France noticed a significant number of patients with an unexplained heart valve disease were taking a drug called Mediator. She contacted the company Servier who denied any relationship between Mediator and the heart disease. By 2008, however, she had assembled a large body of evidence against the drug which she took to the medicine's regulator, but they also dismissed her data. She wrote a book about her findings and then started to receive threatening emails and her department's research funding was suddenly cut. Servier took her to court and her book was banned. She was under intense pressure but stuck to her guns and eventually, in 2010, the book was reinstated, and the drug was also banned by the European Medicines Agency. The drug had first been used in 1976 and it is impossible to calculate how many people died or suffered serious life-changing heart problems over the following 34 years. The whole thing eventually became France's biggest pharmaceutical scandal and made headline news around the world. The key fact, however, is that without the true heroism of a French doctor who had to face vicious personal attacks, the drug Mediator would still be destroying untold numbers of lives. I must add that the drug was never authorised for use in America and the UK and that several other countries like Spain and Switzerland also banned the drug in 2000 when evidence of a link with heart valve disease started to emerge. So, alarm bells really should have been ringing in France and the EU before Dr Frachon became involved, but, of course, the drug company made sure they weren't.

Final Comments

The eight examples of scurvy, puerperal fever, radical mastectomy, bed rest for heart attacks, stomach ulcers, the beta blocker scandal, type 2 diabetes and chronic fatigue syndrome are just the tip of a serious medical problem, but I would be surprised if you have heard of any of them, even though they have resulted in the death or other serious harm of somewhere around 50 million to 100 million people over the last 200 years. It would seem there is a strong desire by medicine to cover up these types of "mistakes", and it would also seem that governments, regulators, and the press and media are also complicit to a large degree. You may think these sorts of devastating medical outcomes are partly historical and could not be happening today, but in Parts 4 and 5 you will be shocked to see even worse current examples. Before then, here are just four others in headline form only. These are probably more well-known.

- The practice of lobotomy from the late 1930s to the mid-1950s destroyed many lives including the sister of President John F. Kennedy. In the UK alone, more than 20,000 lobotomies were performed and most of them caused serious and often devastating outcomes and deaths. Shockingly, it involved severing the connection between the frontal lobes and the rest of the brain and there were various ways like drilling a hole on either side of the skull and then simply inserting a knife to make the cut. The claim was that it was a miracle cure for diseases like schizophrenia and depression. However, lobotomy is now officially viewed as one of the most barbaric and misguided medical procedures of the twentieth century. The man who invented it, Portuguese neurologist Egas Moniz, was, unbelievably, given the Nobel Prize for his work.

- The use of mesh implants for women has destroyed around 8,000 UK lives, although some have suggested that the true figure is nearer to 100,000. Some of the women are unable to work, or even walk and some are confined to wheelchairs. Many will live with excruciating pain for the rest of their lives. The worldwide figures could be well over a million.
- The use of breast implants which has been shown to cause cancer in some patients.
- The widespread practice of tonsillectomy in the mid twentieth century when around half of all people had their tonsils removed. Most of these operations were unnecessary and some caused painful side-effects.

I have a personal interest in tonsillectomy. When I was ten, a visit to the doctor ended with a recommendation that I should have my tonsils removed. My father implicitly trusted doctors and decreed I must have the operation. My mother violently disagreed. Why? Well, she had been in exactly the same position and her parents had made her undergo the operation when she was 17. She endured bouts of pain for the rest of her life because of it and was determined I would not suffer the same fate. It was the only time my parents ever had a serious argument. Eventually, she prevailed and I shall be forever grateful to her. I never did need my tonsils removed. It was just unfounded medical dogma – a bad idea that caused much unnecessary suffering for many people but continued at staggering levels for many years.

Despite escaping the overprescribed practice of tonsillectomy, here is something I did not escape from. It makes me very angry. My first dentist retired when I was 20. Five years later, I went for the tenth routine check-up with my second dentist. He explained that during that time there had been no decay and no need for any new fillings, yet a majority of my back teeth had large amalgam fillings. He had waited five years to be certain that I had no decay so that what he was going to tell me was true. He then said eight words I will never forget: "I should not speak ill of my predecessor, but…" He then went on to explain how, at that time, my original dentist had been one of many throughout the country who had decided to drill out people's back teeth and put amalgam fillings in even if there was no decay. He was clearly very angry about all of this, and I also remember being shocked, even though I could not anticipate what would eventually happen. The problem was the teeth had large fillings with a thin layer of natural tooth around them. Over many years, what happened was that parts of this thin tooth would break off. The first (and probably the second) time this happened it could be refilled, but after another break there was not enough tooth left to hold in the filling. There were then just two options: either have the tooth extracted or fit a crown. Unsurprisingly, I chose a crown each time. This really was a solution that hopefully will last for the rest of my life.

However, since the age of 25, I have never needed a single new filling in any of my other teeth. If I had not had this despicable first dentist, I would probably now have a mouth full of original healthy teeth. Instead, I went through hell with dozens of fillings and refillings and then crowns. Information on the web confirms all this is true, but what I didn't realise was that the main reason it was done was greed. The dentists simply received extra money for every filling they carried out. I am not the only person to suffer from this appalling procedure. Hundreds of thousands of other people would have also been affected, but I suspect very few of them would know the real facts that I was told by my new young dentist. You will also see in Part 4 how the mercury in amalgam fillings can lead to serious health problems and how many countries have now banned them and this is another appalling outcome of what these dentists did. I can never forgive what happened.

If you are still doubting that things could be as bad as I am suggesting, then here is one more piece of evidence. In 2005 one of the most eminent doctors in the world, Professor John Ionaddis of Stanford University in America, reanalysed 49 of the most respected and influential medical papers of the previous 13 years. He showed that 32% of them had subsequently been proven to be wrong or had significantly overstated the benefits of the treatments involved. To this day no one in medicine has been able to contradict the conclusions of Professor Ionaddis, even though a few have tried. These influential papers significantly determined medical practice for over a decade. It is impossible to know how many patients suffered because of this poor science and the reluctance of medicine to regularly keep checking what it does is correct. But remember, these were the most respected and trusted medical papers that were used for widespread treatments of their time. If 32% of them were wrong, it begs the question of just how much trust can be placed on all the other research which still forms the basis for most of the other treatments that doctors use. All this is further emphasised by Dr Richard Horton, editor of the Lancet medical journal, who, in 2016, said, "Much of the scientific literature, perhaps half, may be untrue."

Medicine accepts it does not know the real causes of virtually any disease, and this has to be one of the major reasons why it makes many mistakes that lead to unbelievable outcomes, suffering and deaths. It can also take years and even decades to remove these treatments. However, I need to emphasise one truly important fact. GPs, hospital doctors and other healthcare workers are *not* really involved in either of these shocking facts. It is the relatively small number of key medical "experts" who dictate what doctors are taught and who develop and approve the medical and drug treatments and guidelines they must all religiously follow who are at the heart of it all. GPs and doctors always have and will continue to try to do the very best for their patients, but they simply have to follow the mandatory guidelines imposed on them. I will unapologetically repeat this several more times throughout the book because it is so important to understand where the real blame lies.

One final note. The discord between patients and doctors, like the one involving chronic fatigue syndrome treatment, was once a rare event. But the declining lack of trust that some patients have for medicine is now occurring in other areas, as these three examples show.

When patients use the medically endorsed low fat diet to lose weight, many of them realise it does not work in the longer term. They then may read about and do exactly the opposite – a low carb diet – and find it does work.

Many patients taking statins suffer significant side effects like muscle pain, headaches and poor sleep. Medicine really does claim that these often just result from the patient's perceptions that statins are harmful – the so-called nocebo effect. Those patients affected, however, know this is not correct because they stop taking the statins and the pain disappears; they start again and it reappears. Can they really have no pain and just imagine it? More on this in Part 5.

Hundreds of thousands of type 2 diabetes patients have reversed the disease simply by using a diet that directly contradicts the official diet they are told to adopt by medicine.

Unless medicine starts to address these issues, it will face a growing loss of trust.

Medical research – can it really be trusted?

Statistics-based research

I'll start this section with one of the most famous quotations of all time. It was originally attributed to Benjamin Disraeli, but whether this is true is disputed: "There are three kinds of lies: lies, damned lies and statistics." Whoever did say it was truly enlightened. Statistics inhabit a mythical world where anything is possible. Where anything can be proven and at the same time disproven, and no one can definitively prove who is right and who is wrong. In today's world it seems that everything is judged on statistical analysis, whether it is unemployment rates, hospital waiting times, crime figures and even happiness.

In theory, statistics can be a powerful analytical tool but in cynical or corrupt hands they can have mind-numbingly disastrous consequences. Politics is recognised as the "spiritual home" for statistical chicanery of the worst type. As Winston Churchill cynically remarked, "The first lesson that you must learn is, that when I call for statistics about the rate of infant mortality, what I want is proof that fewer babies died when I was prime minister than when anyone else was prime minister. That is a political statistic." When unemployment was rising, a previous government changed its official definition no less than 20 times in five years to massage uncomfortable figures. This type of statistical manipulation is endemic and so it is little surprise that few people trust "official political figures".

Before the 2015 election the Conservative party and Labour party both issued reports on living standards. The Conservatives claimed that living standards had risen under the coalition government while Labour claimed they had fallen. In a BBC interview a leading economist was asked, "Who was right?" To which he replied, "They are both right!" He went on to explain that each party had simply cherry picked the data that suited their own purposes. The start and end dates for the analysis were different and the Conservatives had, for example, included the value of pensions, savings, house prices and bonus payments, while Labour had concentrated mainly on basic pay. But who is to say what is right and what is wrong in this situation? If you took 100 economists and asked them to do the analysis, you would get 100 different answers. There would never be, and could never be, any consensus, any "right" answer. All this is possible just by "cherry picking" statistical data. There was no covert fraud. Both parties used exactly the same sets of official data. So, imagine what happens when you add in the possibility of data manipulation, changing definitions and actual fraud.

You may be wondering what all this discussion about politics and statistics has to do with medicine. Well, medical research has also become subsumed by statistical analysis with inevitable and disastrous consequences. How did it all start? It started shortly after the end of the Second World War when scientists started to develop new ideas for carrying out medical research. In 1948 the first randomised controlled clinical trial was published in the British Medical Journal and, in 1950, Doll and Hill's epidemiological study on the relationship between smoking and lung cancer was completed. Both relied heavily on statistical analysis of large-scale data. These trials and studies represented a revolution in medical thinking that would ultimately affect the lives of countless millions of people around the world. It is no exaggeration to say medicine fell under the spell of statistics. It was expected that this would allow the causes of most diseases to be determined which would then lead to effective treatments. Probably no one realised at the time how this type of complex, statistical-based research, and the ability to manipulate it so easily, would eventually lead to a world where most research could not be trusted.

Whilst most people know they cannot trust political statistics, most would implicitly trust medical research even if it was based on statistical analysis. They would refuse to believe such statistical chicanery was possible within medicine. But fraud in one form or another can be found in every walk of life. High-profile figures like politicians, bankers, peers of the realm, senior police officers, judges, football managers and comedians usually hit the news headlines when they commit it, but many other individuals are similarly culpable when they complete their tax returns, fill in their monthly claims for expenses or apply for social security benefits. It really should come as no surprise, therefore, to learn that fraud occurs in medical research. But, as you will see in the next three sections, the manipulation, cherry picking, data rigging and fraud that exists within medical research makes even the politicians look like amateurs.

Fundamental flaws in clinical trials

The very design and protocols of clinical trials have several major flaws which have serious implications for patients.

Fundamental flaw 1. A vital requirement of all clinical trials is that neither the patient nor the doctors monitoring them should know who is taking the drug and who is taking the placebo. They should, in the jargon, be "double blind". The problem is, because most drugs have side effects, some patients will experience them, and these people will then know they are taking the drug; a process called "unblinding". This means the doctors monitoring them will also get to know since discussing any side effects of the treatment is an integral part of the trial. But the trials are meant to be "double blind" for a very good reason. Bias by both the patient and doctor, even if this is subconscious, is almost certain and will almost certainly favour the drug. As we have seen, many drugs have small benefits and the bias caused by "unblinding" can account for most and even all of this small "benefit". If you find this hard to believe, then here is one example.

We have seen that antidepressant drugs reduce depression by just 5% more than a placebo, but I also said there was a final twist to this story. Antidepressants are notorious for side effects. One of these is a dry mouth and virtually everyone suffers from this effect. So, in the clinical trials everyone knows exactly who is taking the drug and this makes the bias in favour of the drug extreme. There is, however, a way round this problem. It is possible to add something to the placebo that induces a similar side effect. This is called an "active placebo". When you do this, even the patients taking the placebo think they are taking the drug. And guess what the results are under these conditions? Both the drug and placebo produce almost the same improvement in symptoms of around 25%. This proves two things. Firstly, the clinical trial protocol is fundamentally flawed because active placebos are never used. Many trials are, therefore, biased significantly in favour of the drug by the very design of the trial. Secondly, antidepressants cannot have a true clinical benefit on the level of depression if they perform the same as an active placebo. In other words, the benefits patients experience must come simply from the enhanced placebo effect. We will explore this in more detail later when we will try to understand how a drug that doesn't work any better for clinical depression than an active placebo is nevertheless inexplicably prescribed to 10% of the entire adult population at a cost exceeding $800 million in the UK alone.

Fundamental flaw 2. Some drugs are used predominantly by older people while others are used by all age groups. You might imagine that when a drug is used mainly by older people, such as for arthritis, it would be tested on that particular age group. This would be a logical assumption, but you would be wrong. In fact, drugs are tested on healthy young adults almost exclusively. Why? The pharmaceutical industry uses the following tortured logic when trying to explain this inexplicable protocol. They explain that older people generally have at least one other medical condition, and probably several others, and may be taking several drugs for these. If they did trials on these people, the benefit of the drug could be difficult to measure because of the other problems the patients were already experiencing and because of interactions with the other drugs they were taking. By using young people who have no other underlying medical conditions and are taking no other medication, the "positive effects" of the drug can be seen and measured.

Let me translate all this into plain and simple English. Many drugs have a tiny benefit. But even this tiny benefit would probably disappear if we gave it to older people with other medical problems and using other drugs. So, we will test it on young people where we can demonstrate that this small benefit exists. Then we'll get it approved on this basis and then we can promote its use for millions of older people where it won't work or will work on such a miniscule level that no one can even feel the benefit, but, of course, we'll make billions of dollars. Oh, and by the way, we won't even talk about the nasty side effects that come with the drug.

If the drug industry cannot prove that a drug works for the people who are actually going to take it, then it should never be approved. Why did experts, academics, medical journals, regulators and politicians allow the pharmaceutical industry to get away with this one? You will soon find out.

Fundamental flaw 3. Clinical trials used for drug approval are rarely carried out for more than a year, and often for just a few months. This is a woefully inadequate period given that side effects can take much longer to show up. For example, smoking is considered to be one of the most dangerous things that anyone can do, and yet, for many people it can take up to 30 to 40 years before the serious effects like lung cancer and heart disease start to show up. The real reason why trials only last for such short times is all down to money. Every extra month a trial continues eats into the period of patent protection, which, of course, is when companies make virtually all their profits. The industry has been very successful in fighting off calls for longer trials that would provide greater safety for patients. In practice what this means is that the clinical trial which is meant to show a drug is safe (as well as that it works) does no such thing. The side effects from drugs usually only start to show up when millions of people around the world have taken them for extended periods. So, when anyone takes a new drug, the reality is they are in fact taking part in a real-life drug trial whether they realise it or not. At some point, whether it is after several months or many years, side effects that were not detected during the trials start to show up. By that time many thousands, and probably tens of thousands, of people will have suffered and some of them will have been killed by the drug even though the clinical trial supposedly "proved" it was safe.

If you find all this impossible to believe and feel the regulator would surely not allow it to happen, then here is one final piece of evidence. Once a new drug is approved, the regulator requires companies to carry out additional stage IV trials over the next few years to see if the drug really works and is safe in the real world. This requirement is very revealing. The brutal truth is that when a new drug is approved, no one knows whether it will eventually cause more harm than good or whether it will kill more people than it saves. We will explore many harrowing examples of this problem in the next few sections, but it is so serious that some doctors have made the following suggestion. If you are offered a "new drug" by your doctor, ask if there is an older drug that has been in use for at least ten and preferably 20 years. You are then much less likely to suffer serious or deadly side effects. If you think the new drug must be better and could be worth the risk, then you will also learn in the next section that, for most drugs, this also is simply not true.

Fundamental flaw 4. So, as we have just seen, many of the side effects of individual drugs are detected only after the clinical trial process is finished and the drug is launched on an unsuspecting public. But what happens when someone is taking two drugs? Are any trials done to see if there are any dangerous drug interactions? The short answer to that is no. No trials of this sort are ever carried out. But if you look at any drug leaflet you will see a list of other drugs that you should not take. These drugs are listed because they cause a serious and dangerous interaction with the first drug. Some of these interactions may already be known, but many are discovered simply by seeing what happens to the millions of people who take them. So, to get to this stage, we again have people harmed and killed so that these dangerous interactions can finally be conclusively established. Only at that stage is a position reached where further harm is minimised for new users because the drug leaflet then adds these new side effects.

But what is the outcome when people take not just two, but multiple drugs for long periods (a process known as polypharmacy)? We will examine the deeply disturbing process of polypharmacy in detail later, but it is not unusual for many, mainly older, people to be taking ten or more drugs simultaneously. What happens then? Quite simply – and quite frighteningly – no one knows. Some of the drugs will interact and may not work at all, while at the same time producing damaging, unexpected and life-threatening side effects and harm. Clinical trials are not designed to detect any drug interactions. Polypharmacy, therefore, is like playing Russian roulette with several bullets in the gun.

Fundamental flaw 5. Clinical trials rely on a placebo pill against which the drug is assessed. The placebo, by definition, should contain substances that have been scientifically proven to have zero effect on the disease involved, otherwise a true evaluation of the drug cannot be made. However, a 2010 study highlighted that no regulations exist that specify placebo composition and that with just a few exceptions, the formulation of the placebo is also never reported in the clinical trial results. Does this matter? Absolutely. As you will see in the next section, the manipulation and fraud that occurs in clinical trials is staggering. Given that drug companies can select their own placebo compounds they could (and no one, not even regulators, would know) select a compound that helps to falsely show a better outcome for the drug being trialled. Consider a diabetes drug and a placebo that contained sugar. The sugar would increase the blood glucose levels in the placebo group and make the drug look more effective than it was. Of course, it would be impossible to prove such a trial actually took place, but when you look at all the other data manipulation and fraud the drug companies carry out, there is a real likelihood that the use of inappropriate placebos is likely to be commonplace. If you doubt any of this, then in Part 5 you will see that, as far as vaccines are concerned, not one true placebo has ever been used in any vaccine trial throughout their entire history.

Manipulation, data rigging and fraud within medical research

As already outlined, randomised clinical trials and epidemiological studies form the basis for most medical research. But the trials and studies rely almost exclusively on exhaustive statistical analysis which, as we have seen, can result in all manner of chicanery, bias and manipulation. In addition, the complexity of the protocols for conducting randomised trials leaves further opportunity for manipulation and data rigging and, of course, outright fraud is also on the agenda. We must also not forget "cherry picking" of data which has become a fine art in medicine and medical research. By the end of this section, you will understand that the claims made by medicine that it is "evidence based" are, in large part, untrue.

So, now we can start to look at the limitations of medical research and explore how data rigging, manipulation, bias, fraud and "cherry picking" make many trial results worthless.

Off-label drug promotion – a $150 billion fraud

We have already seen that drugs are tested for a specific purpose and are approved by regulators only for that specific condition. It is illegal for drug companies to promote the use of a drug for any other condition because by definition there is no proof it would work. Pushing drugs in this way is called off-label promotion. There is, of course, a simple and legal solution for the companies. If they are confident a drug would work for another disease, then they can simply carry out new trials to prove it. The cost and even the timescale would be less than normal because they have already done the entire preliminary work in the original trial. But there is still a significant risk that the drug would simply not work. The fact is 80% of drug trials fail to produce positive results and so they cannot be approved for use. So, do the companies have a solution to this terrible dilemma? Well, in fact they have a very simple solution. They just promote the drug to doctors anyway and ignore the law. Weren't we always taught that the simplest solutions were the best?

We have already seen that regulators require further trials to be carried out after drugs have been approved to see how they perform in the real world. The industry has, however, usurped and corrupted the process so it can be used to facilitate off-label drug promotion. They carry out very cheap stage IV trials to "show the drug works on other conditions" and then use various promotional techniques to get doctors prescribing them. Remember, these are not clinical trials. They lack all the rigour of clinical trials, they are not placebo controlled, they are not randomised, and they are not double blind. In fact, they prove just about nothing, but if you get a leading academic to sign a paper and get it published in a journal or present it at conferences or just get your sales reps to promote it to individual doctors, you can be on to a winner. Remember, it is not illegal for doctors to prescribe drugs that are off label; it is only illegal for the drug companies to promote such use. This dispensation for doctors has some logic to it. Imagine a doctor has a patient with a serious or life-threatening condition which has not responded to any approved conventional treatment but there are indications that another drug "might" be effective. Then, with the patient's approval, it could be worth trying this drug rather than just letting them suffer or die. This dispensation was meant to be used judiciously and reserved for exceptional cases.

Here is the story of a drug called Neurontin which illustrates how all of this works in the real world. It came to light because of a whistleblower who worked at a pharmaceutical company called Parke-Davis which was a subsidiary of Warner Lambert which later was taken over by the drug giant Pfizer. David Franklin, a Parke-Davis sales representative, had collected thousands of pages of internal documents and in 1996 decided to turn whistleblower by bringing a case against the company for defrauding government health programmes. He alleged that the company had carried out a massive illegal scheme to promote the drug Neurontin for off-label uses. This involved paying academic experts to put their names on flimsy research papers written by the company which seemingly showed that the drug worked for these other conditions. Eventually, federal prosecutors as well as 47 US states also launched both criminal and civil investigations of their own. Court documents were originally sealed at the company's request, but many of them were released in 2002 in response to media petitions. They showed a well-coordinated plan of incredible dimensions. Neurontin had been approved by the FDA in 1994 as an add-on treatment for epilepsy when other drugs failed to control seizures. There wasn't much money in that, of course, and the company wanted to expand the drug's market. The company's plan was to get doctors to prescribe Neurontin for a number of common but vague conditions like pain, restless leg syndrome and anxiety. If the campaign was successful, huge markets would be opened up.

The studies the company carried out were so small and poorly designed that few scientific conclusions could be drawn from any of them. Medical education and communication companies were then hired to prepare articles about the trials and then find doctors willing to sign them with the implication that they had written them. One of these firms, for instance, was paid $144,000 for 12 journal articles. The second part of the strategy was to see that the articles and the information in them were widely distributed to practising doctors. Then specially trained salesmen would visit doctors' offices to answer questions about the research. Parke-Davis also sponsored educational meetings and conferences all over the country, where the "authors" of the papers and other experts would promote the use of the drug for more than a dozen unapproved off-label uses. These "authors" and experts were reportedly paid tens of thousands of dollars each. But doctors in the audience were also often paid. This would normally be illegal, but by calling them "consultants" the company was able to circumvent the law. These consultant meetings were often little more than vacations for potential high prescribers of Neurontin. The company tracked doctors after the meetings and, according to a New York Times story, the company found an increase of about 70% in prescriptions after these dinner meetings.

As a result of all these efforts, Neurontin become a blockbuster drug, with sales of $2.7 billion in 2003. About 80% of prescriptions that year were for unapproved uses – conditions like post-traumatic stress disorder, insomnia, restless leg syndrome, hot flushes, migraines and tension headaches – and yet there was no good, published evidence that it worked for any of them. In May 2004, eight years after the case began, Pfizer pleaded guilty to illegal marketing and agreed to pay $430 million to resolve the criminal and civil charges against it. That might sound like a lot of money, but it is dwarfed by the $2.7 billion of illegal sales in just one single year.

In case you think I may have cherry picked an isolated example myself to prove a point, the following are just a few of the many fraud settlements paid by the drug companies for the period 2007 to 2012, that anyone can verify as being true. These fines relate to the illegal promotion of off-label drug use:

- Pfizer: $2.3 billion – illegal promotion of Bextra, Geodon, Zyvox and Lyrica (2009)
- Novartis: $426 million – illegal promotion of Trileptal (2010)
- GlaxoSmithKline: $3 billion – illegal promotion of several drugs and two other charges (2011)
- AstraZeneca: $520 million – illegal promotion of Seroquel (2010)
- Eli Lilly: $1.4 billion – illegal promotion of Zyprexa (2009)
- Abbott: $1.5 billion – illegal promotion of Depakote (2012)
- Bristol Myers Squibb: $515 million – illegal promotion of several drugs (2007)

The total of just these seven fines and settlements is $10 billion. You may wonder why the companies continue to carry out such fraud when the fines are so large. Well, in every single case, just as with Neurontin, the money the companies raked in, courtesy of the illegal promotion, exceeded the fines by several orders of magnitude. Who said crime does not pay? It certainly pays for the pharmaceutical industry, and it is little wonder they carry on doing it. In fact, a 2020 study published in the Journal of the American Medical Association showed that 25 of the largest drug companies had paid over $33 billion in fines in the 13 years between 2005 and 2018. So, pharmaceutical fraud is still rampant, and the industry is raking in billions of dollars from it. Alan Cassels, a drug policy researcher at the University of Victoria in Canada, said, "Pharmaceutical companies are simply criminal recidivists which break the law, pay the fine and then break the law again."

So, the proof that off-label fraud exists, and exists on a large scale, is indisputable. But sadly, most cases go undetected and are certainly not prosecuted. Remember that if the whistleblower at Parke-Davis had not spilt the beans, then the Neurontin fraud may never have been uncovered. There is, however, a simple way of assessing the true scale of this unbelievable problem. The actual numbers of drug prescriptions for unapproved uses is about 20% of the total – an incredible 1 in 5 of all prescriptions. Of course, doctors are legally allowed to use off-label drugs but only in special cases. They are not meant to be used for mass prescribing for common conditions like pain and anxiety where there are already numerous other legally approved drugs. The level of off-label prescribing for genuine reasons would be a tiny percentage of total drug prescriptions. A figure of 1% would probably be a reasonable estimate, but I will be very generous to Big Pharma and say it could be as high as 5%. This means that the other 15% of all prescriptions are for unapproved uses simply because they have been illegally promoted by the industry. It also still means that 20% of all prescriptions made by doctors have no scientific basis because no off-label drug has any proof it works. Medicine's claims that everything it does is "evidence based" are shot down in flames by this single incredible scandal.

The global turnover of the pharmaceutical industry in 2019 was $1,000 billion. Around 15% of this, or about $150 billion, is due to illegal promotion. There is not a shred of proof that any of it works. It is indeed a $150 billion fraud, and it is occurring every single year. Patients are paying for this fraud with their lives and their health because there is no proven benefit from these drugs, but the side effects are ubiquitous. Each year, governments and taxpayers are paying $150 billion for drugs that have no evidence they work, but as we will see in detail later, they then pay another $75 billion to treat the side effects of the very same drugs: a staggering $225 billion in total. This is almost certainly one of the biggest ongoing frauds in the entire world.

Hiding inconvenient data

The normal rules for drug approval require two clinical trials to be submitted to the regulator. If these show a positive statistical benefit, the regulator must approve the drug. Now imagine you are a drug manufacturer and the first two trials you have done aren't successful; the drug didn't have any benefit. You have nothing else in the pipeline. You staked everything on this one drug. Well, why not try another two trials. Yes, they are expensive to carry out, but everything hinges on getting a positive result. And bingo, one of them does indeed show a statistical benefit. The "rules of statistics" say as much. If you toss five coins you rarely get five heads but occasionally it does happen. Now you know that if you keep going you are sure to find a second one that shows positive results. Indeed, the eighth trial is also positive. The job is now done. You submit these two trials to the regulator who by law must approve the drug and now you could well have a new blockbuster on your hands. Of course, if all eight trials were examined together the drug would never be approved. But incredibly, the laws governing drug approval do not require this.

Initially, drug companies could do as many trials as they wanted and could keep this secret. So, in the example above, they would just submit the two that worked to the regulator, and no one would even know the other six trials existed. But because of pressure from independent observers and consumer groups, the law was changed so every single trial has to be officially registered before it's started. Has this made any practical difference? The first thing to say is the new law is not retrospective. In other words, all the drugs previously approved do not have to undergo a re-examination and are still widely prescribed. It has certainly made it more difficult for the industry to hide what is going on. But the law on approval has not changed. So, the regulator may still be given just the two trials that showed benefits. They can see there are six other trials and could, if they wanted, demand to analyse them. But as we will see, this rarely happens and the drug is still frequently approved. Also, the new law still does not require the drug company to publish the results of the other trials. So, all that has really changed is that outside observers can now see the numbers of trials performed and can smell a rat whereas previously they might only have been able to guess at such subterfuge or, occasionally, whistleblowers would spill the beans.

Of course, some drugs do have genuine benefits and only two trials are needed to prove this. Nevertheless, this type of subterfuge is commonplace. It is illegal for me to call it *fraud*, as inexplicably all this hiding of data is perfectly legal. So, instead, I will call it "*fraud*". How common is it? The generally accepted figure is that 50% of all trials were originally hidden or are now only available to the regulator and never disseminated to anyone else. What does all this tell us about the efficacy of the drugs that hundreds of millions of people take? It tells us clearly that many drugs do not work or work so minutely they are of little clinical benefit to patients. What is less clear is which ones are useful and which are not. It tells us that a great many people are suffering side effects from drugs with no meaningful benefit. The lenient laws and rules that permit all of this to happen are what surprises people the most.

Surrogate end points

Drugs are developed to treat specific diseases. When statins were developed, they were intended simply to reduce the risk of heart attacks and strokes because high cholesterol on its own has no other detrimental effects on people's health. So, you might expect that when statin drugs were initially tested in clinical trials, they would have needed to show that they did indeed reduce the number of heart attacks. But this is not the case. Statins only had to demonstrate that they reduced cholesterol levels. Cholesterol, in this case, is what is known as a surrogate end point – something that we hope is associated with the real outcome, but it might not be, either not at all or perhaps not very well. I do not want to give the game away here, but in Part 5 there is a special section devoted to cholesterol lowering drugs, where the truth about statins will surprise and shock you.

Here, the key take home message is that the pharmaceutical industry loves surrogate end points. Proving a drug will affect a surrogate end point is quick, cheap and easy. Statins and blood pressure drugs, for example, lower cholesterol and blood pressure in just a few weeks at most, whereas proving they reduce heart attacks might take years. Also, because the trials only take a few weeks, most side effects will not even show up. So, this is a win-win for the industry, and they are constantly trying to get as many drugs accepted on data from surrogate end points as they can get away with. But the problem with many surrogate end points is they are often only loosely connected, or not connected at all, with real-life clinical outcomes, and in some cases, they are in fact associated with increased mortality or other serious side effects.

One tragic example of this was the use of anti-arrythmia drugs to treat patients with heart rhythm disturbances. The drugs encainide and flecainide were approved by the FDA because they reduced these irregular heart rhythms. Most cardiologists and doctors started to prescribe them because, whilst the irregular rhythms were benign in themselves, they were believed to increase the risk of fatal heart disease. But did they really increase heart attacks and deaths, especially when these are the only outcomes that matter to patients? Eventually, the CAST clinical trial (Cardiac Arrythmia Suppression Trial) was carried out to confirm the expected benefits and to get an accurate measurement of these benefits. Imagine the horror when this trial had to be stopped early because not only did the drugs not work at all, but they were killing people as well. In the trial, 9.6% of patients given the drug died compared with just 3.6% given a placebo. These drugs had been used for over five years and given to millions of people worldwide before the trial results led to their abandonment. Dr Peter Gøtzsche estimates that at their peak usage in the US alone, they caused about 50,000 deaths in one year. In just one year the drugs killed the same number of Americans as the total number killed in the Vietnam War. Over the five years they were used the total US death toll would probably have been around 150,000. It is impossible to accurately predict the worldwide deaths, but a figure of 300,000 would be a very conservative estimate.

Surrogate end points can allow the pharmaceutical industry to "get away with murder" quite literally. But in this case the fact that the drug approval was based on a surrogate end point was, of course, only part of the problem. Medical dogma and consensus had also incorrectly assumed that reducing heart arrythmias must also reduce heart attack deaths and this is why they were so aggressively used. It took five years before this was shown to be incorrect. This is just one more example of how medical dogma can also lead to hundreds of thousands of deaths. The problem with most surrogate end points is that they simply allow drugs to be approved and then used very rapidly, even though many of them have little or no benefit as well as serious side effects. A number of cancer drugs have also been approved because they have shown they can reduce the size of tumours. Do you think this would surely save cancer deaths? In Part 5, you will again be surprised at the real outcomes.

The ultimate statistical scam of relative risk exposed

This is an extract from a press release on the "perils" of drinking alcohol: "... regularly drinking two large glasses of wine or two strong pints of beer a day triples mouth cancer risk." Would this increase in the risk of mouth cancer make you think twice before drinking your favourite tipple? Most people assume this means that if they drank at this level, their own personal risk, and that of everyone else who did the same, would triple, but this is not the case. So, how can we assess what this sensational headline really means? Well, the real risk (scientifically known as the absolute risk) of anyone dying from mouth cancer is 1 in 100,000. This figure is for non-smokers. (For smokers, the figure is 3 in 100,000). So, for non-smokers, for every 100,000 people who die, just one will die from mouth cancer. The other 99,999 will die of something else. Two drinks every day triples the risk, so if everyone drank this amount there would be three people dying – an increase of two. So, just two extra people out of 100,000 would die of mouth cancer. This is the real meaning of this sensational headline and one you would probably never have imagined. (Please note I am not advocating alcohol consumption at this or any other level, or even its non-consumption. Alcohol has other effects, some beneficial and some harmful, and every person must make a personal decision.)

Everyone must make up their own minds about the sort of risks they are prepared to take in life, but this seems to be one of the lower risks that we all face in the grand scheme of things, despite the alarming headlines. In fact, if every single adult in the country drank two large drinks every day, the extra deaths attributable to mouth cancer would still be only half the number of people dying in car crashes, and none of us hesitate to jump into a car. Incidentally, while this next fact is not directly relevant to this section, it is something that everyone should consider when they make decisions on alcohol. While it really does slightly increase the risk of cancer, there is also strong evidence it reduces deaths from heart disease. The likely reality is that modest levels of alcohol will not cause excess deaths. The extra deaths from cancer being offset by the lower deaths from heart disease.

Now imagine a reverse scenario. Imagine there are 100,000 people who have two alcoholic drinks each day. As we have seen, three of them in total will die of mouth cancer at some point in their lives. Also imagine that a new wonder drug has been developed that could slash the risk of these people dying by two-thirds. Note that no drug other than antibiotics has come even remotely close to achieving this level of effectiveness, but for the current exercise we will assume that such an imaginary wonder drug has been developed. The drug company would ensure banner headlines around the world proclaiming its new wonder drug slashes mouth cancer deaths by an astounding 67%. Patient groups would demand this life-saving miracle drug be funded and made available for everyone. But if a drug could cut cancer death by this percentage it is going to cost a fortune; think £100,000 minimum for a year's supply per person. But in our 100,000 group of people, this drug will prevent just two extra deaths and, of course, we do not know and can never predict which of the 100,000 will eventually develop mouth cancer, so all of them will have to take it for the rest of their lives if these two individuals are to be "saved". No mention has yet been made of drug side effects. The pharmaceutical industry would, of course, claim no side effects exist. But the reality is that, as with every drug, there really are side effects, and with 100,000 people taking the drug, many more will be killed and injured eventually by the drug's emerging side effects than the two lives that are "saved".

This example gives you an insight into the magical world of relative risk reduction. This is the name given to the statistical scam that converts a miniscule *absolute* risk into an apparently enormous *relative* risk. The absolute reduction in deaths using the new wonder drug is 0.002%, whereas the relative reduction is an eye watering 67%.

Of course, this is a fictitious example of a drug that does not exist and, of course, the financial implications are so extreme it would not be funded even if it did exist. But the key point I want to make is that most drugs are sold based on relative risk reduction claims. Perhaps now you will understand why I titled this section "the ultimate statistical scam of relative risk exposed". The real or absolute benefits of many drugs are usually so small that if doctors and the public knew these figures they would not be taking many of them. Relative risk numbers look so much better and are used simply to deceive people.

Sometimes with complex statistical clinical trials, the maths involved can make relative and absolute comparisons difficult to understand for the average person. There is, however, a simple tool that helps. This is called the "Number Needed to Treat" (NNT). This is simply the number of people who need to take a drug for just one person to gain any benefit. So, in our fictitious example above, the drug would prevent two cancers out of every 100,000 people treated – or one for every 50,000 people. So, the NNT is 50,000. For antibiotics, the NNT is one because every single person treated is cured. The larger the NNT number, the more useless the drug. We will see several real-life examples of this relative risk scam in later sections, and you will be surprised at the high NNT scores of many popular drug treatments.

The large-scale randomised clinical trial is not what it seems

Medicine views the randomised clinical trial as the best proof we have that a drug works. But over recent years a new phenomenon has evolved – the large-scale randomised clinical trial (the large-scale RCT). These large RCTs can involve thousands of patients and are now seen as the ultimate level of proof regarding the efficacy of drugs. They have in fact become something of a religion. Anything other than a large-scale RCT is increasingly viewed as of little value. The pharmaceutical industry has very cleverly convinced the whole of medicine over many years that, in this case, bigger really is better. There is just one problem. The large-scale RCTs hide an inconvenient truth, which is that the trial needs to be large simply because that is the only way it can detect what are in fact the miniscule benefits of many modern drugs. The truth is the validity and value of a trial is in fact inversely proportional to its size.

If you take a drug that works perfectly, such as an antibiotic, you could prove conclusively that it worked by recruiting a small number of patients for your trial – maybe no more than 20. But if your drug only benefitted, say, 1 in 200 patients you would need thousands of people to prove statistically that it worked. So, when a drug has been approved using a large-scale RCT you know that its benefits will invariably be miniscule. Yet the large-scale RCT is now accepted worldwide as the ultimate proof of a drug's benefits. How can so many people be fooled so easily? However you look at it, the large-scale RCT has ushered in a whole generation of virtually useless drugs that provide miniscule benefits to the patients taking them and are more likely to do overall harm when side effects are taken into account. But nothing is likely to change. The academics and senior researchers who advocate their use have reputations to protect as well as close ties with Big Pharma and the monetary gain that brings. But no one has more to gain than the pharmaceutical industry which relies on large-scale RCTs for much of its profits. So, there is no hope in the short term that this dire situation will change. But at least you now know that if you are ever offered a new drug that has been tested in a large-scale RCT, it is highly unlikely you will gain much benefit from it, and don't forget the side effects.

Manipulation and data rigging in clinical trials

The dosage scams

Over half of all drug sales are accounted for by just five diseases. These are cardiovascular disease, cancer, mental problems, diabetes and respiratory disease. We have seen that it is a financial imperative that once a drug comes off patent, and its price typically falls by 90%, that it is replaced with a new version that can command the higher price again. Drugs have been used to treat some of these key diseases for many years, so now we are on "third generations" of some drugs. But finding new drugs is getting more and more difficult, especially finding ones that are better than those already being used. But the new drugs simply must be developed and marketed or the pharmaceutical industry is, quite literally, going to be in serious financial difficulties. So, as a drug company, you have a new drug that, from your initial trials, does not look very promising. You don't have any other drug in the pipeline, so it simply has to succeed. What can you do? You could carry out multiple trials and pick just the two that work as we have already seen, but there are also other methods you can use.

Let us imagine the old drug doesn't have too many side effects so the only way you are going to get the new drug selling well is to show it has better clinical outcomes. You do not have to worry about getting the drug approved by the regulator. All you have to do for this is to submit two clinical trials that show positive benefits compared to a placebo. Even if they are the same, or worse than the old drug, the rules say the regulator must approve it. The more difficult part is to persuade the people, like NICE, who make decisions about which drugs to fund. The drug companies, however, have a simple solution. They carry out further trials where they compare the new and old drugs directly against each other. The trick is to use a low dose of the old drug and a larger dose of the new drug. Not surprisingly, the new drug will then get better outcomes. You then hire a leading clinician to sign a paper that your PR people have written confirming the results – without, of course, giving full details of doses – and get this published in a leading journal. So, the drug has been approved by the regulator and given a glowing report by a trusted clinician. Who would deny patients access to a "better" drug even if it does cost ten times more? Job done and it is all so easy when you know how. You will, of course, need to ensure the full data from the trials is not made available to anyone else but stays securely under lock and key. But this, of course, is the normal practice.

Now imagine that the old drug is reasonably effective but has a number of side effects that are tarnishing its reputation. Simple. Just reverse the protocol. Give a high dose of the old drug so the side effects are maximised and obviously a low dose of the new drug. As if by magic, the side effects comparison will ensure a speedy uptake of your new "safe" drug. The simple fact is when drug companies test drugs, they are four times more likely to report positive results than when the drugs are tested by completely independent researchers. It is difficult to find any description for this type of research other than "fraud". I must call it "fraud" because once again all this is deemed to be perfectly legal.

I'll give you one example of a clever variation on the "dosage scam". Pfizer wanted to promote its antifungal drug fluconazole and devised an innovative method to do so. It compared fluconazole with an older drug called amphotericin B. This older drug was highly effective when given intravenously and this was the established method of administration because it was almost useless when taken orally since it was not absorbed well. You can probably guess that Pfizer compared fluconazole with an oral dose of amphotericin and, low and behold, fluconazole performed markedly better and, of course, it soon became a nice little earner.

Stopping trials early

The protocols for clinical trials specify all the hundreds of different parameters that will apply, such as what outcomes are to be measured, what doses are to be used, how the randomisation will be achieved and how many patients will be recruited. The protocols are supposed to be "set in stone" for good reasons, so that any subsequent manipulation of the results is avoided. By now, you will probably understand that when it suits them, the industry regularly bends the rules. And this includes the well-used scam of stopping trials early. Many drug side effects take time to develop. So, if a trial is scheduled to last 12 months, but the company is monitoring the results as the trial progresses and notices that after six months virtually no side effects have occurred, they may decide to stop the trial at that point. They can then "demonstrate" that the drug is particularly safe. Of course, if the trial had continued for the full duration, the drug's side effects would have started to emerge.

Dodgy subgroup analysis

If a drug shows no overall benefit in a clinical trial, another favourite "scam" companies employ is to start looking at subgroups. So, as the company analyses the trial results in detail, they may find that those people who were born in July see a favourable response to the drug whereas all the others do not. In theory, they could try to market the drug just for people born in July. This would, of course, be ridiculous, because it has only happened due to a statistical quirk – occasionally if you flip a coin, five heads do come up one after the other. If they carried out the trial again, then this time, by chance, it might be people born in February. Of course, no company could get away with marketing a drug using this particularly silly example, but this is a major scam that companies employ regularly, and they invariably get away with it when the subgroup selection is less blatant and obvious.

"Run-in" phase

Some trials use what is known as a run-in phase. This is carried out before the real trial commences and involves giving patients the drug and placebo often in sequence. The reasons for doing this are purported to be to assess how compliant people will be in following the trial protocol and in taking the medication as specified, and to exclude those judged unlikely to comply. But you can perhaps see that this leaves the whole process open to abuse. It gives the researchers the opportunity to pre-assess which patients might benefit most from the drug and which might experience side effects. Those who experience side effects can be excluded on the pretext that they are likely to be poor compliers. Those who reported benefit would, of course, be included.

Any trial that uses a run-in phase must be viewed with extreme suspicion, and the HOPE study is a perfect example. This was a large-scale trial investigating the effect of the drug ramipril on the prevention of heart disease. Following the run-in phase, 10% of the 10,576 eligible patients were excluded. The reasons for exclusion – which included poor compliance and side effects such as impaired renal function and hyperkalaemia – were almost certainly caused by the drug and not the placebo. The results of the trial were hardly impressive. After five years of treatment the absolute difference between ramipril and placebo in overall mortality was just 1.8%. This meagre benefit would, of course, have been even lower if those suffering from serious side effects had not been excluded from the trial. It is even possible that the drug may never have been approved in this situation. Run-in phases can totally distort the benefits of drugs and, in many cases, they can hide even serious side effects.

Ignoring people who drop out of trials

Some people who take part in trials must stop for genuine reasons, such as moving house, but these are relatively rare events. By far the biggest reason people drop out is that they experience unpleasant drug side effects and are not prepared to continue. So, how dropouts are treated can radically affect the outcome and, therefore, the validity of the trial. You will perhaps not be surprised to learn that people who drop out of trials because of side effects are often not analysed in the final trial report thus seriously understating the dangers of the drug. This really is research "fraud".

"Me too" drugs

We have already seen that the industry has several ways of ensuring a new drug gains approval, particularly when they have an old drug whose patent is about to expire. But they also have other ways, and one of the most prolific involves the development of "me too" drugs. These are either old drugs that are being recycled, or that have been modified in tiny ways. This means they already know they will work in much the same way and, therefore, that the development costs and risks of failure are much smaller. Of course, because their outcomes will be similar to existing drugs, they still need to do other rigged trials using, say, the scam of different doses to convince doctors to use them, especially as they will be around ten times more expensive. But these stage IV trials are cheap and there are always experts who will promote them for you for the right amount of money, and most doctors are taken in by this deceit, so you do not really have a problem.

So, what is the extent of this problem? In the five years from 1998 to 2002, 415 new drugs were approved by the FDA. Of these, 14% were truly innovative and 9% were old drugs that had been changed in some way that made them, in the FDA's view, significant improvements. What about the other 77%? Incredibly, they were all me too drugs. The FDA even classified them as being no better than drugs already on the market to treat the same conditions. Around 77% of the pharmaceutical industry's "new drugs" were almost virtual copies of existing drugs.

I will end this section with one audacious example of a me too drug. This requires a basic understanding of the term stereoisomer. Most complex molecules are found in two forms called stereoisomers. These have identical chemical compositions and identical structures. They differ only in that they are mirror images of each other. Invariably, one isomer is active and the other inactive when taken as a drug. The original drug will consist of a mixture of both isomers, but here comes the clever part. The company takes out a new patent on the active isomer and produces a drug containing only that individual isomer. The equivalent dose of each drug will, of course, produce identical outcomes since the active ingredients are themselves identical.

The proton pump inhibitor drug Prilosec, manufactured by AstraZeneca, was the world's bestselling drug in the late 1990s with annual sales of $5 billion. It was due to lose its patent in 2001 and this would have had a devastating effect on the company's profits. So, the company developed the single isomer version which they named Nexium. Of course, they still had another hurdle to overcome. They needed to show that Nexium was better than Prilosec because they intended to charge 30 times more for it. Can you prove that something is better than itself? Absolutely not, unless, of course, you carry out some form of "fraud". The company used 40mg of Nexium and 20mg of Prilosec for the trial and then claimed that Nexium produced better outcomes. This is like a petrol company claiming their petrol was more efficient than a competitor by using two litres of theirs and one litre of the competitors and then claiming their car did more miles before it ran out. Of course, no other industry could get away with such a blatant fraud, but you may have noticed that I used the term "fraud" when examining the Nexium trial. This is because, unbelievably, a drug company is simply allowed to carry out such deception without any rebuttal from the drug regulators.

The laws governing drug approval are at the very heart of the travesties that result from me too drugs. A company only has to prove that a drug has some statistical benefit – however small – and the regulator must approve it. It does not have to show the drug is better than existing drugs and in fact it can be less effective, but it will still be approved and then ultimately used by doctors. How is it possible that law makers allow all this to happen? We will see shortly, but I will give one insight now. In the US, the drug industry employs three lobbyists for every congressman and senator. Incessant lobbying is just one reason why the industry gets its way with appallingly lax laws.

AstraZeneca still had one final hurdle to overcome. They needed to ensure doctors knew about the "benefits" of using Nexium rather than Prilosec. To do this, they allocated $500 million and a series of shady marketing techniques to get the message out and "educate" doctors. That may seem like a lot of money, but Nexium soon became a blockbuster drug with sales of $5 billion each year, so it was money well spent.

Here is one final part of this incredible story. When Nexium started to be used by doctors, Thomas Scully, the head of Medicare and Medicaid in the US, gave speeches explaining that Nexium was a waste of money and doctors should use the old drug Prilosec which cost 30 times less after it came off patent. But as he had no final control over what gets prescribed, he had to sit and watch as the US doctors wasted $800 million every year. When I say that Scully gave speeches, he said, "Any doctor that prescribes Nexium should be ashamed of himself." AstraZeneca complained about him to the White House and on Capitol Hill. Scully says he was put under pressure to "shut up". He hasn't. The fact politicians at the highest level were prepared to turn a blind eye and literally give AstraZeneca $800 million a year instead of standing up to this "fraud" tells us everything we need to know about the power of the pharmaceutical industry. Nexium is a straightforward "fraud", but it still became a blockbuster drug for the second time, and even today it rakes in $5 billion a year from around the world. If you are not shocked and disgusted by all of this, you really should be.

Most drugs don't work for most people

If you still think everything you have read in this section couldn't be true, then consider the statement made by Dr Alan Roses, worldwide vice-president of genetics at GlaxoSmithKline. He said that most prescription medicines do not work for most people who take them, and that the vast majority of drugs – more than 90% – only work in 30–50% of the people. It is an open secret within the drug industry that most of its products are ineffective in most patients, but this was the first time a senior executive had gone public and told the truth. There is also little doubt that even Dr Roses has overstated the benefits of drugs because the BMJ has analysed and evaluated 3,000 of the most important medical drugs and treatments and found that only 11% had solid proof they worked and benefited patients. This published BMJ clinical evidence data remains unchallenged.

BMJ editor Fiona Godlee takes on corruption in science and medicine

When considering the dark forces at work in science and medicine, Dr Godlee said, "I think we have to call it what it is. It is corruption of the scientific process. Medicine and science are run by human beings, so there will always be crooks." She explains how hundreds of papers are being pulled from the scientific record for falsified data, plagiarism and a range of other reasons, and an estimated 70% of retractions are based on some form of scientific misconduct. She has strong words about the overuse of drugs and the influence of the industry. She also explains how medical journals are also part of the problem because they have publication bias, meaning they invariably only publish positive findings and only rarely report the many drug trials that fail. As part of her plan to help change all this corruption, the BMJ have re-analysed several clinical trials involving controversial drugs and treatments. One of them concluded that the antidepressant drug Paxil, which had been used to treat teenage depression, wasn't safe and didn't work, despite the claims of the drug company. However, it took a court case to gain access to the Paxil trial data that the company had refused to release before the true analysis could be carried out.

This is why Dr Godlee said, "It's led me and many others to increasingly question the idea that the manufacturer of the drug could ever be considered the right people to evaluate its effectiveness and safety. This seems to be a very mad idea which has grown up historically, and we have to start questioning it and we have to come up with alternatives, which would mean independent studies done by independent bodies." Dr Godlee says it matters because bad science can be dangerous: "Patients do get hurt. Drugs that shouldn't be available are available. Drugs with harms are used and patients are unaware of those harms. So yes, we know that patients are harmed, and we know that the health systems are harmed as a result of poor science."

Of course, the pharmaceutical industry always dismisses anyone who challenges its drugs and its so-called gold standard clinical trials, but as editor of one of the top three medical journals in the world, Dr Godlee is a more formidable opponent. The world should hope that she can make progress, but I doubt it, because as will be seen shortly, the drug industry really is too powerful and really has gained control over most of medicine. I hope I am wrong.

Finally, here is one example where the pharmaceutical industry really could not dismiss the "fraud" in its so-called gold standard trials. Three drug companies, Eli Lilly, Jansen, and Pfizer, each produced a similar variant of the drug olanzapine to treat schizophrenia. Each one of them had their drug tested against the others. Guess what? They all declared that their drug had the best outcomes. Really? At least two of them (and possibly all three) must quite simply have committed some sort of "fraud" in the trials.

Summary

This section started with a question: "Medical research – can it be trusted?" I think I have proved fairly conclusively that the answer is, in large part, a resounding no. A no that has profound and life-threatening implications for patients caught up in its "dirty web".

Does the pharmaceutical industry really want to find cures?

For most people, this would seem an absurd question. Surely the industry wants to find cures for diseases. Surely they could make huge sums of money if they did. But this is not a silly question. There used to be an "in-joke" in medical research laboratories. It went something like this: "What is the worst thing that can happen during a clinical trial? The first is that we kill someone. The second is that we find a cure!" (Cue embarrassed laughter.) A drug that cured people would be a financial disaster for the pharmaceutical industry. If drugs were invented today that cured every disease, the pharmaceutical industry would cease to exist in around 13 years' time when all the patents ran out. There would be no need for new drugs since the existing drugs would already provide 100% of the cures for everything, and the industry could never survive on the meagre profits available once patent protection was lost. The example of antibiotics shows exactly what happens when a real cure is developed. Antibiotics that were invented 60 years ago are still being used today. Anyone can make them and profits are minimal. No one wants to invest in new antibiotics even though they are now desperately needed.

Even though it is certain that most diseases could never be cured by drugs alone, the key point is the pharmaceutical industry is certainly not looking for, and absolutely does not want to find, cures. Instead, it seeks to develop drugs that simply minimise symptoms and mediate the course of a disease. In this model, drugs invariably have to be taken long term and, in many cases, for life, thus guaranteeing long-term profit streams. It also enables new drugs to be developed that can seamlessly replace older drugs as soon as they come off patent, thus maintaining, or even increasing, this same profit stream indefinitely.

Of course, there are always exceptions to "every rule", and the drug Epclusa is a classic example. Epclusa is an antiviral drug manufactured by the biotechnology company Gilead Sciences to treat hepatitis C. This is a virus usually spread by contaminated blood, and one of the main sources is from unsterilised needles shared by drug users. Epclusa works by preventing the virus from replicating and it has a cure rate of around 95%. This means the number of carriers continues to fall as people are treated, then new transmissions also fall, and this in turn means sales of the drug also fall. At its peak, sales of Epclusa reached $12.5 billion, but these are now falling significantly, and the company's share price is also falling. Gilead Sciences has certainly made many billions of dollars, but when the drug finally loses its patent, profits will not just continue to fall, but will evaporate almost completely. There will then be no opportunity to develop a new drug which you can claim is better than the existing one since Epclusa is already near perfect. Epclusa is a wake-up call to all the relatively small emerging biotechnology companies who may be thinking of developing a similarly effective drug for other diseases.

Of course, large established pharmaceutical companies would never even try to produce such a drug, even though they constantly claim they are looking for cures for disease. My view is if they ever developed such a drug by accident, the information would be put into a sealed vault – never to be seen again. But it isn't just the pharmaceutical industry that don't want to find cures. Major banking and investment companies who provide most of the funding for the industry and who own a large percentage of pharmaceutical shares have equally negative views on cures for disease.

Goldman Sachs is the most powerful investment bank in the world. It is so powerful it was once described as "a vampire squid wrapped around the face of humanity". This is a summary of Goleman Sachs' view on drugs that cure: "Drug companies would stop being profitable if their drugs really cured people, because they would lose their market. In fact, curing people is an unsustainable business model. The bank is, therefore, hesitant about investing in the emerging biotech industry. They accept that drugs like Epclusa carry tremendous benefit for patients and society, but they are unlikely to provide the funding that other biotech companies need to develop such drugs now that they have seen the dire financial implications of Epclusa."

Other investment banks and financial companies will almost certainly have the same views and policies, and this means that very few such drugs will be developed in the future. In fact, even Gilead Sciences has now reverted to pushing the conventional pharmaceutical drug model. Their drug Remdesivir, which was originally developed to treat Ebola, has now been approved to treat COVID-19 even though it does not save any lives, but is simply claimed to reduce the length of stay in hospitals. Goldman Sachs will almost surely be applauding this minimally beneficial drug.

I should add one note of caution. Please do not imagine that drugs could be developed by biotech companies that would cure most diseases if only the necessary funding was available. Nearly all the major diseases like cancer, heart disease, strokes, diabetes and dementia are truly complex and have lifestyle causes. Very few cases will ever be cured just by a drug, but if such funding was available, biotech companies would almost certainly be able to find cures for a relatively small number of quite specific diseases, like hepatitis C, that would still be of tremendous benefit to patients and society. Sadly, not many of them will ever be developed. This is what happens when industries like pharmaceuticals and finance have effectively taken control of medical research, such that profits are the only priority, and patient outcomes and lives are treated as irrelevant. Medicine's elite are also aware of this shocking situation, so why are they not pressurising governments to change the way the pharmaceutical industry operates?

Of course, prevention of disease also represents the same identical financial disaster for the drug industry and the finance industry. Prevention is, of course, what lifestyle medicine seeks to do and, as we will see later, for this reason it is firmly in the crosshairs of the pharmaceutical industry, which is using all its power to try to discredit and destroy all natural and lifestyle interventions. The take home message of this section is simple: if you want to prevent disease or cure it completely, do not expect drugs to provide the answers and, because medicine uses drugs almost exclusively, do not expect that doctors will be able to help you stay healthy or help you cure most diseases either.

The drug industry only spends money if there is a payback

It is essential to understand another critically important fact. The pharmaceutical industry does not spend any money unless there is a payback or profit to be made. How do we know? Because they have said so many times in unambiguous terms. But actions usually speak louder than words. So, let us examine two pharmaceutical actions that prove this in undisputable terms.

Growing antibiotic resistance is one of the key priorities and threats for modern medicine. Unless new antibiotics are developed, modern medicine will cease to exist as we know it. Many routine operations will cease because the risk of death will be so high. In addition, 10 million people will die each year from untreatable infections. What is the response of the pharmaceutical industry to this impending health disaster, bearing in mind the sole reason the industry exists is to develop drugs, including antibiotics? Well, their response is they have stopped virtually all research into new antibiotics. Thirty years ago, 35 drug companies were carrying out research to develop new antibiotics. Today the figure is just three. Why? Because they will never be able to make a profit from their investments. If they did develop a new generation of antibiotics they would be used as a last resort treatment by medicine, and thus in small quantities. This would never generate enough profit to cover the development costs. So, unless governments step in with funding or find other ways of encouraging research, medicine as we know it faces partial extinction. Even now, antibiotic resistance is already a fact of life (or more accurately a fact of death). Untreatable infections currently cause annual deaths of around 7,000 people in the UK, with the global figure standing at 700,000. This is predicted to rise to 10 million annually by 2050. This is more than the total of all cancer deaths added together.

The second example involves the French pharmaceutical giant Sanofi which stopped production of its snake bite treatment - FAV-Afrique - because it did not make sufficient profit. This serum saved countless lives. Médecins Sans Frontières said, "Tens of thousands of people will die unnecessarily from snake bites because of an imminent shortage of serum." This is one of the few truly effective treatments that medicine has in its arsenal, saving virtually everyone bitten provided they can be treated quickly enough, But, unless other benefactors or governments step in, thousands of lives will be lost each year.

I have gone into some detail with these two examples, not to lament on a disgraceful and shameful situation, because this is a fact of life, but so that we are under no illusion that the industry spends money only when there is a profit to be generated. Saving lives has no interest for them. They do not care how many people die because of their single overriding goal of maximising profits.

How dangerous are prescription drugs?

Prescription drugs are the third leading cause of death

Peter Gøtzsche in his book *Deadly Medicines and Organised Crime: How Big Pharma Has Corrupted Healthcare* states that prescription drugs are the third leading cause of death after cardiovascular disease and cancer. After reading this section you will understand exactly why this seemingly impossible claim is indeed true.

Prescription drugs killed around 1 million EU citizens in the five years from 2014 to 2019 (200,000 each year). This is three times as many as the Syrian conflict over a similar period. This is the official figure, and the one thing we know is the real figure is even greater because when a death is classified as being caused by a drug there must be reasonable certainty that it was the cause. But there are many more deaths where a drug might have been the cause but where it cannot be proven beyond reasonable doubt. In addition, as we will see later, there are many deaths caused by drugs that are only uncovered many years later and so do not figure in official statistics. There will also be other drug-related deaths that will never be discovered. So, the real figure is much higher. It's just that no one really knows how high. For the moment I will stick with the official EU figure of 200,000 each year which is horrific enough.

But drugs don't just result in death. It is widely accepted that for every person killed by a drug, 100 others will suffer from other side effects. About 75 of these will experience side effects that they learn to live with, like muscle pain, while around 25 others experience side effects that require medical intervention. These range from relatively minor problems to life-threatening diseases like cancer and heart disease. The annual EU figures are: 15 million people simply have to learn to live with drug side effects and 5 million need to seek medical attention because the side effects are severe. Of these, over 2 million are admitted to hospital, and 200,000 will suffer life-threatening conditions, such as heart attacks or cancer, from which they recover, but, of course, life for these people will never be the same again and most will live under a dark cloud for the rest of their lives.

The EU accounts for just under 20% of world drug consumption. So, the global figures are simply about five times all these individual figures. Please do the sums yourself which I realise are so mind-boggling you will say "this simply can't be true". But whatever your gut instinct tells you, remember these are official minimum figures and the only challenge that can be made is that the real figures are in fact significantly higher. There is one further official figure that puts all this into even more perspective. As well as the cost in human life and suffering, there is a huge financial cost to all of this. EU figures show the annual cost of treating all these people because of their drug-induced side effects is a staggering €80 billion. To put this into perspective, the EU spends around €200 billion on purchasing drugs each year but then spends €80 billion on treating the side effects of the very same drugs. This is almost unbelievable. If it wasn't for the fact these are official figures, you might be entitled to wonder if they had been produced on 1 April.

The removal of drugs and black box warnings

Over many years, an average of 20% of all drugs that had been approved by regulators were subsequently given a "black box warning" or taken off the market, because of serious and life-threatening side effects that were subsequently discovered only when large numbers of people started to take them. The current average figure in the US has, however, increased to 30% because regulators are now allowing an increasing number of fast-track drug approvals. The abandonment of the long-established gold standard clinical trials for this increasing number of drugs has led to less scientific appraisal on the benefits of the drugs and many more serious outcomes. Incredibly, the figure for those specific drugs given this fast-track approval is now a frightening 57% as exposed in a 2017 study. This fast-tracking approval started in the late 1980s and initially it was done for, and restricted to, serious life-threatening conditions which in theory could benefit from earlier use of these drugs. Slowly, however, over three decades, the drug industry has "persuaded" drug regulators to extend this rapid approval to a wider range of more minor conditions which has led to the rapid rise in serious drug outcomes, and these significantly outweigh any minor benefits the drugs may provide. A "black box warning" is the strongest that can be applied to a drug. It tells the doctor the drug is potentially life-threatening and so should only be used in exceptional circumstances and with the patient's formal approval, such as for a life-threatening condition where other drugs have failed and where there are no other alternative treatments. Remember, none of these life-threatening side effects show up in the original trials and many lives are lost before the deadly nature of the drug is then uncovered. Think about this carefully. An average of 30% of all new drugs are so dangerous that, eventually, they have to be given this ultimate black box warning or removed from sale. This is an incredible and frightening statistic.

The grapefruit saga

A few years ago, a major publicity effort was made to warn people of the dangers of eating grapefruit while taking a long list of prescription drugs. Leading medics came on TV and radio and articles were published in newspapers. So, what exactly is the problem? When people take drugs (and indeed when they eat food or take vitamin supplements), not everything is absorbed by the body. For some drugs, the absorption rate may only be around 20%. Of course, the doses given to patients take this malabsorption into account. However, grapefruit has unique properties that increase the absorption rate of a long list of drugs. For example, it may double or triple the absorption level. This effectively doubles or triples the dose of the drug. Why is this important? Believe it or not, this effect has led to a significant number of deaths. If you want to know how dangerous drugs really can be, look no further than what at first glance seems to be an innocuous story involving grapefruit. The fact that doubling, or tripling, the dose of a number of drugs can lead to death is a stark reminder of the "Russian roulette" people play when they take drugs. Paracelsus said, "What differentiates a drug from a poison is the dose." But a sobering fact is that if someone did take grapefruit with one of the implicated drugs and died because of the side effects of the drug, the likelihood is the real reason for the death may never be uncovered except by chance. The death may, purely innocently, be blamed on an unexpected heart attack, for example.

The reality is autopsies are only performed in about 1 in 100 deaths. This is one more simple example of how official drug deaths are always understated.

Suicide

When someone wants to commit suicide, prescription drugs are one of the preferred methods. This is not surprising when you consider how dangerous they can be. Overdoses of everyday drugs, like sleeping pills and painkillers, will often result in death. Incidentally, when we move on to lifestyle medicine, we will explore the scare stories that are printed about the dangers of vitamins. If vitamins are so dangerous, as pharmaceutical silverbacks and lobby groups contend, you might imagine that people would try to commit suicide using them. It is, however, highly unlikely that anyone would ever succeed given the impeccable safety record vitamins have and clearly no one has ever succeeded or these very same pharmaceutical lobbyists would make sure it made headline news around the world. We will see later just how safe vitamin and mineral supplements are, especially when compared to drugs.

Even the most common and widely used drugs can kill people

You may be shocked to learn that aspirin kills around 100,000 people and results in 500,000 hospitalisations each year because it can cause gastrointestinal bleeding which is often impossible to stop. So, one of the most widely taken drugs of all time, and one that most people would assume is perfectly safe, kills many people worldwide. Virtually all other commonly used drugs also cause deaths. As far as aspirin is concerned, the official medical position has been that its benefits for diseases like heart attacks outweigh the risks, although this has been disputed over many years by other medical experts. In the last four years, two major studies involving over 30,000 people have shown no benefit for heart disease risk and have again confirmed the increased risk of bleeding in both the stomach and brain. Even the US Food and Drug Administration currently states that it "does not believe the evidence supports the general use of aspirin for primary prevention of heart attack and stroke". The American Heart Association, however, continues to promote aspirin for some groups of patients as does the NHS. So, anyone offered aspirin really should try to analyse all the evidence before deciding on whether to take this clearly controversial drug for heart disease, because for many people the serious risks really will outweigh any benefits.

It gets worse

All this information on the dangers of drugs is incredible. But what if the real situation is much worse? The side effects of some drugs are well known and, therefore, the deaths and other conditions they cause can be predicted with at least some accuracy. As we have seen, however, these side effects are not normally detected during the initial clinical trials. They are usually exposed by observing what happens in the real world when millions of people take them. Even so, it can take many years for some side effects to be detected because no one is necessarily looking to find them. Some are detected only by chance. For example, if a researcher decides to look at the outcomes for a drug after it has been on the market for five years, he may, by chance, notice an unexpected correlation between the drug and, say, heart attacks that no one expected. If you want a current example of this problem, consider statins. These have been used for nearly 30 years, but it was only about five years ago that researchers found out they increased the risk of diabetes, and four studies showed increases ranging from 30% to 100%.

There are two things to note. If a drug has been shown to be killing people for five years, the official deaths for earlier years are not retrospectively amended to take this into account. This means true deaths from drugs are always under-reported. The other is that many side effects and deaths may never be uncovered because researchers simply just do not look for them, not because of any dark motive, but because they really don't expect them to exist. Also, most of these studies are invariably funded by the drug industry and they are not going to be busting a gut to throw money at studies that would uncover such deaths and other side effects that would drastically reduce their profits.

The final proof

If you still doubt things could really be as bad as I am suggesting, then here are nine real-life stories that are so scary, so dreadful and so evil that when you have finished reading them you will understand that far from exaggerating the situation, the reality is in fact beyond your worst nightmare.

The scandal of beta blockers used during surgery

In January 2014 a report was published in the European Heart Journal online by two researchers: Darrell Francis, professor of cardiology at Imperial College London, and Graham Cole, a clinical research fellow in cardiology. The study they had carried out involved a drug protocol used throughout the EU for people undergoing operations. The protocol involved the use of beta blocker drugs to protect the heart during surgery. The research report, however, concluded that, far from saving lives, the protocol had resulted in the deaths of 800,000 people over the five-year period during which it had been used. The report was on the website for just one hour before it "disappeared". Why did it disappear? The possibility that a universal drug guideline used throughout the EU might have caused the deaths of 800,000 people would have caused panic and alarm in medical circles and the drug industry. You can judge for yourselves, when you know the full story, whether this hasty retraction of the paper had more to do with trying to preserve medicine's reputation rather than any genuine concern for patients' lives.

You may be wondering how 800,000 people could be killed by a universal EU medical guideline. Well, it turns out the chairman of the committee that developed and approved the guideline was Professor Don Poldermans – a man who has now been booted out of his job at Erasmus University in the Netherlands for research fraud; the very research that was used to create these guidelines. Don Poldermans had financial conflicts of interest with several pharmaceutical companies. He carried out corrupt research which included making up some of the results that supported the use of beta blockers. He was also the chairman of an ESC (European Society of Cardiology) committee that subsequently recommended widespread use of these drugs to protect the heart during surgery.

In trying to defend his decision to remove the paper, the editor of the ESC, Professor Thomas Luscher, made the following comments:

> "Jumping to conclusions may be particularly dangerous for both physicians and patients."
>
> "The validity of Professor Poldermans' manuscripts remains uncertain as only one paper has so far been officially retracted."
>
> "A proper clinical trial is needed to assess whether the use of beta blockers before surgery might be beneficial or harmful."

Words almost fail me. To suggest that jumping to conclusions in a situation like this may be dangerous for patients is ludicrous. To suggest that the validity of Professor Poldermans' manuscripts remains uncertain when he was sacked for research fraud is nothing short of laughable. To suggest a proper clinical trial was needed to assess whether the beta blockers that had been in use for five years and given to millions of people might be beneficial or harmful is incredible, especially given the protocol had already been approved by "proper" clinical trials.

It took six months before the guidelines on beta blockers were withdrawn and the use of the drugs was stopped. Subsequent analysis vindicated the original paper by Darrell Francis and Graham Cole who criticised the lamentably slow process that led to the change. They called for improvements to permit guideline experts to perform rapid amendments in such circumstances. Let us not forget that in this final six-month period of drawn-out obfuscation, probably another 80,000 people were killed by this guideline. This is simply unforgivable. The guideline committee was also at pains to point out that people taking beta blockers prescribed by their GP should carry on as normal as there was no evidence that they were harmful in a non-surgical setting. But wait a minute. If beta blockers killed 800,000 people in a surgical setting, can we really be expected to believe that there would be zero risk to everyone else? There must be a serious question mark over beta blockers in general and you might expect that an expert committee might have been set up to at least examine the possibility. Unsurprisingly, this did not happen.

At this stage, I want to compare the beta blocker scandal to another human tragedy. The Grenfell tower fire was a human tragedy which resulted in the deaths of 72 people. It made headline news for months and still makes the news even years after the event. When a tragedy like this happens, governments spring into action, thousands of people protest and hundreds of thousands sign petitions demanding change. Public enquiries and court cases then follow, together with new laws and regulations aimed at preventing this type of tragedy happening again.

So, when 800,000 people in Europe – which is 11,000 times as many as Grenfell – were killed because of fraudulent medical research, wouldn't you expect it to have made front-page headline news around the world, not just for weeks or months, but for decades? But the reality is, I am willing to bet you have never even heard of this gigantic scandal. It did not appear on any national television programme or newspaper, and the internet was also almost totally silent. Because of this there was no public outrage, no petitions, no public enquiries and no court cases or new laws. In fact, as you will see, virtually nothing has changed. We still commemorate and remember the Battle of the Somme 100 years later, whereas the beta blocker scandal, which saw nearly the same loss of life, has effectively been airbrushed out of existence. Rewriting history and censoring major events, like the Tiananmen Square massacre, is something we have come to expect from dictatorships like China and Russia, but it is beyond belief that such a thing could happen in seemingly democratic societies like the UK and the EU.

The censorship of this scandal is, therefore, a critical issue. When it was exposed in 2014, medical journalists would have known about it; it is their job to know. Their editors would then also know. Did they all self-censor? This is difficult to believe on such an explosive story. The truth may never emerge but my guess, and that is all it can be, is that the medical profession and the drug industry would have desperately wanted to keep it under wraps given the scale of the deaths and the reputational damage it would have caused them. But, almost certainly, this had to be a concerted establishment cover up that also involved governments, regulators and media owners, and it worked. Eight years later, almost no one knows anything about it.

In his book *Doctoring Data*, Dr Malcolm Kendrick wrote a searing and detailed account of the beta blocker scandal. He is one of only a handful of people who have had the courage to report on this scandal, and when he did, he was accused by medical experts of using reckless and sensational headlines. But any report or book that covers a medical fraud resulting in the deaths of 800,000 people must, by definition, be sensational. The experts were in effect saying Dr Kendrick should also have self-censored and not covered this scandal just like the media and press. Almost unbelievably, and without any sense of shame or guilt, another professor said that what was needed was "a period of quiet contemplation". All senior medical people and academics knew about this scandal and knew their profession had caused the deaths of hundreds of thousands of people. They clearly felt it was right that the scandal should be censored, and the public should not find out about it. But can such censorship really be justified?

Professor Poldermans did lose his job, but is this sufficient punishment when he committed outright fraud which then caused the deaths of 800,000 people? He would almost certainly have made a fortune from his ties with the pharmaceutical industry, and today he is a free man enjoying life as if nothing had happened. If the scandal had not been censored, it is very likely that public pressure would have led to legal proceedings and a long jail term. This would not only have been legally and morally justified but would have acted as a serious deterrent to any other doctor considering the same sort of fraud in the future. Consider that if one single person is killed in a railway accident, court cases ensue, politicians vow to take tough action and directors can face charges of corporate manslaughter. But, when medicine and medical research are involved, there appears to be complete immunity from prosecution for all concerned regardless of the death toll. How is this possible? What sort of society have we become?

Here is another reason why the scandal should not have been censored. Professor Poldermans carried out clinical trials that showed that giving beta blockers before and after surgery dramatically reduced the incidence of post-operative heart attacks and subsequent deaths from 34% to 3.4%. But after the deaths were exposed by Darrel Francis and Graham Cole, a reanalysis of all the other relevant clinical trials – excluding those conducted by Poldermans – was eventually carried out. This showed that administering beta blockers had precisely the reverse effect of that claimed and resulted in an overall 27% increase in post-operative deaths. Even when Professor Poldermans' expert committee was drawing up the beta blocker guidelines, other researchers and doctors expressed serious concerns that his findings were "simply too good to be true". But because of the strict hierarchical nature of medicine, the expert panel ignored all these concerns. No one could stop it from happening. Dr Malcolm Kendrick, in a blog, asked the question, "Who shall guard the guardians?" In other words, who checks on the expert committees that produce medical guidelines which effectively carry the force of law, such that doctors who challenge or do not follow them can be censored or lose their job.? At present, the answer is no one. If the beta blocker scandal had been exposed and people had been able to openly question how medical dogma and its extreme hierarchical control had been one of the key factors in this tragedy, then some action may have been taken to prevent it happening again. But as you may guess, nothing has changed.

Up to this point, I have concentrated on deaths just in the EU to keep the story as simple as possible, but the reality is the beta blocker protocol was also used in most developed countries like the US, Canada and Australia. The worldwide death toll is impossible to calculate accurately, but a conservative estimate would be around 1.5 million. A staggering thought is that no one realised these deaths were occurring and had it not been for the efforts of the two UK researchers, the death toll would by now be around 4 million. During its use, 1 in 30 of all EU deaths were caused by this protocol.

I will finish this section with one last comment. In the five years between 2009 and 2014 the official figure is that prescription drugs killed around 1 million EU citizens, but this single medical scandal alone means the real figure is nearly twice as high at 1.8 million. The official figures will never reflect this extra 800,000, which is a scandal in itself. But we will see there are even more scandals to be exposed and the real figure is even higher. Maybe now you can see why Peter Gøtzsche's claim that prescription drugs are the third leading cause of death is indeed not just plausible, but a near certainty, and why official drug deaths are grossly understated.

Vioxx

Vioxx is one of a family of drugs known as COX-2 inhibitors. These drugs are used mainly to alleviate pain for people with arthritis, and other drugs of the same type had already been associated with increased cardiovascular risk. As early as 1996 when the drug, which was owned by the pharmaceutical giant Merck, was being developed, the company's own scientists as well as external researchers hired by Merck had established the heart attack risk with Vioxx. But Merck "persuaded" these external investigators to change the wording of their report so the risks were hidden.

Painkillers in general are notorious for causing stomach problems such as bleeding which can be difficult or impossible to control. One of the advantages of COX-2 drugs was that they had fewer such gastrointestinal side effects when compared to other painkillers such as aspirin. Merck came up with what it thought was the perfect plan to maximise the benefits of the drug and hide the very inconvenient problem that it was going to cause heart attacks and kill people.

During the trials, it monitored the gastrointestinal benefits for the specified trial duration, but it only assessed the heart attack outcomes for a shorter period. Naturally, this reduced the apparent risk of cardiovascular events. The other tricks used were to carefully select only patients for the trials who already had a low inherent risk of cardiovascular disease and, in addition, some of the heart attacks that did occur "magically disappeared" from the final reports. There is a catalogue of other "scams" it used to play down the risks and hype up the benefits but these are fairly technical so I won't go into them in any more detail. Almost unbelievably, in 1999, the drug was approved by the FDA despite the disconcerting evidence which was still there, even after the best efforts of Merck to cover it all up. Over the next two years further trials were carried out that showed the increased heart attack risk more clearly. As a damage limitation exercise, Merck issued a press release in May 2001 in which it said, "Merck reconfirms favourable cardiovascular safety of Vioxx." The corruption of the truth was now total.

But in September 2004 Merck withdrew Vioxx from the market voluntarily. Why? Well, rumours about the heart attacks had started to leak out. People who thought their heart attacks (or their relatives' heart attacks) were caused by the drug started bringing law suits against the company. The company clearly knew the game was up and that if it persisted in promoting the drug it would lead to substantial compensation payments that would soon outweigh the ongoing profits. Note that the decision to withdraw it was financially driven and not because of any concern for the lives of the patients taking them. It has been estimated that the drug caused 120,000 heart attacks and about 60,000 deaths. In 2007 the company announced a settlement of $4.85 billion which was paid out to some of the victims or their relatives. Many more, however, never even knew Vioxx was the cause of their suffering. In 2012 Merck was also fined $1 billion in criminal fines and its total legal bill was another $1.2 billion. Put simply, this is another example of the pharmaceutical industry knowingly and callously killing people for profit. As you would by now perhaps understand, no individual was ever charged with any crime.

Despite all this devastation, however, it is highly likely (although it can't be proven conclusively) that the death toll from the drug was in fact much higher than the initial estimates. Independent investigators found out that when Vioxx was introduced in 1999 there had been the largest increase in annual US deaths over the previous 60 years, and then in 2005 when it was withdrawn, there had been the largest fall in deaths. The drug was prescribed mainly to older people and the increase in deaths and the subsequent reduction was concentrated in the over 65s, which mainly involved heart attacks which is exactly what Vioxx caused. In 1999 deaths increased by around 100,000 and then fell by a similar number in 2005. The likelihood, therefore, is that 500,000 US citizens were killed by the drug over its five years of use. Vioxx was also prescribed around much of the developed world but it is impossible to calculate the total number of deaths although it is likely to be well over a million.

Avandia and Seroxat

In 2012 GlaxoSmithKline was found guilty of fraud and fined $3 billion. There were three separate charges. It concealed critical evidence relating to its diabetes drug Avandia, it illegally promoted the powerful antidepressant Seroxat for use in children even though it had not been approved for such use, and it offered lavish entertainment to doctors willing to promote several other medicines for off-patent use. Avandia was first marketed in 2001 but it didn't take long before serious concerns started to be raised about the risk of heart attacks. It subsequently emerged during the legal investigation that GSK knew about the increased risk of heart attack but had not reported these to the FDA even though it was legally obliged to do so. Critics had repeatedly called for the drug to be withdrawn, but it was not until 2010 that it was finally banned. By then it is estimated that it had caused another 120,000 heart attacks and 60,000 deaths.

The promotion of the antidepressant drug Seroxat for use in children marks yet another low point for the company and for the industry in general. The original trial, the now infamous Study 329, showed the drug was ineffective for reducing depression in children and showed a significant increase in the risk of suicide. But when it was published, the study cited that Seroxat was effective with minimal side effects. This "surprising" transformation in outcomes was only achieved by using some of the most blatant data manipulation ever seen in medical research. The study ended thus: "Conclusion: Seroxat is generally well tolerated and effective for major depression in adolescents." GSK also lied to its sales force telling them that Study 329 showed "remarkable efficacy and safety". The exact number of children driven to attempt suicide and those who tragically succeeded is not known, but inquests show clearly that the drug was wholly, or in part, linked to a number of deaths.

The company also illegally promoted other drugs, including Wellbutrin, by handing out cash, as well as everything from Madonna concert tickets and pheasant hunting trips to basketball tickets. Once again, no individual was ever prosecuted. It's true the executives involved were sacked but every single one of them soon found gainful employment in senior positions in other drug companies and one was even given a high-level post within the NHS. So, people who had knowingly caused the deaths of thousands of people and children were welcomed immediately back into the industry and even the NHS. This is truly sickening. Despite the seemingly large fine, $3 billion is far less than the $29 billion profit made from the drugs during the years covered by the settlement. For Big Pharma, crime really does pay. It's no wonder that Sidney Wolfe, a doctor and director of consumer organisation Public Citizen's Health research group, said, "Until more meaningful penalties and the prospect of jail time for company heads who are responsible for such activity become commonplace, companies will continue defrauding the government and putting patients' lives in danger."

Polypharmacy

Polypharmacy is the name that is applied when people are being prescribed multiple drugs simultaneously and for long periods. It occurs most frequently (but not exclusively) in older people. Those in care homes are very likely to be receiving multiple drugs, such as sleeping pills, antidepressants, tranquilisers, statins, blood pressure drugs, osteoporosis drugs, mood stabilisers, antacid drugs and anticoagulants. A Swedish study of 762 people living in nursing homes found that 67% were prescribed ten or more drugs. This is quite normal in many western societies. So, what's the problem? We have already seen that pharmaceutical companies test each new drug on young people who are not taking any other drugs for the very reason that other drugs could interfere with the drug on trial. No trials are ever carried out to see what happens when even two drugs are taken simultaneously. There is no data; there are no clinical trials. So, only God is likely to know what happens when someone is taking multiple drugs. The drugs might not work at all or there could be horrific and unexpected deadly interactions and side effects. No one has any idea. The lack of clinical trials to show that multiple drug taking is effective and safe is another nail in the coffin of the claim that medicine is evidence based. Of course, none of this stops it from happening.

So, why is polypharmacy practised? It is promoted simply in the belief that it must help patients, because each drug in isolation has clinical trials to show it works, and so surely lots of drugs, even though many have small benefits individually, will result in a meaningful overall benefit. It is important to emphasise the word "belief", because that is all it is – there is no evidence. You could also add that the pharmaceutical industry is pushing polypharmacy for all they are worth since it is a nice little multi-billion-dollar earner. Has anyone considered the potential downside and side effects? Not a chance.

So, is there any evidence that it could be harmful? In fact, there is good quality evidence. Researchers in Israel conducted a trial in 2007 in which 190 disabled patients in geriatric nursing departments, with comparable ages, gender and co-morbidities, were split into two groups. One group carried on taking their normal drugs, while the other had the number of drugs reduced by an average of three each. Those on reduced drugs did not suffer any adverse effects, but after one year, there was a significant difference in the number of deaths between the two groups, as well as the referral rate to acute care facilities. The one-year mortality in those who did not have their medications reduced was 45%, and their referral rate to critical care was 30%. The one-year mortality in those who did have their medications reduced fell to 21%, and their critical care referral rate fell to 11.8%. For patients who had their medications reduced, the reduction in mortality and referrals to acute care in a single year were staggering: a 53% absolute reduction in death and a 60% reduction in critical care referrals. The researchers also noted the reduced drug costs and the improvement in quality of patients' lives. These figures represent unbelievably better outcomes for these patients than any drug treatment in the entire history of medicine. So, the best drug treatment ever discovered appears to be stop taking the drugs. Of course, some drugs do work and cannot be stopped, like insulin for people with type 1 diabetes. But clearly there are drugs, or drug interactions, that are causing serious harm to the elderly. Blood pressure lowering drugs, for example, can cause sudden reductions in blood pressure on standing up (postural hypotension) and this can lead to falls which in turn can lead to broken hips.

Another study in 70 patients where the number of drugs was reduced from 7.7 to 4.4 per patient showed that 88% reported global improvement in health and most had improvement in cognitive function. A review in the Journal of the American Medical Association also came to the following conclusions about polypharmacy: "The finding that simultaneous discontinuation of many drugs is not associated with significant risks and apparently improves quality of life should encourage physicians to consider testing this in larger clinical trials across a variety of medical cultural settings. Polypharmacy may have different faces in different countries or clinics but there is no doubt that the problem is global."

In fact, I have not yet found any study that shows polypharmacy has any benefit. So, why are bigger and more definitive studies not done to confirm these alarming findings, so action can then be taken to reduce drug prescriptions for older people? Well, it shouldn't surprise you that the pharmaceutical industry is not likely to fund studies showing that the more drugs you take, the shorter your life will be, as well as reducing your quality of life. Without industry funding, such a study would be financially beyond most researchers. However, one experiment has in fact been carried out. It was not actually a clinical trial but a public health experiment and it turned out to be the largest and longest one ever undertaken in the world to assess the effectiveness and safety of polypharmacy.

In 2004 the UK launched the Quality and Outcomes Framework (QOF). Its aim was to detect patients with early signs of disease and markers for future diseases, such as high blood pressure and high cholesterol. These patients would then be prescribed drugs with the aim and expectation that many serious future diseases, like heart attacks, chronic kidney disease, strokes and diabetes, would be prevented. In fact, it was projected that 30,000 lives would be saved each year and that this in turn would significantly reduce hospital admissions and pressure on critical care services. In 2004 doctors were paid £15,000 a year to carry out all the extra patient testing, prescribing and follow ups. This sum has increased significantly over the years and the scheme has so far cost an incredible £30 billion. About half of this sum was spent on drugs.

This all sounds very promising, but there was one major problem. No one had ever checked what the real outcomes were. Presumably everyone just assumed that giving all these drugs must surely be working and saving lives. Then, in 2016, a group of researchers from Michigan, York and Manchester Universities carried out a detailed study comparing the data on mortality for chronic diseases in the UK with those in similar countries which weren't using a QOF-type protocol. The results showed there was no meaningful difference in the number of deaths. The expected saving of 30,000 lives each year did not materialise and the number of hospital admissions did not fall but continued to rise by around 5% each year. QOF has, therefore, been a complete £30 billion waste of money. But this is not the only problem. What the study didn't do was to compare the non-fatal drug side effects and the quality of life of the two groups. We have already seen that drugs produce significant numbers of non-fatal (as well as fatal) side effects. In the UK around 500,000 people require medical attention for drug side effects each year and about 200,000 are admitted to hospital because they are so severe. So, it is clear that those taking all these drugs see no improvement in mortality and life expectancy, but they do suffer from drug side effects that result in a significantly poorer quality of life.

Very few people have ever heard of the Quality and Outcomes Framework. Even fewer knew that the millions of healthy people who had no symptoms of any disease had no idea they were taking part in what was a poorly designed experiment, because there was no pilot study to see what the effects might be. Also, when the study that showed there were no benefits was published, virtually no one, including investigative journalists, knew anything about it because the whole thing was effectively kept secret. This is perhaps not surprising when as a country you have just wasted £30 billion and reduced the quality of life of millions of people. The Quality and Outcomes Framework is yet one more example of how medicine gets so many major issues wrong. It is a major embarrassment for medicine, the government, regulators and the drug industry. It is so embarrassing that it is unlikely that anyone will ever admit they were wrong. It is still being kept under wraps and the protocol is still being used. Millions of people are being given multiple drugs with no overall life-saving benefit but are suffering from non-fatal side effects. In addition, it is costing over £2 billion each year. It's all quite appalling and unbelievable.

So far, all the information has been about the overall outcomes for large numbers of people in trials and experiments. But how does polypharmacy affect real people who are caught up in its dirty web? This is what happened to Peter Gøtzsche's father who was 88 at the time. He was hospitalised for dizziness shortly after his medication was increased. He was then given even more medication which resulted in confusion and an inability to communicate. He was soon transferred to a nursing home where his conditions were so severe it led to him being listed as DNR (do not resuscitate). Peter Gøtzsche convinced his father's doctor to stop all medications. He then hired a private nurse to give him an organic diet rich in fruits, vegetables, nuts, seeds and grains. Within three days the nurses on the ward did not recognise him because he had made such an incredible recovery, and the next day he was discharged. He was back to his old self and was able to enjoy playing card games again with his friends. He died several years later while relaxing peacefully at home.

Peter Gøtzsche also relates the story of another woman aged 88. She was admitted to hospital after developing diarrhoea and dizziness. Her family were shocked at the rapid decline in her health and the emergence of several new symptoms. She was delusional and they couldn't wake her. They then discovered she was being given several new drugs. Shortly after, a psychiatrist then diagnosed Alzheimer's and prescribed another drug called Aricept. Her daughter-in-law stopped her taking this and several other drugs which had dramatic effects. She soon regained her pre-hospitalisation level of health. This clear insight into the dangers of polypharmacy led her daughter-in-law to become an advocate for other patients and families affected by it. There are so many similar examples of the devastating effects of polypharmacy that it would take many books to record them all.

I have had personal experience with my father of how drugs can induce falls when standing up (postural hypotension) and the subsequent broken bones, and how this is followed by a rapid and severe deterioration in health from other new conditions which develop in hospital. My father was one of the most communicative people of his age that I have ever known. He had no symptoms of memory loss or confusion. Yet within a few weeks of being admitted, I could barely communicate with him. A doctor even asked me how long he had had his memory problems. When I told him my father had perfect memory, I could see he didn't really believe me. Sadly, this story didn't have the same happy ending as the two stories related by Peter Gøtzsche. My father deteriorated rapidly and then finally caught a hospital acquired infection and died a few days later. Unfortunately, at the time, I hadn't even heard of the term polypharmacy, otherwise I would have tried to do something about it. Since then, I have heard many similar stories of older people admitted to hospital who then develop serious and new conditions. Very few people are as lucky Peter Gøtzsche's father. Modern medicine doesn't work well for old people.

Surprisingly, the devastating consequences of polypharmacy are more widely understood, and are being challenged, than I would ever have thought possible. In 2019 the charity Age UK issued a report with the title "More Harm than Good" about the consequences of polypharmacy and the fact that older people are being let down by a healthcare system that is allowing medicines to do more harm than good. It wants the government to take full account of the harmful effects of inappropriate multiple medications on older people in its planned review of NHS overprescribing.

The British Medical Journal also launched its "Too Much Medicine" initiative in 2017 which aims to highlight the threat posed by overdiagnosis and the waste of resources on unnecessary care. They are just part of a movement of doctors, researchers, patients and policy makers who want to deprescribe, raise awareness of and find solutions to the problem of too much medicine. Many other organisations around the world, including the Academy of Medical Royal Colleges, have urged similar initiatives to allow doctors to reduce over-prescribing and the harm it causes. Even the previous Health Secretary Matt Hancock said he was "incredibly concerned" by the rising trend of doctors prescribing pain pills, sleeping tablets and antidepressants. He said, "The disturbing findings that 1 in 8 adults are taking super-strength addictive opioid painkillers proves to me that we are in the grip of an over-medication crisis." However, despite all these initiatives and despite all the damning comments and evidence, little has changed and the devastation of polypharmacy continues virtually unchanged. The reasons for all of this will soon become clear.

The American opioid tragedy

Opioids are highly addictive drugs. Heroin is an opioid and using it is, of course, illegal. But pharmaceutical-based opioid drugs, if prescribed by a doctor, are legal. The pharmaceutical drugs are approved for pain relief and typical approved uses include serious accident victims and terminal cancer patients to alleviate the severe pain in the last few weeks of life. Of course, using the drugs for these relatively small numbers of people and short periods of time could never generate huge profits which are the overriding priority of the drug industry. As is usual in these circumstances, the industry had a clever plan to radically increase sales of opioid drugs. The company Purdue Pharma, with its drug OxyContin, was at the centre of the American plan to increase sales in the mid-1990s. Other companies then followed the same route with their own opioid drugs. The plan was to claim there was an epidemic of chronic pain throughout America, and that the best way to treat this "epidemic" was by prescribing powerful opioid drugs that were both safe and non-addictive. None of these claims were true, but the drugs were still approved by the Federal Drug Agency and then doctors were persuaded, pressurised and incentivised to start using them. It was, for example, implied that they would be guilty of negligence if they did not prescribe them, even if the level of patient pain was small and could have been treated with other conventional painkillers. In his book *American Overdose*, author Chris McGreal details the complex sequence of events of the opioid tragedy from the 1990s to the present day. In her book *Dopesick*, Beth Macy concentrates mainly on the individual human devastation caused by the drugs. These books are a sad, but compelling read. A reviewer said, "*Dopesick* will make you shudder with rage and weep with sympathy." I will, however, just concentrate on the tragic and devastating outcomes.

Up to 2020 over 750,000 deaths have resulted from opioid use. A further 650,000 deaths are predicted to occur in the next ten years. Currently, official figures show there are 2.6 million people who are addicted to opioid drugs, but other experts suggest the real figure is nearer 5 million. The addiction means most of these people cannot hold down jobs. Their only aim in life is to find the money to buy more and more drugs. Addiction overrules everything. Children of addicted parents go hungry because whatever money the family has is spent on drugs. Many children end up living with grandparents or going into foster care. Crime often becomes commonplace as the only way to buy the drugs. Addiction is devastating not just for those addicted but for complete families. Between 2.6 and 5 million people are addicted but around 10 million lives in total have effectively been destroyed. The financial costs to the US economy are also mind-blowing. A committee of government economic advisors calculated the total cost at $504 billion in 2015.

The American opioid crisis was declared a national public health emergency in 2017. The rules for prescribing opioids were tightened in 2016. But in the 20 years before they were changed, three-quarters of all addictions and deaths came from opioids prescribed by doctors. When they were changed, prescriptions reduced and this forced some of those already addicted to switch to street drugs like heroin and fentanyl. Street drugs now account for 68% of deaths overall, and new prescriptions by doctors account for 32% of deaths. The presidential commission report on opioids says, "We have an enormous problem that is often not beginning on street corners, but in doctors' offices and hospitals in every state in our nation... this crisis began in our healthcare system."

Federal scientists first warned of the coming opioid crisis in 2006, but no action was taken by regulators, government and medical organisations until 2016. This inaction resulted in hundreds of thousands of deaths and millions of lives effectively destroyed. This is a sad but recurring theme for these types of human tragedy. But let's not forget it is the pharmaceutical industry which lies at the heart of this disaster. They aggressively marketed opioid drugs using lies, while at the same time concealing their highly addictive nature. But it is only in recent years that they have started to pay a price for all of this. Some are paying compensation to individual states, while others are being charged with offences like illegally bribing doctors to overprescribe opioids. Purdue Pharma, who started this whole tragedy, have declared chapter 11 bankruptcy and the Sackler family which owns it has recently negotiated a deal with the US Department of Justice in which they will pay $8 billion to opioid victims. The New York Times noted, however, that "it is unlikely that the company will pay anything close to the $8 billion negotiated in the settlement deal, because it is in bankruptcy and the federal government will have to take its place in a long line of creditors".

Given that the opioid crisis has cost the US hundreds of billions of dollars and that Purdue made $30 billion in illegal opioid sales, it is no more than a slap on the wrist for the Sacklers. But there is one more crucial point. Part of the deal is that the Sackler family will be immune from any liability and prosecution relating to future opioid deaths and, as we have seen, there are likely to be over half a million more deaths over the coming years. One attorney said, "Criminal liability is not something that should be sold. It should not depend on how rich you are, it's not right." Robert F. Kennedy Jr. said, "This deal sets a disastrous precedent of officially anointing a separate system of justice for the 1%. This is a gangster family that has knowingly killed thousands of Americans for profit." Margarida Jorge, a campaign director for an advocacy coalition, said the deal was "a betrayal to the families of more than 750,000 Americans who have lost their lives. The Sacklers will still come out ahead, with the fine making up only a fraction of the profit one of the country's richest families made from peddling poison to Americans in pain". Robert Weissman, president of the advocacy group Public Citizen, said, "For there to be accountability for the corporate fuelled opioid addiction epidemic, which has taken hundreds of thousands of lives, there must be prosecution of those members of the Sackler family who, along with other executives and owners, were responsible for Purdue Pharma's deadly deception."

We have already seen that drug companies have been fined tens of billions of dollars for fraud but that the fines have been only a fraction of the money these illegal sales generated. The Sacklers are just one more example of how true justice never happens for the pharmaceutical industry and shows just how powerful they are. All those involved really should be imprisoned for life for the devastation they have caused and the millions of deaths they have caused. The whole process of litigation against all the companies involved will take years to complete and the final costs for the entire drug industry is expected be in the tens of billions of dollars. The total will be just a fraction of the trillion dollars that the whole opioid scandal will finally cost. I suspect that, apart from Purdue, all the other companies that sell opioid drugs will survive this process and, in a few years' time, they will be hugely profitable again. Will it make them change their ways? Of course not. The drug industry prospers and survives only by overpromoting mainly mediocre or even useless drugs, while covering up, or downplaying, their dangers. Even now, some drug companies see a new opportunity to substantially increase sales and profits. Having addicted millions of people, the industry is now developing new drugs to help alleviate the addiction. Of course, this new generation of drugs will almost certainly not work very well, and they will also have their own serious side effects that will only emerge years later. This will eventually enable them to develop yet more drugs and increase sales accordingly. Remember also that over the next ten years another 650,000 Americans are projected to die from opioid drugs and doctors will kill 200,000 of them with their prescriptions. You simply couldn't make this up – it is crazy and sickening. Beth Macy, author of the book *Dopesick*, makes a simple but profound comment: "Patients should employ a healthy scepticism the next time a pharmaceutical company announces its latest wonder drug."

So far, this section has concentrated on America, because this is where the opioid tragedy started. As the scandal unfolded, medical organisations in Britain and other western counties really did believe this sort of disaster could not occur here. Sadly, this is not the case and opioid drug use has been escalating rapidly in the UK. Opioid prescriptions are being issued to 5 million people each year, and over 500,000 people have been taking them for at least three years. In the last ten years prescriptions have gone up by nearly 250%. The future does not look good. Some people are accusing the drug industry of using the same promotional techniques to doctors that they used in America. Could a national emergency be declared at some point in the UK, and how many people will be killed by these drugs? Only time will tell.

Thalidomide

Until about ten years ago, I would surmise that virtually everyone on the planet including myself thought thalidomide was just an awful rare tragedy, and that when people realised what was happening, the drug was immediately taken off the market to avoid any further harm. How wrong could I be? Given what I already knew about the pharmaceutical industry, perhaps I should have known better. This is the true, horrific and tragic story of thalidomide. I should add that if you search on the web, you can find much more detailed descriptions and stories.

Thalidomide was developed by the German company Grünenthal. It was used as a mild sleeping pill, a tranquilliser and for morning sickness. It was first licensed in the UK in 1958, but reports of very rare and devastating birth defects soon started to emerge. Some physicians started to criticise the drug and the company's response was to hire private detectives to keep an eye on them. One physician had found 14 cases of extremely rare birth defects related to the drug. Grünenthal threatened him with legal action and sent letters to about 70,000 German doctors declaring thalidomide was a safe drug. They did this even though they knew about the birth defects and also about 2,000 cases of serious nerve damage which they also kept quiet about. Grünenthal harassed this doctor for the next ten years. An FDA scientist who refused to approve thalidomide for the US market was also harassed and intimidated, not only by the company acting as the US agent for thalidomide, but also by her bosses at the FDA who still wanted the drug approved for use.

The immense power of Big Pharma is illustrated by the thalidomide court cases. They started in 1965 in Södertälje, the home town of Scandinavia's biggest drug company, Astra. Astra had manufactured thalidomide for Grünenthal, but the victims' lawyers had enormous difficulty finding experts who were willing to testify against Astra. In the USA, the company that had distributed thalidomide, even though it wasn't approved by the FDA, had hired every expert there was on birth defects to prevent them from testifying for the victims. In Germany the court cases were a complete farce. The company's lawyers even argued it wasn't against the law to damage a foetus, as it had no legal rights. Three years into the trial, Grünenthal threatened journalists for what they had written and the trial ended with a ridiculously small settlement, about $11,000 for each deformed baby. No guilty verdict was ever rendered, no personal responsibility was assigned, and no one went to prison.

The UK behaved like a dictatorship state. The journalists weren't allowed to write about the court cases and people at the highest positions in the country, including the prime minister, were more interested in defending the company and its shareholders than in helping the victims. After a stalemate that lasted for ten years, the national scandal couldn't be held back any longer and the company distributing thalidomide, Distillers, which also sold liquor, faced a public boycott. A chain of 260 stores actually did boycott Distillers and Ralph Nader announced that if the victims didn't get a similar compensation to that awarded in the United States, a US boycott would also be launched. It took 16 years before the incriminating evidence that had been described in an article that the Sunday Times was forbidden to print finally came to public knowledge. But even this only happened because of a case in the European Court of Justice, where the Sunday Times' unpublished article was finally made public. As in Germany, no one was found guilty and no one was even charged with a crime.

Until it was banned from sale, Grünenthal ignored all the reports of deformity and nerve damage and didn't take any action. It was a classic case of profits before patients. It didn't matter how seriously malformed the children were and how many there were, as long as the company managed to keep the reports secret. If you look on the web you can find a long and detailed article by Harold Evans of the Guardian detailing how Grünenthal and German federal officials colluded to hatch a high-level plan to terminate the German legal trial. The victims were pressurised to give up their claims in exchange for what turned out to be a totally inadequate financial settlement. The victims were treated callously and any financial redress was totally inadequate given the level of disability. Even today, many victims are still driven to begging on the streets in numerous countries including Spain. Grünenthal meanwhile flourishes. In 2015 it had revenues of over €1.2 billion.

In total, 10,000 children were deformed. People with such serious handicaps would today need and receive around €2 million in compensation to provide the level of care needed over their lifetimes. Herein lies a major reason why governments around the world wanted to "brush the whole thing under the carpet" for as long as they could because the cost of compensating all these people would be €20 billion in today's money. Grünenthal could never have paid this sort of sum, so the money would have had to come from governments themselves.

We have seen how, as a result of research "fraud", beta blockers caused the deaths of 800,000 people in Europe alone. We have seen how the drugs Vioxx and Avandia both caused the deaths of at least 60,000 people because the companies covered up the fatal side effects. There are countless more examples of callous life-taking "fraud". But because thalidomide is so indelibly engrained into the collective human psyche, I'll hazard a guess that you are still more outraged at what you now know happened with thalidomide than with any of the others. Thalidomide wasn't the first example of a pharmaceutical company and its directors putting profit before human life and disability, but it must surely have been the most callous and evil example at that time. It seems almost inconceivable that any human being could knowingly destroy thousands of children's lives. Those involved should have been sent for trial in The Hague, charged with crimes against humanity and imprisoned for life. But as we have seen, no one was even prosecuted and no personal responsibility ever assigned. The company and its directors survived unscathed and even prospered. When people talk about man's inhumanity to man, they usually reserve such comments for people like Hitler or the leaders of ISIS, but some of those who run pharmaceutical companies are surely guilty of crimes that are just as heinous.

Much of what we now know about thalidomide has only recently been uncovered because documents previously hidden for over 50 years have finally started to come to light. But if you think that thalidomide is the ultimate horror story, then you need to prepare yourself for what you are about to read. Politicians around the world vowed that "thalidomide would never happen again", but now we know that drugs have caused three other similar birth defect tragedies. Two of these have only been uncovered in the last ten years and the numbers of damaged babies significantly exceed those from thalidomide.

Accutane

In the 1980s there was a second drug scandal involving birth defects similar to thalidomide. This involved the drug Accutane which was used to treat acne and was manufactured by Hoffmann-La Roche. It had been known for years that the drug caused birth defects, not just by the company, but by regulators and by doctors alike. In the US, the FDA estimated that around 1,000 deformed babies were born, and that the drug also caused about 1,000 miscarriages. Another 6,000 women became pregnant while taking Accutane and had abortions to avoid the risk of the severe birth defects associated with the drug. The worldwide figures are not accessible. The drug remained on the market despite many prominent politicians and doctors demanding it should be banned. Instead, regulators placed black box warnings on the drug stating it should not be used by pregnant women. Later, women even had to sign consent forms to get it. Roche finally withdrew the drug in 2009 after numerous costly law suits and adverse publicity. But generic versions are still available in most countries and birth defects are still occurring even today.

Primodos

Primodos was manufactured by the German company Schering, now part of the drug giant Bayer. It was used as a pregnancy test. It started to be prescribed in the mid-1960s. The first alarm bells came in 1967 when severe defects, such as heart faults, spina bifida and physical deformity, were reported. A paediatrician called Dr Elizabeth Gal did research at Queen Mary's Hospital that showed a link between Primodos and severe birth defects. She fought a ten-year battle to get the drug removed from the market but said she was stonewalled at every turn. In 1970 its licence as a pregnancy test was revoked but inexplicably the drug continued to be promoted and used. In 1975 a warning appeared on the package stating it should not be taken during pregnancy because of the risk that it may cause malformations. In 1977 the drug regulator confirmed this association. It was finally withdrawn in 1978; 11 years after the serious side effects were first reported. A Sunday Times article asked why it had taken so long to take the drug off the market.

Some of the families affected started to campaign for truth and justice. They had found nine scientific experts who were willing to testify that the drug was the cause of their birth defects. But just as with thalidomide, every single one of them was then hired to carry out other research work for Schering. The company claims that "the timing was purely coincidental". What this meant was that the scientists could not testify for the families because of their conflicts of interest. The families' cases collapsed and they were also denied legal aid to explore other avenues.

In the 1980s the German prosecutor seized documents and was contemplating a prosecution against Schering. This never went ahead, but the documents were kept in secure storage. Then in 2017 an investigative journalist uncovered and gained access to them. These showed that Dr William Inman, the UK's principle medical officer on the safety of medicines, had evidence in 1975 that there was an incredible 1 in 5 risk of birth defects for those women using Primodos, but inexplicably he didn't take it off the market. In fact, he destroyed the information to thwart any claim against the company. Not surprisingly he also failed to pass this critical information on to the families. What we also now know is that in Korea, Primodos was used to promote abortions. So, the fact that it caused severe defects is hardly surprising.

It has taken 50 years for this scandal to be brought into the public domain, and without the work of one dogged journalist it may never have come to light. When all the evidence emerged, it gave the families hope that they might at last have a chance of achieving the justice they deserve. But sadly, and almost unbelievably, an expert working group of the UK Commission on Human Medicines published a report in November 2017 which concluded that there was no "causal association" between Primodos and severe disabilities in babies. They recommended that the families involved should be offered genetic testing to establish if there was a different underlying cause. Given all the evidence available, this is a shocking outcome. It shows what can happen when medicine is allowed to become its own judge and jury. I really do believe that if this had gone through a normal independent legal process, then true justice would have prevailed.

Valproate

Valproate is manufactured by the French pharmaceutical giant Sanofi. It was first marketed in 1967 for the treatment of epilepsy, but was subsequently used for bipolar disorder and migraines. Two studies published in 2017 by French health authorities showed the drug was responsible for severe malformations in babies and it also caused autism and developmental problems. Another study showed it increased the rate of autism by 900%. In the UK, this drug tragedy has resulted in 20,000 children developing these devastating conditions. The worldwide figure is impossible to calculate accurately, but because the drug was widely used, a figure of half a million, and maybe even more, is quite possible.

Starting in 2017, doctors were told not to give valproate to girls and women of child-bearing age unless there were no alternatives and unless they had discussed the serious risks with the women involved. But just as with thalidomide, Accutane and Primodos, the increased risk of birth defects, especially for spina bifida, has been common knowledge for years. It was widely known by regulators in the UK even in 1973 that the drug caused birth defects, but they waited over 40 years before alerting the public to the risks. In medical circles it was widely known in the 1980s. The autism connection came to light about 20 years ago. Babies exposed to the drug in the womb have a 35% risk of developing severe developmental disorders, and an 11% risk of congenital malformations.

There are 26 different drugs available to treat epilepsy, but it is only in the last five years that doctors have been told not to prescribe valproate to women of child-bearing age unless all other drugs have failed to control the condition. Why was this simple decision not made decades ago? Why were hundreds of thousands of children allowed to suffer serious deformities? Perhaps we can gain an insight from the public review held at the European Medicine Agency in London in September 2017, which was set up to examine this tragedy. Joanne Cozens, chairwoman of the Organisation for Anti-Convulsant Syndromes (a patient support group representing children and parents caught up in this tragedy), criticised the actions of Sanofi and the regulators, and accused medical experts of being complicit in allowing thousands of children to suffer deformity. She said, "Sanofi have a loyal bunch of clinical experts promoting valproate and resisting warnings. I can see a few of you in the room today. You know who you are and we don't trust you anymore because you are complicit in avoidable injury to children."

Documents from 1973 show that regulators decided not to warn patients directly of the harms for fear: "It could give rise to fruitless anxiety." Health professionals were told at the time that "this compound is teratogenic in animals, meaning it could harm the human foetus", but the Committee on the Safety of Medicines said the warning "should not go on the package inserts so that there would be no danger of patients themselves seeing it".

I am almost lost for words. Here we have one more drug-induced medical scandal. We have seen so many of these that it is difficult to decide which is the most heinous. But valproate must surely be at or near the top of the list, simply because it involves around half a million children around the world who have been devastatingly harmed for their entire lives by those they should have been able to trust. And let's not forget the families involved. Parents have had to give up everything to become full-time carers for their damaged children, living on meagre state handouts with no compensation and fearful that, when they die, their children will not get the level of care they need. In total, around 1.5 million family lives have been effectively destroyed.

In 2010 families in England and Wales were about to bring a legal case against Sanofi. Three weeks before the trial was due to start, their legal aid was suddenly and inexplicably withdrawn. This meant the trial collapsed. The families were, of course, devastated, but they had no idea what was to follow. Sanofi claimed it had spent millions of pounds in legal costs to prepare for the trial and would have had a legal right to charge the families for this incredible sum. Of course, they would have known that the families could never repay it since most of them were already living off minimal state handouts, but they had a much more cunning plan. They said if the families signed letters promising never to sue again, they would not be billed. Of course, they had no choice but to agree, even though they knew they would never be able to achieve the justice they deserved.

What happened after the review in 2017 at the European Medicine Agency was concluded? There was some additional tightening of the rules for the use of valproate and the way the dangers were communicated to women of child-bearing age. And that is all. Was anyone held to account? Was anyone charged with any crime? By now you may understand that was never going to happen. This was the final chance for the families to see any sort of justice achieved. It is impossible to understand the extent of the despair they must feel. The whole tragedy is shocking beyond belief.

Summarising the birth defect scandals

A common picture emerges when drug-induced birth defects start to occur. When the first links between a drug and child deformities are uncovered, the company denies any link and the individuals who expose what is happening are either attacked or stonewalled. The company never admits liability even when the facts become indisputable. They make statements like "the sale of the drug was in compliance with prevailing laws" and "the evidence for a causal link between the drug and congenital deformity is weak". The company uses every tactic available to prevent claims against the drug being made. For example, hiring every expert witness to work for them, so they are unable to help the families and testify against the company. Regulators and governments are invariably complicit in this cover up, instinctively supporting the drug company at the expense of the families and children involved. Many years and even decades go by before any decision is taken to ban or restrict the drugs. Countless deformities occur in the intervening years. Even senior medical people are culpable because the deformities at some stage become common knowledge within medical circles. Why don't doctors demand that studies be carried out quickly to find out the truth, so if a drug is indeed responsible then it can be quickly removed?

The families and children involved are invariably treated callously and inhumanely, and usually denied access to crucial information and legal aid that would enable them to seek compensation through the normal court justice system. So, not only are families destroyed by these avoidable deformities, but many parents have to give up work and normal life to become full-time carers surviving on minimal state handouts. Despite the claims that a thalidomide tragedy would never happen again (and these would have been genuine at that time), devastating birth defects caused by prescription drugs have occurred continuously over the last 50 years and continue to occur even today. Much of this has been covered up until recently. It is almost impossible to believe this has occurred with such regularity and over such prolonged periods. Evil is perhaps the strongest single word that can be applied to a human being, and when the truth emerged about thalidomide, I thought nothing could be more evil. But I was wrong. The devastating stories of the drugs Accutane, Primodos and valproate show unequivocally there are many more evil people within drug companies, regulators, governments and medicine than anyone could ever have imagined. Another really scary thought is how many more scandals might still be "under wraps"?

The nine devastating drug outcomes just examined are not isolated events. There are sadly many others and here are just two more outlined cases.

Hormone replacement therapy drugs were estimated to have caused around 200,000 deaths from cancer in the US between 1990 and 2003. In 2003 when this evidence emerged, treatments were significantly reduced. The fall in prescriptions saw a 12% reduction in the number of breast cancer cases. The drug company Pfizer, which bought the main producer of HRT drugs in 2009, continued to maintain the drugs were safe, but by 2014 it had paid out $1.6 billion to settle cancer claims. One woman was awarded an incredible sum of $76 million in a court case, partly because the evidence showed Pfizer deliberately promoted a treatment it knew could cause cancer.

The drug Trasylol was used to stem bleeding in various types of open-heart surgery between 1993 and 2007. However, a study eventually showed it caused kidney failure and led to increased deaths. In the US it was withdrawn by the FDA in 2007 and was also temporarily suspended in other countries. In 2009 it was removed worldwide. In the US alone, the deaths were estimated at 22,000 by the doctor who carried out the study. Total world deaths are unknown but must be at least 50,000. Another devastating fact is that the drug's manufacturer, Bayer AG, had in fact conducted its own study and found almost similar outcomes but had failed to report this to the FDA.

This section started with the question: "How dangerous are prescription drugs?" I'll let you make up your own mind.

The pharmaceutical industry's money tree

The previous sections have given a vivid picture of medical research and drugs. Here is a summary. Most research simply cannot be trusted; there is so much data manipulation, cherry picking of data, statistical "scams" and outright "fraud". The drug industry has been fined tens of billions of dollars for illegally promoting unproven drugs and for hiding lethal side effects of drugs that then killed tens of thousands of people before they were eventually banned from sale. While some drugs do work reasonably well for some people, the benefits of many of them are small and most drugs don't work at all for most people, and this is before we try to balance all this against their many, and often lethal, side effects. Drugs are the third leading cause of death and the side effects and deaths are certain to be higher than the official figures suggest. The majority of new drugs are not breakthrough drugs. Around

70% are just slight variations on the old drugs they are intended to replace. Sometimes they are marginally better and sometimes they are worse than the older drugs even though they usually cost between ten and thirty times more. Drugs are rarely tested on the people who are going to take them, so the truth is no one really knows what will happen when millions of ordinary people, particularly older ones, take them. It is, therefore, not surprising that 20 to 30% of all drugs are eventually given the ultimate black box warning or banned from sale because they are killing people or causing serious side-effects. Another 20% of drugs prescribed by doctors (off-label drugs) have no proof they work. In addition to all of this, there is an almost exponential increase in nearly every single disease and the drugs used to treat these diseases only rarely prevent or cure them. Most drugs simply minimise the symptoms and just slow down the decline before premature death occurs.

Given all these facts, why have drugs become the mainstay of medicine? Why have governments and regulators passed lax regulations that allow the pharmaceutical industry to get away with all of this? Why are the press and media not challenging any of it? Why, in many cases, are they helping to cover up drug scandals that have killed hundreds of thousands of people? Why is no one really promoting non-drug approaches that would provide better outcomes for patients and cost virtually nothing?

Let me give you the briefest insight into what is to follow with one simple historical event. Thirty years ago, when Peter Gøtzsche was working as a doctor, he attended a one-day planning meeting with a pharmaceutical company. When this was over, he was handed a blank envelope by a pharma representative. When he opened it later, there was a thank you note for his help and a $1,000 note. In today's terms, allowing for inflation, this would be equivalent to around $2,500. Given that attending a meeting was just a normal part of his job at the hospital, he was quite surprised to receive anything and particularly shocked by its unexpected largesse. The implication was obvious. If you work with the drug industry, you can expect significant financial rewards on top of your medical salary even though you are not working directly for the pharmaceutical company. So, perhaps you can see where this is leading.

We have seen the drug companies spend large sums of money on medical research and they make sure everyone knows about it. But what they don't advertise and in fact keep cleverly under wraps is that they spend over twice as much on what they euphemistically call "marketing and administration" than they do on drug development. The former editor of the New England Journal of Medicine and the US Securities and Exchange Commission have estimated that the industry spends 35% of their total turnover on marketing and administration, and just 15% on drug development. Marketing and administration consist of three main things: administration costs, advertising and other marketing costs, and, what the industry calls, "education" costs. It is the education costs which are crucial to this section. These represent around 20% of turnover. In 2019 global drug sales were just over $1 trillion meaning the drug industry spent $200 billion on "education" worldwide. So, the crucial question is what exactly is this colossal sum spent on? The answer is probably the most important key to understanding why your doctor knows virtually nothing about lifestyle solutions to health.

The $200 billion is spent in two ways. Firstly, millions of individuals and thousands of organisations receive money either directly or indirectly from the drug companies. Secondly, the companies spend a significant sum on their own representatives, external PR companies and external lobbyists whose sole job is to promote the pharmaceutical industry and its drugs to the tens of millions of people and organisations involved in healthcare. It is impossible to accurately calculate how much is given to each group since the drug industry is desperate to cover up and play down this incredible sum. A realistic assumption would be that $100 billion is spent on monetary payments and the same sum is spent on "educating" people about the industry and its products. The total sum is so incredible that the exact split doesn't really matter. The key is to simply understand the real motives for doing all of this, because they are not, as the industry would have everyone believe, simply done to help "educate" everyone.

So, now we can start to analyse this incredible pharmaceutical money tree in more detail. I'll start with a list of the main monetary beneficiaries and then look at each one in more detail and discover the real motives behind them all. The main recipients are:

- doctors
- key medical opinion leaders
- medical researchers
- medical organisations
- medical journals
- major charities
- patient groups
- medical schools
- pharmaceutical lobby groups
- information controllers
- politicians and governments
- drug regulators
- the media and press

In total, all these people and organisations receive around $100 billion each year. I should add that while this is a worldwide figure, most of it is spent in the developed world. It is impossible to find out how much they receive individually, but there are a few clues. Recent legislation in the USA – the Sunshine Act – commonly known as "Dollars for Docs", required the drug industry to list all its payments to every individual doctor. In the first 16-month period these totalled $3.49 billion. An estimate for all doctors around the world would be between $10 billion and $20 billion each year.

So, now we can ask the second crucial question: when the industry gives $100 billion each year to all the lucky recipients listed, what is the payback? We have already seen that the industry only spends money when there is a payback. They really do not do this with any altruistic motive even though that is what they claim. If they really wanted to be altruistic, they would simply spend the money on developing antibiotics and continue producing snake bite serum and thereby save millions of lives. But, of course, they don't. Many years ago, the pharmaceutical industry knew most of its drugs were ineffective for most people. They knew they would struggle to find new drugs that were any better than the existing ones when these lost their patents. They knew they had to get doctors to prescribe drugs to many more people if they were to hit their ever-increasing profit targets, and they needed to keep increasing drug prices. They knew that even many of the drugs that did work provided quite modest benefits even after the trials and data had been manipulated, and this included downplaying the risks and side effects.

So, they were left with just one solution. They simply decided to financially incentivise everyone who was involved in healthcare, with the aim of ensuring pharmaceutical drugs would be accepted as the best and in fact the only effective way of treating sickness and disease. Of course, it is all dressed up to look like altruism and given the fine sounding name "education", but however it is dressed up, it is quite simply "bribery". Given that it is legal (unbelievably) for the drug industry to give such enormous sums of money to these recipients, then I cannot call it bribery, so instead I will call it "bribery". Of course, all of this happened slowly and very cleverly over several decades in such a way that most of the people involved never really understood how they were being led into a world where drugs would be accepted as the only way to treat every disease and where the idea of preventing disease by natural means was dismissed, ignored and even treated with outrage and censorship. The drug industry really has achieved its incredible plan. So, now we can look at how this "bribery" works in the real world with our real-life beneficiaries.

Doctors

Doctors are required by law to undertake what is called "continuing medical education" (CME). As part of this, there is a requirement to attend seminars each year that update a doctor's knowledge of new treatments, drugs and other medical developments. Unlike virtually every other profession where necessary training is paid for by the employer, doctors are required to pay for this CME themselves. However, many years ago, the pharmaceutical industry decided they would invite doctors to attend free medical seminars and even provide free travel and accommodation. Most doctors take up this incredibly generous offer. Of course, the industry maintains this is purely for educational purposes and doctors swear that even though they accept these free invitations, they in no way affect their professional judgement or prescribing habits. Neither of these assertions is correct. For many years, not only the doctor, but his wife and family, would be invited to attend seminars in five-star hotels in exotic locations, like Lake Garda, with all travel, hotel and other expenses, such as spa treatments, paid by the company. Such "blatant bribery" attracted the ire of independent industry watchers and eventually, the outcry became so fierce laws were introduced to curb these excesses. Now, only the doctor can receive free attendance, travel and accommodation. But don't be fooled. Determined global corporations always find ways around rules and regulations introduced by hapless governments. So, now, as an example, the company may, during the event weekend, "employ" the doctor on a short-term consultancy basis where his views will be sought on various issues. Can the drug industry really gain anything meaningful from such interviews? The answer, of course, is they gain very little because this is simply a means to an end. The fees for this short consultation simply allow the doctor to effectively bring his wife and family for "free". Problem solved – job done. And all this is now perfectly legal again.

We know the industry must get a payback on all this expenditure and for this to happen the doctors involved must change their prescribing habits. This is exactly what happens because these seminars are used to promote specific drugs, and prescriptions rise after the seminar. How do we know? Well, as we have already seen, when pharmaceutical companies are charged with serious fraud – and this happens regularly – the federal investigators will acquire every single memo, email and report relating to the drug in question. These internal documents reveal clearly the sums that are spent on these events and show the increase in sales of the drugs that were promoted and the extra revenue this brings. This is always more than the cost of the seminars. If it wasn't, they would be stopped. Doctors always maintain they are not influenced by the industry but these internal company reports show clearly this is not the case. Those GP practices that didn't attend particular seminars usually see no increase in prescriptions for the drugs promoted. If these drugs really were the best for the patient, then this should be common knowledge within the profession and all doctors would be switching to them, not just those who attended the free seminars. Doctors may genuinely believe their clinical judgement is not affected, but many patients are receiving drugs not because they are the best for their condition, but because the doctors subconsciously or unwittingly are influenced by what they are told in these seminars.

By paying for the entire event, the pharmaceutical company not only increases sales of its promoted drugs but also gets to control the overall agenda. So, they can also ensure that anything that would compete with, or be a threat to, their drugs is excluded. There is, for example, substantial evidence on the benefits of fish oil for preventing heart disease, but doctors never get to hear about it because they have unwittingly and effectively given the industry complete control over seminar agendas. These seminars are not usually organised and run by the pharmaceutical companies themselves because this would simply appear to be biased commercialisation. They are organised instead by ostensibly independent medical education companies that appear to give the whole thing an air of respectability and independence. But when your entire business relies 100% on fees from the drug industry there is no independence. You become an extension of the industry and simply follow their agenda.

Here is a key point. What would happen if doctors decided to pay for these seminars themselves rather than just accept the free industry invites, either because they wanted to learn about other possible treatment alternatives or because they thought they were effectively being "bribed" to increase the use of specific drugs? Would anything really change? Absolutely not. The key medical decision makers would simply block data on alternative treatments and say there was no proof any of them worked. They would also only allow the same types of drugs and official medical treatments to be promoted that the industry would do in their own CME seminars. So, the fact that doctors get these free seminars really makes little difference to what happens to their patients. They simply have to follow official rules.

Free CMEs are the key funding that doctors receive from the industry. There are just a few other relatively minor ones. Surgeries can be provided with free lunches in return for a short meeting and a few words from a pharmaceutical representative which often involve the promotion of a specific drug, and free gifts can appear if prescriptions for a particular drug hit certain levels.

Key opinion leaders in medicine

Who are the key people the drug industry really needs to surreptitiously dominate in their plan to control medicine and healthcare? The industry actually has an acronym for them. KOL stands for key opinion leaders in the various medical disciplines, such as cardiologists, oncologists and gastroenterologists as well as key academics. These are the people who doctors and GPs will recognise by name and whose opinions they will trust. So, how does the industry "influence" these people?

One of the surest ways to rise to the top of your chosen medical discipline is to get involved in medical research. Get papers published and your prestige and standing will increase. Eventually, as you rise through the ranks, you will have other researchers doing most of the work while you take most of the credit. There is just one problem: medical research is expensive. I'm sure you can guess where this is heading. Yes, never fear, the pharmaceutical industry is ready, willing and able to help the next generation of KOLs to reach the top. There are, of course, conditions relating to this largesse. If a research study found negative results for a drug and was nevertheless published, the "would-be" KOL would find their funding dried up and their dreams of reaching the top would never materialise. But, of course, this rarely happens as the "unwritten rules" are well understood by all concerned. If you want to be really useful to the industry you could, as well as doing research that demonstrates the efficacy and safety of drugs, also do studies that show lifestyle treatments, such as homeopathy, acupuncture and vitamins, have no benefits. Combine these two and your path to the top is almost guaranteed. It is really a form of "grooming" to ensure each new generation of KOLs is on board with the pharmaceutical model of healthcare while at the same time helping to destroy all other modalities that stand in their way.

Why are KOLs so important to the industry? When you reach the top of your chosen discipline, you will sit on committees involved in setting medical guidelines. Each new guideline will invariably involve extending the prescribing of drugs to ever greater numbers of people. I have only ever seen one guideline that recommended reducing drug prescribing. When a new drug is developed, an endorsement from a KOL will persuade many doctors to switch to this new, and invariably much more expensive, drug which can be worth billions of dollars to the industry. Many leading KOLs will also sit on pharmaceutical industry regulatory panels and can ensure the laws relating to the drugs they produce are never too onerous.

Once they reach the top with the help of pharma funding, the industry then needs to keep them on board throughout their careers. How do they do this? A leading cardiologist will, for example, be asked to critically review the results of a clinical trial for a new blood pressure lowering drug. The premise is that they will use their expertise and knowledge to evaluate the drug against other existing treatments. If they find the new drug is indeed better or safer, then their final study report will be invaluable to the company and sales will rise accordingly. Given it can take many weeks just to read the thousands of pages of a clinical trial, this type of work requires months of work and great dedication. So, the fees will be commensurate and a figure of around $100,000 is not uncommon. In theory, such critical assessments of drugs by leading specialists should be beneficial for patients and medicine as it stops pharma companies simply hyping up their product if left to their own devices. By now, however, you may sense there is another big "but" coming, and sadly, reality falls far short of these lofty ideals. Hundreds of such papers written by leading specialists were retracted when it was discovered they had not been written by the author but by the PR department of the drug companies. The KOLs had effectively just added their signatures and walked off with their "$100,000 cheques". Indeed, one single academic published in excess of 200 such papers over just a few years – a world record I believe. This, of course, would be an impossible feat unless the papers had already been "pre-written". When this fraud was discovered, you might imagine the pharmaceutical companies and doctors involved would face serious criminal charges and even jail sentences. This didn't happen and as far as I am aware the doctors didn't even have to pay back any of their fraudulent income. Instead, we simply had the ubiquitous and meaningless platitude of "steps have been taken to prevent this sort of thing happening again" from medicine's elite. There is no doubt that both the companies and doctors involved are more circumspect now about how these reports are produced but don't be fooled. The company still has a controlling role. Draft copies will go back and forth until the company is happy with the wording and the outcome. If a KOL did produce a critical report, the company has the absolute right not to publish it so it would never see the light of day anyway and the doctor would, of course, never be asked to do such work again. The company would simply find another doctor prepared to come up with the "positive report" they required.

There are, of course, other ways in which leading KOLs can be rewarded and "incentivised". We have already seen, for example, how Big Pharma provides free seminars to doctors to fulfil their continuing medical education obligations. At these seminars the lectures are usually given by key medical opinion leaders. Typical fees for just a single lecture are around $10,000 plus free travel and all expenses. Many KOLs do multiple lectures each year and a minimum six-figure sum is easily attainable. But such sums are for the average KOL. The most influential and most senior experts can command much higher figures. Here I'll refer back to the Dollars for Docs information from the US. The three top earning doctors received the following payments from the pharmaceutical industry for promoting drugs at medical seminars in just 16 months:

- Suijata Narayan – $43.9 million
- Karen Underwood – $28.5 million
- Sanjay Yadav – $23.1 million

In a single year they received more from the drug industry than they would from their entire remuneration as a doctor over their 40-year medical career. Only a small number of chief executives from the biggest global corporations earn such sums. They are quite simply obscene given that, first and foremost, these people are supposed to be doctors. In the five years since it was first published, Dollars for Docs has shown that over 2,500 doctors have received more than half a million dollars and more than 700 of them received over a million dollars. There is absolutely no reason why the top experts in the UK should not be earning similar sums. But, of course, this can't be confirmed because there are no similar laws on disclosure.

The huge amount of money the drug industry gives to key opinion leaders to promote drugs to doctors raises the question: if these drugs really are so effective, why do they need to be pushed so hard? Surely if a drug worked really well, doctors would know about it from professional meetings and medical journals and would actually be mandated to use them from organisations like NICE. The drugs that are promoted in this way invariably have limited benefits.

Medical researchers

The pharmaceutical industry funds around 70% of medical research. The next biggest providers are governments, followed by various public and corporate donations and other fund-raising events. The pharmaceutical money is spent in several ways. The companies carry out research in-house using their own researchers. Alternatively, they pay independent companies to carry out research for them. They also give money to universities and other institutions which allows them to carry out fundamental medical research.

In practice, when an industry provides 70% of research funding, it gives them an unprecedented level of power and control. The independent research companies the industry uses are independent in name only. If these companies were to produce damaging findings on drugs, their future would be bleak. Funding and commissions would dry up and very few could survive. These companies know full well that their very survival depends overwhelmingly on pharmaceutical money. Hence you will see them offering competing adverts touting for business. These adverts emphasise how the company places great emphasis on expediting the trial process and "ensuring" successful outcomes to maximise overall financial benefits for the drug company. Nowhere will you find mention of drug safety or similar concerns. As far as universities and other institutions are concerned, the end result is much the same. Research detrimental to the industry rarely happens. If it did, their funding would also simply dry up. "Everyone knows the unwritten rules of the game."

You might think the other 30% of research spending would surely be independent but this is also not the case. Governments fund around two-thirds of this other research, but politicians are not medical experts and have no idea what the money should be spent on. They rely on their key medical advisors to help define the research priorities which are then rubber stamped and funded. Of course, as we have seen, these KOLs are committed to the pharmaceutical industry, so most of the research involves drugs or the development of more testing and screening options for patients which leads inevitably to even more drugs being prescribed. The same applies to major charities as we will see shortly. So, quite simply, the pharmaceutical industry has a virtual monopoly over medical research. This is the main reason why so little money is spent on finding the real causes of disease, and why so little research is carried out on lifestyle solutions to health.

Medical organisations and societies

Organisations and societies covering most medical disciplines, like cardiology, oncology and haematology, usually receive funding from the pharmaceutical industry, and this money is often used to fund annual meetings and other main events which are attended by hundreds of senior doctors. One example gives an idea of the extent of the funding and involves the American Medical Association which received over $40 million in a single year from pharmaceutical advertisements in its publications which was more than double the amount it received from all its subscriptions. The drug companies also provide free lunches and dinners at key events and often create what resembles an exhibition hall that displays their drugs and services together with friendly sales people eager to ply the doctors with free gifts.

Medical journals

Doctors read medical journals or at least the summary reports. They rely on them to provide unbiased information which will in turn influence the treatments and drugs they use. Medical journals used to be run as independent organisations publishing research based on merit and quality and, therefore, fulfilled this important role. But today many journals are either owned wholly or partly by pharmaceutical companies. The editors of such journals, whilst still ostensibly independent, know full well they will only remain editors if the "right" scientific papers are published. For those journals not owned by the industry, there is a perfectly legal way of exerting the same kind of power and influence.

Papers published in journals cannot be copied or reprinted without approval. Reprints can be obtained legally by paying a fee per copy and this can be expensive. If a drug company wants a particular drug study to be published, but the journal is likely to reject it because the quality of the study is poor, the company can "incentivise" publication by guaranteeing to purchase several thousand reprints in advance. This can represent a major source of revenue for the journal. To give one example, the Lancet receives 45% of its entire revenue from reprints. It represents a major dilemma for the editors. Do they only publish high-quality, rigorous studies and reject everything else and, therefore, lose significant income in the process which may affect the very viability of the journal? Several former editors of journals have spilt the beans. Dr Marcia Angell in her book *The Truth about the Drug Companies* has this searing indictment: "It is no longer possible to believe much of the clinical research that is published, or to rely on the judgement of trusted physicians or authoritative medical guidelines. I take no pleasure in this conclusion which I reached slowly and reluctantly over my two decades as an editor of The New England Journal of Medicine."

Major charities

Charities such as The British Heart Foundation, Cancer Research and Diabetes UK are major beneficiaries of pharma funding. If you thought that organisations like these were funded only by public donation and charity raising events, think again. Many of these organisations carry out medical research, so Big Pharma needs to ensure it is the "right sort of research". Research into prevention of disease is, of course, frowned upon as is research into lifestyle treatments and, of course, these wouldn't be funded. Research involving drugs is naturally encouraged and well funded, as would research into new diagnostic testing that enables earlier detection of disease or mass screening programmes that enable more people to be diagnosed as sick, since these would both lead to more drugs being prescribed. These unwritten rules are, of course, well understood by all concerned, and the pharmaceutical model of treating sick people with drugs prevails, even within these "independent" charities. These are big businesses. The directors earn big salaries with big pension obligations to be funded, and they are invariably professional career managers. Maximising income is their main priority. If this means working with the drug industry, well, everyone else does it, and they are encouraged to do it by governments, so what's the problem? The problem is, of course, that drugs become the only option people and even doctors are ever aware of, even though there are much safer and more effective ways of staying healthy and treating disease.

Patient groups

Patient groups are very different to the large charities. They don't carry out research or any type of clinical analysis. Their main function is to lobby on behalf of the patients they represent. This lobbying is usually aimed at governments and usually involves demands for more funding for their specific cause. This can involve demands for more testing or more screening, but, predominantly, it involves demands for more spending on drugs and, specifically, newer drugs. You can perhaps see why the pharmaceutical industry is very interested in patient groups. Here we have independent organisations with very vociferous sets of supporters all demanding more expenditure on newer expensive drugs. For the industry this is like all their Christmases arriving together. The industry is now a prolific funder of patient groups. Additionally, and crucially, the industry "educates" those running the organisations about the benefits of their drugs, especially new drugs. You can guess that side effects are glossed over and benefits exaggerated. The people running these groups are rarely professional managers and usually have limited scientific training. So, you can go over the top in talking up your product.

As long as these organisations have sufficient funds and know about your "new wonder drugs" the beauty is you can leave it entirely in their hands, knowing the intense pressure they, and their supporters, bring will often change government policy and more spending on your drugs will ensue. A textbook example of this process was with the drug Herceptin manufactured by Genentech. This was a new and hugely expensive cancer drug initially approved by the FDA in 1998. It arrived in the UK sometime later, but the National Institute for Health and Care Excellence (NICE) looked at all the evidence and concluded that the modest benefits of the drug, its huge costs and the serious side effects such as heart attacks did not warrant any funding and that older and cheaper existing drugs were just as effective. But the fight by cancer patient groups to get NICE to approve the drug was in full swing. Then one woman managed to ask a direct question to Tony Blair on live TV about why the government was withholding funding for this "new wonder drug" that "could save patients' lives". Of course, Mr Blair would have known nothing at the time about this specific drug, but promised to look into it. The next day the papers had explosive headlines, such as "Government withholds funding on life-saving cancer drug". The dice was loaded and the government, fearing serious adverse publicity, overruled NICE and insisted Herceptin be funded, albeit only for certain types of cases.

What are the facts about Herceptin? It reduces the risk of breast cancer deaths after three years by 3%. But it increases the risk of heart attacks by 2.1% – a net gain of just 0.9%. Hardly the results you might have been expecting from a "wonder drug". But what is really sad about this whole story is that almost certainly more patients would die on Herceptin than the best of the older drugs. The older drugs might have reduced cancer deaths by only 2%, but they almost certainly didn't cause heart attacks, so overall there would be fewer deaths. The patient groups, of course, won the day, and the patients, although they didn't know it, were more likely to die, but the pharmaceutical industry was laughing all the way to the bank, while unsuspecting tax payers funded this hugely expensive intervention. Incidentally, if you still doubt that many drugs only have tiny benefits, look no further than chemotherapy drugs for proof. A 2% reduction in risk of death is the typical sort of benefit you can expect. One detailed study in Australia, which examined all chemotherapy studies carried out over a six-year period, found that the drugs increased five-year cancer survival rates by just 2.2% on average.

Patient groups are an essential part of the pharma game plan to continually increase drug sales – particularly new and obscenely expensive ones. When a specific patient group does not already exist, drug companies have even been known to establish one themselves, placing carefully selected leaders at the top. This is another example that demonstrates the extreme lengths to which the industry will go in order to increase its sales, as well as the lax laws that continue to allow this sort of flagrant activity to take place.

Medical schools

Medical schools receive funding from Big Pharma. As you can imagine, this gives them a great deal of influence over what is taught. Unsurprisingly, drug treatments loom large. In fact, learning about drugs takes up around 60% of the total medical curriculum. Prevention of disease barely features. Even though food is the most important factor in staying healthy, over their five-year course, students are taught about it for just two days, but even then, most of it is not scientifically correct as you will discover in Parts 4 and 5. This is all part of the industry's plan to ensure the supremacy and universality of drugs is maintained and that everything else that affects health is marginalised and even discredited.

One simple story illustrates how insidious this whole process has become. A friend recently visited the doctor to find there were two final-year medical students there obviously gaining hands-on experience in a GP surgery. The doctor explained to them that obviously it would be normal to take the patient's blood pressure for the particular condition involved, but for this patient, she wasn't going to. This was because the patient suffered from extreme white coat hypertension. In case you don't know, this is a condition where someone has normal blood pressure but this goes up significantly when, and only when, they are placed in a stressful position like seeing a doctor. What was shocking was that neither final-year student knew what white coat hypertension was. I believe the doctor looked shocked and asked the patient to explain the details to the students. How could this be possible? White coat hypertension is very common. I also have it even though my own blood pressure is absolutely normal, so you would expect every doctor and every student to know about it. It can easily be confirmed by using a 24-hour blood pressure monitoring device. If someone has the condition, they would generally not need blood pressure lowering drugs because 99.999% of the time they don't have high blood pressure. Can you guess where this is leading? There are some estimates that around 20% of people who have their blood pressure tested in a doctor's surgery will have a high reading just because they have white coat syndrome. If students are not being taught about it, then, as doctors, they will simply prescribe blood pressure lowering drugs to all these people even though they don't need them. These patients will then also suffer unnecessarily from the drug's side effects. Whatever money Big Pharma gives to medical schools could be repaid handsomely by just this single "syllabus oversight". Blood pressure lowering drugs are one of the most prescribed medicines of all time. Around 20% of prescriptions are unnecessary but are earning Big Pharma billions of dollars worldwide. To misquote an old saying, "Money corrupts, but lots of money corrupts absolutely."

Pharmaceutical lobby groups

Most countries have lobby groups that promote their industry's interests. In the UK, two of the most prominent ones are Sense about Science and the Nightingale Collaboration. These organisations, of course, deny they are lobby groups. Instead, they portray themselves as totally independent bodies whose aim is simply the promotion of good science, despite the fact they have received funding from companies like Coca Cola. They effectively help to endorse industries like Big Pharma, Big Food and Big Ag, as well as others like Big Chemical that provide products such as emulsifiers, preservatives and colourings for processed foods. These groups try to provide positive information on things like drugs, GMO crops, artificial fertilisers and processed foods, but one of their main focuses is something rather different. Many of their campaigns involve attacking those people who are trying to expose the truth and the damaging side effects of these products, like the fact GMO crops cause cancer or processed foods cause obesity. The tactics they use are well established and range from vicious personal attacks as well as the use of dodgy, biased and cherry picked "science". Lifestyle medicine is portrayed as quackery and those who promote it as quacks. We will learn more about these groups and the threat they pose later, when we turn our attention to lifestyle medicine and its incredible potential.

Information controllers

The control of information and data by governments, internet companies, global corporations and the global elite is a major concern and is becoming a serious threat against democracy itself. Whilst most people understand that dictatorships like China, Russia and North Korea control and censor the information their people can access and have no qualms about rewriting history to suit their purposes, the idea that all these things are happening in even the most democratic places, like Britain, the US and Europe, is still not widely understood.

The internet is now the main source of information for the vast majority of people. When it was invented, its aim was to provide unregulated access for everyone and enable people to learn and communicate freely without restriction. It's difficult to pinpoint exactly when censorship started to emerge, but whatever the initial causes, it has escalated exponentially to such a degree that many people and organisations, particularly those involved in natural health, now face a near Orwellian level of control. The latest version of censorship is to eradicate what is now called "fake news", "misinformation", "health fraud" or a number of other similarly vague definitions. In the three years since I wrote the prequel to this book, information control has seen more significant and devastating changes than any other section in the book. In fact, these new levels of control and censorship represent perhaps the greatest threat to lifestyle medicine I have ever witnessed. These attacks are being led by social media companies, internet providers and pharmaceutical lobby groups and all this is reinforced by conventional media groups. Here are a few examples of the type of censorship and control that are now being employed.

Facebook now removes articles and posts it deems to be "misinformation" and natural health is at the forefront of this savage attack. Much of this is done by robots which are programmed to look for any content that does not conform to conventional medical drug-based practice. People and natural health organisations could at one time challenge these decisions with real people, but now even this is becoming difficult or even impossible to do. Some Facebook accounts for organisations and individuals who promote natural health solutions have been closed down completely with no ability to appeal.

Another well-used tool of information control and censorship involves internet search engines, which effectively means Google, since it controls over 90% of the market for online searches. When people type a subject into their search engine and the results come up, how many will go past the first or occasionally the second page? Very few will do so. So, getting on that first page is crucial to anyone or any organisation that uses the internet to promote their business or disseminate information. This used to depend solely on the number of hits each site had. If someone, for example, typed in "natural ways to treat arthritis", there are many lifestyle organisations and practitioners who would provide advice. The one with the most hits would come up first on the web page search and other sites would also be ranked accordingly. But this is now changing and sites promoting natural solutions to health are selectively having their ranking downgraded by Google. To give you one example, Dr Joseph Mercola is a US doctor who has had many years of experience in using natural solutions for many health issues. His internet site was the most visited natural health site ever with 1.9 million hits each month. The site has been in existence for over 15 years and was genuinely helping people to improve their health. If it hadn't, it would not have got such an incredible level of support over so many years. But then, in June 2019, Google changed its algorithm for natural health content and started manually lowering website rankings. Within a few weeks the number of people visiting the Mercola site fell by 99%. Not only that, but in its place near the top of the web page appeared sites like WebMD and Healthline which now seem to dominate natural health-related Google searches, even though these companies never promote any natural solutions. These companies in fact only promote drugs and conventional medical procedures and much of their funding comes from pharmaceutical adverts. WebMD alone receives $700 million a year from drug adverts. So, people who want to learn about natural solutions for health are directed to sites that only promote drugs. Would it then also surprise you to learn that pharmaceutical companies now indirectly own many of the major medical websites like WebMD, MedicineNet and Medscape which are now owned by a private investment firm KKR, which has major financial and managerial ties with drug companies.

Big Pharma and other global corporations such as Big Food and GM companies also use shadow organisations that effectively control information about their products and the ability of individuals to access all facts. Wikipedia, for example, is a major reference point for many people. But if you want to find out true information about drugs, lifestyle medicine or GM crops, for example, Wikipedia is the last place you should look. You probably know Wikipedia articles are regularly amended by accredited authors as new information arises – it is a fluid system. Corporations liaise with and fund many of these accredited people to write appropriate content and to continually monitor the various entries and to change them back to "their version" if anything "unfavourable" appears. Independent researchers and other professionals who can spot dodgy and incorrect content and who try to correct them haven't a chance against these professional industry shills.

We will see classic Wikipedia misrepresentations of facts in subsequent sections but here is one example. This involves the beta blocker scandal which killed 800,000 EU citizens and which has already been covered in detail. If you type in Don Poldermans, the professor who was responsible for the research fraud that caused all these deaths, you might wonder what all the fuss is about. There is no mention of any deaths, which is incredible. How can you omit to mention 800,000 deaths? This is rewriting history on a grand scale. It exactly mirrors the official history of China, where the Tiananmen Square massacre "never happened". In addition, the main reasons quoted for Don Poldermans dismissal is that he did not obtain written consent from some of the trial participants, the data were not collected according to the trial protocols, and in several cases the trials had fabricated data. But the facts are simple. Don Poldermans' trials claimed beta blockers reduced death rates during operations by 34% but the truth was they increased deaths by 27%. His data manipulation must have been staggering to achieve such an incredible turnaround. Simply saying that "in several cases the trials had fabricated data" must be one of the biggest travesties of the truth, ever. Finally, at the very end and without any sense of shame, the article says, "The initiation of a perioperative course of beta blockers seems to increase mortality by 27%." The word "seems" is ridiculous and misleading given that leading medical experts have confirmed this figure. No one reading this article without prior knowledge would have any idea that 800,000 EU citizens had been killed by fraudulent research. They might even think Don Poldermans had been harshly treated and had lost his job for a "few minor technical infringements". This type of biased downplaying and omission or rewriting of facts is the norm for Wikipedia articles on drugs and medical scandals. Of course, this sort of bias is even more savage when it involves lifestyle solutions to health. Many of these are simply ridiculed and many more are just deleted. If you run a Wikipedia search for some high-profile lifestyle experts, you will no longer find them because their pages have also simply been removed. All this is appalling censorship of democratic free speech and even Larry Sanger, the co-founder of Wikipedia, has made it clear that the information so many people have relied on over the years is now too corrupt to be trusted. YouTube is also censoring natural health organisations and even respected doctors who promote it, and has removed hundreds (probably thousands) of such videos.

These examples are just the tip of a huge iceberg. It would take too many pages to list all the ways in which access to natural health solutions are being controlled and censored, as well as the ways in which drugs are being promoted in their place, not just by internet and media companies but by politicians, regulators, global corporations, media organisations and a host of other groups like Advertising Standards Authorities. It is in effect an all-out war against lifestyle medicine as we will see in Part 4. Unless this control and censorship can be curtailed, future generations will never be able to stay healthy. Their destiny will simply be a lifetime of sickness and disease treated only with drugs that have minimal benefits and their own serious side effects. I haven't seen a doctor or taken any drugs for 25 years and am much healthier now than I was 30 years ago, but future generations will never know how to do this. If you want find out about lifestyle solutions to health, you really should not try to do it by internet searches. Books by reputable lifestyle advocates are one of the very few things that have so far remained completely uncensored.

Henry Kissinger once said, "When you control the food supply, you control the people." Today, it's more "when you control information, you also control the people".

Politicians and governments

The first priority of politicians and political parties is to get elected. Nothing can be achieved without power. To do this, politicians need money to help fund electoral and political campaigns and major donations by global corporations are crucial. In the US, Big Pharma is the biggest single political donor, easily outfinancing the insurance industry, the finance sector and utility industries. Information is available in America about this funding but is not easily accessible in many other countries. I will, therefore, concentrate on the US where the sums are staggering. In 2018 the drug industry gave $24 million to senators and members of the House of Representatives. The highest paid politicians usually sit on regulatory committees that affect the industry, which provides a clue as to the real motives. The highest paid member of the Senate received $538,000, and for the House of Representatives the figure was $452,000. You can imagine that the drug industry expects something in return for all this largesse, because as we have already seen, it does not spend any money unless there is a payback. Many people would look at the money given to politicians and call it outright bribery, but in fact it is all perfectly legal courtesy of the laws passed, unsurprisingly, by the politicians themselves.

A very recent figure showed an even more incredible payment. In 2020 President Biden received a staggering $8.7 million from the pharmaceutical and health products industry. In other less democratic societies, including some African countries, nearly every politician wants to be the Minister for Health. Why? Very few of these countries have independent drug advisory bodies, and the decision on which drugs a country uses are often ultimately made by the minister. This opens the door for massive financial inducements and it is well known that many African politicians have millions of dollars hidden away in Swiss bank accounts.

As well as direct financial donations to politicians, Big Pharma also uses lobbying as a major technique to gain influence over government health agendas, and they invariably employ professional lobbyists to represent their interests. There are 535 elected politicians in both US Houses, but in 2018 there were a staggering 1440 pharmaceutical lobbyists – nearly three for each politician. The industry spent $260 million just to lobby and influence these 535 politicians – an average of half a million dollars for each one of them. Lobbying is common in most countries. The cost worldwide is not known but is probably several billion dollars. Through political lobbying, the industry also achieved a crucial victory when it convinced senior politicians that by allowing doctors to work with them, pharmaceutical companies would be able to develop better drugs and treatments. This meant they could legally pay doctors huge sums of money without being accused that it was mere bribery that could affect medical judgements. Governments now actively encourage medicine and the drug industry to work together.

Big Pharma uses lobbying to help promote a rosy picture of the industry. They will promote the idea that the industry is relentlessly seeking new treatments and cures for diseases like cancer and dementia and that breakthrough drugs are close to being found that will transform medicine. They will explain that drugs are powerful things that occasionally cause some harm, but overall the benefits exceed the harm and, therefore, when bad outcomes happen, politicians should never be too critical as this could delay the new and exciting drugs that are being developed. They will, of course, never mention that in the last 50 years very few breakthrough drugs have ever been developed despite identical claims that they were imminent in each of those years. They will never admit that drugs are the third leading cause of death, that 20% of all drugs have either been taken off the market or given the ultimate black box warning because they are doing more harm than good, or that another 20% have no scientific proof they work.

But, of course, all this money and lobbying works. Lord McNair said, "UK officials are pretty much brainwashed by their pharmaceutical advisors into peddling pharma friendly nonsense." All governments allow lax and industry friendly laws to be passed. It is impossible to know whether politicians are simply taken in by all the positive but biased information they are exposed to or whether the enormous sums of money themselves are a key driver even if this is, in some respects, subconscious. It is probably a combination of the two. But the industry also has one more card up its sleeve if needed to keep politicians "on side". If a country considers imposing much stricter rules regarding certain types of drugs, the industry simply threatens to move some of its operations abroad. The rules are then quietly shelved. On top of all this, once they are in power, governments need a thriving economy to fund all the promises they made to get themselves elected. Big multinationals are big employers and usually have many well-paid employees who contribute considerably to government tax revenues. Big multinationals based in your country are also a "political status symbol" and they are encouraged in every way possible. The pharmaceutical industry represents over 1% of global GDP. But most of the companies and their headquarters are in Europe and North America; here it represents around 2% of GDP. Indeed, the industry is not just viewed as financially important but is considered in many countries as strategically important. No government can afford to alienate such a powerful industry, particularly one that generates so much money. Governments will indeed go out of their way to protect it.

I should add one other thought. Politicians are just like the majority of ordinary people who have been falsely led to believe over many decades that drugs are the only option for treating disease. This provides a further reason for them not to be too restrictive of the industry. Governments are, therefore, highly influenced by and supportive of the pharmaceutical industry, but they have a major problem because of the corruption that exists in the industry and medical research. "Fraud" is commonplace and this in turn causes deaths and serious harm to millions of people. Governments have to be at least seen to put patient safety first, but the lax legislation that allows so much of the "fraud" to continue tells a different story. Laws have been tightened in response to various scandals that have been exposed, but there are invariably hidden loopholes the companies can exploit. Even the most powerful country in the world, the US, has shown it is virtually impotent when it comes to effective legislation that might reign in the industry's lethal excesses. As an example, there has never been a single successful prosecution for fraud where the company has not actually made more from the fraud than the fine that was imposed on them, as we have already seen. Typically, they make between five and ten times more from the fraud than the fine. When GlaxoSmithKline was fined $3 billion in 2012, they had in fact made fraudulent sales of $29 billion. Most independent commentators would say that if you really want to stop future fraud, then the fine should equal the amount of the fraud with say 50% on top. So, in the case of GSK the fine should have been $45 billion instead of the $3 billion imposed. A fine of that magnitude really would stop future fraud in its tracks but, of course, it wasn't and drug companies continue to commit similar frauds at will. Alternatively, jail sentences could be imposed on senior executives for serious fraud. This too would also stop future fraud in its tracks. But it just doesn't happen. The simple fact is governments talk tough on issues surrounding patient safety and they punish fraud with what will seem, to the public, to be incredibly large fines, but in reality, it has absolutely no deterrent value for the reasons outlined. It's all just a smokescreen. The industry is just too powerful and viewed as too important to be punished and regulated as it should be, and so companies continue to flout the law with impunity. There is little likelihood that this will change anytime soon.

There is, however, one threat to the industry that is real, current and dangerous. This is lifestyle medicine which has answers and treatments that work better than drugs for most diseases. It is the ultimate threat to Big Pharma. The industry has, therefore, made attacks on lifestyle medicine via its paid advocates, one of its absolute priorities, and has lobbied organisations and governments remorselessly to convince them there is no proof it works and that it "may" even be dangerous. Most governments have now joined the attacks on lifestyle medicine and there will be much more on this in Part 4. So, you can see that all the money the industry pays to politicians and the extravagant and incessant lobbying they use really does pay off. Sadly, it is patients who pay for these lax laws because of the millions of dangerous and often lethal side effects from drugs that should never have been approved in the first place, together with the fact most people are denied knowledge of safe and effective natural solutions to health that would enable them to stay healthy.

It is important to add that all the other major industries like Big Ag, Big Chemical, Big Data, Big Food and Big Finance also adopt identical "bribery" and lobbying tactics but there is one other potential benefit that politicians may gain particularly if they adopt lenient laws affecting them. Once they leave politics, senior government ministers can be offered lucrative positions in these companies. The money offered usually dwarfs their political salaries. The former prime minister David Cameron would have earned around £150,000 a year but he has since earned an estimated £7.2 million for part-time work at Greensill Capital bank, and the former Lib Dem leader Nick Clegg now earns around $650,000 a year with Facebook. However, if a minister ever introduced draconian laws against such industries and companies, it is unlikely they would be offered such jobs once they leave public service.

Drug regulators and medical advisors

The major drug regulators in the US, the EU and the UK are now, in large part, funded by fees paid by the industry for drug approval services. In the US the industry funds 65% ($670 million) of regulators costs, in the EU the figure is 89% and in the UK, it is 86%. Regulators are staffed at the management level, mainly by people who have close ties and financial links with the industry or who have previously worked for them. The movement of people between the two, referred to as "revolving doors", is commonplace and well documented. A 2016 BMJ study found that 15 out of 26 FDA employees who specialised in haematology and oncology who left the agency ended up with jobs within the drug industry. Another study found that 11 of 16 FDA medical examiners who worked on 28 drug approvals also ended up working for the industry. In 2021 it was revealed that nine out of the last ten FDA commissioners went on to work for the pharmaceutical industry or to serve on a drug company's board of directors.

Governments also have medical experts who advise them on key policy decisions because most politicians and particularly Health Secretaries have virtually no medical knowledge and rely almost exclusively on this advice. Sir Patrick Vallance started his career as a clinical academic and consultant physician in the NHS. Then, in 2006, he joined the drug giant GlaxoSmithKline and in 2012 he became their president for research and development. In 2017 he left the company and became the UK's chief scientific advisor. This is another classic example of "revolving doors". After his government appointment, it was uncovered that he owns £600,000 of shares in GSK. The then Health Secretary Matt Hancock admitted he did not know about this, but claimed that Sir Patrick would not let this influence his judgements in any way. I know what I think, but you can make your own decision.

Donald Light at the Netherlands Institute for Advanced Study said, "The pharmaceutical industry has shaped the rules of the drug regulators, funded their operations, and lobbied them constantly in a classic pattern of regulatory capture." Dr David Healy in evidence to the House of Commons Health Select Committee also criticised the regulators for having "undergone regulatory capture and advancing the interests of the drug companies rather than the interests of the public". This whole system leaves the door wide open to monetary corruption. In addition, as we have just seen, governments are hugely influenced to promote their pharmaceutical company's interests. For all these reasons, drug regulators have simply become organisations that, in the main, promote the interests of the industry they are meant to regulate. Here are four examples that show the extent of this catastrophic situation.

In 2009 nine FDA scientists wrote to President Obama about widespread corruption in the FDA at the highest levels, including several commissioners. The scientists were frustrated and outraged and gave many examples of the corruption, which they described as systemic and violating the law. They noted there was an atmosphere at the FDA in which the honest employee fears the dishonest employee, and that senior officials had suppressed or altered scientific findings and conclusions, had abused their power and authority, and had engaged in illegal retaliation against those who spoke out. Even after going to the highest level they could, it got the whistleblowers absolutely nowhere. This, perhaps, is not surprising given the government's own overriding financial priorities.

In 2012 a former FDA scientist, Ronald Kavanagh, spoke out about what was happening at the agency. He explained that drug reviewers were clearly told not to question drug companies and that their job was to approve drugs. If reviewers asked questions that could delay or prevent a drug's approval – which, of course, was their job as drug reviewers – management would reprimand them or reassign them. Obviously in such an environment people will self-censor. Sometimes reviewers were literally instructed to read only a 100 to 150-page summary and to accept drug company claims without examining the actual data, which on multiple occasions were found to directly contradict the summary document. On other occasions they were ordered not to review certain sections of the submission, but invariably that was where the serious safety issues would be.

When a drug has been approved, the companies are usually required by law to carry out several phase IV trials once data starts to emerge from real-life outcomes and they are given specific time limits to complete them. This is to confirm the drug works and that there are no major unexpected side effects. The reality, however, is that in a majority of cases the industry simply does not meet these legal requirements or time limits and the regulators just allow it all to happen.

In 1990 the FDA spent an average of 2.8 years evaluating the effectiveness and safety of drugs before giving approval. In 2018 this time frame was just ten months, so it is little surprise that many more drugs now produce dangerous side effects. The drug industry wants faster approval to maximise its profits and the regulator has simply made the change meaning patient safety is again being sacrificed. Now, in 2022, the time frames are falling even further and many drugs are accepted on just one clinical trial rather than the two that have been required for decades.

So, it is clear there is systemic corruption at the highest levels within drug regulators and that we have reached the appalling stage where regulation has effectively become a virtual extension of the drug industry marketing machine, promoting its interest at the expense of public safety. Many people die simply because of this appalling situation.

The media and press

The media and press rely heavily on advertising revenue as a source of income. In the US, where the direct advertising of medical drugs is permitted, the figures are mind-blowing at around $10 billion per year. In the rest of the world the figure is probably no more than $10 billion in total because only over the counter drug advertising is permitted. It is nevertheless still a significant sum. The drug industry, therefore, has significant influence over these media companies and if they ever did anything harmful to the industry, a temporary withdrawal of advertising would be very damaging. This is unlikely to happen because, for many other reasons which we will now explore, the media and press also usually follow a pro-pharmaceutical agenda just like governments, regulators and medicine.

The media and press are disseminators of information, but health correspondents do not read complex medical reports about drugs, so they need contacts that provide such information in a form that both they and the public will understand. Enter the pharmaceutical industry, which, as we have seen, is always ready to help "educate" everyone and, in the process, they can take full control of the information on which the media base their articles and programmes. The industry rarely promotes its own drugs to the public, of course, instead it relies on trusted and highly remunerated leading academics and clinicians who do the job for them. These experts naturally command instant respect, authority and integrity. So, when they present new drugs or cancer breakthroughs to the media, would any medical correspondent dare to doubt them or ask searching questions? It just doesn't happen. The reality is the PR people at Big Pharma prepare the carefully scripted press release and not the academics. This will, of course, paint the rosiest picture possible about the drug's effectiveness and even severe side effects will be glossed over with a catchall phrase like "the drug is generally well tolerated". There will usually be a statement to the effect that this represents a breakthrough in treatment and a major step in the quest to find a complete cure for the disease in question. These "breakthroughs in treatment" and "cures" have been promised and reported for decades but real patient outcomes in cancer, Alzheimer's and Parkinson's, for example, have barely changed in decades. This process can deceive both the journalists and the public on a gigantic scale, as these two examples illustrate.

In 2012 a new cancer drug was launched. It didn't have a direct effect on the cancer itself but worked by enhancing the effect of another chemotherapy drug that was already being used. Newspapers headlines proclaimed that "the drug increased life expectancy by a staggering 30%". But what were the real facts? The first drug increased average life expectancy by three months. The new drug, launched with "wonder drug status" to front page banner headlines, did indeed increase life expectancy by a further 30%, which, in this case, turned out to be one extra month. So, in total, these two hugely expensive drugs increased life expectancy by four months, and even this heroically assumes there was no data manipulation to make the results look better than they really were. The headlines carefully avoided spelling out this disappointing truth. A 30% increase in life expectancy sounds so much better than one month. The PR team at the drug company used the wonders of statistics to promote a minimally effective drug into a front page headline-grabbing drug and, of course, the devastating, debilitating and life-changing side effects of the two cancer drugs were never even mentioned. But, of course, the press and media swallowed the whole story hook, line and sinker as I'm sure did most of the general public.

In July 2015 a new Alzheimer's drug hit the headlines. It is manufactured by Eli Lilly and called solanezumab. The headlines were unequivocal. The Daily Telegraph reported: "In a landmark announcement, pharmaceutical giant Eli Lilly said that solanezumab has been shown to put the brakes on the disease for people with mild symptoms and prevented mental decline by a third". The Daily Mail proclaimed: "Landmark drug to stop Alzheimer's disease has been unveiled ... solanezumab has been shown to slow or even halt the illness". The reality is, by comparison, rather disappointing. The drug had previously failed to demonstrate any benefits in two big studies, but was now being retested in a different patient group. These new interim studies showed the drug may have had very small effects on some measures of cognitive function but not others. At an Alzheimer's Association Conference in Washington, an Eli Lilly consultant acknowledged that the observed effects from solanezumab wouldn't even be noticeable to patients or their families. The director of the Alzheimer's Therapeutic Research Institute in California also said, "The cognitive measures do not have a direct relationship to clinically apparent benefit." So, why bother to present provisional results that don't even demonstrate that the drug had any noticeable effect? One answer could be that the Big Pharma PR machine simply wants everyone to think a "breakthrough" is yet again just around the corner, thereby keeping everyone on board with the drug model of medicine. But a few seasoned commentators also smelt a rat. They surmised that the press releases may have been more about revitalising a flagging Eli Lilly share price just before the lucrative annual executive bonus award was calculated, rather than about informing patients.

There are, of course, other ways the media can be influenced. James Murdoch, for example, used to sit on the board of directors at GlaxoSmithKline in a "media advisory role". Why did GSK want this? Well, quite simply, they used this situation to "indoctrinate" one of the most powerful media tycoons on the planet. It would, of course, have been done with the utmost subtlety and finesse so he wouldn't realise he was just being used to ensure that the Murdoch empire provided "sympathetic coverage" of the company and the pharmaceutical industry in general. He would be fed the same types of stories that patient groups are given, hyping up the benefits of new generations of drugs so he could "encourage" his editors to give full prominence to such "wonderful" developments. But, crucially, he would also be told that occasionally "mistakes" happen with powerful and beneficial drugs and that it was important not to overreact with critical reviews so "patient perception" of the overall benefit of drugs was not damaged. This paid off handsomely when GlaxoSmithKline was fined $3 billion in 2012 for serious fraud which killed tens of thousands of people. Media coverage in the Murdoch empire was virtually non-existent.

Medical leaders, most of whom have close ties with the pharmaceutical industry, seriously promote the idea that the media should only report on health issues that are supported by science. This was exemplified in 2012 when Sir Paul Nurse, who was a senior geneticist and president of the Royal Society, was a guest editor on BBC Radio 4's Today programme. He used this opportunity to get the message across that the media could do significant harm in respect of the public's perception of healthcare if they reported unproven stories and information. He was very clear in his thoughts. He said the media should always check with senior medical people before reporting anything to do with health, to ensure it was correct and based on science. This may sound logical and seem a sensible thing to do, but in reality, it amounts to censorship on an unbelievable scale with damning consequences. It would give medicine's key decision makers near complete control over what is published and, if there is anything they don't want to be covered, they can find some excuse to delay or prevent it from being reported, even if it is true. We have already seen, for example, how 800,000 EU citizens were killed by fraudulent medical research but there were no media reports of any kind even though it was all true and scientifically proven. This story should have made headline news around the world, but it would have been damaging to medicine and I have no doubt that senior medical people played a significant part in the "establishment's" decision that somehow persuaded the media to censor this entire scandal.

This section has shown how the media and press, just like almost everyone else, has become a virtual extension of the pharmaceutical and medical complex's agenda to promote drugs and discredit all other treatments.

Summary

The pharmaceutical industry has gained a near monopoly of control over every individual and organisation that can affect its business. This has been planned and implemented over the last 60 years, slowly and almost without anyone being aware they were in effect handing over complete control of the medical agenda to the drug industry. No other industry has achieved such a level of control. They have used every technique in the book from disguised or outright "bribery" within medicine, charities, patient groups, regulators, politicians and medical researchers, from the most intense lobbying and "education" agenda of any industry in the world, from threats targeted at governments, and from outright "fraud", data manipulation and data control.

But the incredible truth is it is society as a whole that is paying for all the drug industry "bribes" that allow all of this to happen. Let me explain with a simple example. As we have seen, the drug industry funds continuing medical education for most doctors in most parts of the world. The total cost of this largesse is probably between $10 billion and $20 billion just for this one group of beneficiaries. This sort of money would almost certainly enable new generations of antibiotics to be developed. Even today, 700,000 lives each year could be saved by developing new antibiotics, but instead the drug industry prefers to give it away to doctors who are already exceptionally well paid. No one seems to think there is anything wrong with this perverted but legal allocation of money.

We have seen that in total the pharmaceutical industry gives away $100 billion each year to a long list of lucky recipients and then spends another $100 billion in promoting its drugs to all of them via an army of representatives, PR companies and lobbyists. But again, it is society as a whole that is paying for this because of the unnecessarily inflated prices everyone is paying for drugs. Big Pharma has simply increased its prices to a level where it can still deliver exceptionally high profits to keep its shareholders very happy, but then still has "a spare $200 billion" to "bribe" and influence everyone. In other industries, similar "bribes" and payments are illegal and punishable with fines and imprisonment. Why has the drug industry been excluded from these sensible laws?

It is perhaps the greatest confidence trick in the history of the world amounting to around $10 trillion (in today's money) over the last 60 years. What really needs to happen is that all governments would legislate to prevent the drug industry from "giving" any more money to *anyone*. The prices of drugs would be mandatorily reduced by this then surplus $200 billion and governments could use this to fund truly independent research free from pharmaceutical bias, "fraud" and manipulation. Given that well over half the drugs currently on sale would not pass truly independent research, they would be taken off the market giving annual worldwide savings of around half a trillion dollars. Of course, this sensible and eminently logical solution will never happen.

The perfect storm

In the last six sections we have seen how:

1. Medicine's rigidly hierarchical structure is dominated by ego, reputation and dogma. For the elite who control medicine with a rod of iron, any new science that challenges the conventional dogma is invariably resisted, and often ridiculed, until the evidence becomes so overwhelming it can no longer be resisted. This can take years and even decades. Tens of millions of people have paid for this medical dogma and ego with their lives.
2. The pharmaceutical industry has gained almost total control of medical research and the entire medical agenda, thanks mainly to its incredible money tree. This means that everything other than drugs stands side-lined or discredited even though it works, in many cases, far better than conventional drug-based medicine.
3. The very science of so-called evidence-based medicine and its reliance on statistics-based trials is so deeply flawed and corrupt that much of it is not worth the paper it is written on. Nowhere is this more apparent than in medical research and the prescription drugs that result from it.
4. Drugs are incredibly dangerous. They are the third leading cause of death, while for many of them, their benefits are tiny or even unknown because of data manipulation, bias and "fraud".
5. Healthcare data control and censorship have rocketed to levels that really mean true democracy no longer exists.

Combine all these things and you have the perfect storm. When the thalidomide scandal broke in the 1960s, politicians and regulators introduced tough new rules that were supposed to prevent such a thing ever happening again. Clinical trials were mandated to ensure drugs were both safe and effective. At first the pharmaceutical industry was alarmed because of the cost and the onerous restrictions. But they soon realised it could be a blessing in disguise. They could simply pass on the huge cost of the trials in higher drug prices and, because of the prohibitive cost, no one else would be able to carry out such trials, thus giving them a complete monopoly on "medical proof" and medical treatment. Lifestyle medicine proponents would simply never have the money to be able to show that what they were doing worked, at least according to these new rules.

The new laws inadvertently handed the pharmaceutical industry a monopoly on healthcare and the means to fully exploit that monopoly. The patent laws which were introduced also enabled the industry to exploit its pricing powers to the full and allowed it to become the most profitable industry ever. It has ruthlessly used this monopoly of both power and money to corrupt and control everyone that could affect or damage its business. This has delivered us into a disturbing world and a disturbing era of medicine, where crimes just as, or even more, heinous than thalidomide occur almost as regular events, where no one, including the most powerful governments on the planet, can seemingly do anything to stop it and indeed their actions seem to support it, and where press and media censorship facilitates its perpetuation. Just who, for example, has the power and who is pulling the strings to ensure a medical scandal that resulted from research fraud and caused the deaths of 800,000 people remains virtually unreported throughout the entirety of the world's media and press?

Of course, we must also remember modern medicine really can perform near miracles, such as its life-saving accident and emergency treatments and the incredible success of antibiotics. It is this life-saving part of modern medicine that everyone is familiar with, whether it be the countless "soap operas" with their life-saving hero doctors, or real-life doctors performing heroic operations in war-torn countries, or individual "miracles" like the footballers Fabrice Muamba and Christian Eriksen who both had heart failure on the football pitch and were quite literally brought back to life because of immediate medical intervention. With the high profile that such events receive, and the public's constant exposure to them, it is little wonder they see medicine in such a positive and "god-like" light, and why many believe only doctors can help them when they become sick.

So, we have this incredible dichotomy in medicine. We have the genuine life-saving and life-enhancing part which saves millions of lives, the part that everyone is familiar with. But we also have the wide scale, pharmaceutical-driven "fraud", "bribery" and data manipulation that are endemic within medicine and medical research that also result in untold harm and millions of unnecessary deaths. This part is largely unknown to virtually everyone on the planet. Earlier I asked the questions: how can the almost endless stream of premeditated medical disasters keep happening and how can these things be suppressed or censored so that virtually no one knows anything about them? I still don't know who really pulls the strings, for example, on press censorship, but this is my personal take on the overall situation.

The pharmaceutical industry's annual $100 billion "bribe" to everyone who is even remotely involved in medicine and health, and their $100 billion "education" agenda, coupled with unswerving hierarchical medical dogma is the crucial part. But everyone's perception of doctors as the modern equivalent of swashbuckling, life-saving heroes is indelibly ingrained into the human psyche. Remember, politicians and the media are no different to everyone else in this respect. So, when an individual medical scandal strikes that threatens to tarnish this "magical aura" surrounding medicine, what do politicians and the media do? Do they expose it in all its gory detail and risk undermining the public's trust in medicine and pharmaceuticals or do they downplay it or, even worse, censor it completely? I believe this must also be part of the story.

A simple comparison with another scandal which only came into the public domain in 2018 sums up the dilemma of whether to expose or cover up the truth. In 2010 Oxfam sent staff to Haiti to provide help in the wake of a serious earthquake. Then, in 2011, it emerged that some staff had paid survivors of the earthquake for sex. Oxfam said it immediately launched an internal inquiry and four members of its staff were dismissed. It also said it had publicly announced the enquiry, but the charity commission said it was not given details about the sexual abuse allegations and that if it had been it would have acted differently. Oxfam did not warn other agencies about the fact that some staff had used prostitutes, even though at least one of those dismissed went on to work for another charity. Many more details also eventually emerged like the fact there had been previous sex scandals like the one in Chad in 2006, which also had not come into the public domain.

I don't need to go into any more details about this particular scandal, however, because the key point is there were many people who wanted to play down its extent because they understood that Oxfam helped so many people in the developing world and feared if it became headline news it would seriously damage its reputation and reduce its donations and ability to carry out this immensely important work. However, when the details started to emerge in 2018, the consensus amongst the media, governments and most other organisations was that Oxfam should not be able to "trade off" the good things it does against the bad things, and that the truth should simply be told. When it comes to medical scandals, however, that have killed hundreds of thousands of people (and are far more serious than the Oxfam scandal, shocking though it was), the same media groups, governments and other organisations think that, with a few exceptions, the right thing is to censor them or play them down. They obviously believe medicine and the drug industry should be able to "trade off" the good against the bad and censor the bad. Can this really be justified? If such medical disasters really were rare events, then I guess philosophers could debate whether, for the overall good of society, such censorship should be allowed. But the fact is they are not rare events. They are common and recurring and have caused millions of deaths, and censorship in this situation simply means no one is ever called to account, action to prevent them reoccurring never happens, and the same tragic loss of life occurs decade after decade.

We live in an Orwellian world where the drug industry is simply out of control. It has too much power and too much money. It has gained almost total control of medical research and healthcare to promote its own interests, while at the same time it has scandalously attempted to discredit and censor all other options that would enable people to stay healthy. Our current medical system has been masterfully orchestrated by the drug companies so it appears to be science-based but this is simply untrue for most diseases. The people who you would normally expect to reign in such power – governments, regulators and the media – have been skilfully manipulated, indoctrinated and "bribed" to endorse this entire sordid and sickening process.

While all this is happening, the shocking and exponential increase in virtually every disease is continuing unchallenged. No one is asking why it is happening, and little meaningful research is being done to find out. An ever-increasing number of sick people represents a financial bonanza for the pharmaceutical industry. Are they behind what is effectively censorship of this worldwide disaster? Of course, it can't be proven, but I believe they are. Can any of this ever be stopped? Everything is so entrenched, and the vested interest groups are so powerful that nothing is likely to change anytime soon. Maybe there will be a medical catastrophe that is so terrible it cannot be censored or hidden from the public. Maybe more doctors will start to challenge the situation, particularly as they approach retirement, when they will have little to fear from the inevitable backlash they would face for exposing the truth. But failing such a disaster or medical rebellion, it is only when enough people realise what is happening, when they fully understand their children and grandchildren are becoming seriously sicker every year with diseases that once barely existed, as well as the fact the

NHS will simply never be able to effectively treat these ever-increasing numbers, that public pressure will finally provide the impetus for change. Disease prevention really should be medicine's number one priority.

A brief history of the pharmaceutical industry and the key influence of "philanthropy"

John D. Rockefeller was, and still remains, the richest and most powerful industrialist the world has ever seen. His wealth in the early 1900s was nearly 2% of American GDP. In today's terms that would equate to around $400 billion, which is significantly more than the wealth of today's richest billionaires like Bill Gates who has around $130 billion. Rockefeller owned companies in many industries like media and chemicals, but his key money maker was oil refining. Standard Oil was the largest corporation in the world at that time and controlled 90% of all oil in the US. He built his vast business empire by ruthlessly creating monopoly positions which involved destroying competitors. This often involved the use of illegal actions and these eventually resulted in detailed federal investigations into the operation and practices of Standard Oil. Finally, in 1911, he was charged with corruption and illegal business practices. The US Supreme Court found him guilty and they sentenced that the Rockefeller oil trust be dismantled and broken up into 34 different companies. I should add that corruption on this scale deserved a prison sentence, but no doubt Rockefeller was too powerful, too rich and too influential for that to happen.

In anticipation of this devastating trial outcome, Rockefeller had already made plans for an ambitious new venture in order to minimise and even reverse the negative public and political opinion from the Standard Oil scandal. He used a trick called "philanthropy" whereby part of the illegal gains from his oil business were used to set up the Rockefeller Foundation. Because this was meant to be a totally philanthropic organisation aimed mainly at improving the development of new scientific medical treatments, he knew it would be granted special tax exemptions. In effect, it became a tax haven. But the reality was the Rockefeller Foundation was simply the front for a new global business venture that aimed to ramp up the newly emerging development and use of synthetic chemical drugs in which it would have huge investments and achieve huge financial profits. The Rockefeller Foundation also attracted other industrialists like Edward Carnegie. They had all built their vast business empires by ruthlessly creating near monopoly positions. Their vision was to create a similar monopoly position within healthcare. It is clear that being found guilty of corrupt practices was not going to stop him doing it all again, especially when he could hide behind the mask of philanthropy.

In the early 1900s, a range of natural treatments like herbal products, newly discovered vitamins, homeopathy, osteopathy and chiropractic were used by doctors to treat patients alongside the newly emerging drugs. These natural products and treatments were widely used and were a serious threat to the new chemical-based drugs that Rockefeller intended to promote, so he set out to destroy them. The Rockefeller Foundation employed Abraham Flexner to write a report which was published in 1910 and called for the standardisation of medical education and the adoption of "modern principles" like laboratory research and the patenting of medicines. Flexner was paid to visit all US medical schools to promote these ideas. At the same time, the Rockefeller Foundation used the media companies it owned to spread the message to the general public and politicians. It also heavily financed the American Medical Association to give it more power and influence so that it would also promote the ideas in the Flexner Report. The medical schools that ignored these ideas and still taught how natural solutions could improve health soon found their funding reduced, and within a few years they eventually disappeared. Rockefeller's crusade caused the closure of more than half of US medical schools, fostered public and press scorn for natural medicines, and led to the incarceration of many practising physicians. The use and availability of natural products like herbs and vitamins was also curtailed by government legislation. Rockefeller had achieved his first main objective of destroying the competition.

The second objective of developing new drugs and persuading doctors to use them soon gained traction. Many of the chemicals that would provide the basis for these new drugs originated from Rockefeller's own chemical companies. Over the following decades, Rockefeller and his descendants invested heavily in the newly emerging pharmaceutical industry and made huge profits from what was meant to be a philanthropic organisation. The Rockefeller Foundation's investment in the drug industry still exists today as does their continuing profit stream. Of course, they still maintain their philanthropic donations, but can corruption really be offset by philanthropy? This is something that everyone has to make their own judgement on.

After 1910 the development and use of drugs continued to grow, and over the next few decades these did bring benefits in treating some of the key diseases at that time. The first antibiotic, which later became known as penicillin, was actually discovered by accident in 1928 by Alexander Fleming. It was the most significant medical discovery in this period but wasn't a drug, and actually originated from a natural mould. It finally became available as a treatment in 1942. But new drugs, like streptomycin which, in conjunction with two other drugs, was effective in the treatment of tuberculosis, also radically changed the way medicine was able to treat patients with, up to then, often incurable diseases. There was, however, another side to these breakthroughs. Many of the drugs also caused serious and lethal side effects, partly because there were virtually no laws governing the development, testing and use of these chemical-based drugs. Nevertheless, up to the 1960s, medicine became convinced as to the overall benefits of the new world of pharmaceutical drugs. I should add that many other non-drug medical breakthroughs were also made in this period. These included hip surgery, radical changes in anaesthesia, open heart surgery, heart transplants, neo-natal intensive care, and the identification of smoking as the primary cause of lung cancer. So, this period was indeed a golden age for medicine, but it is also important to add that, during this time, it was doctors who controlled the use of drugs. The drug industry produced new drugs and promoted them to doctors, but it was the doctors who made the final decisions. I make this point because all this was soon to change. Another key fact is that natural lifestyle treatments really would have had a significant effect on health and disease treatment, as you will see in Part 4, but, of course, Rockefeller had effectively eliminated their use by medicine.

A significant turning point in drug use came with the thalidomide tragedy when the devastating consequences of this and other chemical drugs started to be exposed. As we have already seen, this resulted in major changes to the way drugs were tested and approved and also to the introduction of new patent laws and drug pricing. The profitability and power of the drug industry rose considerably after these changes were fully implemented and this encouraged plans to radically increase drug sales and profits even further. Up to this point, drugs had been used just to treat people who had become ill. But just treating sick people would not lead to an increase in drug use and it would be a dead end for profits which was the industry's top priority. So, in 1975, the chief executive of Merck, which was the largest drug company in the world at the time, proposed that the future prosperity of the pharmaceutical industry "would require expanding the market for its products beyond merely treating the ill to include the healthy as well". The plan involved expanding drug use by "creating" new diseases as well as changing the definitions of existing diseases so nearly everyone could be labelled as sick and, therefore, needing drugs. Of course, this plan would need to be carried out circumspectly and in such a way that the general population would not understand that healthy people were slowly being labelled as sick.

This drug industry plan to label "everyone as sick" deserves some extra analysis, because its key aim was simply to increase sales and profits and not to improve people's health. It has been an amazing success, and in the 30 years between 1980 and 2010, drug revenues increased an incredible 25-fold. It involved creating a significant number of blockbuster drugs – those that have annual sales of over $1 billion – and these increased from just one to over 100 in the same period. It all started in 1984 with the Glaxo drug Zantac which was originally used just to treat stomach ulcers. But Glaxo then employed more sales people and got them to promote it for a much wider range of conditions that it claimed were treatable. One of the key ones was heartburn which they said affected around half of the entire American population at some point. The company recruited a famous star to say the drug had cured her condition. They also employed senior medics to endorse its benefits and finally used extensive marketing and publicity campaigns. Zantac's annual sales then soared to $2.5 billion which made it the bestselling drug of all time. "Disease mongering" was the term used to describe the drug industry's plans to convince healthy people they were all essentially sick from something, and also that those who already had some slight symptoms were in fact "very ill". Natural human changes, like the menopause, were literally classed as a "disease" that needed universal long-term hormone replacement treatments. Some of the existing treatments like blood pressure drugs and statins, however, turned out to be the most profitable changes of all.

What happened was that the industry aimed to achieve continued reductions in the limits by which they were prescribed and to "persuade" the regulators to approve them. Blood pressure drugs, for example, were initially given only to those with high blood pressure – typically 180/110 and over – but today in the US, anyone with a reading over 130/85 can be prescribed them, while in the UK the figure is 140/90. Because a significant number of people exceed these figures, it has resulted in an incredible increase in drug use and industry profits. Incredibly, however, as you will see in Part 5, there are no overall health benefits for most of these patients. Similar increases in use were made for many other drugs like statins. In this case, however, it was simply approved for people with incredibly low risks of heart disease and once again there was no proof it gave any benefits whatsoever. Prozac, which is used to treat depression, is just one of many other similar examples with shaky outcomes but huge profit increases. A detailed expose will be made of all these key drugs in Part 5.

The plan to label everyone as sick, however, has now reached a new turning point. Our Future Health is a UK research programme that aims to transform the prevention, early detection and treatment of diseases. Some of its funding is from the government and charities like Cancer Research UK, but around two-thirds is from the drug industry. It aims to initially recruit 3 million volunteers to take part in the research programme. Its first stated aim is to learn how to prevent diseases. However, we have already seen copious evidence that disease prevention has never been adopted by medicine for nearly any disease. The major drug companies have also provided most of the funding for this research and they will never develop any treatments to prevent disease since it would ultimately cause the entire industry's extinction. When you look at Our Future Health's programme in detail, you will see that while the word prevention is used, virtually everything is simply about things like early detection, improved testing and changing the course of disease progression. The main outcome of this research will simply be earlier disease detection, which will radically increase the number of sick people. This will provide another profit bonanza for the drug industry since drugs will then be prescribed much earlier. Will early detection help patients? Early detection of diseases like Alzheimer's and Parkinson's will have no effect whatsoever, since there are simply no effective treatments and telling people they have them will result in despair which could actually shorten their lives. Early detection has also been ongoing for many years for things like routine blood pressure and cholesterol testing, but heart disease is still the biggest killer. If all those involved really wanted to improve people's health and life expectancy, they would simply have used all the funding to find the true causes of disease and then use this to prevent them. Sadly, this research will achieve little or nothing other than a profit bonanza.

Quite simply, the world has reached a situation where the pharmaceutical industry effectively controls much of human health, even though its main objective is simply to escalate sales and profits. But most importantly, this whole process of pharmaceutical domination was started by John D. Rockefeller, one of the most corrupt, as well as the richest and most powerful, industrial tycoons the world has ever seen.

I'll end this section with something of a déjà vu. What is your impression of the Bill and Melinda Gates Foundation? Most people, including the media, believe it is a wonderful philanthropic organisation that gives billions of dollars to good causes. A typical headline is "Bill and Melinda Gates the most generous humans ever". But if you were ever to inspect some key academic journals, you would find that political scientists and development scholars are actually quite sceptical about the Gates Foundation and its power to control many global health institutions, as well as questioning its spending priorities. They believe it is too big and powerful to scrutinise. The reality is that, with around $50 billion currently at its disposal, the foundation is so powerful it is effectively defining the path that medicine and medical research takes for certain types of disease like viral infections. The foundation now spends almost as much money on global health as the World Health Organization. Its guiding principle is that "it is driven by the interests and passions of the Gates family". The Lancet medical journal said, "Is this governance really good enough?" Should a non-medical, computer industry founder really be deciding the course of certain aspects of medicine, especially when this is simply driven by his own passions and has no official scrutinisation? This is also particularly unfair because his foundation's $50 billion of funds, which are all invested in company shares, make huge profits but actually pay zero taxes. Of course, Bill Gates isn't the only billionaire philanthropist who benefits from no taxes. Over the past 15 years, the number of philanthropic foundations with $1 billion or more in assets has doubled to more than 80. Just in the US, these philanthropists gain an estimated $40 billion every single year by paying no taxes and diverting it from the US Treasury. Quite simply, it is the public that either has to pay more taxes to make up for this loss of revenue, or they simply have to accept that the government can't fund the key things they want, like better investments for their children's education.

Here is one devastating example of why Bill Gates' power to control is challenged by some key academics and political scientists. Polio was a disease that, by the start of the twenty-first century, had been significantly eliminated in most countries and there were few deaths at that time. Nevertheless, Bill Gates became passionate about eliminating the disease and his foundation has since contributed significant sums of money for a global attempt to finally eradicate it completely from the remaining countries like India and Pakistan. This may sound wonderful, but the governments involved were in fact devastated by this. Why? Because the death toll and health burden from other diseases like diarrhoeal infections were over a thousand times higher than that from the relatively few remaining cases of polio. An estimated 130,000 children under five died each year in India compared to about 100 from polio around the time the Gates Foundation got involved. The governments could do nothing about it because they didn't dare challenge Bill Gates for fear of losing future donations. They were effectively compelled to emphasise polio eradication against their will and watch huge numbers of their children die unnecessarily from preventable diseases because of "one man's obsession and passion". It is highly likely that Bill Gates simply wanted to go down in history as the man who finally eradicated polio. I should add that, while it has been recently eradicated from India, it is still active in Pakistan, Afghanistan and Nigeria. Despite the huge sums of money spent, it is unlikely its eradication can be achieved in countries like Afghanistan for obvious political reasons. Also, the huge numbers of diarrhoeal deaths of young children remain unchanged, but if their governments had been able to spend this money, tens of thousands of children's lives would have been saved. It really is a terrible indictment of Bill Gates.

One other point that is worth noting is there are other rich philanthropists who provide a significant proportion of the Gates Foundation's funds, with Warren Buffet alone contributing nearly $30 billion since 2006. Most people believe Bill Gates has provided all the money but this is not the case. His total contributions to the foundation are $36 billion over the last 20 years and he has probably contributed just over half of the funds. In comparison his own personal fortune in 2021 still stands at $130 billion – up by $23 billion during the 2020 lockdown. But there is another salutary fact you should be aware of. In 1998 Microsoft was charged in a US antitrust law case for illegally maintaining its monopoly position in the PC market by restricting the way computer manufacturers could use other internet software. In 1999 the judge found Microsoft guilty and ordered the break-up of the company into two separate software divisions; this was immediately appealed by Microsoft. The appeal court did not change the basic guilty verdict, but did rule it was no longer seeking to break up the company and would instead seek a lesser antitrust penalty. I won't go into the details of the settlement because they are not relevant. The important point is Microsoft was found guilty of unlawful monopolisation in the same way John D. Rockefeller and his company Standard Oil were found guilty. They both made their fortunes, in part, by breaking the law, and both of their philanthropic organisations were, therefore, partly funded by illegal profits. Of course, some people would say does this really matter now since these funds are being used beneficially. But as you have just seen, there are a significant number of highly respected, dissenting voices and very concerning ways in which the money is being spent.

Parts 5 and 6 explore in much more detail the worrying evidence about Bill Gates' influence on medicine as well as other vital health factors like agriculture and food. You really will be shocked at what you read, but let me add one other fact for you to ponder before then. The Gates Foundation has spent $10 billion over the last ten years on developing and promoting vaccines. At the World Economic Forum in Davos in 2019, Bill Gates forthrightly told an interviewer that he expected to make a 20-fold return on his investment in global vaccines. In other words, he expected to make $200 billion of profit. Note also that he called it an "investment" rather than philanthropy, which is what it should be. So, when he ecstatically and forcefully promotes vaccines for virtually everyone and every viral disease, is he being purely philanthropic or does making profit play the major part? Most billionaires like Bill Gates may in part be philanthropic, but their desire to exert control has always been there. It was the main reason for their business and financial successes. It is clearly still there now and will probably never disappear and, of course, profits play a vital role in all of it.

A final thought

I'll hazard a guess that you are in a state of shock after what you have read in the last 60 plus pages, since it will challenge everything you thought you knew about medicine and drugs. You must be thinking, can I really believe everything I have just read? So, let me give you a final compelling piece of evidence that demonstrates it is indeed all true. The pharmaceutical industry is accepted as one of the most litigious in the world. They have an army of top lawyers at their disposal. Anyone or any company that threatens their business, profits or patents in any way will find themselves swiftly in court facing huge claims for damages. But there is one group of people they have never sued even though they have probably done more damage to the industry than anyone else. These are the people who write books exposing the truth about the drug companies. These books are hugely damaging both financially and in terms of reputation. There are many people who won't take any drugs, including me, because of what they have read and learnt. The industry, therefore, faces a reduction in profits, but the reputational damage is even more significant. Yet the lawyers have not been set loose.

Consider the title of just one of Peter Gøtzsche's books: *Deadly Medicines and Organised Crime: How Big Pharma Has Corrupted Healthcare*. Many people would consider even this to be libellous. But it gets much worse. The centrepiece of the US Organized Crime Act of 1970 is the Racketeer Influenced and Corrupt Organizations Act, in which racketeering is defined as the act of engaging in a certain type of offence more than once. The list of offences that constitute racketeering include fraud, bribery, obstruction of justice, obstruction of law enforcement, tampering with witnesses and political corruption. Peter Gøtzsche says that Big Pharma does so much of this all the time that there can be no doubt that its business model fulfils the criteria for organised crime. Referring to the drug industry he also says, "The morally repugnant disregard for human life is the norm."

All this is explosive and deeply damaging. Imagine having your company and industry described in this way and being labelled as racketeers. The Racketeering Act was in fact introduced to bring to justice serious criminal activity and corrupt organisations like the Mafia. Peter Gøtzsche, therefore, is effectively comparing drug companies to the Mafia. But the industry has simply taken it on the chin as they have with hundreds of other similarly damaging revelations and accusations. People like Peter Gøtzsche are their true nemesis, but the simple fact is they would not dare to litigate against him because everything he says is true. I'm sure he took legal advice and his lawyers must have been confident they could defend all these potentially libellous statements. The drug industry's complete lack of litigation on any of them shows they are all true, however unbelievable they may seem. Peter Gøtzsche also cites a former vice president of the world's largest drug company, Pfizer, who said, "It is scary how many similarities there are between the drug industry and the mob. The mob make obscene amounts of money, as does the industry. The side effects of organised crime are killings and deaths, and the side effects are the same in the industry. The mob bribes politicians and others, and so does the drug industry..."

Peter Gøtzsche is one of the world's leading experts on medical research. Twenty-five years ago, he established the Nordic Cochrane Centre and co-founded the highly respected Cochrane Collaboration where he was a director. He has published more than 50 papers in the big five medical journals – BMJ, Lancet, JAMA, NEJM and Annals. It is also compelling evidence against Big Pharma that hundreds of other respected doctors, academics and investigative journalists have also written similarly damning critiques and books. Here are just a few titles of some of the other books written by doctors which give a graphic indication of their content:

- *Pharmageddon* by David Healy
- *Too Many Pills: How Too Much Medicine Is Endangering Our Health* by James Le Fanu
- *Can Medicine Be Cured? The Corruption of a Profession* by Seamus O'Mahony
- *Bad Pharma* by Ben Goldacre
- *The Great Cholesterol Con* by Malcom Kendrick

- *The Myth of the Chemical Cure: A Critique of Psychiatric Drug Treatment* by Joanna Moncrieff
- *The Truth About the Drug Companies: How They Deceive Us and What to Do About It* by Marcia Angell
- *Stats.con: How We've Been Fooled by Statistics-Based Research in Medicine* by James Penston
- *Selling Sickness: How the World's Biggest Pharmaceutical Companies Are Turning Us All into Patients* by Alan Cassels
- *The Rise and Fall of Modern Medicine* by James Le Fanu
- *Our Daily Meds: How the Pharmaceutical Companies Transformed Themselves into Slick Marketing Machines and Hooked the Nation on Prescription Drugs* by Melody Peterson

After this devastating section, prepare to have your spirits lifted...

Part 4

Lifestyle Medicine – The Truth You Can Believe

Lifestyle medicine really does have the potential to transform your health and life expectancy and in this section, we will look at the evidence and explore how it works.

Are most diseases preventable?

I have made a very bold claim that many of the major non-communicable diseases, like heart disease and cancer, are in large part preventable. So, unless I can convince you that this is indeed possible, you will be entitled to dismiss everything else I am going to say about lifestyle medicine. So, here it goes. We have seen how the science behind much of modern medicine is so deeply flawed it simply cannot be trusted. Even the randomised clinical trials medicine describes as the "gold standard" in medical research are themselves riddled with flaws and are manipulated to such a degree that many are not worth the paper they are written on. So, I won't quote clinical trials to make the case, even though some do exist. Instead, there is a much better way of proving that prevention is not just possible, but is indeed entirely logical. This involves simply looking at the history of disease and its progression. It involves looking at what happens to real people in real life as opposed to the "make-believe world" of clinical trials where drugs are almost never tested on the people who are actually going to take them.

If we look at drugs like Vioxx and Avandia – each of which caused at least 120,000 heart attacks and 60,000 deaths – the original clinical trials showed the drugs were safe. Had doctors simply relied on these "gold standard" trials, then Vioxx, as an example, would still be in use today, and would by now have caused half a million heart attacks and a quarter of a million deaths. The fact that it didn't and was withdrawn from the market after it had killed "just" 60,000 people is down to one simple fact. Researchers began to look at real-world events; they started to count the dead bodies that were piling up and the patients in hospitals recovering from heart attacks. They looked at what was happening to real people who were taking the drugs and the evidence was indisputable. Tens of thousands of people were being killed or seriously harmed each year. It showed the utter folly of the clinical trial process as it currently exists and its devastating consequences, and it showed how simple observation of real-life events could reveal the truth.

The drugs were approved by clinical trials but they weren't "unapproved" by new clinical trials, even though medicine claims these trials are the only type of proof it accepts. The clinical trials were shown to be wrong by simply observing real events. Quite simply, however, medicine dismisses nearly every lifestyle and natural solution to health because the evidence is based on real-life outcomes, yet, when it suits them, it ignores its "gold standard" clinical trials in favour of these very same outcomes for real people. This hypocrisy is staggering. So, now we are going to look at the outcomes for real people by examining the history and progression of several diseases and we'll start with the single biggest killer: heart disease.

A hundred years ago, heart disease was much rarer. In western Europe and the US, it increased steadily up to about 1930, then escalated ten-fold over the next 20 years – a 1000% increase. By the 1950s it was the leading cause of death and half a million US citizens were dying each year. This single example of disease progression is compelling and informative. How is it possible to explain such a dramatic escalation of a disease without there being some significant environmental or lifestyle cause? It certainly can't be explained by genes. The exact causes may be unknown or debatable, but there simply have to be lifestyle or environmental reasons. In fact, when the world's leading scientists started to look at the possible causes of this devastating epidemic in the 1950s, they concluded it was caused by significant changes to people's diets over the same 20-year period. Much more on this later when you will discover that, while the overall logic is correct, the experts did in fact chose the wrong dietary cause.

Some people did try to suggest that high levels of heart disease may have always existed but no one realised what they were and, therefore, there is nothing to explain. But this hypothesis does not stand up to scrutiny when we look at the history of heart disease in other parts of the world. By 1960 every doctor was being taught about heart disease – it was, after all, the single biggest cause of death in the west – and medical education is universal. So, every single doctor and pathologist in the world would know exactly what the symptoms and markers were, and would have recognised them if they were occurring. But at that time, other parts of the world, such as Eastern Europe and South East Asia, still had very low levels of heart disease. Then, at various times over the next 50 years, these regions also saw exactly the same sort of rapid rise that the west had seen nearly 100 years ago. Today, for example, Ukraine has more heart disease as a percentage of its population than the US did in the 1950s. China also had little heart disease 50 years ago but it is now escalating so rapidly that experts are predicting not just a human catastrophe, but, in the longer term, dire economic consequences for the whole Chinese economy. For many decades, experts who study heart disease trends have also been able to successfully predict when this modern epidemic would start to occur and escalate in country after country. This always coincides with rising living standards and the adoption of western diets and western lifestyles.

There are many other clues. France has one of the lowest rates of heart disease in the world. The UK has nearly three times as many as France, while the Ukraine has 20 times more. The Japanese also have a low rate of heart disease, but when they move to other countries, the rate invariably increases significantly. The same used to apply to the Chinese who 50 years ago had very low rates of heart disease, but when they emigrated to another country they too soon acquired the heart attack rate of that country. The large Chinese community in San Francisco suffered this huge rise in heart disease in the 1960s and 1970s, well before China itself succumbed to the current run-away epidemic.

The American Heart Association states that 80% of heart disease is preventable. Many natural health doctors would say the figure is even higher. The NHS says 35% of heart disease could be prevented just by one single lifestyle change: exercise. The World Health Organization also says 80% of heart diseases could be prevented. There are many more examples, but hopefully I don't need to elaborate further since this is really an open and shut case. Heart disease has undergone exponential growth from low levels. This occurred at different times in different countries and regions until it is now the leading overall cause of death around the world. Changes in lifestyle and environment simply have to be the predominant cause. I have not yet discussed what causes it, but the key message is simple and logical. If the causes can be found, it must be possible to reverse this epidemic and bring heart disease back to the same low levels that once existed. This is what history unequivocally tells us.

I should add one further point. While much of the rest of the world is in the grip of an escalating heart disease epidemic, in the west, where it all started, two specific areas of progress have been made. The number of people dying from heart disease has fallen because of much better and quicker emergency medical treatments. Also, cigarette smoking, according to leading medical organisations, more than doubles the risk of heart disease overall. Sixty years ago, 65% of the entire adult population of the UK smoked; today the figure is just 15% and this huge 70% reduction is likely to be the biggest single reason for the fall in heart disease and deaths. Despite these two significant successes, however, heart disease still remains the leading cause of death in the UK and other western countries. All this means that there is something very wrong with the medical approach to heart disease and this will be explored in detail in Part 5.

I have gone to some lengths to prove that the prevention of most heart disease is indeed not just possible, but completely logical. But most other diseases are also increasing alarmingly and these too have to have major lifestyle and environmental causes. I should add that pharmaceutical drugs are also an increasingly significant cause of many diseases as already outlined. Just two drugs – Vioxx and Avandia – caused 240,000 heart attacks, and drugs overall are the third leading cause of death.

Five major diseases account for around 70% of all deaths in western countries. These are heart disease, stroke, cancer, diabetes and dementia. Heart disease, stroke and cancer alone account for 62%. We have just explored the overwhelming evidence that it must be possible to prevent most heart disease, but there is strong evidence that lifestyle and environmental factors are a major cause of all the others as well, which we will now briefly explore.

Sixty years ago, the number of cases of type 2 diabetes was around 200,000, now it is over 4 million and the numbers continue to rise each year. Type 2 diabetes used to be called *age-related diabetes* because it only used to affect older people; now, children as young as eight are developing the disease. Embarrassingly, medicine had to stop using the term "age-related diabetes" and instead had to think up the new name "type 2 diabetes" once these alarming trends started to occur. Medicine itself acknowledges that this is a disease caused by poor lifestyles which include poor diets and a lack of exercise and, therefore, it must be preventable. This is both a human and financial catastrophe. Around 10% of all hospital admissions are for diabetes and the outcomes it causes, like limb amputations, heart attacks and liver disease. Furthermore, 10% of the entire NHS budget is spent trying just to minimise its symptoms often with little success as well as treating its devastating consequences. Yet despite the fact it is preventable, it is set to escalate even further, which is nothing short of a scandal.

As far as cancer is concerned, even the most conservative medical organisations state that a third of all cancer is preventable by adopting a healthy lifestyle. Cancer Research UK says the figure is 40%. Other experts confidently put the figure at 50%, while a high-profile study by researchers at Stony Brook University in New York concluded it was 90%. Very recently, the American Cancer Society has accepted that genes cause less than 5% of cancer risk and that 95% are caused by epigenetic factors like diet, smoking, environmental pollutants, drugs, stress, obesity and physical inactivity. We will explore these in more detail and look at the reasons for the difference in figures in the section on cancer. But what is clear is medicine, overall, accepts that a significant proportion of cancer is preventable. Most lifestyle medicine practitioners would also put the figure up to around 90% depending on the type of cancer involved and there is strong evidence to back this up. For example, just as with heart attacks, there are significant differences in the rates of cancer in different countries and regions. Countries with low levels often see increases in cancer as their economies become more industrialised and they become more westernised. There is also a large and consistent body of evidence that shows how immigrants moving from countries with low cancer levels to those with high levels, soon develop the same higher cancer rates. This in turn casts serious doubt over the ideas proposed by some experts that many cancers are down just to chance or are caused by faulty genes and it, therefore, means that if it was possible to determine all the many potential causes, then most cancers would also be preventable.

Most of the evidence that was presented for the prevention of heart attacks also applies to strokes, so I won't go into any more detail on this now. In addition, I will also cover Alzheimer's in its own section because the evidence is much more complex.

Another key point is that in the 1950s and 1960s, obesity, and particularly childhood obesity, was so unusual that I remember being truly shocked at the age of 11 when I saw for the first time an obese boy at my new school. I still have the school photos to prove it. You only need to look at films and TV programmes from that period to confirm that childhood obesity was rare. But the current "epidemic" in which 20% of children are now obese has been getting progressively worse for so long that it seems to have lost its ability to shock, and many people even think it is quite normal. As we will see later, there are many factors involved in the current obesity epidemic, like diet, exercise, environment, chemicals, bacteria and certain drugs. Medicine confirms that obesity has lifestyle causes, and that it is a significant risk factor for diseases like heart disease, stroke, cancer and diabetes. Sixty years ago, it barely existed and the current epidemic has nothing to do with genes. If it was possible now to go back to the lifestyles and diets of that time, obesity would almost disappear again. But this can only happen now, when all the individual causes are known and communicated to people and when they are adopted. More on this in Part 5.

So, there is irrefutable evidence that a significant proportion of the major diseases could be prevented. But the other key fact is we are also literally in the midst of an epidemic of these chronic and degenerative diseases. Their escalation has been increasing over decades but very few people know how serious the whole thing is becoming. How many people, for example, know that around half of all UK children have now been diagnosed with at least one chronic disease, when 60 years ago it was probably no more than 1 in 20. What is medicine doing about this whole tragic situation? Shouldn't they be declaring a national emergency in every affected country and demanding funding for research to uncover the real causes of these epidemics so they can be reversed and enable most people to become healthy again? One problem is medical research is effectively controlled by the drug industry and involves developing drugs to simply treat diseases, which means research into their causes is almost non-existent. But there is one other key fact why literally nothing is happening. Medicine has, for many years, claimed that most of the increases in major diseases are linked to the long-term trend of rising life expectancy, since older people are more likely to develop diseases like heart attacks, cancer and strokes. It has consistently tried to use this "get out of jail card". But whilst older people are more likely to develop these types of disease, there are two key facts that show clearly this only plays one part, and in fact a significantly reducing part, in the huge increases in disease prevalence that the western world is now facing.

The first is that average life expectancy in the UK has barely changed since 2010. It has effectively stalled, and future projected increases are also being dramatically scaled back. Despite all of this, however, incredible increases in diseases, like strokes, cancer and diabetes, have occurred in the last decade, are still happening, and are projected to carry on occurring. Overall life expectancy on its own cannot explain any significant part of this. The second is that if increased life expectancy really was the major cause of the exponential increase in diseases, then only older people would be affected, but the facts are quite shocking. We have seen that half of all children have at least one chronic disease and younger adults are also seeing significant increases in the major diseases like stroke, heart disease, cancer and diabetes. Type 2 diabetes never used to affect people below about 60, but now children as young as eight develop the disease. Strokes are now occurring in people as young as 20, and a US study showed that strokes in the age range 20–44 went up by 60% over a recent 12-year period.

There are a wide range of other diseases that are increasing exponentially in children as well. These can cause serious disabling outcomes and include asthma, food allergies, learning difficulties, skin conditions, ADHD, obesity, autism and IBS. None of this escalation in so many diseases can be explained by overall changes in life expectancy, by genes, or by excuses like "they may have always been there but we just didn't know". Autism in children is increasing exponentially. Official figures from Northern Ireland show that in 2008, 1.2% of schoolchildren had the diagnosis but this increased to 4.5% in 2021. This is a 275% increase in just 13 years. Because autism affects males disproportionally, it means that 1 in 15 boys now have this devastating condition. Asthma is reaching epidemic proportions and 10% of children are now affected. Childhood cancers are increasing. They are up by 40% in the last 16 years, and are still increasing faster, in percentage terms, than any other age group. Mental illness in young people is escalating so fast it might even eclipse the human catastrophe of diabetes.

Surely the powers that be should be sounding alarm bells and carrying out urgent research to find out the true causes of these catastrophic increases in nearly every disease, but this is not happening. In fact, scurvy and rickets, once consigned to the history books, are also making a big comeback, and the fact that these Victorian and pre-Victorian diseases are returning now is nothing short of a national scandal especially when the causes are already known with 100% certainty. Something very sinister is happening.

In America there is an organisation called the Children's Health Defense (CHD) which is headed by Robert F. Kennedy Jr. Its purpose is to spread the message about the staggering and frightening increase in virtually every childhood disease and to fight for action to reverse this generational catastrophe. Approximately 54% of children in the US now have at least one chronic disease and this figure is continuing to increase. The organisation is, however, probably fighting an uphill battle since most people have got so used to these diseases which have increased insidiously and without publicity such that many of them now seem to think they always existed and that it is normal for so many children to be so sick and treated just with drugs. One of the articles published by the Children's Health Defense is titled "Chronic Illness in Children – Who is Sounding the Alarm?" This is the vital question, because no one officially involved in healthcare, whether it be medicine, charities, regulators or governments as well as the press, seems concerned. No one is demanding action to find out why children are experiencing such a devastating and historically unprecedented burden of chronic illness. I should add that the Children's Health Defense is also experiencing some of the most vicious attacks and censorship that has ever been experienced in a democratic society. The reasons for all of this will be explored later.

In case you still need even more proof that most of these increases in almost every disease have to be preventable, consider the incredible variations in life expectancy that occur between individual regions and social strata within society. These facts are shocking, compelling and almost unbelievable. But looked at in another way, it is also a cause for optimism. A study carried out a few years ago showed that the average life expectancy for boys born in Knightsbridge was 95 years, and for boys born in Tranmere in Merseyside it was 67 years. So, boys in Knightsbridge would, on average, have 28 more years on the planet than those born in Tranmere. Whilst this is deeply sad and shocking on one level, it shows conclusively on another level just what is possible in terms of enhanced life expectancy. Girls have similarly increased life spans in Knightsbridge although the figures are "more modest" at around 20 years compared to Tranmere. There are numerous other studies worldwide that measure variations in life expectancies and they all show similar results albeit not so drastic as the comparison between Knightsbridge and Tranmere. Looking at the overall average outcomes of these studies, a healthy lifestyle can realistically add around ten years to the average life expectancy in the UK of around 81, while an unhealthy lifestyle can reduce it by around ten years.

Given that heart disease, strokes, cancer, type 2 diabetes and dementia account for around two-thirds of all deaths, then clearly the inhabitants of Knightsbridge and other similar districts and regions must be delaying or even avoiding most of these diseases, while the inhabitants of Tranmere are succumbing to them much earlier. Could it be that the wealthy residents of Knightsbridge along with other affluent areas have access to special life-saving drugs or surgical techniques that no one else knows about? Absolutely not. It would indeed be the greatest scandal in the history of the world if this was the case. No, the reason is related simply to the lifestyle and environment for both groups and even health experts educated in conventional medical systems agree this is the only way to explain such facts. There are, however, many complex reasons for all of this which will be explored in more detail shortly. The fact is I have never seen any medical people even try to claim that medicine, via the treatments, drugs and surgery it uses, influences in any way whatsoever the huge gulf between the health and life expectancy of the people of Tranmere and Knightsbridge. So, why do they then ignore all the evidence and revert back to treating people just with drugs and surgery? Why don't they actively and seriously demand and carry out research to find out which lifestyle and environmental factors are involved in these incredible disease and life expectancy variations? Lifestyle factors which clearly and conclusively work far better than anything that medicine uses.

When mortality statistics like those for Knightsbridge and Tranmere make it into the public sphere, poverty pressure groups express outrage and demand more funding for healthcare in these deprived regions. But more healthcare expenditure is not the solution. Lack of medicine is not the cause. Instead, society should be putting enormous effort into finding out the true causes of disease, and working out how to prevent them, thereby allowing most people to have longer and healthier lives. But, of course, as we have already seen, only 1% of all medical research is directed at finding the causes of disease. Prevention is simply not on the agenda for medicine, Big Pharma and governments. No one is systematically researching it and no one is actively promoting it. There is no money to be made from it. Indeed, prevention spells disaster for all of them in terms of employment, profit and government revenue. Solutions to all these devastating issues will, therefore, simply not be realised by "the establishment". But this is where lifestyle medicine comes into its own. Practitioners and doctors who study and advocate lifestyle solutions to health have been exploring the true causes of disease for decades and have achieved incredible results with their real-life patients. Of course, they are usually ridiculed, attacked and marginalised by the "establishment juggernaut", but, as we will see, an incredible amount of evidence exists; knowledge that would allow a significant majority of people to prevent, in large part, most major diseases. But, of course, you will not find any of this from conventional medical or government sources. Put quite simply: lifestyle and environmental factors lie at the very heart of most diseases and their effect on life expectancy is profound. A long and healthy life is something most people could achieve. This is what we will soon explore in detail. I must, however, keep repeating that a wide range of drugs can also be a key cause in many diseases.

Here is another incredible piece of evidence. The US spends significantly more on medicine and drugs than any other country in the world. It spends $3 trillion per year (18% of its entire GDP) on healthcare, while the average for similar major European countries is around 10% of their GDP. Yet, the US has the lowest life expectancy of all the major developed nations, the fewest people alive over the age of 65 in percentage terms, the highest rate of children's deaths and illnesses, and it is the only country in the world where overall life expectancy has started to fall. The latest annual figures show that, per head of population, the US spends $11,000 on healthcare. The average EU figure for the top ten wealthiest countries is around $5,500, and for Turkey the figure is $1,300. Despite these huge differences in medical expenditure, average life expectancy in 2019 was 78.8 in the US, around 82.5 in the EU and 78.9 in Turkey. So, the US has a lower life expectancy than even Turkey, even though its medical expenditure per person is over eight times more. All this clearly shows that spending more on medicine is not the solution for human health and life expectancy that most people believe, and it gives yet another type of proof that lifestyle and environment have to be the real key factors.

Have you heard about blue zones? The National Geographic writer and researcher Dan Buettner has investigated and identified what he calls "blue zones": regions of the world where residents regularly live to 100 plus. They include Okinawa, Japan; Nicoya, Costa Rica; Ikaria, Greece; Barbagia, Sardinia; and Loma Linda, California whose Seventh Day Adventist community is known for its longevity. What do these blue zoners have in common? Genes will play a part for some of them, of course, but environment and lifestyle are key, says Buettner. A plant-based diet is a key common denominator, as is an active lifestyle. But that's not all. Other things blue zoners share include strong social networks and beliefs, plus healthy ways of dealing with life's stressors. Drugs and conventional medicine seem to play only a minor role in their lives and polypharmacy is something they are unlikely to have ever experienced.

Buettner has identified nine key denominators:

- Move naturally and often.
- Live with purpose – having a sense that life is worth living and finding your reason to get up in the morning can add years to your life.
- Stress less – find ways of coping better with life's inevitable ups and downs.
- Eat less – eat until you are 80% full.
- Eat a plant-based diet – don't necessarily exclude meat; just cut it down.
- Enjoy a glass of wine – all blue zoners (except Seventh Day Adventists) drink alcohol regularly but *moderately.* Despite the continued warnings from medicine, an enjoyable glass of wine a day seems to do these centenarians no harm whatsoever.
- Have faith – being religious is common to many blue zoners, but having a spiritual dimension to life is what seems to be crucial. Meditation and yoga are good alternative options.
- Put loved ones first – make time for family and friends through regular visits, shared activities and celebrations. Maintain that vital sense of connection.
- Find your tribe – mix with people who support and reinforce your goals.

It can all be summed up in Buettner's words: "Eat your vegetables, have a positive outlook, be kind to people and smile."

Finally, here is another interesting, although unusual, corroboration from an entire country. This occurred in Cuba in the 1990s after the collapse of the Soviet Union. Soviet funding for Cuba also collapsed and Cuba was plunged into crisis and poverty became widespread. Fuel and food were in short supply. Everyone was forced to either walk or use bicycles and processed ready-made foods largely disappeared. The diet of necessity consisted of simple, natural home-grown foods and there wasn't even a great deal of that. If such a thing was to happen in the UK, poverty action groups would be up in arms and predicting a dire health catastrophe. But what happened? The death rates for chronic diseases like heart disease, stroke and diabetes plummeted to 50%. But by the end of the 1990s, Cuba's economy started to recover. People started to use cars again and their diet also reverted to "normal". What happened? Heart attacks, strokes and diabetes all increased again to around pre-crisis levels. I am certainly not suggesting we need a crisis with widespread poverty to reduce chronic disease levels, but the Cuba experience simply adds a different and graphic type of proof of what is achievable. We do not need to abandon our cars to improve our health; driving and exercise are not mutually exclusive. But we do need to increase our physical activity and we do need to significantly reduce highly processed foods and eat far more natural food. But before moving on to the key factors that affect health and life expectancy, I want to give one simple but compelling example of how lifestyle medicine can achieve incredible success. This is not a major life-threatening disease but its effects can be completely debilitating and bring utter misery to those who suffer from it.

Cystitis

Cystitis is largely preventable. But if there was ever a graphic example of how medicine has strayed from its true path and its fundamental principles and at the same time betrayed women on a grand scale, look no further than cystitis for the proof. Medicine can cure most cases of bacterial cystitis with antibiotics. So, you might ask, what's the problem? Well, the medical cure comes with a guaranteed period of debilitating symptoms and intense pain while waiting for doctors' appointments, then waiting for the antibiotic to work and sometimes waiting for a different antibiotic if the first one fails. It is no "free lunch". Neither does it prevent reoccurrence. Many women suffer from repeated and devastating attacks. Increasing antibiotic resistance is also now adding to the problems.

This is a story of Angela Kilmartin, a housewife and former opera singer; a woman who had no medical background or medical training, yet she has helped millions of long-suffering women overcome this debilitating condition. Between 1966 and 1972, she had 78 attacks of cystitis each of which was treated with antibiotics and some with operations. She was incontinent, feverish, passing bloody urine and fainting from the pain. Thrush from the antibiotics often caused equal misery, but nothing was offered to stop the attacks happening in the first place. Cystitis savagely affected her life and relationships and destroyed her career. Unable to guarantee stage appearances, she was forced to give up a promising career in opera and instead decided to take revenge upon cystitis. She has been free of the disease since 1976 when she developed a comprehensive prevention plan and has since written seven books on cystitis which have helped millions of women overcome this dreadful disease. It has been estimated that 60% of women experience the misery of recurrent cystitis at some point in their life. Around 4 million women develop the disease every year in the UK. There are over 4 billion women in the world and whilst the work of Angela Kilmartin has helped a few million of them, the vast majority still know nothing about how to prevent cystitis and neither do their doctors. Every year, millions of women go through the same wretched process that plagued Angela Kilmartin. A visit to the doctor, a course of antibiotics, one week of hell and then blessed relief and cure, until the next time and then the time after that. Amazingly, no one seems to think there is anything wrong or strange in this incredible, repetitive process.

When I was studying chemistry and physics, I was taught that science was all about the "why" question. Why does an apple fall to the ground? Why is the sky blue? For researchers in virtually every field of science, the "why" question is the driving force behind virtually everything they do. But when we look at cystitis, medicine hasn't even asked the "why" question. Angela Kilmartin did, and in doing so helped millions of women. She achieved what the very best brains in medicine around the world had failed to do because she asked the right question. She then researched methodically and with single-minded determination until she had the answers. Remember, she had no medical or any scientific training or background of any kind. How did this begin? Well, after 78 attacks of cystitis over five years and the unremitting misery they brought, she suddenly had her "eureka moment". This thought suddenly came into her mind: "why do I keep getting cystitis?" This may seem such an obvious question when you see it written down and when you understand the whole story that it actually sounds strange that she didn't ask the question much sooner. But no doctor or even the greatest brains in medicine had ever asked the question either, and that was because, as far as medicine is concerned, women simply get cystitis and doctors can cure it with antibiotics – period. What more did anyone need to know?

As soon as she asked the question, she was filled with hope. Even though she wasn't a scientist, it was clear there had to be a cause, and once that was understood, it was logical that there had to be a way to prevent it. She read all the existing evidence, uncovered the real causes of cystitis and then, using herself as a guinea pig, worked out the solutions. I won't go into the details but they involve simple, but well-tried and tested ways of preventing the bacteria that cause cystitis from entering the urethra. Here are two telling quotes summarising her books:

"Angela Kilmartin has done more than hospitals full of doctors." – Woman's Journal

"Angela Kilmartin is almost a legend in the world of urology." – Dr David Delvin

This is what Geoffrey Chamberlain, president in 1994 of the Royal College of Obstetricians and Gynaecologists in London, had to say about her book *The Patient's Encyclopaedia of Urinary Tract Infection, Sexual Cystitis and Interstitial Cystitis*:

> Cystitis is a bane of womankind. From its mildest form of irritation to the severe disease of a life-threatening illness, cystitis has been with us for many centuries. Like other commonly occurring conditions, it has perhaps been put to one side by formal medicine; doctors hand out a pocketful of antibiotics and a bit of advice on extra fluids. It was not until Angela Kilmartin started her pioneering work on actually identifying the details of this disease that it came into a medical spotlight.
>
> This book outlines the work she has done for many years to help women with cystitis. It is an excellent account of the background science of the subject and gives very good advice on how to prevent cystitis. There is also a very important section on non-bacterial cystitis, for this is a mystery still to some doctors. Angela Kilmartin again dissects the problem and gives first rate advice on its management. This book is a must for any woman who has ever had the miseries of a urine infection. It is well produced and will help women. I recommend it thoroughly.

All of this is, of course, incredibly positive, but there is a darker side yet to be revealed. The work of Angela Kilmartin is well known within senior medical circles as confirmed by the president of the Royal College, so it is all the more surprising, and disturbing, that if you look on the NHS website under cystitis you will find not a single mention of any kind on how to prevent cystitis. Not one word. It would be so easy for the NHS to provide a link to this book and recommend it, and save millions of women the misery of cystitis, at the same time reducing the pressure on overworked GPs, and saving on drug costs. So, why has this not been done? Why has this pioneering work seemingly been airbrushed out of existence by medicine's elite? I cannot give a definitive answer, but I can give some clues as to what is likely to be going on in the minds of those responsible.

You might imagine that medicine would welcome such pioneering work and the millions of lives it could transform. But the reality is this is a complete embarrassment to medicine, to its credibility and to the inflated egos of those involved. Single-handedly, a housewife has uncovered the true causes of cystitis, a condition that accounts for around 3% of all GP visits by women, and worked out how to prevent it, while the best brains in medicine sat on the side-lines uninterested and unconcerned. To recommend this book would effectively be an admission of one of its key failings as a profession, which emphasises treatment and virtually ignores prevention. The old saying "prevention is better than cure" continues to by-pass medicine.

Somewhere in the back of their minds will also be the thought that, if they were to promote this book, there would be countless other health experts with solutions to other intractable medical conditions such as TATT and IBS, as well as the big killers, heart disease and cancer. Promoting this book would open a crack in the door that they would never be able to close. It would give people the opportunity to see there was a real alternative to medicine's "pill for every ill". They will not allow this to happen no matter what level of human misery and suffering it causes. I must add that if Angela Kilmartin had written her book today, I am absolutely certain the current president of the Royal College would not dare endorse it in the way Geoffrey Chamberlain did in 1994, because if he did, he would face ridicule and attack from his colleagues for promoting an "unproven" lifestyle treatment.

No one in medicine's elite will be formally asked to explain why they are allowing women to suffer unnecessarily in this way. The invincible aura that surrounds medicine and its treatments means the media and press never challenge such things. But if they had to try to explain it, I know exactly what they would say – it would go something like this... "But, of course, this is all anecdotal evidence. It hasn't been proven in large-scale clinical trials. More long-term research is needed before we could consider such treatments." Ah yes, that old "you haven't done a clinical trial and more long-term research is needed" routine; the perfect way to kick every natural treatment into the long grass. It always comes to medicine's rescue when they are in a tricky situation. Of course, when antibiotics were first developed, clinical trials hadn't even been invented, but this didn't stop medicine from using them to treat cystitis then, and it doesn't stop them using them now. This was, of course, the right thing to do, because even without clinical trials, it was absolutely clear antibiotics worked. But exactly the same thing can be said of the protocols developed by Angela Kilmartin which have helped millions of women. The irony, however, seems totally lost on medicine's elite and never ceases to amaze me. Also remember, 20% of all drugs prescribed by doctors have no clinical trials backing them up – the so-called off-label use promoted by Big Pharma. The hypocrisy is breath-taking and the actions of medicine's elite are indefensible, but, of course, no one would ever dare challenge them.

I need to repeat yet again that GPs and doctors are not involved in this very sad situation. They could only find out about this effective solution for cystitis if they were taught about it at medical schools, at their seminars for continuing medical education or if it became an official treatment. Of course, this is all controlled by the elite medical decision makers which means doctors will never find out about it. Finally, we have the pharmaceutical industry masterminding and overseeing the whole devastating process and making sure, via their "money tree", that no simple natural cure or prevention of any kind ever gains the slightest credence that would threaten its drug-dominated model of healthcare. The whole thing is almost unbelievable.

Essential background information

Before moving on to lifestyle medicine's main weapons, there are four pieces of essential background information that will help to set the scene.

Human evolution

The first type of life on the planet evolved around 4 billion years ago. These were single cell microorganisms that first developed in the oceans and later moved onto the land. Multi-cell organisms developed around 800 million years ago and this led ultimately to the evolution of millions of different animal species, most of which eventually evolved or became extinct. Humanoid-like beings first evolved about 7 million years ago. Around 2 million years ago Homo erectus evolved and 200,000 years ago Homo sapiens. There were also many different species in the genus Homo during this evolutionary period like Homo habilis and Homo neanderthalensis. But the key message is our ancestors have been around for at least 7 million years. The evolution of the human species resulted in changes to height, weight, movement and, most importantly of all, brain size.

How did our ancestors live and what did they eat? Our human ancestors, who evolved initially in Africa, clearly lived a basic life although they did indeed produce artwork and over time developed more sophisticated tools and lifestyles. The lifestyle of hunter-gatherers epitomised the way our ancestors existed and this involved a nomadic way of life where small groups of people moved around their region using temporary shelters. Finding food was a major part of life and this involved significant levels of physical activity. Food was basically plant-based together with animals and fish whenever these could be caught. Plant-based food consisted of vegetables, fruits, nuts, seeds, roots and other edible parts of plants. Huge varieties and numbers of plants were eaten often varying with the season. The key point to all of this is that, over 7 million years, human evolution and the human genome have been directly linked to completely natural foods. Natural plants and animals contain thousands of compounds like vitamins, minerals, amino acids, fats, proteins, fibres and compounds like polyphenols, oligosaccharides, bioflavonoids, anthocyanins and glucosinolates which are essential for the body to operate effectively and efficiently. The body has developed receptor sites that recognise these types of compounds allowing them to be efficiently absorbed and utilised.

Around 10,000 years ago the hunter-gatherer way of life started to change because of the development of farming. This happened in many areas of the world over a period of 2,000 or 3,000 years. Farming communities did not move around their regions like hunter-gatherers, but had to produce sufficient food in relatively small areas. This meant they tended to concentrate on a few key crops and a few types of domesticated animals. These included easy to produce crops like wheat and barley, peas and lentils, and milk and cheese together with a few meats and fruits when in season. This increasingly restricted diet laid the foundation for many of today's chronic diseases although at the time it did not have the same devastating effect because of mitigating circumstances like the incredible levels of physical activity involved in manual farming and the fact that all the foods were still natural, like full grains, as opposed to much of the highly refined foods of today like white bread. Nevertheless, this radical change of diet compared to the natural diet of hunter-gatherers over 7 million years of evolution turned out to be the first stage in the current epidemic of chronic diseases like heart disease, strokes, obesity and type 2 diabetes.

Around 250 years ago another profound change occurred: the Industrial Revolution. This led to huge additional changes in lifestyle. Instead of relatively small rural villages, urban conurbations emerged in conjunction with factories and eventually huge cities with millions of inhabitants. Once again, major changes occurred to sanitation, food, water, housing and hygiene. The changes to life expectancy and disease were exceptional over such a relatively short length of time. Average life expectancy in some tenement slums in the 1800s was just 15 years. The key point again is changes to lifestyle have caused the most profound changes in health, disease and life expectancy. Of course, I am not suggesting that mankind should go back to being hunter-gatherers. Modern life is incredible, but mankind is now suffering from diseases that barely existed throughout our 7 million years of evolution. Not only that, but many disease numbers are escalating exponentially and affecting ever younger people and children. The key point is that looking at our history and evolution provides the basis for understanding why this is happening and how it could be reversed.

In other words, we could have most of the wonderful opportunities that modern life offers, while still increasing our life expectancy and health, and at the same time, avoiding or delaying many of the chronic modern diseases.

Life is miraculous and so complex that the human body will never be fully understood

It would be possible to write thousands of books to explain in detail what is already known about how the human body works. But the reality is even this incredible level of knowledge represents the equivalent of no more than a handful of sand in a desert. Even within this huge – but in relative terms, small – level of knowledge, there are many aspects where, even now, scientists disagree on fundamental issues, and despite the huge advances in research, medicine still does not know the causes of almost every disease. Many leading experts say life is so complex that even with all the scientific advances that are occurring and the exponential increases in computer technology, we will never fully understand how the human body works.

I am going to outline just four very different aspects of the body which give just the briefest insight into its incredible complexity and the countless trillions of bodily functions that occur each second. All of these require even more trillions of complex interactions that link everything together and keep the body working in harmony. This is vital in understanding how lifestyle medicine works and how it works in harmony with life as opposed to synthetic chemical drug treatments which are alien to the body, and which, with a very few exceptions, are like throwing a spanner into the most sophisticated and complex machine ever made, and then wondering why there are so many calamitous repercussions.

Cells. The cell is the basic living unit of the human body as well as all other organisms on the planet. There are over 200 different types of cell in the body including various nerve cells, skin cells and muscle cells. Cells group together to form tissue, groups of different tissue make up organs, and different organs group together to form organ systems like the respiratory, circulatory and musculoskeletal systems. The basic cell is incredible. Imagine a single cell that has been magnified many millions of times. On the surface would be millions of openings which open and close to allow a continuing stream of materials to flow in and out. If you were to enter one of them you would be bewildered by the incredible technology and complexity. There would be endless corridors branching out in every direction. Some would lead to the central memory bank in the nucleus and others to various types of assembly and manufacturing plants. The nucleus itself would be a huge sphere inside of which would be miles of coiled DNA molecules. Huge numbers of raw materials, as well as products produced in the assembly plants, move along the corridors in an incredibly organised way in what are effectively containers called vesicles. There are clean-up crews called lysosomes that get rid of unwanted or damaged molecules. There are memory banks, decoding and operating systems and energy generators called mitochondria to name just a few of the complex control systems. The whole thing would be like a gigantic automated factory carrying out almost as many functions as all the manufacturing activities added together from around the entire world. All this occurs in something that is just one-thousandth of a millimetre in diameter.

Despite this incredible complexity, a cell can divide and replicate its entire structure in just a few hours. The way the cell divides is, in itself, a feat of mind-blowing complexity. The human body has around 10 trillion cells, and each cell type has a different lifespan. Bone cells are renewed about every ten years, red blood cells every four months, skeletal muscle cells every 15 years, while gut and tastebud cells last around three days. The shortest is a type of white blood cell called neutrophils which has a life of just four hours and the longest are neurons and certain eye cells which last a lifetime. An incredible 2 million new red blood cells are formed every single second. In total, over the entire body, 230 billion new cells are created every day. Replacing all these cells and the body parts they form requires a huge variety of basic raw materials and these, of course, come from the food we eat and drink. One of lifestyle medicine's key aims is to define diets that provide optimum levels of all of these vital foods that allow the complex bodily functions to operate optimally. As well as food, things like positive thoughts, physical activity, sleep and vitamins and minerals also play a significant role.

Genes. After looking at cells it is appropriate to consider the nucleus of the cell. Inside the nucleus is the DNA which is a long chain molecule that provides all the information for the body to develop, survive and reproduce. DNA looks like a twisted ladder and the rungs contain the genes that are coded instructions for building the tens of thousands of proteins, hormones and enzymes that make up the human body. There are 3 billion molecules of DNA that make up the genes in each cell nucleus.

I am not going to elaborate any more on the incredible complexity of DNA and genes and how they work. Instead, with this brief background information, I want to concentrate on the Human Genome Project. Back in 1990, the US and several other countries provided $3 billion for this project and the aim was to decode every one of the 20,000 different genes in a human body. The belief of most of the world's leading scientists was that once completed it would lead to a revolution in medicine that would ultimately lead to effective and, in some cases, personalised treatments for many diseases like cancer and multiple sclerosis. They believed many diseases were caused by defects in specific genes and once these could be identified, gene-based designer drugs would then be made that would literally transform disease treatment. As the project neared its completion, news headlines like "Scientists find genes to combat cancer" and "Gene therapy offers hope to victims of arthritis" were omnipresent. When the first draft of the project was completed in 2000, President Bill Clinton declared from the White House: "We are here to celebrate the completion of the first survey of the entire human genome. Without doubt this is the most important, most wonderful map ever produced by mankind." Since then, a further $3 billion on average has been spent each year on the many aspects of genetic research. These include speeding up the gene sequencing process. The original single genome project took 13 years in total and cost $3 billion. Now it takes just seven days and costs under $1,000. In total, around $60 billion have been spent on gene research to date.

So, have we seen the predicted revolution in medicine and the expected miracle treatments? Sadly, the answer is no. The Human Genome Project and subsequent gene research is indeed one of mankind's most incredible scientific achievements, but we now know that the human body is almost infinitely more complex than the world's very best scientists could ever have predicted. Part of this complexity is that genes do not act independently and with specific properties as originally thought. In fact, they are just one small part of a complex network of interactions that also have different functions in different tissues. Phillip Gell FRS, emeritus professor of genetics, sums up the problem succinctly: "The heart of the problem lies in the fact that we are dealing not with a chain of causation but with a network that is a system like a spider's web in which a perturbation at any point of the web changes the tension of every fibre right back to its anchorage. The gap in our knowledge is not merely unbridged but in principle unbridgeable and our ignorance will remain ineluctable."

The historian of science Evelyn Fox Keller also explains that we are in "one of those rare and wonderful moments when success teaches us humility … we lulled ourselves into believing that in discovering the basis for genetic information we have found the 'secret of life'. We were confident that if we could only decode the message in the sequence of chemicals, we would understand the 'programme' that makes an organism what it is. But now there is at least a tacit acknowledgement of how large that gap between genetic information and biological meaning really is."

Some scientists and lifestyle practitioners did in fact predict right at the start that the human genome would have little effect on most diseases. You only have to look at identical twins with a well-known breast cancer gene to realise the gene alone does not cause the cancer, and that is why one identical twin can die of cancer aged 30 while the other lives to 85 and never develops the disease. You can also look at how it is possible to reverse a disease like type 2 diabetes just by changing diet. How would this be possible if a faulty gene was the cause of the disease? So, the key message is that, with a few exceptions like sickle cell anaemia and cystic fibrosis, genes alone do not cause diseases to happen. Some of them may play a part, but that part is once again a tiny element of an almost infinitely complex process. Even the American Cancer Society has recently accepted that genes cause less than 5% of cancer risk and the other 95% are caused by epigenetic factors like diet, smoking, environmental pollutants, drugs, stress, obesity and physical inactivity. So, after 30 years and over $60 billion spent on research, the project has achieved almost nothing in terms of people's health and it almost certainly never will. The problem remains that medicine's sole aim is to find ways of treating diseases. Finding out what causes them and then preventing them from happening in the first place does not seem to be part of the medical agenda. Fortunately, this is lifestyle medicine's main goal.

Speech. This is one of those things we all take for granted and rarely even think about. But speech involves over 100 different muscles in the throat, larynx, mouth and lips, as well as lung functions and one of the most complicated rapid motor systems in the body. The brain controls all of these functions via the central nervous system and then local nerve fibres which connect to all the sound producing muscles. The resulting brain activity is like a carefully tuned orchestra; each instrument generates a specific sound and those sounds are coordinated to produce the overall symphony. But the complexity is much greater than this simple outline implies. I have just read a 16-page research paper on just one of the 100 or so muscles that control speech. The complexity is such that I can only understand about half of it and the paper also outlines the huge areas of knowledge of this one muscle that we still don't understand. So, even though speech is probably one of the simplest bodily functions you could imagine, it is incredibly complex and even though the basic principles are understood, the detailed complex interactions are not. In comparison, organs like the liver, kidneys, heart and, of course, the brain itself are probably many billions or even trillions of times more complex. This is before we can even start to understand how the brain can control and coordinate all these major organs at the same time as well as countless other functions, like walking, sight, hearing, balance, emotions, thoughts, smell, taste, touch, writing, memory function, problem solving and the immune system to name just a few.

Microbiome. The human body is made up of 10 trillion cells and it also has 20,000 different genes. But in fact a healthy body actually contains over 100 trillion cells and 200,000 different genes. Why this huge difference? Well, we are in fact home to around 100 trillion mainly friendly bacteria. They are on every surface, like skin and intestines, but the vast majority inhabit the gut. Gut bacteria are usually referred to as the microbiome. There are thousands of different types of bacteria in and on the body, and in total they have around 200,000 different genes. So, in terms of the number of cells and the number of genes in our body, we are just 10% human. Every person has a unique microbiome and as we will see in the next section, it plays one of the most incredibly vital parts in our health and our ability to prevent and control disease.

The key points from this section are that the human body is so complex that we will never be able to fully understand exactly how it works, and genes are almost certainly not going to provide solutions to the epidemic of chronic diseases. But despite this almost infinite complexity, it is still possible to work out the main causes of disease. The lifestyle we each lead is the predominant factor but things like prescription drugs and dangerous chemicals are also playing an increasingly significant role.

How life expectancy has changed over the last 170 years and its main causes

In 1850 average life expectancy in the UK was 41 years – in 2018 it was almost 82. These figures are the overall average for men and women. On average, life expectancy increased by two and a half years in each of the intervening decades. Life expectancy increased in every single decade but there were some variations. The lowest increase was around two years and the highest around four years. So, what are the reasons for this doubling of life expectancy? Medicine does accept that lifestyle and environmental factors like improvements in sanitation, clean water, housing, nutrition and hygiene played a part, but if you read any encyclopaedia, conventional medical literature and media coverage, you will see medicine is given credit for the lion's share of the increases. Amongst the main reasons cited are: the control of infectious diseases with vaccines and antibiotics, the use of other drugs and surgical treatments and a major reduction in infant mortality. But this is where the accepted medical version starts to diverge from reality. Let's look at some of the real facts.

In 1850 infectious diseases were the leading cause of death and these included typhoid, cholera, diphtheria, whooping cough, typhus, tuberculosis, smallpox, pneumonia, measles, scarlet fever and diarrhoea. Some of these are caused by viruses, like measles and smallpox, and others are bacterial infections, like diphtheria and typhoid. There was, however, a great decline in mortality in all of these diseases which started in the mid to late nineteenth century and continued through the first half of the twentieth century. By 1950 the death rate for many diseases had declined to incredibly low levels. Whooping cough deaths had fallen by 99% compared to 1850, while measles and scarlet fever deaths had fallen by almost 100%. From 1900 to 1943, deaths from diarrhoeal infections fell by 93.5%. But there were no vaccines or antibiotics available during this great decline for these diseases. In fact, up until 1950 there were only two vaccines that were given to large numbers of the overall UK population: smallpox from 1796, and diphtheria from 1942. Typhoid and cholera vaccines were developed in 1896 and 1900 respectively but were not widely used. The typhoid vaccine, for example, was mainly given just to British soldiers in foreign countries and the small number of other foreign travellers. The first antibiotics only became widely available in the late 1940s. There will be much more detail on all of this later where you will also see that even the most famous vaccine of all time – smallpox – does not live up to its legendary status. The key point is the major part of the incredible decline in deaths involving infectious diseases, and thus the increase in life expectancy, occurred without vaccines and without antibiotics, so medicine's claim that vaccination was the single most useful health intervention that has ever been introduced surely deserves some challenge especially in developed western nations. In fact, even today, medical students are taught that, during the great decline from 1850, deaths from infectious diseases for which there were no vaccines or antibiotics at the time (which means most of them) declined solely due to improved social conditions.

Reductions in child mortality were also a major factor in increases in life expectancy in the developed world. In the UK in 1850, over a quarter of all children under the age of five died (274 out of every 1000). By 1950 the deaths had fallen to 44 out of 1000 – an 84% reduction. Almost identical declines occurred in all other developed countries. Much of the information in this section comes from the US, because many detailed studies were carried out there to examine the reasons for the incredible decline in child deaths, but the conclusions are still completely applicable to the UK. There was consensus in the US amongst public health professionals and contemporary scholars in that era that public health programmes, like providing clean water supplies, building sanitation systems, expanding the birth registration system and pasteurising milk, played a central role in the decline in infant mortality. Another key factor was the subsequent efforts to educate mothers on infant care and the important role that hygiene played, like frequent bathing, keeping their own hands clean, avoiding contaminated water, milk and other foods, and breast feeding wherever possible. Even in 1999, the CDC (Centers for Disease Control and Prevention) also described sanitation, water purification, the Children's Bureau and milk purification as the major public health achievements behind the decline in infant mortality. The CDC is very "pro-medicine", so the fact it does not quote any conventional medical procedures in the list of reasons for the decline in deaths gives stark proof that they did not meaningfully exist at that time. The reality is there were no childhood vaccines or drugs, no paediatric surgery or intensive care technologies, and no treatments for diarrhoeal disease and pneumonia which were the two leading causes of infant deaths. It is true that some of these treatments started to be developed in the 1940s, but they were only available to a small number of children until their use started to ramp up significantly in the 1950s. So, quite simply, the 84% decline in UK child mortality between 1850 and 1950 resulted almost solely from social and lifestyle changes. This alone contributed to more than half of the increase in overall life expectancy during the same period.

For the rest of the population, there were a number of life-saving drugs, like insulin (which started to be used in the mid-1920s), and other medical treatments and surgery that helped to reduce deaths mainly from 1900 to 1950, but even medicine does not claim they played a decisive role in the overall increase in life expectancy. In fact, as we have seen, medicine was also a major cause of death in western Europe and the US in this period. Puerperal fever which was caused by doctors' contaminated hands and equipment led to the deaths of tens of millions of mothers shortly after giving birth. Bed rest for heart attacks also caused around 10 million deaths. Other medical treatments of that time, like lobotomy, bloodletting and the use of poisons like mercury and arsenic, also caused devastating outcomes and deaths. While it is impossible to find accurate statistics, it is not impossible that overall medicine caused more deaths and serious outcomes than it saved. What is absolutely clear is that improvements in lifestyle and environmental factors like sanitation, clean water, housing, nutrition, hygiene and other living conditions were the key reasons for the increase in life expectancy in the 100 years up to 1950. Life expectancy rose by 41 years from 1850 to 2018. But by 1950 it had already increased by 25 years. This accounts for 60% of the total, and medicine overall played only a small part in it.

I should add one further factor that also played a significant part. The working conditions resulting from the Industrial Revolution were appalling and led to serious diseases and premature deaths. Here are just a few examples. Cotton mills produced fine particles of cotton that caused lung diseases which progressively worsened and eventually became fatal particularly in the cardroom section. An article in the Lancet medical journal in 1863 noted that "a carder seldom lives beyond 40 years of age. Many have to give up working much younger". At its peak, the cotton industry employed over 2 million people, so the effect on overall health and life expectancy would have been significant. In addition, the machinery (as was the case in all other industries) had no safety barriers or screens and many people died from horrific accidents. Mining and quarry accidents and deaths were common as well as the resulting lung diseases. Copper workers suffered from TB and bronchial conditions. In some industries the outcomes were much worse. Workers in the pottery industry, who manufactured the flint that reduced product breakages, had an average life span of just two (yes, two) years after staring their job. This was due to the lung disease silicosis which was caused by flint inhalation. However, new industrial laws, together with the impact of more compassionate industrialists, like Sir Titus Salt and the Cadbury family who built safer and healthier villages and factories for their employees, also started to make important reductions in mortality and improvements in health.

After 1950, the story becomes much more complex. Antibiotics became widely available and did indeed save many lives, as did other drugs like cortisone and streptomycin. Life-saving accident and emergency services improved markedly and many other types of surgery were developed for serious and disabling conditions. Paediatric surgery was developed as well as intensive care systems and child mortality has been reduced from 44 in a 1000, to 4 in 1000 today. Nearly all of this 4% reduction in deaths is due to medical advances. Many new vaccines (like the measles vaccine) were introduced, which significantly reduced the incidence of viral diseases, but in developed countries like the UK, and in terms of lives saved and overall life expectancy, they did not achieve much because the death toll from most infectious diseases had already declined to exceptionally low levels due to improvements in living conditions well before most vaccines were introduced. As an example, according to official figures, 4,500 measles deaths have been prevented in the UK since the measles vaccine was first developed in 1968. This may seem significant but it averages at just 92 each year, and whilst every life saved is important, it is essential to balance this against the side effects of the vaccines which will be explored in more detail in Part 5. Whilst vaccines have reduced the numbers of people who become infected, could stopping people from developing such viral diseases, from which nearly every healthy person recovers, also be counterproductive and have consequences in the longer term? This will also be examined.

Of course, living standards and lifestyle conditions have also continued to improve for most people since 1950. Cigarette smoking has also declined by a staggering 70% and, given that it reduces a smoker's life expectancy by an average of at least ten years, it would have increased overall life expectancy by over three years. Both of these, together with the fact that increasing numbers of people are learning for themselves how to prevent disease and stay healthy, mean that lifestyle solutions are still playing a significant role in increased life expectancy.

There is no doubt that medicine has saved many lives since the middle of the twentieth century with its incredible accident and emergency services, antibiotics and several other key drugs. The 4% reduction in child mortality alone would have increased overall life expectancy by around three years. But given that drugs are the third leading cause of death, it is still causing many deaths as well. What it also hasn't done is prevent the huge increases in the numbers of people developing virtually every single disease as well as the fact that young people even in their early twenties are now suffering and dying from diseases like strokes that never before affected anyone of their age group. Given these facts, it is perhaps not surprising that since 2011, life expectancy has now effectively stalled, and for some groups has even declined.

To summarise the life expectancy situation: between 1850 and 2018 life expectancy increased by 41 years. Between 1850 and 1950 it increased by 25 years (60% of the total) and nearly all of this was due to improvements in sanitation, water quality, hygiene, food and other living conditions. Between 1950 and 2011 it increased by 16 years (40% of the total). Medicine and lifestyle both contributed to this increase, but it is impossible to say by how much, although the reduction in smoking and the reduction in child mortality each contributed over three years. From 1850 the overall reduction in child mortality is the single biggest contributor to the doubling of life expectancy in the UK, accounting for around half of the 41-year increase. Lifestyle changes accounted for 85% of this and medicine 15%.

After 2011 life expectancy has effectively stalled. No official bodies have yet been able to come up with definitive reasons, but one of the most commonly touted explanation is that it is austerity after the 2008 financial crisis that led to constraints on health spending, social care and other public spending which then resulted in stalling and even falling life expectancy for some groups. But the outcomes for many European countries cast serious doubt on this often "political" idea. Some countries like Germany and Sweden that adopted no austerity also experienced a slowdown in life expectancy. Other countries like Greece, Spain and Ireland introduced severe austerity policies (many times greater than the UK), but actually saw an increase in life expectancy. So, whilst it may play a part, austerity on its own simply cannot explain changes in overall life expectancy. My own view is that the incredible increase in the numbers of people developing virtually every disease and the fact that young people are developing them and dying at ever younger ages has to be one of the main causes. All of this will be explored in more detail later.

This is the moment to consider another crucial aspect of life that is perhaps just as important as life expectancy itself, and that is healthy life expectancy. Healthy life expectancy means exactly what it says. It is the age before which good health is maintained and people can live a normal life, doing all the things they enjoy like walking, dancing, gardening and going on holiday. But it is the age at which many wide-ranging diseases then start to take hold, significantly affecting normal life. These include heart disease, strokes, Alzheimer's, cancer, arthritis and Parkinson's disease. Average life expectancy in the UK is currently 81, but average healthy life expectancy is just 64. This means that the average person spends the last 17 years of their life (21%) with diseases and conditions that significantly affect their lives. Healthy life expectancy has in fact been declining for a number of years and there is no obvious reason why it will change anytime soon. Medicine has been unable to do anything about this devastating decline in the final chapter of life, but lifestyle medicine really can transform healthy life expectancy and increase it significantly, just as it does for overall life expectancy.

How can you prove that something works to treat disease or promote health?

I'm sure most people believe it must surely be possible to prove conclusively whether a drug or any other treatment actually works or not, how well it works and whether it is safe. However, one only needs to look at the huge numbers of scientifically approved drugs and procedures that have had to be subsequently removed from use or significantly curtailed because they don't work or are dangerous to realise that such "proof" is far more complex and difficult to achieve than most people could ever believe. Medicine, of course, claims clinical trials are the only thing that can prove a treatment really works. They are the "gold standard" of proof and nothing less is acceptable. As we have seen, the drug industry states that the randomised, double blind, placebo-controlled clinical trials cost over $2 billion for the two trials that supposedly provide this definitive proof. So, as well as the fact that even these billion-dollar trials are frequently found to be incorrect, it also means that no one in lifestyle medicine could ever afford to carry them out to prove that what they do works. Consider how much it would cost to prove the benefits of just one single vitamin. Vitamin D has multiple effects and it plays a part in around 100 of the body's main functions which enables them to operate optimally and control overall health and disease prevention and treatment. These include maintaining healthy bones, improving immune response for viral infections like flu and Coronavirus, reducing the risk of heart attacks, strokes, kidney disease, Crohn's disease, colorectal and ovarian cancers and rheumatoid arthritis, to name just a few. But a clinical trial is only designed for, and can only determine, one single outcome. This means that at least 100 sets of two clinical trials would be needed to prove all of vitamin D's benefits, meaning it would cost over $200 billion for just this one vitamin. But there are hundreds of essential natural compounds like vitamins, minerals, amino acids and plant- and animal-based compounds that affect human health, and each of them have multiple functions. There are also countless other key factors that affect health and disease, like diets, exposure to thousands of chemicals, exercise, sleep, mental positivity and hundreds of types of gut bacteria. It would probably take the entire wealth of the world to prove that all these things worked using the clinical trial process. This, quite simply, can never happen.

But the absence of clinical trials doesn't mean these natural substances and other lifestyle factors don't work, because other types of evidence do exist. Can these provide 100% proof? No, nothing can provide 100% proof, because as we have seen, even clinical trials have been proven to be wrong on countless occasions, but the evidence for lifestyle solutions is nevertheless compelling. Despite all of this, and based solely on the fact there are no clinical trials, medicine simply ridicules and dismisses out of hand every natural solution for health and disease treatment. Given such an unequivocal and uncompromising position, you might imagine that everything medicine does must surely be based on clinical trials. So, let's look initially at how well medicine adheres to its own "gold standard" scientific principles. First, do clinical trials give "gold standard evidence"? Second, does medicine use only clinical trials to provide the proof for everything it does?

As we have seen, clinical trials are artificial experiments that only rarely test the people who are going to take the drug or treatment. We have also seen numerous examples of the fundamental flaws in clinical trials, as well as the data manipulation, bias, cherry picking of data and "fraud" that is endemic. We have also looked at the increasing use of trials that are based solely on surrogate end points which often result in no meaningful improvement in people's physical symptoms, or in critical outcomes like life expectancy. All this means no one knows what the real outcomes for new medical drugs and treatments will be until they are given to huge numbers of people in the real world. This is one of the reasons why there are so many medical catastrophes, why so many deaths occur and why most drugs have no benefit at all for most people. Medicine should be demanding and ensuring that clinical trial protocols are improved so they actually start to live up to their so-called gold standard claims and reputation, but, of course, this doesn't happen. But the fatal flaws in clinical trials and medicine's refusal to demand improvements is only one part of the problem because, despite medicine's claim that everything it does is based on science (which means clinical trials), this also is simply not true.

So, which parts of medicine are not based on clinical trials? We have already seen that 20% of all drug prescriptions have no clinical trials to back them up – the so-called off-label drugs. This has been happening for decades usually because of illegal and fraudulent promotion by the pharmaceutical industry who have been fined tens of billions of dollars for it all. In addition, cancer drugs represent 15% of the entire turnover of the drug industry, but only a few have ever been tested in a placebo-controlled clinical trial. Each new drug is, of course, tested, but only against an existing cancer drug, but these are not proper placebo-controlled trials. Medicine claims the reason for this is that it would be unethical to give half the patients in a trial a placebo which they believe would have no effect on the cancer and thus give them worse overall outcomes. There are, however, possible ways around this. People with terminal cancer are still given chemotherapy drugs that are supposed to extend life. But many people refuse to take them because the side effects are so severe they can effectively destroy what life is left. It would, therefore, be quite possible to carry out trials on terminal patients where the drug's real effectiveness was measured by comparing it to a true placebo without running into these ethical issues, but such trials are not carried out. We have already seen that most chemotherapy drugs have tiny benefits, typically just 2%, but the drugs also have severe side effects. Could it be that the drug industry doesn't want to do these trials in case the drug performed worse than the true placebo. This is a real possibility given the severe side effects of the drugs and the potential "placebo effect" from the placebo pill. It is a risk they clearly won't take. But whatever conclusions you draw from all of this, the simple fact is medicine does not use its "gold standard" of proof on most cancer drugs. Just these two examples mean that around 35% of all drugs by value have no clinical trials to back them up.

Polypharmacy was covered in Part 3. It is a treatment regime where mainly older patients are given multiple drugs (typically between five and ten) per day. Clinical trials will have been carried out on the individual drugs, but no trials have ever been carried out to assess the outcomes when these drugs are taken together. Does each drug then work as expected or do drug interactions minimise the benefits or even stop them completely? Are there serious or even potentially lethal side effects from the interactions? Quite simply, no one knows. Interestingly, the drug industry clearly understands that many drugs don't work well when taken together because individual drug trials are carried out mainly on young healthy people who are not taking any other drugs. The reason for this, according to the industry, is that older people usually are taking at least one other drug and this could interfere with the new drug on trial and distort the trial outcome. So, it is a simple fact that even taking just two drugs together can lead to serious outcomes and you only have to look at drug leaflets to find this out. But taking five to ten polypharmacy drugs together? Quite simply, there are no trials, and no one knows whether there are any real benefits, or how dangerous they are. Polypharmacy accounts for another 20% of all drug prescriptions and there is simply no evidence on whether it works or is safe.

Another amazing fact is that no vaccines have ever been tested against a true placebo. For vaccines the placebo should basically be a dilute saline solution, but in fact the "placebos" that are used are either existing similar vaccines, or they contain similar active chemicals that are used in the vaccine itself. These chemicals which are usually known as adjuvants are intended to stimulate the immune system to recognise the dead or partial virus in the vaccine, but the key message is that these chemicals are one of the key causes of vaccine side effects. Putting them in both the vaccine and the placebo means they both have the same detrimental outcomes which then simply hides the side effects of the vaccine. This is another shocking revelation that will be covered in much more detail in Part 5. But again, what this means is that the clinical trials for another significant part of medicine do not follow the "gold standard" rules. In total, and quite amazingly, over half of all drugs that are used do not have truly scientific clinical trials.

Very few surgical practices have ever been tested in clinical trials. They are often developed out of necessity, in a trial and error form. Surgery is carried out and then the outcomes evaluated. This usually leads to changes in practice which are expected to improve outcomes. This process often develops over a number of years. At some point, a particular surgery becomes accepted as a standard treatment, and specialist surgeons are then trained to treat increasing numbers of people. At this stage it may seem unthinkable that the surgery could be causing any harm. Knee surgery is a prime example of this, but some years ago a trial was carried out in which some of the patients were given normal knee surgery, and the others were taken into the operating theatre, given the normal anaesthetics, but then just their skin was cut in the same place that the deep operational incisions would have been made and then stitched up as normal. The actual physical outcomes of the two groups were then independently monitored and analysed. Some of those in the true surgery group did indeed see improvements in their conditions and physical movements, others saw no meaningful change, while a final group saw their conditions worsen. The key result, however, was that there was little difference in overall outcomes for the surgical and non-surgical groups. Before this trial, surgeons would probably never have believed that there could be such little overall benefit. The reality is most surgical practices have not been tested in clinical trials, so their true benefits or dangers are also not known. Consider the use of mesh implants for women. It is true that, in this case, some trials were carried out but the study period was so short that no significant side effects showed up. It was only several years after mesh implant surgery had become common practice that serious and devastating outcomes started to emerge. Trials that are too short to detect side effects are a common flaw in much of medical and drug research. Of course, there are some treatments like hip replacements that have overwhelming benefits. Nevertheless, surgery – just like drugs – has a long list where there are no "gold standard" clinical trials to back them up, and for medicine to then dismiss lifestyle treatments for the same reason is outrageously hypocritical and unscientific.

We will now look at the sort of proof lifestyle medicine can provide. Many natural substances have been tested in trials by medical researchers against standard drug treatments. The herb berberine, for example, was tested in two separate trials against metformin, which is the world's top blood sugar lowering drug for treating type 2 diabetes. Berberine reduced blood sugar by almost exactly the same amount as the drug and did so without any side effects. Medicine accepts this type of trial (testing one drug against another drug) for cancer treatments, but stubbornly refuses to accept it for berberine and other natural compounds. These trials aren't placebo-controlled but, without a hint of shame, medicine accepts one but not the other. A major advantage of natural solutions is that there are rarely any side effects which means people can try them to see if they work without risk, unlike drugs.

The key type of evidence for lifestyle medicine, however, is simply about real-world outcomes for real people. So, what does the average person want from a treatment? They simply want to be cured, or if that is not possible, they want to see a significant improvement in symptoms so they can lead a relatively normal life. Alternatively, they simply want to prevent disease from happening in the first place. Does the average person care about whether the treatment has gone through a $2 billion trial or is the end result the only thing that matters? I'm absolutely sure the outcome is all that matters for nearly everyone, and that is why many people do try lifestyle solutions to see how they work. But let's go back one step and ask why some people actually try them. After all, over many decades, medicine has been portrayed as the pinnacle of mankind's achievements. The NHS is revered by nearly everyone and most people's trust in doctors is absolute. All this means that if you have a health problem, you simply visit your doctor and expect him or her to solve it for you. The problem comes when this doesn't happen. When someone develops pain or a skin condition, like psoriasis, they visit their doctor who (unless there is an exceptional and serious diagnosis) will invariably prescribe a painkiller or a steroid drug. The problem is these drugs will not cure the disease, neither will they eliminate all the symptoms and, of course, most of them will also cause significant side effects. The drugs will usually reduce the symptoms but in many cases not to a level the patient expects, or to a level they can tolerate. Some people do simply accept this and try to learn to live with the condition because they trust medicine so implicitly, but other people will not be prepared to simply accept poor outcomes and the continued suffering this entails. They will be more inquisitive. They may discover a book or go on the web to try to find out more about their condition, where they will learn about, for example, hemp oil supplements which, when they try them, usually work significantly better than conventional painkillers. or about vitamins, probiotics and natural creams that can help with psoriasis with no side effects compared to the serious risks in using steroids, like weight gain. Coincidentally, the National Institute for Health and Care Excellence has just issued a startling recommendation that doctors should stop using several painkilling drugs for certain conditions because there is new evidence that they don't work and they have serious potential side effects. This is clear proof that the original clinical trials were wrong (yet again), but in this case the consequences are serious, including deaths.

There are, as we will see shortly, conventionally trained doctors who use lifestyle treatments, as well as independent nutritionists, organisations like Diabetes.co.uk and Food for the Brain Foundation, plus therapists like acupuncturists, physiotherapists, homeopathists and chiropractors. All of these practitioners and organisations can provide specific lifestyle treatments and advice to help with patients' conditions. There are tens of thousands of them in the UK. If medicine achieved what patients wanted, none of them would be needed. The fact they exist, and in such numbers, is a telling reminder of the severe limitations of medicine for many health conditions. Of course, once people have tried a natural solution and found it often works better than drugs, they may at that stage investigate further and start to read about how lifestyle medicine can help with other conditions, how it can actually prevent diseases from happening in the first place and how it can also increase life expectancy.

There are many treatments that lifestyle medicine has been using for years. During that time, many thousands of people around the world have benefited from most of them and "proved" that they work, except, of course, medicine will never accept this type of proof. We have already seen that a Southport surgery in Merseyside has either reversed type 2 diabetes or brought it under good control in hundreds of patients just by changing their diets. This surgery has saved over £50,000 on diabetes drugs as well as transforming its patients' health and significantly reducing their risk of serious diabetic complications like amputations, blindness, heart attacks and liver disease. Nearly every patient has also achieved significant weight loss. To ignore and dismiss this huge body of evidence from an NHS surgery and its doctors would be shocking and yet, this is exactly what medicine has done. Imagine if the entire town of Southport then adopted this protocol and thousands more patients were cured. Medicine really would still dismiss it and say something like "we don't know what would happen if there was a control group". Even if the entire county of Merseyside, and 100,000 patients were cured, they would still not accept it as proof and probably say "stop all this nonsense now – there are no clinical trials". If it wasn't so tragic, their position would be laughable as well as untenable.

Even the British Medical Journal has effectively mocked medicine's immovable hard-line position. As they point out, parachutes have never been tested in a placebo-controlled trial, so according to medicine, there is no proof they work. A clinical trial would require, say, ten people to be taken up in an aeroplane, five would have a genuine parachute and five would have a dummy parachute that didn't open. They would all jump out. There would, of course, be five deaths and five lives saved. But this would then conclusively prove that parachutes work according to medicine's rigid trial protocol. You might think this is silly and ridiculous (which it is), except for the fact that this is the only way medicine would ever approve any lifestyle solution. To make things even more appalling, remember that medicine does not adhere to its own rigid trial protocols for well over half of all the drugs it uses – including every vaccine – as well as huge swathes of surgery. Now imagine that a senior doctor was up in a two-seater plane and the pilot said they were going to crash and that the doctor should put a parachute on and jump out immediately. Without a clinical trial, the doctor should surely ignore this advice and stick to his rigid principles. Do you think he would sit there and die, or would he put the parachute on and save his own life? The simple fact is it is absolutely clear – even without clinical trials – that parachutes work. The thousands of real-life outcomes for countless lifestyle solutions provide exactly the same sort of proof.

If hundreds or thousands of real people try a lifestyle protocol, like a dietary change, and their condition significantly improves or is cured it would also provide better proof than most clinical trials. Why? Because of the extent of the "fraud", data manipulation and statistical "scams" that are commonplace in these trials, as well as the fact most drugs aren't tested on the people who are actually going to take most of them, so no one knows what the real-life outcomes will be. But as well as its standard get out of jail card of "there are no clinical trials", medicine still has two other rebuttals it usually makes in these circumstances. First, it would say there could be other reasons for the health improvements, rather than the dietary change they all used. It would emphasise that "association is not causation" which is another well-used "get out of jail card". Whilst this is theoretically correct, the odds that, say, 1,000 people who tried the dietary change and saw improvements, just by chance, happened to do something else, like start exercising or reducing their stress levels, independently and all at the same time, which then caused the improvement is, to say the least, extremely unlikely. The odds would be miniscule, and, of course, it would still be another lifestyle change that had actually caused the health improvements. Secondly, medicine could say the benefit may simply be down to the placebo effect. This again is possible, but given that lifestyle solutions are safe and cheap with virtually no side effects, would it really matter (unlikely though it would be) if it really was just the placebo effect and people were cured or saw their condition significantly improve?

Having outlined all this important background information, it is now time to examine in detail the ways lifestyle medicine can radically improve our health and life expectancy.

Lifestyle medicine's main weapons

The human body is supremely complex and for everything in it to work perfectly in the way that nature and 7 million years of evolution intended it to work, the lifestyle you lead is key. This section outlines the seven key factors that, working synergistically together, would help most people live a long and healthy life, minimise the risk of developing most non-communicable diseases and rapidly help the natural immune system to defeat inevitable viral diseases like colds, influenza and COVID-19.

The mind profoundly affects our health

We have already seen how powerful the mind can be in relation to our health when we looked at the placebo effect. Just an idea implanted in our mind that something we are going to do, like taking a pill, will improve, say, our depression, will indeed do just that – even if there is nothing in it but a bit of dried vegetable extract. Of course, this doesn't work for every disease (like infectious diseases) but when it does, it can produce benefits that are as good as, or almost as good as, drugs and, of course, there are no side effects. But the very nature of the thoughts we have in everyday life and the state of our minds are just as – if not more – powerful than even the placebo effect. Even medicine tacitly understands that something medically significant happens when it uses the term stress as a risk factor for many diseases such as heart attacks. The problem is stress in a medical context is so limited it cannot significantly help people who want to prevent such diseases. Of course, the real problem here is that there are no drugs to treat stress and that is why medicine rarely promotes it. It has acknowledged that stress is important, but that is about as far as it goes. It's just an unnecessary distraction compared to the real business of dishing out pills. In spite of this negative bias by medicine's elite, a surprising number of scientific studies have been carried out and the findings are revealing and quite profound. The studies have looked at many different aspects of how the mind affects our health including relationships and social contact, being happy or sad, being optimistic or pessimistic, as well as the conventional medical view of stress.

One American study published in the British Medical Journal in 2001 was entitled "The Hound of the Baskervilles effect: natural experiment on the influence of psychological stress on timing of death". This is quite a weird and obscure name for a scientific study but the findings are actually much easier to understand than the title. In China and Japan, the words "death" and "four" have almost identical pronunciations and so the number four invokes discomfort and apprehension, very much like the way we view the number 13, except that for the Chinese and Japanese the effect is greatly magnified and much more traumatic. The study found that cardiac deaths peak on the fourth day of each month for Americans of Chinese and Japanese descent, and that this pattern is not seen amongst the native US population. The study used computerised US death certificates to examine more than 200,000 Chinese and Japanese deaths and the deaths of 47 million US citizens from 1973 to 1998, making it one of the largest and most comprehensive studies of its kind. So, here is a real, scientifically measurable and proven effect, which is that Chinese and Japanese people die more often on the fourth day of each month. The reason for this seems to be simply that they consider the number four to be unlucky which in turn presumably engenders feelings of anxiety and fear. And although no one can fully explain it in mechanistic scientific terms, its effect is so powerful that it can change when people die. Witch doctors in countries like Haiti have also caused healthy people to die by cursing them and telling them they would die. Fear then did the rest. I also remember a case about 40 years ago of a man who was given a terminal cancer diagnosis. He was given about 12 months to live. Just over a year later he died. But for some reason the doctors decided that an autopsy would be carried out. What they found came as a complete shock. There was not even a trace of cancer; neither could any other cause of death be established. He died, it seemed, because he knew he would. When his medical records were checked, his original X-ray did not show any cancer either. It is possible that somehow the wrong X-ray had been inadvertently used for the diagnosis. These various examples are unexpected and difficult to believe, but, as Albert Einstein said, "Not everything that can be measured matters, and not everything that matters can be measured."

The INTERHEART study was a large study involving 52 countries and 29,000 people which examined risk factors for heart disease. As part of this study, psychosocial wellbeing was measured and its effect was significant. The lead researcher Annika Rosengren, professor of cardiology at Gothenburg University, said, "Collectively, these measures were responsible for about one-third of the risk of the population studies. Persistent severe stress makes it two and a half times more likely that an individual will have a heart attack compared with someone who is not stressed. The INTERHEART study shows that stress is one of the most important factors in heart attacks in all ethnic groups and in all countries."

The mainstream response to this study was predictable, and best encapsulated by Professor Sir Charles George, medical director of the British Heart Foundation. He did say that the results "suggested" that stress might have more of a role as a cause of heart attacks than many people had previously thought, however, he then went on to say that the findings were the result of people's own "self-reported" stress which may not be reliable. In such a casually dismissive fashion, the evidence about stress is simply swept under the carpet by medical experts, but they should not have done so and here is the reason why. The only way the effectiveness of drugs for conditions like pain can be assessed and then approved is by simply asking patients to assess how well they work and their views are then simply accepted. So, why were similar views simply dismissed in the INTERHEART study with the claim they may be unreliable? This is just one more example of medicine's determination to dismiss every health solution that doesn't involve drugs.

In the early 1960s the town of Roseto in Pennsylvania had significantly less heart disease than its neighbouring town of Bangor. Roseto's community of 1,600 was made up almost entirely of immigrant Italians while the 5,000 people in Bangor were an ethnic mix. The head of medicine Stewart Wolf and sociologist John Bruhn set out to investigate what would later become known as the "Roseto effect". They looked mainly at men aged 55 to 64 since this age group suffered a high incidence of heart disease in the wider population. In Roseto the rate was close to zero. There were two other statistics that caught the eye. In Roseto the crime rate was zero and applications for public assistance were also zero. So, what did all this have to do with heart disease and longevity? Further investigation revealed that nearly all the men had hazardous jobs in the local mines and their diet was appalling by conventional medical standards. But the way they lived was very un-American. Three generations of a family lived under the same roof, with the elderly being the most venerated. Rosetons also appeared to do everything together: evening walks, social clubs, church festivals. The sense of community was palpable even though, by any standard, the whole town was poor. The research of Wolf and Bruhn covered a 50-year period from 1935 to 1985. They discovered that the Rosetons very low rates of heart attack started to "normalise" from 1965 onwards and this coincided with increased prosperity for the town when its residents started to move from the old town centre to the newly built suburbs which slowly destroyed the community bonds that used to exist. By 1985 there were no differences in longevity or heart attack rates between the two towns. In their book about the Roseto effect, Wolf and Bruhn wrote, "People are nourished by other people." In essence, Roseto was a demonstration of the old homily that a problem shared is a problem halved. People supported each other and no one felt completely isolated, despairing or stressed. A sense of community and sharing was even more important in determining health than were other lifestyle choices such as diet and even smoking, factors that would normally contribute to heart disease. Roseto isn't unique. Many other studies have noted the importance of community in helping people live long and healthy lives. The Amish, for example, whose community spirit is legendary, continue to benefit from good health and longevity. They even use conventional medicine only sparingly.

If community and a sense of belonging is a safeguard against disease and also benefits longevity, what happens when people feel social isolation? Two major studies in California and eastern Finland set about finding out and these involved over 20,000 people. The conclusions are stark. Those people lacking in social relationships and who felt lonely were nearly three times more likely to die of heart disease and other causes than those who felt connected. Researchers from Brigham Young University in Utah were intrigued by this research and set about analysing all the individual studies they could find. In total they analysed 148 studies that included 308,849 people who were assessed for an average of seven years. They were astonished by the impact of social interaction, community and relationships on our mortality. Living with a partner and being socially active with lots of friends increases your chance of living longer by an average of 50% compared with someone who lives alone and is isolated. Yet doctors rarely mention this when advising their older patients about healthy old age. The researchers estimated that isolation was as devastating as smoking 15 cigarettes a day and twice as harmful as being obese. They described it as one of the biggest, and yet generally unrecognised, causes of nearly all diseases. The crucial role of social interaction was first noticed years ago amongst children in orphanages and custodial care. Those who had little or no human contact often died suddenly and this observation dramatically changed the way children in care were treated. Today, there is enormous emphasis placed on contact and social interaction.

Tim Smith, the lead researcher in Utah, said, "Physicians, health professionals, educators and the media take risk factors such as smoking, diet and exercise seriously. The data we present makes a compelling case for social relationship factors to be added to that list." But as you will perhaps realise, this has not happened. A recent US study has also linked the development of dementia with the increasing levels of loneliness affecting the elderly. The researchers showed that loneliness can trigger inflammatory responses in the brain, which in turn can lead to neural changes associated with dementia. Other studies have made the same conclusions. Isolation and loneliness can significantly affect the lives of young children. Those who endure loneliness are far more likely to suffer from heart disease as an adult.

How old do you feel? Recent research published in the Journal of Gerontology shows that it is more important than you may think. In fact, it turns out to be even more important than how old you actually are. Feeling younger than you are can actually keep your mind sharper for longer. But if you start to feel older than your actual age, your brain will also follow suit and age more rapidly. The study involved nearly 6,000 people aged between 65 and 98 with normal cognitive function. The researchers found that just feeling older made patients 18% more likely to suffer cognitive impairment. It also meant they were 30% more likely to eventually develop dementia.

Optimism is a major factor in living a longer life and preventing disease, while pessimism does exactly the opposite. A new study published in 2019 confirms what many other studies and other experts have advocated for many years. Previous studies had reported that optimistic individuals are less likely to die prematurely or suffer from chronic diseases. The 2019 study indicated that the group with the most optimistic people (upper quartile) had a 15% increase in life expectancy compared to the group with the most pessimistic (lower quartile). This would mean in the real world, where average life expectancy is nearly 82, that the most optimistic people will live around six years longer and the most pessimistic people will live around six years less than the average person. This must also mean that the optimists delay the serious diseases like heart attacks that result in most deaths and that pessimists succumb to them sooner. There are many other aspects of our "mental and emotional state" that affect our health and longevity, and that have been the subject of scientific studies. Here are some key points of just a few of them.

Overall, people with religious beliefs have positive health and longevity outcomes, although a recent study has shed new light on this. Those people with positive spiritual beliefs – such as God always loves them and forgives their shortcomings – have the best outcomes in terms of health. Those who have negative spiritual beliefs – such as believing that God's punishment is the cause of their illness or who otherwise believe in a "fire and brimstone" God – actually see their health worsen.

People who lead destructive lives also fare badly in terms of health. "Neighbours from hell" or those who take pleasure in dominating and humiliating others are typical examples.

Of course, those on the receiving end are also badly affected in terms of health. On the other hand, people who like to help and are kind to others will have this repaid by better health and longevity. Playing music and singing also have significant and positive effects on our emotions and this also applies to other creative hobbies like painting.

Perhaps unsurprisingly, medicine seems sceptical that "positive" thoughts and emotions can enhance health and increase longevity, probably because it would undermine the "pill for every ill" concept. Despite this scepticism, positive emotions really do have incredible benefits and there is overwhelming evidence to support it. Here are some key examples of these emotions that affect our health and longevity either positively or negatively:

Healthy Emotions	**Unhealthy Emotions**
Happiness	Cynicism
Positive mindset	Pessimism
Optimism	Laziness
Conscientiousness	Resentment
Purposefulness	Negative thoughts
Hard working	Anger
Caring	Self-centredness
Resilience	Despair
High self-esteem	Loneliness
Satisfaction	Self-pity
Love	Dissatisfaction
Hope	Fear
Forgiveness	Superstition

Of course, there are also many "external" factors that affect our mental state and thus our health.

Positive Factors	**Negative Factors**
Close relationships	Physical and mental abuse
Supports from family and friends	Broken relationships
Social activities	Bullying boss
Educational attainments	Racism
Music	Social isolation
Singing	Forced migration
Creative hobbies	Money worries

If you can tick most of these positive and healthy boxes and very few of the negative ones, you are well on the way to a long and healthy life. You might feel after what you have read that if you've got your emotional life and stress under control there is not much more you need to do. But that would be a mistake. Most of the scientific studies have looked at heart disease and the message here is clear. Your very thoughts, emotions and stress levels really can reduce your risk by around 30–50%. Given that heart disease is still the biggest killer, this is, of course, of great significance, but what about other diseases?

The studies all show our mental state has an effect on virtually every disease but the extent is less well defined and may not be as high as for heart disease. The biggest factors for type 2 diabetes, for example, are likely to be a poor diet and lack of exercise. As far as cancer is concerned, the few studies that exist do show a link with our emotions and stress, and many people in lifestyle medicine think this link is highly significant as we will see later, but the true extent is unclear and, of course, there are many other factors involved. So, the message is clear. Work hard on optimising your emotions and stress levels, but the other factors we are about to examine are all vitally important and even more important for certain aspects of health and disease control.

How do positive emotions actually work in reducing the risk of heart attacks and increasing life expectancy, and indeed how does the reverse happen with negative emotions? The human body is, as we have seen, so complex it is impossible to say with absolute certainty. But part of the answer is that thoughts are not just confined to the mind. We can experience some of them in our bodies. Think about "butterflies" in the stomach when you are anxious, or blushing, or the intensity of the fight or flight response to a sudden fright. Positive emotions cause the body to manufacture and release hormones that have a positive effect on our health and happiness, such as serotonin. Negative emotions can produce excess hormones, like cortisol, that can cause a number of conditions like affecting sleep. Adrenaline is a hormone that rapidly activates the body's sympathetic nervous system so it can respond to "fight or flight" situations. However, recurring levels of anxiety and fear can result in continuously high levels of adrenaline which can affect blood pressure, heart rate, breathing and many other factors which all increase the risk of heart disease. So, while the exact reasons are not all known, the facts are simple and logical. Positive emotions are a major factor in helping to prevent disease and increasing life expectancy. Negative emotions do the reverse.

We have already seen that diseases like heart attacks are many times higher in countries like Ukraine compared to countries like France. France is noted for its social interactions and its "relaxed" way of life, whereas life in Communist and former Communist countries is dire by comparison. Countries like Ukraine and Russia have very low average life expectancy (around 73 years), and many other places are also effectively ruled by dictators and people are helpless to do anything about it without risking their lives. Despair, fear and pessimism prevail, while positive thinking and positive emotions rarely exist. It is little wonder that life expectancy is low (around 67 for men in Russia) and that diseases like heart attacks are high. Of course, there are still many other factors like diet and physical activity that also play a significant role, but negative emotions are possibly one of the key causes in these countries. Indeed, even in the west, this almost certainly played a part in our overall health in the 1930s and 1940s. We have seen how heart attacks rose by 1000% between 1930 and 1950. But this was when the Great Depression and World War II were occurring and these must have had a significant impact on people's mental and emotional health and almost certainly played a part in the increase in heart disease. Having made this point, changes in diet were almost certainly the major cause and this will be examined in detail in Part 5.

Food – the key factor in our health

I'll start this section with an extract from an article by the Alliance for Natural Health International in relation to the physical, mental and emotional problems the current Coronavirus pandemic is causing worldwide and about what food can do to help restore societal wellbeing:

> One of the key levers you can use to reset or reboot your resilience is food. Plain and simple. Food is not just a fuel or energy carrier, a mere delivery system for calories, it's a rich source of "information" that informs every cell and action in our bodies, including turning on and off genes. That's why it really matters what food you eat, when you eat it, how you prepare it and what state of mind you are in when you eat it. It's the flow of information that you ingest, provided your gut is healthy enough to assimilate it, that determines a lot more of our experience of life than many realise. This seems like a bold claim, but consider that food was our first and, for a significant time, our only medicine and it will make sense why so many of our biochemical processes and pathways are reliant on molecules we must eat in our food. Your food has the power to create health, alter your trajectory if you're heading down a disease pathway, reset your metabolism, put out the fire of inflammation, turn on powerfully protective cellular mechanisms and so much more. All of which helps to create a level of resilience and flexibility in your mind and body that allows you to meet the challenges of modern life with far less stress and damaging outcomes.

The food we eat is the most important lifestyle factor in maintaining health and avoiding disease. All the other factors that will be explored are vitally important and add specific and crucial benefits, but the food you eat really is the key. There is, however, nothing that involves more controversy and disagreement than that of diet. Which diet is best for our health? There are quite literally hundreds and maybe thousands of them including all their variations. Take your pick from just a tiny selection:

- UK government dietary guidelines
- US government dietary guidelines
- All the other dozens of government dietary guidelines (they all have differences by the way)
- The Paleo diet
- The Stone Age diet
- The low GI diet
- The Atkins diet
- The Mediterranean diet
- The Cretan diet
- The vegetarian diet
- The vegan diet
- The low carbohydrate diet
- The low fat diet
- The high protein diet
- The Weight Watchers diet
- The South Beach diet
- The 5–2 diet
- The 6–1 diet

- The alternate day diet
- The cabbage diet
- The bread and beer diet (sorry, I couldn't resist it. I made this one up – or at least I hope I did)

Confused? It's probably not surprising. However, there is one vital point. I don't know anyone who doesn't agree that diet is a crucial factor in our health, and that includes even those in medicine who are most sceptical about the influence of lifestyle on health. So, if everyone agrees that diet is crucially important, why is there no agreement on what constitutes the best diet for our health? Why are people left to make near impossible choices? Why are there major disagreements even within the official medical community? Why have no researchers ever carried out definitive research to establish at least a reasonable assessment of an "optimum diet"? The brutal truth is there are numerous and powerful vested interest groups that will make sure this never happens because it would threaten their entire businesses. Genuinely independent research would spell disaster for the sugar industry, the processed food industry, the chemical companies that supply all the processed food additives and the soft drink industry to name but a few. And don't forget, the pharmaceutical industry needs sick people; it doesn't want everyone on a healthy diet which would precipitously reduce its drug sales.

Governments, nevertheless, still issue their dietary guidelines. So, can you trust these? Sadly, if you want to stay healthy, they are the very last thing you should ever look at. Why? Because these guidelines are simply the end result of intense lobbying by powerful organisations, industries and companies. The sugar lobby demands sugar levels are not set too low; the artificial sweetener industry promotes its widespread use even though it can be just as dangerous as sugar; the dairy lobby wants the recommendations to include substantial amounts of its products even though many people have allergic reactions to dairy products; the grain industry lobbies for high levels of wheat and corn, even though there is strong evidence that the highly refined grains that most of them are turned into are almost as dangerous as sugar. Even the dieticians in the NHS – who actually draw up the dietary guidelines for the government – receive sponsorship for their conferences from the likes of Coca Cola, and so, even they are compromised. The whole thing ends up being a misleading and unscientific compromise, depending simply on the influence of the various industries and companies involved. Even harmful foods still end up being included in the guidelines. But there is one other key factor that makes them unreliable. This is the absolute, but misguided belief in the need for low fat in the diet. We will explore this in much more detail later.

One important fact is the key nutrient types the body needs. There are two main groups: macronutrients and micronutrients. There are four macronutrients: fat, protein, carbohydrates and water and these have their own main roles. They provide energy and allow the body to grow, repair itself and function perfectly. Micronutrients include all vitamins and minerals and are just as essential for life even though they are needed in much smaller quantities. One other fact we now know with certainty is that there is no single diet that works perfectly for everyone. This is because of the unique and complex differences in the human body, in the way people live their lives, as well as other factors like their emotions, levels of physical activity and crucial differences in their microbiome.

So, if you can't rely on government dietary guidelines and there are so many other confusing options as well as understanding that there is no absolute one size fits all diet for everyone, what can you do? Don't panic. The first step is to eliminate the extreme diets and certainly nearly all the celebrity diets. Many of these can be harmful because they are so restrictive. They should certainly not form part of a long-term healthy diet. But that still leaves many options. The situation is, however, not nearly as impossible as it may seem. Most of the truly reputable diets agree on a number of key things, such as:

- Plant-based foods, particularly vegetables, are universally accepted as one of the keys to good health.
- Fruits are mostly good, but minimise those high in sugars, especially fruit juices like orange juice.
- Fish is widely recommended.
- Certain organic meats, like chicken, lamb and beef, can be eaten in moderation. It's important not to burn them.
- Natural fats like olive and coconut oils, lard, butter and cheese, and fats in foods like seeds and nuts.
- Other important foods are pulses, seeds, herbs, beans and mushrooms.

There are, however, disastrously unhealthy foods that you should really try to give up, or at least cut down drastically. These include sugar, high fructose corn syrup, synthetic low calorie sweeteners, highly refined products like white flour and white bread, hydrogenated vegetable oils, trans-fats and industrialised foods that contain dangerous chemicals. Nearly all of these are found in processed and particularly ultra-processed foods and these should be drastically minimised. They don't just contain these unhealthy foods like trans-fats, hidden sugars and chemicals galore, but they also have low levels of essential nutrients like vitamins, minerals and fibre because of the incredible levels of industrialised manufacturing that are used to make them. How dangerous can ultra-processed foods be? A February 2021 study found that those with the highest intake of ultra-processed foods were, on average, 58% more likely to die of cardiovascular disease compared to those with the lowest intake, 52% more likely to die of ischemic heart disease, and 26% more likely to die from any cause. As noted by the authors, "These findings should serve as an incentive for limiting consumption of ultra-processed foods and encouraging natural or minimally processed foods."

There is another important point relating to fats. As well as saturated fats, the other two key types are omega 3 and omega 6 fats. Omega 3 is found naturally in foods like fish, nuts and seeds like flax and chia, while omega 6 is found naturally in foods like poultry, eggs, walnuts and seeds like pumpkin and sunflower. Both of these are essential for good health. However, throughout most of mankind's history, the ratio eaten naturally has been around 1:1. But when vegetable oils like sunflower, corn and soybean were developed and manufactured, they started to be used extensively. Natural oils and fats like lard, butter and olive and coconut oils were quickly replaced by these omega 6-based vegetable oils because they were cheaper. They are used almost universally in processed foods and even most restaurants and cafes. Before I learnt about lifestyle medicine, I (and probably most other people) also started to use sunflower and corn oils for cooking thinking they must be healthier than the saturated fats that were being officially demonised. All this has resulted in the average person now eating up to 20 times more omega 6 than omega 3. This really is a major health issue, not just because of the high level of omega 6, but because these vegetable oils are subject to damage and oxidation due to the industrial processing used. Studies have shown they significantly increase overall mortality and are a major cause of all inflammatory diseases like obesity and fatty liver disease. Most lifestyle medicine advocates would recommend a significant reduction in vegetable oils, but would also recommend not to reduce your fat intake overall. Just try to replace as many vegetable oils as you can with fats like lard, butter, avocado oil and extra virgin olive oil for cooking, and fats like flaxseed, walnut oils and olive oil for non-cooking use. Also keep eating the natural and essential omega 6 foods like eggs, poultry, walnuts and seeds like pumpkin and sunflower. Of course, the food industry companies who make vegetable oils claim they are perfectly safe, but this, of course, is exactly what the tobacco industry also claimed about cigarettes for over 30 years.

All of these key facts could form the basis of a healthy diet for nearly everyone. A remaining controversial part is deciding on the remainder of the diet and what to do about things like carbohydrates. When I look at specific diseases like heart disease and type 2 diabetes in more detail, the importance of diet, and in particular the controversial role that carbohydrates and fats play, will be analysed in much more detail. While the foods we eat are a vital part of lifestyle medicine, there are a huge number of options with a wide range of benefits, and understanding all of this is important to enable you to choose your own diet. If there is something you really don't like, don't feel you should eat it just because it's classed as healthy. There are usually many alternatives that have similar health-giving properties. So, most people can work out a healthy diet that they really do enjoy. Quite simply, I have never enjoyed food throughout my entire life as much as I do now, even though nearly all of it consists of natural foods with a significant proportion of vegetables. One of the keys is to find things that add flavours and tastes you really enjoy. You do not have to suffer to be healthy. However, even though I have outlined many of the key facts, this is something that really does need additional reading. I will make recommendations at the end of this section.

You may be wondering if there is any real proof that the food we eat can radically affect our health. Well, quite simply, throughout the book, you will find information on a number of large-scale observational studies – the ones that follow large groups of people over many years and assess the effects of their various lifestyles – that do indeed show that healthy lifestyles, including diet, result in less disease and increased longevity. Clinical trials, however, are less numerous for the simple reason that Big Pharma controls most medical research and it is not going to fund any trial that promotes natural solutions. Nevertheless, some trials are carried out. The examples I am going to quote relate to extra virgin olive oil, nuts and oily fish. The results are impressive and compelling. Eating nuts, extra virgin olive oil and oily fish (or fish oil supplements) can significantly reduce the number of heart attacks and other cardiovascular diseases (CVDs) by around 30%. Here is a summary of the paper published in the British Medical Journal by Dr Aseem Malhotra, one of Britain's leading cardiologists:

> Changes in diet can rapidly improve outcomes of CVD as demonstrated by several randomised trials. In the DART trial, 2,033 survivors of heart attacks who were advised to eat fatty fish had a significant 29% reduction in all-cause mortality compared with control patients. The survival curves separated within months. Likewise, in the GISSI prevention trial, 1g of omega 3 fatty acids significantly reduced all-cause mortality and cardiovascular mortality in 11,324 heart attack survivors. Survival curves separated early with a significant reduction in total mortality after just three months of treatment.
>
> The PREDIMED primary prevention randomised controlled trial found that an energy unrestricted diet, supplemented with extra virgin olive oil or nuts achieved an impressive 30% reduction in major cardiovascular events in over 7,500 high-risk individuals initially free of CVD. This reduction occurred within three months. Furthermore, this solid clinical trial evidence builds on a wealth of existing data from observational, cohort and secondary prevention studies. It also provides further strong causal evidence that simple diet interventions can rapidly and powerfully reduce CVD outcomes. It is the abundant alpha linoleic acid, polyphenols and omega 3 fatty acids found in olive oil, nuts and oily fish that rapidly exert positive health

effects by attenuating inflammation, atherosclerosis and thrombosis. Conversely, the consumption of trans-fats commonly found in fast food can rapidly increase C reactive protein and other inflammatory markers within weeks.

A 30% reduction in cardiovascular events such as heart attacks, as well as significant reductions in overall mortality, simply by adding extra virgin olive, nuts and fish oils to a diet might seem implausible, but here is not just one, but three impeccable, randomised clinical trials that prove just that.

Another study published in the New England Journal of Medicine examined the outcomes of two of the largest epidemiological studies ever carried out: the Nurses' Health Study and the Health Professional's Follow-Up Study. It examined the specific outcomes related to nut consumption. This also confirmed a 29% reduction in deaths from heart disease for those who ate a daily handful of nuts, but it also showed an 11% lower chance of dying from cancer. Over a 30-year period, all-cause death rates were reduced by 11% for those who ate nuts once a week, and up to 20% when eaten every day. A new 2021 study has also shown that people over the age of 50 who eat nuts five times per week also have improved cognitive function.

I have concentrated on these three foods so you can see the wide range of powerful evidence that exists on their incredible benefits. However, similar evidence exists for many other healthy foods and here is one of the most important types. I've said that plant-based foods like vegetables are one of the keys to good health so here is some of the evidence. The BROAD study and several others show plant-based diets reduce the risk of heart attacks by 40% and strokes by 29%. They also form the basis for tackling many other diseases like type 2 diabetes and obesity.

Sadly, the response of medicine's elite to all this evidence is predictable for all the reasons we have already explored in detail. There is no recommendation that people should start using these incredibly beneficial foods. But despite medicine's stance, I include extra virgin olive oil, nuts, fish oils and a range of vegetables in my diet every single day and my heart health, like blood pressure and heart rate, is just as impressive as it was when I was in my early thirties and at the peak of natural health.

Finally, here are my key book recommendations for essential reading on healthy foods and diets:

- *Reset Eating* by Rob Verkerk and Meleni Aldridge
- *Low GL Diet Bible* by Patrick Holford

Exercise

Yes, the dreaded word: exercise. There is, I'm afraid, no easy way to say it. Physical activity is really important to your overall health and longevity. Can I hear the agonised groans as I write this? Do I have to start running long distances or even marathons, you might be thinking. Well, actually, marathons are probably one of the worst things you could do. The human body was not really designed to run marathons as Pheidippides found out to his cost after he ran from Marathon to Athens and promptly died. I have never had so many colds and muscle problems or felt as tired as when I used to run marathons myself. After about three years, I saw the light and reduced my runs to a more sensible distance.

Running is excellent, but for many people this is not possible, nor is it necessary, because walking is also an excellent form of exercise. The only problem is it doesn't necessarily get the heart working much faster, which, as we will see, is important. You could, of course, simply go out and walk faster to get your heart rate up. But this may take away some of the pleasure of the walk and not everyone will want to do it. This is where a recent exercise discovery could help. "High intensity interval training", or HIIT for short, was developed for busy working people with limited time for exercise. Fifteen minutes of HIIT can give the same health benefits as an hour of normal exercise. What is it and how does it work? It simply involves a number of repeated, short bursts of intense effort of around 30 or 40 seconds, interspersed with slower recovery periods lasting around two to four minutes. It can be used for most types of exercises such as running, rowing and biking. Ideally, it requires the short bursts to be carried out at, or close to, your maximum capacity. If you are running, for example, you need to do fast sprints. However, unless you are already a fairly serious athlete, doing something like this would be pretty dangerous. But it really can be modified for all levels of fitness. You would probably not get all the potential benefits, but you would certainly get many of them. So, if your preferred exercise is walking and you haven't done anything more strenuous for a while, it is vital that you start slowly and build up slowly. Do perhaps half your walk as normal to allow your muscles to warm up. Then stride out at a faster pace for say 20 paces, slow down again for a short period and then do the same again. Over a few weeks or even months, slowly build up the number, the intensity and the duration of the higher intensity walking. Because you are walking and you will not be going "flat out", these can be increased to say ten on each walk. They don't need to last any longer than about 40 seconds, with slower recovery periods in between of around two or three minutes. Depending on what suits you and what you feel capable of, you could do less or even more. The key thing is simply to get walking and eventually reach a total of around two and a half hours each week with an average of something like 30 minutes five days a week.

There are many other types of resistance exercise, like weight training, press-ups and sit-ups, that are also very beneficial but there are so many good guides I won't go into any more detail. The choice of exercise is very personal – the main thing is to get motivated. Just remember that aerobic exercise – exercise that gets the heart beating faster – is very important. There are many other activities like dancing that are also very good for your health. One more key thing people should do, particularly as they get older, is to retain flexibility by doing various stretching exercises. Again, there are many possibilities like using a range of yoga positions. It all depends on your individual preferences.

But is there any proof that exercise really works and improves our health and longevity? Well, cast your mind back to the very first page when I said that around 30% of all the major chronic diseases could be prevented simultaneously by just one lifestyle intervention, and that you should not dismiss this seemingly ridiculous claim because the evidence comes from none other than the NHS itself. Well, that intervention just happens to be exercise. The NHS and medicine rarely advocate lifestyle solutions to health because of their close and financially rewarding ties with the pharmaceutical industry. So, when they do recommend a lifestyle solution, you know the evidence is overwhelming and indisputable. Here – word for word – is what the official NHS website has to say:

> Step right up. It's the miracle cure we've all been waiting for.
>
> It can reduce your risk of major illnesses such as heart disease, stroke, type 2 diabetes and cancer by up to 50% and lower your risk of early death by up to 30%.
>
> It's free, easy to take, has an immediate effect and you don't need a GP to get some. Its name? Exercise.

Exercise is the miracle cure we've always had, but for too long we've neglected to take our recommended dose. Our health is now suffering as a consequence.

This is no snake oil. Whatever your age, there's strong scientific evidence that being physically active can help you lead a healthier and even a happier life.

Research shows that physical activity can also boost self-esteem, mood, sleep quality, and energy, as well as reducing your risk of stress, depression, dementia and Alzheimer's disease.

"If exercise were a pill, it would be one of the most cost-effective drugs ever invented," says Dr Nick Cavill.

Given the overwhelming evidence, it seems obvious that we should be physically active. It's essential if you want to live a healthy and fulfilling life into old age.

It is medically proven that people who do regular physical activity have:

- up to a 35% lower risk of coronary heart disease and stroke
- up to a 50% lower risk of type 2 diabetes
- up to a 50% lower risk of colon cancer
- up to a 20% lower risk of breast cancer
- a 30% lower risk of early death
- up to a 63% lower risk of osteoarthritis
- up to a 68% lower risk of hip fracture
- a 30% lower risk of falls – amongst older adults
- up to a 30% lower risk of depression
- up to a 30% lower risk of dementia

To stay healthy, adults should try to be active daily and to aim for at least 150 minutes of physical activity over a week through a variety of activities.

For most people, the easiest way to get moving is to make activity part of everyday life, like walking or cycling instead of using the car to get around. However, the more you do, the better, and taking part in activities such as sports and exercise will make you even healthier.

For any type of activity to benefit your health you need to be moving quick enough to raise your heart rate, breathe faster and feel warmer. This level of effort is called moderate intensity activity. One way to tell if you're working at a moderate intensity is if you can still talk but you can't sing the words to a song.

If your activity requires you to work even harder, it is called vigorous intensity activity. There is substantial evidence that vigorous activity can bring health benefits over and above that of moderate activity. You can tell when it's vigorous activity because you're breathing hard and fast, and your heart rate has gone up quite a bit. If you're working at this level, you won't be able to say more than a few words without pausing for breath.

If you are not truly amazed by what you have just read, I'll be very surprised. I've heard many people who advocate lifestyle medicine eulogise about the benefits of exercise. But, for once, I have to congratulate the NHS for doing exactly the same and in such a clear, unambiguous and scientific manner. This, however, is where the praise ends. I have to point out that something is very, very wrong. Why? Look at the list of benefits that exercise brings. It contains all the big killer and life-destroying diseases. We are looking at a potential 20–50% reduction in risk. Imagine a world where there were, on average, 30% fewer cases of heart attacks, strokes, diabetes, dementia, Alzheimer's, depression and some major cancers. As well as saving millions of premature deaths around the world and reducing the anguish of diseases like dementia and Alzheimer's, it would transform the NHS, which would be able to offer far better and timelier care for the much-reduced number of other sick people and it would not be so financially distressed.

Remember that currently there are no drugs or medical treatments available that can prevent any of the diseases listed (except for heart disease, and even these have a limited benefit). But exercise can actually prevent, on average, around 30% of all of them simultaneously! This is truly sensational information. The scandal is (I will almost guarantee) that neither you, nor virtually anyone else, knows anything about it. The information may be on the NHS website but it is not being promoted. There are no big publicity campaigns, no media coverage; doctors are not using this incredible information to recommend exercise on any significant scale. Not many people by themselves would find this information on the NHS website because it is not easy to find and I only found it by accident when I was researching this section.

However, if a drug had been developed that could prevent a third of all the major chronic diseases, it would be headline news around the world for months. It wouldn't be hidden away in a hard to find section of the NHS website. It would be promoted so widely that literally everyone would know about it. It would be proclaimed as the greatest medical breakthrough since antibiotics were discovered, and indeed, it would be exactly that. However, whilst the incredible benefits of exercise are on the NHS website, they are not being promoted and quite shockingly, virtually no one knows anything about them. Surely everyone should know these incredible facts. Some really would ignore it just like those who smoke ignore its consequences, but there is little doubt that most people would then choose the path to incredible health by adopting it.

When I read the NHS article and then found out that not one of my friends and acquaintances knew anything about it either, I was so angry I started writing letters to every medical organisation in the country asking why virtually no one knew about this potentially life-changing information. The replies simply kept quoting the existing and failing policies and never answered my questions. It was then I decided to write an open letter to all Members of Parliament. I also wrote three separate letters to the Medical Royal Colleges and the National Institute for Health and Care Excellence but did not receive a single reply. I believe the information and questions are so important I will reproduce in full the letter to the House of Commons and the final letter that I sent to the Medical Royal Colleges and NICE.

To all members of the House of Commons

18th March 2018

Dear Member of Parliament,

Heart disease, strokes, dementia, cancer and diabetes: these are the major life-taking and life-destroying diseases that people most fear. They account for nearly two-thirds of all deaths and a major part of the NHS is given over to dealing with them. Even those people who survive will often live with a dark cloud hanging over them for the rest of their lives.

But how many people know that nearly a third of these diseases (on average) can be prevented by physical activity? The answer is virtually no one. You may be surprised and shocked to know that even most doctors and medical students don't know either. This is why I am writing to you directly in the hope that you will apply pressure to change this inexplicable situation. The attached open letter to the Medical Royal Colleges and the National Institute for Health and Care Excellence explains everything but let me add a little more detail here first.

Eighteen months ago, I discovered, by chance, the section on the miraculous benefits of exercise on the NHS website. I learnt that exercise is the most effective scientifically proven tool available for combating disease that has ever been discovered – with the possible exception of antibiotics. Ever since, I've been trying to understand why almost no one knows anything about it.

I have written to all the organisations involved in healthcare asking why exercise has effectively been side-lined. These include the Department of Health, NHS England, Health Education England, Public Health England, and the General Medical Council. In each case I was told that wide-ranging policies are in place to promote exercise. But how can this be true when no one knows about its very specific and miraculous benefits and when only 14% of the population do any meaningful exercise?

But learning that even doctors and medical students are not taught about exercise except in a vague qualitative way was the most shocking discovery. Medical curricula and guidelines are controlled by the Medical Royal Colleges and NICE so I wrote to them asking if they could defend why they are not seriously promoting physical activity as a major medical treatment.

Neither of them replied. I then wrote to the Department of Health asking if they could apply pressure and persuade them to respond. But I was told that these organisations are independent of government and there was nothing they could do to help. That is why the only way forward was to write the attached open letter. I am asking you to take action because this is no small thing. The scope for saving and transforming lives is enormous.

Each year a million people and their families face the devastating consequences of a diagnosis of one of the main life-taking and life-destroying diseases. Given that, on average, exercise could prevent nearly a third of all these diseases, it means 300,000 people each year are developing serious diseases that could be prevented. In addition, around 10 million people suffer from depression and exercise could prevent up to 30% or 3 million cases.

Medicine really should be embarrassed that it is not taking decisive action to prevent all of this, but I care more about people's health and lives than medicine's embarrassment. I hope you do too.

I hope you will ask some serious questions and help bring about change.

Yours sincerely,

Anthony Armstrong

Final comments

In case you have any lingering doubts as to how powerful exercise can be, consider these two quotes from the 2014/2015 House of Commons Health Select Committee report on exercise:

"We know of no other intervention with greater promise than physical exercise to reduce the risk of virtually all chronic diseases simultaneously." University of Bedfordshire

"If physical activity were a drug then the ranges of its benefits on mental well-being, mental illness, heart disease, obesity, diabetes and osteoporosis is such that no politician would dare withhold those benefits from the public. At a time when the NHS struggles to cope with the pressures of mental illness, obesity and diabetes, it is financially irresponsible to fail to promote physical activity." Transport and Health Study Group

Also, please don't be put off by the word exercise, or think that most people won't do it because it sounds like something that only serious athletes can do. A brisk 30-minute walk five times a week will achieve most of the benefits outlined.

I also need to tell you that the organisations involved will probably use the following arguments to defend the current status quo. They will say there are several medical initiatives in place to promote exercise. These will include the NHS Diabetes Prevention Programme and social prescribing. They may also say that Public Health England has the remit to promote exercise and that it also has a number of ongoing initiatives like One You, Couch to 5K and Active10.

Please do not be lulled into a false sense of security by these sorts of arguments. At the very most the total number of people involved in all these individual initiatives is no more than 2 million. This may sound a lot but it is only 4% of the entire adult population. These programmes are better than nothing but they are not the solution that will change the health of the other 48 million adults who are not involved in any of them.

An open letter to the Academy of Medical Royal Colleges and the National Institute for Health and Care Excellence

2016 was a transformational year for my health. It all started when I came across the following information on the NHS website about the benefits of exercise:

Step right up. It's the miracle cure we've all been waiting for. If exercise were a pill, it would be one of the most cost-effective drugs ever invented.

It is medically proven that people who do regular physical activity have:

- *up to a 35% lower risk of coronary heart disease and stroke*
- *up to a 50% lower risk of type 2 diabetes*
- *up to a 50% lower risk of colon cancer*
- *up to a 20% lower risk of breast cancer*
- *a 30% lower risk of early death*
- *up to a 63% lower risk of osteoarthritis*
- *up to a 68% lower risk of hip fracture*
- *a 30% lower risk of falls – amongst older adults*
- *up to a 30% lower risk of depression*
- *up to a 30% lower risk of dementia*

But this discovery was down purely to luck. I was actually looking for other information and came across the section on exercise only by chance – probably a one in a million chance. I was amazed by what I read. That exercise can simultaneously reduce the incidence of all these diverse, life-taking and life-destroying diseases, and by such staggering percentages, is nothing short of incredible. I should add that I have been running for over 30 years but I did this because I actually enjoyed it and the challenge it provided. I knew exercise was good for me in a vague sort of way, but such vague recommendations by medicine and politicians provide no real motivation. The fact is, over recent years, my level of exercise had been declining significantly. It was becoming all too easy to allow bad weather or any other excuse to put me off. But the information on the NHS website has changed everything. The message is so powerful and clear that it has empowered and motivated me to significantly increase the exercise I do. I now run more often, for longer and faster and I am not put off by bad weather. This will clearly lead to better health and significantly reduce my risk of developing all these diseases.

But what if I hadn't found it? Clearly my level of exercise would be continuing to decline and my health would now be on a downwards spiral. Does it seem right that my health and my ability to prevent serious disease should depend simply on luck, on a chance discovery of a hard to find section of the NHS website? Can you understand why I feel so angry? And what about the other 50 million adults in the country who also don't know and are, therefore, similarly uninformed and unmotivated? In fact, I haven't been able to find a single person who knows about the specific benefits of exercise listed by the NHS. The experts we should have been able to trust have let us down badly.

For the last year I have been trying to understand how it is possible that this life-changing health information has been communicated to virtually no one. I have written to the Department of Health, NHS England, Health Education England, Public Health England and the General Medical Council seeking answers. All the replies claimed that effective policies were in place to promote exercise. But clearly these are hollow claims. Even more disturbing was my discovery that even doctors and medical students are not taught about exercise except in a vague qualitative way. The General Medical Council advised that NICE and the Medical Royal Colleges were the main decision makers governing what doctors are taught, what techniques and treatments they use and the guidelines they follow. That is why I wrote to you asking if you could defend this whole disturbing situation. You chose not to reply and that is why, finally, I was left with little option but to write this open letter.

I want to use this letter to issue a challenge to you. Debate this issue in front of an independent panel and see if you can convince them why it is right that medicine is effectively ignoring the most powerful scientifically proven medical discovery since the development of antibiotics. On one side of the debate would be a single member of the public with no medical training and on the other would be the finest medical brains in the country. To make things even easier for you, I will spell out my case now so you know exactly what you will be facing and can prepare your arguments in advance. Surely, I wouldn't stand a chance. Except, of course, you will never take up this challenge because you will understand that you cannot defend the indefensible; no matter how many experts you mobilise.

This is my case. The first part outlines what should be happening, and the second explains why.

All doctors, medical students and other health professionals should be taught explicitly about the quantitative benefits of exercise and learn about the most appropriate forms of exercise for their patients. This should start to happen within weeks because all the necessary information already exists. Medical guidelines should be drawn up requiring doctors and health professionals to communicate the specific benefits of exercise to all patients, to use it as a first line treatment for all the key diseases by issuing a "prescription for exercise", and even prescribe it for otherwise healthy people so that they stay healthy.

Doctors should reinforce the message by telling their patients that exercise is the most important scientifically proven thing they can ever do to stay healthy and that it will achieve more than any other treatments that medicine can prescribe. This initiative should be accompanied by wide scale media and press coverage and would continue as the reduction in heart attacks, strokes and other diseases started to occur. Once this became clear, many more of those who initially refused to join in might finally be convinced.

The reasons why you should be doing all of this are logical and compelling:

1) One of the founding principles of the NHS says, "It should support individuals to promote and manage their own health." Given that you know about the miracle of exercise, but virtually no one else does, then you have failed to follow your professional principles and those of the NHS. It also means you can benefit from it personally while effectively denying it to others. Does this seem right?

2) You might try to claim that medicine is taking exercise seriously by citing examples like the NHS Diabetes Prevention Programme and the use of social prescribing for exercise. But these are reaching only a tiny fraction of the population.

3) You may also argue that Public Health England has been given the role of promoting exercise. But this is nothing more than an excuse and a lame one at that. PHE can never promote exercise effectively. It has no direct contact with the public and most

people haven't even heard of it or know what it does. Its remit is so wide ranging that it doesn't have the resources or means to get the message across. But it is the results that are damning and speak for themselves. Around 50 million adults need to be informed about exercise but after many years PHE has probably reached no more than 2% of them. This is not a criticism of PHE. They have been given a role they simply cannot fulfil.

There are about 100,000 GPs and health professionals in surgeries and health centres around the country. Contrast this with a few dozen or so people at PHE who are likely to be dealing with exercise. Doctors and other professionals have direct contact with the public. In addition, they remain the most trusted profession bar none. A positive message about exercise from a doctor will do more than all the other initiatives that have ever been undertaken over many decades. Quite simply, doctors are the only route by which the benefits of exercise will ever be realised. It seems that even PHE understands this problem which is probably why they launched the initiative called "Moving Healthcare Professionals". This is designed to inform doctors about the benefits of exercise. There is just one huge problem. They say the aim is to change the culture of healthcare professionals within a generation! A 30-year timescale for something so important is frightening. Ten million people will have developed serious diseases unnecessarily by this stage.

4) If a drug had been developed that could prevent around a third of all the major chronic diseases simultaneously, it would be headline news around the world, not just for months but for years. It would be promoted so widely that everyone would know about it. It would be proclaimed as the greatest medical breakthrough since antibiotics were discovered, and indeed, it would be exactly that. Of course, such a drug does not exist, but exercise, which can achieve all these things, is given no such accolade. Why is exercise treated differently?

5) Exercise costs nothing whereas allowing disease to happen and then treating it costs billions. Public Health England estimates that our lack of exercise is costing £7.4 billion annually. This sum could help to transform the NHS.

6) Exercise also makes people happier and boosts self-esteem, mood and energy.

7) The failure to promote exercise effectively and the endless debates, reports and initiatives hide a brutal truth and some chilling statistics. Each year a million people and their families face the devastating consequences of a diagnosis of one of the major life-taking and life-destroying diseases, like heart attacks, stroke, dementia, cancer and diabetes; diseases that exercise can help to prevent. Given that exercise can, on average, prevent nearly a third of them, it means that 300,000 people each year are developing serious diseases that could have been prevented and, of course, many will eventually die from them. Even those who survive will often be incapacitated in some way or live under a dark cloud for the rest of their lives. In addition, depression affects at least 10 million people each year and up to 30% or 3 million cases are preventable.

8) You, as the key decision makers in medicine, alone hold the key to changing this shocking situation. You are the ones who can change medical curricula and inform

doctors. You can issue mandatory guidelines to ensure the effective communication of this life-changing information about exercise. You can issue guidelines requiring doctors to use exercise as a first line treatment for virtually every major disease.

9) When I first learnt about the benefits of exercise from the NHS website, I remember feeling shocked that something so simple could achieve so much. One of the friends I told about it initially laughed at the idea because it seemed so implausible that the claims made about exercise could be true. Even when he had read the evidence, he said, "If all this really is true, why is my doctor not telling me about it?" And this one simple question really does go to the heart of the problem and it explains succinctly why no meaningful progress is ever made.

10) Just as I was finishing this letter, a further incredible piece of research was published. It showed that exercise can give people in their seventies and eighties the immune system of 20-year olds. In fact, it is highly likely there isn't a single disease or health issue that exercise couldn't significantly improve.

Finally, here is one simple example of a press release that would literally start to transform the nation's health within weeks.

The Miracle Cure

If a drug had been developed that could prevent around 30% of nearly all the major life-taking and life-destroying diseases, like heart attacks, stokes, diabetes, dementia, major cancers and mental illness, everyone would expect medicine and doctors to use it. Indeed, it would become medicine's major priority because it would be the greatest medical breakthrough since the discovery of antibiotics.

Sadly, such a drug doesn't exist. But a simple lifestyle change that we could all do can achieve exactly the same results. It has been called a miracle cure and that is exactly what it is. Its name? Physical activity.

The evidence continues to mount and is now indisputable. Physical activity really can prevent up to 30%, on average, of all these diseases. It could achieve more than any other treatments that medicine currently possesses. Each year, 300,000 cases of the most serious diseases could be prevented as well as 3 million cases of depression. This is why medicine now feels compelled to ensure that every man, woman and child in the country gets to know about this miracle.

Starting next week everyone visiting their doctor or other healthcare professional will be given a single sheet of paper that details all the benefits of physical activity together with recommendations for their age group. Of course, we all have choices on how we lead our lives but you owe it to yourself to take up these recommendations. And remember, serious diseases can devastate entire families not just the person involved. The NHS would also be transformed and would be able to give better and timelier care to all its other patients.

Joint press release by:

The Medical Royal Colleges, The National Institute for Health and Care Excellence, The Chief Medical Officer, The British Medical Association, The British Heart Foundation, The Stroke Association, Cancer Research UK, Diabetes UK, Alzheimer's Research UK.

If all these bodies issued such a joint press release, it would make headline news across the entire country. It would start a nationwide dialogue that would lead to a greater uptake of exercise than has been accomplished over the last decade. And crucially it would cost nothing. Why has something like this never even been considered, let alone implemented?

I hope I have given you due cause to reflect, and that you will consider implementing these changes. What is needed is a revolution in thinking. The whole of medicine needs to be galvanised behind the concept of promoting exercise so that people will be motivated to take control of their own health just as the founding principles of the NHS envisaged.

Anthony Armstrong

Before I sent the letters to every MP, I knew they could not directly take up my case and that only my own MP could actually do this. But I hoped that if they fully understood what was happening, they might at least raise the issues at an appropriate time and press for action. I did in fact receive 14 replies. Three of them were sympathetic to my case and encouraged me to ask my own MP to help me make progress, but four were very worrying and implied that everything that could be done in respect of exercise was surely being done – this in spite of the damning evidence I had provided. My own MP did in fact take up the case very earnestly with the Secretary of State for Health and I was able to exchange several letters with his help. Despite all of this, no progress has been made because those in power simply keep repeating that robust policies are in place. The fact that they are not having any significant effect seems to fall on deaf ears. Those in power never answer difficult and embarrassing questions. As I already indicated, the Medical Royal Colleges and NICE simply haven't replied to any of the letters I sent.

So, we have the amazing situation where medicine's key decision makers know about the profound benefits of exercise, and many of them really do openly declare they use it to help protect themselves from developing all these life-taking diseases, but they don't even tell their own doctors and medical students about it, let alone the general public.

The microbiome

We have already seen that the average human is a host to around 100 trillion bacteria. These bacteria are on every surface of the body both inside and out and, as an example, there are around 10 billion microbes on just one of your hands. When some people read about this for the first time, they are shocked and even upset that every part of their body is covered in billions of "bugs". Many people regularly use antibacterial soaps to help kill them off, and many use antibacterial mouthwashes. This is because we have been led to believe over many decades that bacteria are dangerous. Of course, there really are some dangerous and even potentially deadly bacterial species, but most of the bacteria on and inside a healthy body are beneficial and actually enable us to control and even prevent the really bad ones from causing serious outcomes. These friendly bacteria really are an essential part of the body's natural defence systems. So, whilst there are a few situations where antibacterial soaps can be beneficial, in the majority of cases, soap and water is the best way to keep yourself clean and healthy. We have probably all seen adverts for products that say "kills 99.9% of household germs". But what about the 0.1% they don't kill? These are often dangerous bacteria that have become immune to antibacterial products or have found ways to temporarily avoid them by forming spores, for example. What happens then is they can multiply rapidly because there are no good bacteria left to crowd them out and this can be a key factor in many serious diseases.

Most of these 100 trillion friendly bacteria actually reside in our gut and are known as the microbiome. Here they perform critical functions such as helping to break down food, promoting a healthy digestive environment, reducing inflammation, creating certain vitamins, helping us to absorb key minerals and producing metabolites that play a major role in regulating our immune system. Dangerous bacteria are dealt with in two main ways. The friendly bacteria occupy virtually all the surface area of the intestine walls meaning there is little space for the dangerous bacteria that have entered the body to settle and then reproduce. But our friendly bacteria can also produce a range of substances (some, incredibly, are like antibiotics) that either kill or damage the invading bad bacteria. They are also our first line of defence against other invading pathogens such as viruses and fungi and it has been estimated that over 70% of our immune system takes place in our stomachs. There are thousands of different bacterial species in and on the human body.

Whilst most of this section is devoted to the vital microbiome, our friendly bacteria also have a range of other benefits like keeping our skin healthy by eating dead cells. They can also produce chemicals on certain parts of the skin that suppress the growth of harmful pathogens. Quite amazingly, the number of species of bacteria could be much greater than anyone may ever imagine. Consider one recent study that found 1,400 different bacteria in just 90 belly buttons. These had never before been found on the human body and many were new to science.

Our good bacteria have, over millions of years, formed a symbiotic relationship with mankind. We provide a safe and viable place for them to live and reproduce, and they look after us in numerous ways like protecting us from dangerous invading pathogens and playing a key role in our natural immune system. Here is just one amazing example. During birth, babies get their first vital friendly bacteria from the vaginal wall. The vagina normally contains a specific range of bacteria but during pregnancy this undergoes radical changes. What happens is the body helps to increase specific types of bacteria that will give the baby optimum protection as well as all the other benefits like helping it to absorb food. For example, it creates significant quantities of a bacteria called Lactobacillus johnsonii which can produce compounds that kill bad bacteria that may threaten the baby. These bacteria only exist in small quantities in the vagina outside of pregnancy. This single example shows the unique complexity and the almost unbelievable natural abilities of the human body that evolution has developed over its 7 million years.

It is often said you are what you eat, but what you digest and absorb is just as important. The health of your digestive tract profoundly affects your overall health and we now know our friendly bacteria play a crucial role in this. So, problems such as indigestion, irritable bowel syndrome, ulcers, Crohn's disease, colitis and diverticulitis, candidiasis and chronic fatigue all have links to a poorly functioning digestive tract which is related to a damaged microbiome. A healthy microbiome clearly plays a crucial role in controlling all these obvious gut-related conditions. But what we are learning about the microbiome has been described by some scientists as one of the greatest discoveries of mankind and has the potential to literally transform our lives and our health. We now know with reasonable certainty that a disturbed microbiome plays a significant role in a huge range of other serious diseases. These include obesity, mental health, cancer, Parkinson's, Alzheimer's, autoimmune diseases, asthma, eczema and autism to name just a few.

Even as far back as 1885, Louis Pasteur hypothesised that if animals could be raised in sterile conditions, they would probably not be able to survive. However, Bernard Wostmann and his team proved that Pasteur's hypothesis was wrong when they developed methods for breeding animals in germ-free conditions. Nevertheless, they discovered that, even though they didn't die, they still had devastating outcomes, because even with a perfect diet, these bacteria-free animals had stunted growth and smaller hearts, lungs and livers, lower cardiac output and many other serious imperfections. When they received intestinal microbiota from animals raised under normal conditions, however, nearly all these devastating conditions were reversed. Microbes really are essential for animal and human development and health.

The Human Genome Project was famously described as the greatest discovery of mankind, but even after $60 billion of research over 30 years, it has achieved almost nothing. By comparison, the microbiome is already producing some spectacular outcomes even though these are just a drop in the ocean compared to its ultimate potential. But now we have to remember one very sad and disturbing fact. You will not learn about any of this from medicine because, as we have seen, they do not promote natural lifestyle solutions to health. You have also seen copious evidence that medical dogma can resist new ideas from gaining acceptance for many decades. The drug industry will also discredit all lifestyle solutions unless it can benefit from them itself. It is, of course, aided in this attack and in the suppression of data by regulators, highly incentivised researchers, governments and most of the press and media. So, as a member of the public, you will never learn anything positive about the microbiome from any of these official bodies. If you want to benefit from it and reduce your risk of developing distressing conditions like IBS, as well some of the most serious diseases that affect mankind, you will need to develop your own plan and I will outline the key things you can do shortly. Thankfully, there are also dozens of books that can help.

I am now going to examine, in more detail, various aspects of the microbiome, and I'll start with a spectacular success story. Warning! If you are about to have a meal and are squeamish, read with care. Have you heard of something called a faecal transplant? It made headlines on the BBC News programmes nine years ago and it is exactly what it sounds like. I won't go into the detail of how the faeces of one person are transferred to another person, but the "active ingredient" being transferred is actually friendly bacteria. Why was such a procedure ever contemplated? To explain it, we need to consider the bacterium, C. difficile. This makes the headlines periodically due to the number of deaths it causes. C. difficile is a potentially deadly bacteria which releases toxins that can cause severe and uncontrollable diarrhoea. The problem mainly manifests itself in a hospital or care home setting after repeat doses of antibiotics that are used to treat an infection that the patient has contracted. An amazing fact is that over 2 million healthy people in the UK have these "potentially" deadly C. difficile bacteria in their gut, but they are kept at safe low levels by our vast army of friendly bacteria. After several courses of antibiotics, however, the friendly bacteria can be largely wiped out, while the C. difficile bacteria survive because they are often resistant to all antibiotics. They are then able to multiply rapidly, and the huge increase in toxins they release causes severe, uncontrollable diarrhoea which can be life-threatening. Over 1,600 people die in the UK each year from C. difficile. In the US, the figure is 30,000 according to The New York Times.

The 2013 research into faecal transplants that made headline news used donors whose faeces contained the six strains of bacteria that, in animal studies, had been shown to be most effective in combating C. difficile. In total, 20 patients who had a resistant C. difficile infection were treated. After the first round of treatment, 14 patients saw complete resolution of symptoms. The remaining six were given a second round of treatment and a further four had complete remission. So, in total, 18 out of 20 patients (90%) experienced a complete resolution of symptoms. The friendly bacteria so inelegantly introduced, multiplied and effectively crowded out or destroyed most of the C. difficile. Such a cure rate is not possible with conventional medical treatments. This research was carried out in a Massachusetts hospital and, unusually, was funded directly by the hospital. It was almost certainly only intended to be seen by other experts involved in this potential treatment, but due to its bizarre and headline grabbing potential, when it leaked out, it became a major storyline in many countries. Why am I explaining this? Well, I suspect that medicine would rather the general public had never heard anything about it, but because of the media coverage, the NHS obviously felt it necessary to write a clarifying statement relating to this trial on its website. After covering the basic facts accurately, it then went out of its way to downplay the hugely impressive trial results which, of course, is the normal response from medicine to every natural solution that works:

> The study was a small feasibility study, meaning it does not provide robust proof that the technique is effective or safe. It did not, for example, have a control group, so we don't know how many people would have got better on their own. Larger, more robust, clinical trials are needed to prove its effectiveness and safety before it is known whether the experimental pill could have the potential to be developed into a new treatment. Nonetheless, the study did show that the capsules appeared feasible, initially safe and somewhat effective.

Don't you just love the words *somewhat effective*? It must be one of the greatest understatements of all time. The simple fact is natural bacteria cured 18 out of 20 people with a life-threatening and resistant infection for which all other medical treatments had failed. Rather than "somewhat effective", this is what they should have said:

> This has the potential to become one of the biggest breakthroughs in modern medicine, and we will pressurise the government for funding for a large-scale clinical trial to finally confirm what is almost certainly an incredible success, so that it can be approved rapidly and then save thousands of lives.

To dismiss the study because it is small shows a failure to understand the significance of the results (or, more likely, this was quite deliberate). A success rate of 90% on an intractable infection like C. difficile can't leave much doubt that the treatment really worked. The odds that there was some other explanation, like all the patients might just have got better at the same time without any treatment, would be astronomically high. In fact, it was simply nonsense. When results are so statistically significant, there is little need of a control group.

Seven years later and I'll be surprised if you have heard anything more about it, but behind the scenes, some encouraging things as well as some deeply disturbing things are happening. The first is that faecal transplants are actually being used in a number of countries. In the UK, NICE approved their use in 2014 for the treatment of C. difficile when antibiotic treatments had failed. However, despite this tacit approval, only a relatively small number of transplants actually take place and many hospitals have never used them at all. Over 1,600 deaths still occur each year and the real tragedy is that around 1,400 of these could be prevented. In the US, the Federal Drug Agency in 2013 initially placed draconian rules on the use of transplants to treat C. difficile. It classed the treatment as an experimental procedure and only a handful of doctors throughout the entire country were allowed to use them. However, after intense pressure from some doctors and the public it relaxed the rules (whilst maintaining its experimental status) so that anyone for whom all antibiotic treatments had failed could, in principle, be treated with a faecal transplant. But just as in the UK, the numbers actually being treated are relatively small. I say relatively, because the actual number for 2018 had grown to around 10,000 which suggests that 9,000 lives were saved. This may seem huge, but the fact is around 500,000 Americans develop C. difficile each year and an estimated 30,000 deaths are still occurring. This means that another 27,000 deaths could be prevented each year. So, why is this not happening?

Clearly much of medicine has not embraced this almost miraculous treatment which results in a 90% reduction in deaths. Many doctors apparently know little about it and this may in part be because the medical seminars which are part of their continuing medical education are effectively controlled by the drug industry who would never allow this treatment to be given any official recognition unless they can gain control of it themselves. It is again important to remember that regulators nearly always side with the drug industry and they continue to make life difficult for those carrying out faecal transplants by issuing draconian rules covering their use. All this is epitomised by one single tragedy.

In 2019 a US patient died because the faecal transplant he was given contained a resistant E. coli bacterium. Any death is, of course, sad, and action should be taken to try to prevent it from happening again, which, in this instance, is entirely possible because the faecal samples simply need to be screened for this deadly bacterium before use, and in fact that is what is now happening. But we should also remember that over the last eight years in the US, a conservative estimate is that 40,000 lives have been saved by this treatment. Would you personally make any major change to a treatment plan that has saved 40,000 lives and caused just one death? The real tragedy is the Federal Drug Agency should be promoting faecal transplants and thereby saving another 27,000 lives each year. Instead it is going to try to use this one death as an excuse to ensure future faecal transplants are given solely to the pharmaceutical industry. The FDA's aim is to class faecal transplants as a drug, and the pharmaceutical industry will then be allowed to patent them. They will then charge many thousands of dollars for a single treatment. When I mentioned this situation to a friend, he said that if all this really is true (which it is), then surely the FDA should be charged with crimes against humanity in The Hague. It is hard to disagree, but, of course, it will never happen.

In the US in 2021, medically prescribed drugs officially caused 187,750 deaths according to the FDA and there are also 19 million hospitalisations each year. Yet the FDA would never introduce tougher regulations on the drug industry despite the fact it causes 187,750 times more deaths than this one faecal treatment that it is now using as an excuse for radical change. There couldn't be a more graphic illustration of the power the drug industry wields over medicine, regulators and governments; where money is the only thing that matters, and where human life is seemingly irrelevant.

There is also a devastating possibility that, if the drug industry is allowed to patent a treatment for C. difficile, then it will eventually be given patents for all the other uses of friendly bacteria that are likely to be developed. It means people would then be able to receive these friendly bacteria only via the drug industry after they had developed a serious disease, because the industry will only ever use bacterial treatments to treat a disease – not to prevent it. It means people would not be able to use them to stay healthy. This, of course, is all part of the pharmaceutical master plan to ensure that as many people as possible become sick and develop diseases, and then ensure that when this happens, their only option is to use pharmaceutical drugs and treatments. It is a distinct possibility that natural probiotic supplements and friendly bacterial foods, like kefir and sauerkraut, could eventually also be banned from sale because the regulators could claim they break the drug patents. The only thing that can stop this from happening is if enough people object and force the FDA to allow faecal transplants to continue to be used as a donor-sourced treatment, just like blood transfusions and organ donations, and to keep it out of the greedy hands of the pharmaceutical industry.

I have quite deliberately spent a great deal of time exploring C. difficile faecal treatments because the whole story is so important. It encapsulates in one example the tragic process whereby effective natural solutions to serious health problems are ignored, supressed or discredited unless they can be taken over by the drug industry. It also outlines the final devastating end game that drug regulators and the drug industry are planning.

Stop the press! Just a few days before I finished writing this book, the following information became available and I just had to insert it here. The FDA has just approved the first faecal transplant classed as a pharmaceutical drug to treat C. difficile. The "drug" is called Rebyota and the company is Ferring Pharmaceuticals. It is, of course, not a drug but just faecal microbiota from natural stools. Its price has not yet been disclosed but it really will be very expensive. All the potentially devastating outcomes that I have outlined will now start to occur. One of the key ones is that only those Americans who can afford it will now get treated. Those who can't may well just die, whereas previously the non-profit OpenBiome had provided stool samples at basic low costs for everyone. It will now have to cease when Rebyota becomes fully operational. I had to add this despicable information here – just one more example of how the FDA puts pharmaceutical profits before human life.

But now we need to move on to other aspects of the microbiome. An incredible amount of fundamental research into the link between the microbiome and a huge range of other diseases is being carried out by biotech and drug companies, universities and many other research organisations. These include irritable bowel syndrome, irritable bowel disease, Crohn's disease, asthma, eczema, obesity, Alzheimer's, Parkinson's, multiple sclerosis, cancer, heart disease, mental health, viral infections including Coronavirus, weakened immune systems, allergies, sleep problems, motor neurone disease, diabetes and rheumatoid arthritis. Much of this research is in the early stages but even now there is reasonable certainty that most of these diseases really can be significantly helped and even prevented by a healthy microbiome.

I'll give you just a few pieces of evidence, and the first is about the microbiome and cancer. Scientists at Imperial College London carried out a study in 2019 comparing patients who took antibiotics before starting an immunotherapy course for cancer against those who didn't. Those who had taken antibiotics had an average survival time of just two months compared to 26 months for those who had not been on antibiotics. The researchers believe that the staggering difference in life expectancy is due to the damage the antibiotics caused to the microbiome and its subsequent reduction in the body's immune response. These findings strongly suggest that improving and strengthening the health of the gut microbiome really could help the natural immune system fight, and even prevent, cancer more effectively.

A study in the US which was published in the journal Pediatric Research evaluated 75 infants who were randomised and received either a probiotic supplement or a placebo during the first six months of life. The study then followed them until they reached the age of 13. At that point, attention deficit hyperactive disorder or autistic spectrum disorder were diagnosed in 17% of the children given the placebo. In those given the probiotic, the figure was zero. Admittedly, this was another relatively small trial but the results are once again so significant they should be acted upon. Surely a medical profession that cares about children's health would be demanding that more urgent trials be carried out so these devastating conditions could perhaps be significantly reduced.

Fifty-seven children aged three to seven took part in a 2015 study called the Pro-Child Probiotic Study, which examined the effect of probiotics on coughs and colds. Half of them were given a probiotic supplement and 50mg of vitamin C for six months. Those taking the probiotics had nearly a 50% reduction in symptoms, a 33% reduction in the number of colds and a 45% reduction in absenteeism from school. Once again, these are incredible results when compared to the tiny benefits of many drugs.

Normally, 30% of people who take antibiotics develop diarrhoea. There are 63 trials with a total of 12,000 patients where probiotic supplements were given during the antibiotic course. These reduced the incidence of diarrhoea from 30 in every 100 to 17 – a 43% reduction in cases.

A 2016 study published in the Paediatrics Journal showed that children who thumb-suck have less frequent allergies and this is thought to be because the constant flow of germs fine-tunes the immune system during their development. On the same theme, there are several independent studies that show the same benefits for children raised on animal farms where their interaction with the animals diversifies their microbiome.

More than 120 leading British scientists in conjunction with the All-Party Parliamentary Group for the Human Microbiome have written a letter to the Health Secretary urging officials to investigate the link between Coronavirus and a bad diet. They say there is a growing body of compelling evidence that shows a clear link between poor gut health and suffering from severe COVID-19.

Obesity and weight gain are increasingly being linked to the microbiome. There are numerous examples and different types of evidence, and I will outline just a few of them:

1) There is clear evidence that children and adolescents born by caesarean deliveries have higher BMIs than those born by natural childbirth. During normal vaginal births, the baby acquires a wide range of crucial friendly bacteria that are present in the birth canal, but these are not present in a C-section delivery.
2) Mothers who take antibiotics before birth have disturbed microbiomes which are then passed on to their offspring and this also leads to a higher BMI. The differences in the type and number of bacteria that are transferred onto and into babies during birth is almost certainly one of the significant causes of their subsequent weight variations.
3) The Avon Longitudinal Study of Parents and Children followed 14,500 children and found that those who took antibiotics in the first six months of life developed higher BMIs.
4) Studies involving mice have shown that when those of normal weight are given a faecal transplant from obese mice, they see significant weight gain. When obese mice are given a transplant from those of normal weight, they then lose weight.
5) In 2015, a woman in the US had a faecal transplant from her daughter (who was healthy but overweight) to treat a serious case of C. difficile. The treatment worked and her life was saved, but, over the next year, she gained over 16 kilos in weight. The doctors concluded that it was the daughter's microbiome that made both women obese. Because of this, they recommended that overweight people should be excluded from future faecal donations.

There are many other serious outcomes that are related to caesarean deliveries and their lack of natural vital microbes that cannot be passed on to babies during birth. Around 80% of all MRSA infections in babies occur in those born by C-section. Similarly, they result in an increase in a wide range of other conditions like allergies, obsessive compulsive disorder, type 1 diabetes, coeliac disease and even autism. In fact, even the Center for Disease Control in the US has stated that if no C-section deliveries were carried out, then 1 in 12 of all autism cases would not occur.

Consider Japan and South Korea where most of the population regularly eat fermented foods like kimchi which play a major role in optimising the microbiome. These two countries have the highest life expectancy in the world and even though there are currently no scientific studies, many independent experts believe fermented foods really can play an important part in longevity.

Finally, a study carried out by the China-Canada Institute examined the microbiota of over 1,000 very healthy people up to the age of 100 with no underlying health conditions. It showed that the overall microbiota composition of the healthy elderly group was similar to that of people decades younger. As Greg Gloor, the principal investigator, said, "The main conclusion is that if you are ridiculously healthy and 90 years old, your gut microbiota is not that different from a healthy 30-year-old in the same population."

Medicine would, of course, say that none of these trials or studies give definitive proof because there are as yet no $2 billion placebo-controlled clinical trials. These will, of course, never happen unless the pharmaceutical industry funds them, and they would only do this if they can produce a bacterial-based drug that can be patented and which would then make huge profits. So, at the moment, medicine will do absolutely nothing about any of the incredible evidence showing the microbiome plays a crucial role in so many diseases. But this evidence is, in every other way, almost unchallengeable. Helping to strengthen and look after your microbiome is completely safe. It will help you in so many ways like reducing your risk of developing disabling conditions like IBS, as well as the near certainty it will help protect you from developing serious diseases like cancer, Alzheimer's, Parkinson's and all the other conditions that have been outlined. You really could start benefitting from an improved microbiome today.

People who advocate lifestyle medicine have known for decades that achieving an optimum level of friendly bacteria and helping them thrive and multiply by providing them with the right food and environment is critical not just to our gut health, but to many other serious and apparently unrelated conditions and diseases. People who adopt lifestyle medicine have been able to benefit from this knowledge for many years. I started taking probiotic supplements about 20 years ago, and predictably at that time, conventional medicine ridiculed them. This is just another example of how natural lifestyle can help you stay healthy decades before medicine will even contemplate such changes. It epitomises lifestyle medicine. Key factors like good diets, physical activity, mental positivity and, of course, the microbiome always produce multiple benefits for nearly every serious health condition and disease.

So, what is a healthy microbiome and what can you do to improve your own? A healthy microbiome contains many thousands of different types of bacteria. The more strains of bacteria you have, the healthier you will be. The microbiome should also be "in balance" which means it shouldn't be overrun by a few specific types of bacteria. Scientists have taken faecal samples and compared the microbiomes of many different people from communities around the world. We no longer have true "hunter-gatherers" but some of the closest descendants such as the Hadzabes in Tanzania have the most diverse microbiomes in the world. They rarely suffer from any of the serious chronic diseases that plague western society even though they would, in many countries, be classed as living in extreme poverty. Some of the least diverse microbiomes are found either in people who have taken repeat doses of antibiotics and other drugs like PPIs and antacids, or those who eat lots of ultra-processed foods, sugar, artificial sweeteners and refined carbohydrates. But even most of the healthiest western people have usually got significantly less diverse microbiomes than the Hadzabes. Here are some of the key things you can do to help develop a really healthy, diverse and balanced microbiome:

- Eat a wide range of the foods that our friendly bacteria thrive on, like vegetables, fruits and seeds.
- Significantly reduce or eliminate the foods the bad bacteria thrive on, like ultra-processed foods, sugar, processed trans-fats and refined carbohydrates.
- Take a wide range of probiotic supplements or fermented foods like sauerkraut and kimchi and fermented drinks like kefir and kombucha. These contain many dozens of different strains of bacteria that can add diversity to your microbiome. If you have never taken fermented foods before, it is important to introduce them gradually, starting perhaps with just a teaspoon and then building up to the recommended intakes over a few weeks. You may have noticed that I have not mentioned or recommended yoghurt, and the reason is most popular brands contain significant amounts of sugar as well as a limited range of bacteria – some with as little as two strains.
- Eat more prebiotics which are foods that feed your friendly bacteria. Good bacteria need plenty of soluble fibre, like oats, nuts, apples and berries, and insoluble fibre, like vegetable and fruit skins, legumes, flax seed and root vegetables. Some of the very best non-digestible fibres are found in specific foods like onion, garlic, asparagus, artichoke, broccoli, oat bran and seeds like quinoa. Inulin which is found in chicory root can be bought as an extracted powder and is exceptionally beneficial.
- Eat a rainbow of natural foods every day and try to consume around 30g of fibre overall.
- I have already mentioned the Alliance for Natural Health International's book *Reset Eating* which is a really healthy overall diet and is perfect for maintaining a healthy microbiome.

It is very clear from all the evidence available that antibiotics can cause devastating and even life-taking changes to the microbiome, but, of course, in some cases, they are essential. The key thing to remember, if you do have to take them, is to then work hard to restore your microbiome as soon as possible. Take a range of probiotic foods and supplements during (and after) the course of antibiotics, ideally an hour before or two hours after each tablet. Other drugs are also implicated in damaging our microbiome and allowing dangerous bacteria to thrive. These include PPI drugs, antacids, corticosteroids, and some anti-inflammatory drugs. Heavy metals like mercury and aluminium are also implicated. Living a healthy lifestyle will mean you are unlikely to develop the conditions these drugs are used for and thus avoid the serious microbiome complications they can cause.

I should add one important note. If your microbiome has been seriously damaged and bad bacteria have multiplied and become a dominant force, and then you take fermented foods, probiotics and prebiotics to help restore the balance, you may effectively start a "gut war". The good bacteria start to destroy the bad ones and "die off" occurs. This can create a short-term toxic effect before the dead bacteria are flushed out of the body. Some people can become constipated, others get loose stools and it can take several days or even a few weeks before the microbiome returns to normal. The extent of all this depends on the type of bacteria involved and how easy it is for the good bacteria to kill and replace them, Of course, doing nothing could lead to serious diseases, but it's important that you are prepared and can understand what might happen.

Another factor that can seriously affect the microbiome is stress. This may at first seem strange, but if I tell you that the microbiome communicates with the brain via the central nervous system and vice-versa, then it becomes more understandable. In fact, the microbiome has been called our "second brain", such is its importance. It contains around 100 million neurons which are critical in the communication process with the brain. Scientists were recently amazed to discover that 90% of the communication came from the gut to the brain and not the other way around. A disturbed microbiome from, say, indigestion or damage to friendly bacteria can affect our mood and emotions and even our mental well-being. Even the production of key feel-good hormones like serotonin depends on a healthy microbiome, and in healthy people, 95% of the serotonin resides in the gut and only 5% in the brain itself. But things like stress, fear and anger can also work the other way around and disturb our friendly bacteria. So, while a positive, non-stressed mental outlook is good for our health overall, it is also really important in helping to maintain a healthy microbiome.

There are three key messages from this section. Firstly, healthy microbiomes are one of the key factors that could reduce the epidemic of modern diseases. People who adopt healthy lifestyles that promote and sustain our friendly bacteria achieve incredible improvements in health. Secondly, there is a worrying risk that at some future point when the billions of dollars of current official research on friendly bacteria is completed, which will confirm just how effective they are, the drug industry may be given monopoly control over "bacteria-based drugs". Then, quite shockingly, it will only be used to treat disease and not to prevent it. Thirdly, antibiotics really are miracle drugs but they can also kill our friendly bacteria and this is also one of the causes of the epidemics of chronic diseases that are escalating around the world. It can all be summed up in the title of Michael Blaser's book *Missing Microbes: How Killing Bacteria Creates Modern Plagues*. Our friendly bacteria really are one of the keys to a long and healthy life. At present, everyone really could achieve these benefits if they wanted to.

Here is one final fact. For many centuries the human body has been linked to five vital organs – the brain, heart, lungs, liver and kidneys. The microbiome, however, is so vital to human health that it really should be classed as the sixth vital organ.

Vitamins, minerals and other natural compounds

Vitamins, key minerals and other natural compounds like amino acids are, quite simply, essential for human life and without them you would die very quickly. But they also play a major part in preventing most diseases as well as treating and even curing them. Medicine really does accept much of this but its view is that we can get everything we need simply from a balanced diet and supplements are simply not needed. In this section, however, I want to explain why relying on food alone is a dangerous assumption and is becoming ever more difficult to achieve, and why most people really should consider the use of key vitamin and mineral supplements. I will explore why the foods that most people eat are deficient in vitamins and minerals and also look at some of the spectacular benefits that result from eating enough of them.

Scientists measure the vitamin and mineral content of natural foods like vegetables, fruits, grains and meats. Records are available from early in the twentieth century. They paint an alarming picture of how the levels have been declining for decades. Why? The official report of the Rio Earth Summit concluded, "There is deep concern over continuing major declines in the mineral values in farm and range soils throughout the world." This statement was based on data showing that over the last 100 years, average mineral levels in agricultural soil have fallen worldwide by 72% in Europe, 76% in Asia and 85% in North

America. So, why is this happening? Most of the blame lies with artificial chemical fertilisers. We know that plants absorb 70 to 80 different minerals from the soil, but the number returned to it by commercial fertilisers can be counted on the fingers of one hand. Every crop that is cut or animal that is sent to market makes a further mineral depletion of the soil in which it was grown. Organic waste that, in former times, would have been composted and returned to the land during periods of crop rotation, thereby rejuvenating the soil and rebuilding the mineral levels, are nowadays mostly consigned to landfill or incinerated.

There are other ways in which chemical-based farming prevents crops from taking up trace minerals left in the soil. These relate to the beneficial interaction between the bacteria and fungi in the soil and the plants that are growing. This delicate balance is significantly compromised by the presence of chemicals in pesticides and herbicides and further depletes mineral absorption. Most of the food we eat is mineral deficient due to the combined effect of soil mineral depletion and the reduced absorbability of those minerals that remain. The examples below give an indication of the reductions in the average mineral content of 27 vegetables and 17 fruits, between 1940 and 1991:

- potassium down 16%
- calcium down 46%
- magnesium down 24%
- copper down 76%
- iron down 27%
- zinc down 59%

Specific foods fare much worse than these averages suggest. In 1948 100g of spinach contained 158mg of iron, but today that has plummeted to just 1mg. A University of Colorado study shows a similar overall picture with an average 50% decline in nutrient content over the last 100 years. Vitamin levels have also seen significant falls, and these are also associated with practices such as "green harvesting" and the breeding of faster growing and bigger fruits and vegetables. Between 1950 and 2000, for example, the vitamin A level in apples fell by 33% and by 51% in bananas. Vitamin C levels are down by an average of 30%. Believe it or not, some supermarket oranges have tested with zero vitamin C. Grains and meats are also similarly affected. In 1900 wheat was 90% protein, but today it is just 10%. All this is happening in plant-based foods like vegetables, fruits and grains and if all this isn't bad enough, when they are included in highly processed foods, the vitamin, mineral and other vital nutrient contents suffer even more serious declines. White bread, for example, contains virtually no nutrients and is almost pure carbohydrate – in essence, it is like eating sugar. In summary, your vitamin and mineral intake is almost certainly significantly lower than previous generations and it is continuing to fall. The current reality of agriculture means, of course, this trend is not going to change – in fact it will escalate even faster.

But there is yet more graphic proof of just how disastrous things have become. Minimum levels called reference daily intakes (RDI) have been established in various countries for the main vitamins and minerals. How were these minimum levels set? Well, as an example, the level for vitamin C was established solely in relation to scurvy. A trial was carried out in the UK at the end of the Second World War involving conscientious objectors and another trial in the US at the Iowa State Penitentiary involving prisoners in the 1960s. All those involved were given restricted diets that contained virtually no vitamin C. The researchers waited until scurvy developed and then gave low doses of vitamin C which they slowly increased until the disease was controlled and reversed. A level of around 10mg per day was found to prevent scurvy in the small number of prisoners involved. But there are significant variations in the way people absorb and utilise vitamins so, to ensure that the recommended minimum level would be sufficient to prevent scurvy for everyone in the country, the RDI was initially set at 60mg. The key point is the official RDI is based solely on preventing this one disease. Other vitamin and mineral RDIs are based on a similar single disease logic like vitamin D and rickets, vitamin B1 and beriberi, and vitamin B3 and pellagra. Others are based on intakes that simply maintain existing levels within the body.

The first thing to understand is there is a huge difference between the bare minimum RDI levels that can prevent these few very specific diseases and the much higher levels that nutritionists believe (and that numerous trials prove) are necessary for promoting optimum health and helping to prevent or treat a wide range of other serious diseases. Here are the current RDIs approved by the Federal Drug Agency for several of the key vitamins and minerals:

Vitamin C	90mg
Vitamin D	20mcg
Vitamin B6	1.7mg
Vitamin B12	2.4mcg
Magnesium	420mg
Zinc	11mg
Calcium	1300mg
Folate	400mcg

So, are people achieving even these minimum levels? Many studies have been carried out and they reveal an alarming picture. A majority of people are achieving levels that fall below even these bare minimums for many vitamins and minerals. A study of 2,000 adults showed that more than 90% were consuming inadequate amounts of folate, while vitamin C and magnesium intakes were low in more than 50% of the group and virtually everyone had inadequate iron consumption. In a study of 433 men and 876 women in low-income groups, 25% of men and 16% of women were so deficient in vitamin C that they were at high risk of developing scurvy. Studies on vitamin D show that between 25% and 90% of people are deficient depending on their age, sun exposure, ethnicity and diet. The problem is, of course, at its worst in winter when the sun is not strong enough to generate any vitamin D. So, given that a substantial percentage of the population have vitamin and mineral levels that fall below the absolute minimum levels that medicine sets – the levels below which it expects specific diseases to occur – what action is medicine taking? I'll give you one guess. The answer is almost nothing. Scurvy and rickets are obvious examples of how totally preventable serious diseases are being allowed to proliferate because of medicine's inaction. But vitamin and mineral deficiency is linked to many other diseases like heart disease, skin problems, cancer, dementia and mental illness. All this, of course, is disputed by medicine's elite who continue to maintain that you can get all the nutrients you need from a balanced diet. This medical position, however, is untenable because the vitamin and mineral content of even a "perfect balanced natural diet" has at least halved in the last 100 years and around 50% of people on average are not even meeting medicine's minimum levels. If everyone ate huge varieties of organic whole natural foods like our hunter-gatherer ancestors did, we may not need vitamin and mineral supplements but this is becoming increasingly difficult in our modern world, where synthetic fertiliser-fed plants, GMO seeds and ultra-processed foods reign supreme for huge swathes of the population.

In the last 100 years, medicine has only rarely recommended or used vitamin and mineral supplements to treat disease or to help people stay healthy. I am going to explain how this has been a tragedy for mankind by outlining some of their incredible benefits. I would, however, need to write several more books to cover every vitamin, mineral and all the other natural compounds that affect our health in full detail. As I write this section, I can see on my bookshelf, a 323-page book just on vitamin B12 and a 311-page book on magnesium. Every vitamin, mineral and all the other natural food compounds have multiple effects on a vast range of bodily functions and play a major role in promoting good health and treating and preventing most diseases. So, I will look in some detail at one vitamin, vitamin D, to provide an insight into what they can achieve. I will give many examples of its incredible benefits and outline some of the studies and trials that have been carried out. I will then examine most of the other key vitamins and minerals in Part 5 where more information will be provided about their effect on specific diseases.

I will start with vitamin D. This is present in a number of foods like fatty fish, eggs and mushrooms but at low levels, such that food alone cannot normally provide adequate amounts for the body to function optimally. Most of our vitamin D comes from exposure to sunshine and this has been mankind's main source for millions of years. Of course, once industrialisation ramped up in the nineteenth century, huge numbers of people started working indoors typically for 12 hours per day. They had virtually no sun exposure and their diets were also devastatingly unhealthy. Levels of vitamin D declined catastrophically and this led to an epidemic of rickets which, in some of the tenement slums, affected up to 80% of children. But things started to improve during the twentieth century when working conditions improved and working hours declined. People had more free time and were increasingly able to spend more time outdoors. As a child, I vividly remember spending nearly all of my free time playing outside with friends. By the middle of the twentieth century, rickets had declined so significantly that doctors were confident it had been completely eliminated in the UK.

But then the idea that sun exposure could cause skin cancer started to take hold within medical circles. People were increasingly advised to stay out of the sun or completely cover their body and use total sun block lotions. Many people, particularly women, religiously followed these recommendations, but this advice has almost certainly led to serious medical conditions, such is the importance of vitamin D for dozens of key bodily functions. Some experts say it could even have reduced average life expectancy by around two years and even cases of rickets are now increasing again. So, can the official medical recommendation for virtually no direct sun exposure really be such a sensible thing? Nearly every natural health practitioner recommends safe sun exposure despite medicine's unchanging position, and given the millions of years where mankind has been naturally exposed to the sun (without any sunscreen lotions), the benefits of sensible exposure are logical and in line with our evolution. Burning should, of course, be avoided, but sensible sun exposure will help to transform your health. Taking vitamin D supplements, however, particularly in winter, can also achieve the same transformation as we will now explore. Another key fact is that older people in care homes, for example, may simply be unable to achieve any meaningful sun exposure and supplements are the only realistic option. I should add that vitamin D is available in two forms – D2 and D3. Vitamin D3 is the one you should take because Vitamin D2 is a poorly absorbable form.

Numerous epidemiological studies have previously found associations between blood serum vitamin D levels and rates of breast cancer, but a 2018 analysis in the journal PLOS ONE of two randomised trials has revealed an even greater benefit. As vitamin D levels increased, cancer rates fell and those women with levels above 60ng/ml had an 80% lower risk of breast cancer compared to those with less than 20ng/ml. This is a staggering result given that it is the most common cancer worldwide, and affects 55,000 women in the UK each year. The study also showed a clear dose response, meaning that every increase in vitamin D levels resulted in a corresponding reduction in cancer risk. The highest serum levels used in the trial can only be achieved by either significant sun exposure or taking very high doses of vitamin D – typically around 250mcg per day.

In 2014 researchers from the University of California and the Naval Health Research Center at San Diego analysed the evidence from five studies involving 4,443 breast cancer patients. The women who had circulating blood levels of 30ng/ml of vitamin D were twice as likely to survive their breast cancer than those with a lower level of 17ng/ml. The researchers said that taking vitamin D supplements should become part of the daily regimen of every woman suffering from breast cancer.

An International Pooling Project published in PubMed analysed the results of 17 studies which examined the effect of serum vitamin D, 25(OH)D, levels on bowel cancer. It concluded that "higher circulating 25(OH)D was related to a statistically significant, substantially lower colorectal cancer risk in women".

A four-year randomised control trial involving 2,302 healthy post-menopausal women over 55 was carried out and published in JAMA in 2016. In the trial, half the women were given a vitamin D and calcium supplement, the other half received a placebo. All the women were subsequently monitored for every type of cancer (except skin cancer) and the results showed that those taking the vitamin supplement had a statistically significant 35% reduction in cases compared to the placebo group. I should add that while this is again a staggering result, the level of vitamin D used was only 50mcg. In the 2018 breast cancer trial, giving 250mcg resulted in an 80% reduction and if this level had been used in the JAMA trial, it is likely that the risk reduction would have been higher than the 35% figure.

Another 2016 study in the peer reviewed journal PLOS ONE showed that doubling the circulating vitamin D levels from 20ng/ml to 40ng/ml resulted in a 65% reduction in all invasive cancers.

These are just five examples of the type of evidence for the amazing effects of vitamin D in helping prevent cancer and also reduce the death rate from those who already have it. So, what does medicine say about them and why does it steadfastly refuse to use vitamin D? The official medical position is that there is "insufficient evidence". The Scientific Advisory Committee on Nutrition, for example, looked at possible links between vitamin D and cancer and concluded they "didn't find enough evidence to draw any firm conclusions". Preventing 80% of breast cancers and up to 65% of all cancers overall (depending on doses used) would be one of the greatest medical achievements the world has ever seen. Medicine should be demanding government funding to carry out more confirmatory trials. But sadly, it is not going to happen for all the reasons already explained.

I'll now outline several other diseases and conditions that have evidence for the benefits of vitamin D. In 2017 researchers in Colorado studied the effects of vitamin D supplements on care home patients over the course of a year. Those who took around 100mcg per day reduced their risk of developing acute respiratory infections by nearly half.

A study published in Endocrine Abstracts examined the outcomes for older patients admitted acutely to hospital in relation to their serum vitamin D levels. Those in the lowest quartile had longer hospital stays averaging 34 days compared to ten days for those in the highest quartile. The lowest quartile also had lower mental test scores, lower mobility scores and an increased risk of falls. Even more significant was that 32% of patients died in the lowest quartile versus 14% in the highest quartile.

In the US, the Atlanta study examined how vitamin D levels affected the outcomes for patients in surgical intensive care units. The average length of stay in intensive care was 13 days for those patients with serious vitamin D deficiency, seven days for moderate deficiency and five days for normal levels. The death rates for the same groups were 12% and 11%, while none of the patients with normal vitamin levels died.

Another study carried out at the Harvard School of Public Health looked at the effect of vitamin D levels on the development of adult type 1 diabetes. Those patients with the highest level, over 100nmol/L, had a 44% lower risk of developing the disease compared to those with levels below 75nmol/L. One of the researchers, Dr Kassandra Munger, said, "It is surprising that a serious disease such as type 1 diabetes could perhaps be prevented by a simple and safe intervention." But then the researchers played down their own findings, saying, "It is premature to recommend universal use of vitamin D supplements for prevention of type 1 diabetes, but the possibility that many cases could be prevented by supplementation with 25–100mcg per day is enticing."

This type of downplaying of evidence is actually quite common by researchers who carry out studies that produce positive outcomes from lifestyle treatments. They will know that seriously promoting natural solutions would not go down well with their superiors and the pharmaceutical industry and could ultimately affect their careers. But despite this desperately sad situation, the actual results speak for themselves. It is worth adding that when researchers carry out trials on existing drugs and find they don't work as expected or produce unexpected side effects, they also downplay their findings. In this case they usually say the trial might have been flawed in some way, because they know their careers also depend on playing down any negative drug outcomes.

The Harvard School of Public Health also carried out a study on vitamin D and heart attacks. It followed 18,000 men for over ten years and showed that those with the lowest levels in their blood had twice the level of heart attacks.

Just under 70,000 people are admitted to hospital each year in the UK due to serious attacks of asthma and around 1,200 die from it. But a recently published study shows that taking vitamin D supplements halves the number of serious attacks. This means it could prevent nearly 35,000 hospital admissions and potentially 600 deaths per year. Medicine has responded in time honoured fashion. While describing the study as encouraging, they have called for more clinical trials before any recommendations can be made on whether supplements should be prescribed. This, of course, is not unexpected. This tactic has been used many times to delay any decision that would mean giving any credence to a vitamin supplement. The admissions and deaths, therefore, just keep occurring.

A study published in Nature in 2016 showed that serum vitamin D deficiency in mid pregnancy was associated with an increase in autism-related traits in six-year-old children. On the same theme, a 2019 study showed that giving mice vitamin D supplements during pregnancy prevented autistic traits in their offspring. So, whilst these don't provide definitive proof, they do indicate that vitamin D could play a part in reducing the incidence of autism.

According to a study published in the European Journal of Clinical Nutrition, increasing serum vitamin D levels to 50ng/ml could extend a healthy lifespan by over two years.

A 2010 Japanese study published in the American Journal of Clinical Nutrition found that school children taking vitamin D were 58% less likely to catch influenza. By contrast, antiviral drugs like Tamiflu reduced rates of infection by only 8%. Even annual flu vaccines only occasionally reduce infections by more than 50% and in 2015 the figure was just 3% according to Public Health England, with the overall average probably around 35%. Further confirmation of vitamin D's impact on flu came from research in 2018 which analysed the data from 25 separate studies which showed that people with low serum vitamin D who then took supplements reduced their risk of infection by half. There are literally thousands of studies in PubMed about vitamin D and the human immune system and the vital role it plays in our health, including a whole range of viral infections from colds through to COVID-19. COVID-19 will be covered in more detail in Part 5, but I'll outline a few tantalising examples of the impressive benefits of vitamin D now.

Over 170 scientists, academics and doctors from around the world have sent an open letter to all governments, public health officials and doctors calling for the use of high dose vitamin D to help reduce the risk of infection, severe disease, hospitalisations and deaths from COVID-19. In 2020 188 research papers were analysed and showed that higher vitamin D levels are associated with lower rates of infection and lower levels of severe cases, hospitalisations, intensive care and deaths. Most of these doctors take vitamin D themselves and their recommendation is for a daily intake of 100mcg.

Researchers in Cordoba, Spain, carried out the first clinical trial on vitamin D and Coronavirus which was published on 29 August 2020. The trial involved 76 patients admitted to hospital with the disease. Fifty of them were given the vitamin. Of the 26 patients who didn't receive the vitamin, 13 (50%) were eventually admitted to an intensive care unit (ICU) and two of them died. Only 1 of the 50 patients (2%) receiving the vitamin was admitted to ICU and none of them died. A featured letter in the British Medical Journal stated that "although this was a small trial the ICU results are so dramatic that they are statistically highly significant". I should add that the trial used a special form of the vitamin called calcifediol which is around three times more active than ordinary vitamin D. When people take vitamin D supplements or get sun exposure which also produces the vitamin, the liver then eventually converts it to calcifediol which is the active form the body uses. Calcifediol was used in the trial because it has an almost immediate effect which is important for this disease. If a drug had been developed that achieved this level of success, it would have been proclaimed as a miracle breakthrough in the battle against COVID-19. But once again, because this is a natural product that cannot be patented and little profit can be made, then nothing has happened. I would be amazed if you have ever heard anything about the incredible results of this trial because once again the whole story has also been suppressed by almost every media group.

When President Trump developed Coronavirus, his team of doctors gave him vitamin D and zinc supplements. Why would they do this unless they could see there was incredibly strong evidence that they worked? Once again, the press and media never reported it even though they went out of their way to emphasise all the drugs he was taking. Dr Anthony Fauci, who is America's leading epidemiologist, did an interview which was available on YouTube. In it he mentioned that he took 150mcg of vitamin D every day. Dr Fauci promotes only vaccines in his official capacity, yet he took the vitamin himself but never recommended it to anyone else. I am sure he now regrets making this public knowledge and I will be surprised if YouTube isn't asked to delete it to help protect his medical reputation.

I could fill many more pages with other evidence of vitamin D, but hopefully I have given enough examples to show its incredible and wide-ranging benefits. Instead, I will just list a few of the other diseases or conditions it has been shown to help. These include: blood pressure, skin diseases, inflammatory bowel disease, obesity, autoimmune diseases, emotional wellbeing, dementia, heart disease, stroke, Crohn's disease, insulin levels, arthritis, lung function, multiple sclerosis and depression. There are literally hundreds of studies and trials for these diseases, but medicine still ignores them all. No doubt they would use their conventional get out of jail card if they were ever forced to explain why. I'm sure you know the answer by now: "There are no large-scale clinical trials." As already explained, vitamin D plays a part in over 100 bodily functions. To prove that it worked for each one of these would cost over $200 billion. All the key medical decision makers know full well it is impossible to fund such trials. This gives them the perfect excuse by which they can follow Big Pharma's aim to reject every lifestyle solution to health and disease and thus enables them to promote only drugs. One other fact that needs to be emphasised is that certain pharmaceutical drugs can significantly reduce the absorption of vitamin D which can ultimately lead to the serious diseases and medical outcomes that have just been outlined. The main culprits are: blood pressure lowering drugs, diabetes drugs, proton pump inhibitors and anti-epileptic drugs. Anyone taking these drugs really should take additional vitamin D supplements to help maintain their disease resilience.

Here is another fact relating to vitamin D. It involves a group of doctors from a number of countries who formed an organisation called the Vitamin D Council. These doctors have spent most of their medical careers exploring the wide-ranging benefits of vitamin D and prescribing it for their patients. They have effectively become worldwide experts and have achieved incredible medical outcomes. Of course, medicine and regulators dismiss and discredit everything the Vitamin D Council does and recommends in exactly the same way they do for virtually all the other evidence on vitamin D. But then an even more drastic attack took place on the Vitamin D Council. For many years, anyone could type in an internet search for their website and read their recommendations regarding vitamin D and also learn about them on Wikipedia. Now, their site has been removed from the web, and if you type the name on Wikipedia there are "no results". It is just one more example of how the "establishment" is using censorship on a grand scale to try to destroy simple and effective lifestyle solutions to health and disease prevention.

However, something positive has also occurred. The Vitamin D Council had its headquarters in the US, but now a new organisation called the Vitamin D Society has emerged in Canada. Many of the doctors involved were originally part of the US organisation. This means that anyone can now access their recommendations again, but I wonder how long it will be before this is also subject to complete internet censorship. Let's hope that Canada, where the population has one of the highest levels of vitamin D deficiency in the world, will resist this inevitable onslaught and help protect its population from a host of preventable diseases.

I have already made it clear that medicine has rarely used or recommended that people take any type of vitamin supplements and this includes vitamin D. Then in 2016 a clinical trial was carried out which showed that taking a daily 10mcg supplement of vitamin D improves musculoskeletal health which means it can radically help prevent skeletal deformities in children and muscular weakness and frail bones in adults. Medicine could not dismiss this trial (even though admitting that a vitamin worked was probably done through gritted teeth) and the official position is that people should now take 10mcg each day particularly in winter. It is, however, important to note that this low level will not affect all the other diseases that have been examined. So, the dilemma for most people is do they believe the official medical position which only acknowledges that vitamin D affects rickets and musculoskeletal health and denies there is any conclusive proof that it benefits other major diseases? Do they, therefore, just take the official daily recommended dose of 10mcg or do they take the 100mcg that is recommended by most vitamin D experts after looking at the immense body of evidence, trials and studies that exists on all the other diseases like cancer and viral diseases especially given that this level is widely accepted as being completely safe? Whilst every vitamin and key mineral is essential for life and good health and whilst they all work synergistically together, most experts would single out vitamin D as a stand out "superstar". You really should consider it.

Finally, here is a list of some of the other key vitamins and minerals. Just like vitamin D, they all have many trials and studies that show their benefits for a range of conditions and diseases. Most of them will be examined in more detail in some of the key remaining sections of the book which look at individual diseases and how they can be treated.

- vitamin A
- the twelve B vitamins
- vitamin C
- vitamin E
- vitamin K
- zinc
- magnesium
- calcium
- selenium
- chromium
- iodine

There are some other key points I want to make. Probably the first key thing that everyone should take is a high-quality, high dose multivitamin each day (but please check it is not made by a drug company). This will contain all the key vitamins and minerals the body needs. Of course, it will be necessary to take additional supplements depending on your individual needs and any specific health condition you either have or are concerned about. If you decide to take around 100mcg of vitamin D3, for example, you will need to take perhaps three or four 25mcg capsules because the multivitamin will probably only contain around 15mcg.

One final point. Sometimes it may be better to follow what doctors do, rather than what medicine's elite say. Some years ago, a survey was done in the US which asked doctors and nurses if they took supplements. The results were surprising. Around 78% of doctors and 82% of nurses admitted to taking them in an anonymous survey. Some took them regularly, others just when they had specific problems like a viral infection. The vitamins most commonly taken were vitamin C, vitamin D, a multivitamin and fish oils. In the UK, Dr Hilary Jones, who makes regular TV appearances related to health, also wrote an article about the views of his medical friends and colleagues regarding supplements. He said that most of them do not believe powerful drugs are the only answer for every health concern and many of them are only too aware of the side effects of drugs and often take them only if they think there would be an immediate benefit. They do, however, believe in the effectiveness of carefully selected supplements and take them in private even though they might never admit it, simply because they are intimidated by the fear of peer group criticism. So, the "you can get all the vitamins and minerals you need from a balanced diet" message that is preached by medicine's elite seems to cut little ice with many doctors. This is all extremely enlightening but also very sad, because many doctors take supplements but dare not recommend them to their patients because they would face potentially serious disciplinary action and reputational damage.

Minimising chemical exposure

Chemicals are a ubiquitous part of the modern world. In the UK there are thousands of food-related chemicals and a quarter of a million tonnes of them are used in food manufacture every year. Four hundred million litres of pesticides and herbicides are deployed.

Countless other sources of chemicals and heavy metals emanate from transport and industries such as plastics, household cleaners, fire resistant furniture and cosmetic manufacturers, as well as energy generation. An incredible 350,000 chemicals have been globally approved.

All of these can find their way into our bodies in one form or another. It has been estimated that there are around 100,000 different chemicals circulating in our blood system. You may be surprised to learn that virtually none of them have ever been tested for their safety or their effects on the human body, and chemical exposure is playing a significant role in the increasing epidemic of modern diseases. Advocates of lifestyle medicine maintain it is involved in a host of diseases like cancer, Alzheimer's, children's brain development, infertility and respiratory diseases. Chemical manufacturers, the regulators who are supposed to control them and governments invariably maintain there is no proof they are harmful. Well, they would, wouldn't they? This, of course, is exactly what the tobacco industry did for decades. Once again it would be possible to write many books about all these chemicals and their effects on the human body, so I can only outline just a few of them, but these will include some of the most infamous and controversial ones.

Herbicides, pesticides and insecticides. The US company Monsanto first produced the glyphosate herbicide Roundup in the 1970s. Roundup, together with the genetically modified crops that it is now used on, has resulted in more public anger, mass demonstrations and petitions than any other in modern history. In 2013 "The March Against Monsanto" involved over 2 million protesters in over 50 countries. Why? Because there was evidence that it caused cancer in significant numbers of people. Lawsuits against the company then started in 2017 and Monsanto was subsequently found guilty and fined millions of dollars. Despite the reputational and financial damage these court cases caused (and to the surprise of nearly every financial expert), Monsanto was bought by the German company Bayer at a cost of $66 billion. The deal was completed in 2018, but incredibly, by 2020 there were another 100,000 Roundup cancer lawsuits awaiting trial. To minimise further business damage, Bayer agreed a settlement of $10 billion to resolve most of these claims. Some plaintiffs' attorneys, however, refused to accept what they believed was an inadequate settlement and new court cases started again in 2021. I should, however, point out that even though Bayer and Monsanto were found guilty and agreed to pay these incredible settlements, they both still deny there is any proven link between cancer and Roundup. Even after 70 years, the tobacco industry has also never admitted that smoking causes lung cancer, and both Monsanto and Bayer will probably adopt the same strategy with Roundup. Shockingly, despite all these trials and the guilty verdicts, Roundup is still being sold legally in huge quantities and without any requirement for a cancer warning label.

A short summary of some of the events leading to these lawsuits is enlightening. In 2012 French and Italian researchers led by Professor Séralini carried out a study on rats, comparing one group eating genetically modified (GM) maize treated with Roundup to a second group eating naturally grown maize. This study was almost identical to the one used by Monsanto to "prove" that Roundup was safe. There was, however, one crucial difference. The Monsanto study lasted just three months while the Séralini study lasted two years. The death rate in the new study for those fed on GM Roundup maize was nearly twice as high as those fed on natural maize, whereas in the original Monsanto trial there was no significant difference. The life expectancy of the rats used in the trials was two and a half years and the three-month trial used by Monsanto is equivalent to less than ten years for a human. Cancer in humans can take many years to develop and progress (and many months in rats). So, it is no surprise the Monsanto trial did not show any significant effect from Roundup.

Using short trials is a well-used "scam" by pharmaceutical and agro-chemical companies attempting to prove their products are "safe". The Séralini trial was not perfect, but the connection between Roundup and cancer was still very clear and it should have led regulators to demand that more trials be conducted so action could be taken against Roundup. This did not happen and independent organisations like Corporate Europe Observatory and Testbiotec accused the European Food Standards Agency of bias in favour of the GM industry. The key regulators in the US and the EU continued to maintain there was no substantive proof that Roundup was dangerous.

Then, in 2015, the World Health Organization's International Agency for Research on Cancer classified glyphosate as "probably carcinogenic in humans" based on epidemiological studies, animal studies and in-vitro studies. The regulators, however, still continued to maintain their positive approval of glyphosate. Nevertheless, 21 countries from all five continents have now banned or severely restricted glyphosate as well as many individual US states, and many more countries like Germany (even though it is the home of Bayer) are phasing it out over the next few years. The very latest country (in 2022) to ban its agricultural use was India. Recently, Mexico also issued its intention to prohibit genetically engineered corn for human use and the glyphosate that it uses by 2024. Why? Because Mexican officials say it poses threats to human health as well as vital pollinator populations: "We have to put the right to life, the right to health, the right to a healthy environment ahead of economic and business interests." Quite shamefully, the Biden administration is now applying strong arm pressure on Mexico to reverse its decision for just one reason: to protect the sales of its GMO corn producers. Only time will tell whether they succeed.

Roundup is not the first Monsanto chemical known to cause human harm. In the 1950s DDT was used as a pesticide but in 1962 a ground-breaking book – *Silent Spring* by Rachel Carson – examined the disastrous relation between agricultural chemicals like DDT and diseases like cancer. As usual she was attacked by the pesticide industry but her work eventually led to the establishment of the Environmental Protection Agency and a decade later DDT was banned from sale in the US. Many other countries then followed with similar bans, but it was only in 2001 that it was finally removed from sale for all agricultural uses worldwide. Its effects, however, are sadly still being felt. Girls exposed to DDT before puberty, for example, are five times more likely to develop breast cancer in middle age according to the president's cancer panel. A ground-breaking 2021 study also shows DDT is linked to increased breast cancer risk generations after exposure. The granddaughters of women exposed to DDT during pregnancy in the 1960s were over twice as likely to develop obesity and twice as likely to have earlier first menstrual periods, both of which are linked to increased breast cancer risk. This generational link is truly alarming. But DDT also remains in the environment for many years and a recent Finnish study examined the effect of DDE (the breakdown product of DDT within the human body) and found that high maternal blood levels nearly double the risk of autism.

I must also add that Dr Stephanie Seneff, an MIT researcher, has also demonstrated a remarkably consistent correlation between autism and Roundup, and a separate study by the University of California and the California Department of Health Services also showed that pregnant women living near farms where a range of pesticides were used had up to a six-fold increase in the risk of their children developing autism. It is almost certain that every one of the hundreds of synthetic, chemical-based herbicides, insecticides and pesticides (and not just those made by Monsanto) will be having varied but detrimental effects on humans as well as all other animal species.

In Roundup, for example, some of the other chemicals which actually make up 60% of the product have been shown to be far more actively toxic to human cells than glyphosate itself. The latest research has shown that one compound – POEA – is over 1,000 times more toxic than glyphosate. These findings expose the alarming fact that regulators only assess the single, so-called "active" ingredient in all such products, and "assume" all the other chemicals the product contains are safe. They also don't require the manufacturer to even list them all, which is unbelievable. It is a staggering betrayal of the supposed science that regulators claim to use in assessing these products and it is placing all human and animal life at an unknown level of risk and harm. Professor Séralini, for example, carried out separate trials that showed Roundup had toxic effects on the hearts of rats and rabbits. Other prominent researchers believe it affects many other diseases like diabetes, autism, infertility, Parkinson's disease and Alzheimer's.

Other pesticides like chlorpyrifos are linked to many of these diseases but are also known to cause significant neurodevelopmental harm in children. It was first used in 1965. It was then eventually banned in the EU in 2020 (55 years later), when it was stated that there is no safe exposure level. Even now, however, it is still being used in many US states even though organisations like the American Academy of Pediatrics have stated its use puts developing foetuses, infants, children and pregnant women at great risk.

The weedkiller Paraquat, made by Syngenta, has regulatory warnings that a tiny amount (around three drops) will cause death. It was first marketed in the 1960s and has since caused tens of thousands of deaths worldwide. It is now banned in the EU, but only since 2007. Its use is restricted in the US but it is still available in many other countries. It is so lethal it is used by people wanting to commit suicide. In Taiwan there are around 160 Paraquat suicides each year. When South Korea (which has one of the highest suicide rates in the world) banned Paraquat, the suicide deaths fell by around 1,200 after the first 12 months. It has also been linked to Parkinson's disease and several lawsuits have recently been launched against Syngenta in the US. The lawyers for the plaintiffs say they will present internal company records that show Syngenta has known for decades that Paraquat causes Parkinson's disease although they chose to hide this information from regulators and the public. One of the evolving problems is that so many weeds are now becoming resistant to chemicals like Roundup that many farmers have no choice but to try other herbicides like Paraquat, despite its potentially fatal consequences.

It is absolutely impossible to even hazard a guess as to how many lives (particularly children) have been affected and how many cancer cases, other serious diseases and deaths have been caused worldwide by these thousands of chemicals since they were introduced around the middle of the twentieth century. It is, however, likely to be more than anyone could ever imagine. Just a handful of them have subsequently been banned or had their use restricted, but even these now banned chemicals will probably affect future generations because of their devastating generational effects.

There are two key take home messages to all of this. Regulators invariably side with global cartels and cannot be trusted to act primarily in the interests of protecting human life and health. The only way people can minimise their risk of harm from these ubiquitous and dangerous products is to avoid GM foods and the chemicals they contain wherever possible. Try to eat only natural organic plants, vegetables, fruits and grains as well as animals and fish reared on natural foods. Finally, avoid using Roundup or other industrial weedkillers or insecticides. Doing this will not only help minimise your own risk of developing serious diseases but it will help future generations to live healthier and longer lives by reducing the control that manufacturers of these chemicals exert around the world. If you ever see petitions or campaigns against them or any of their dangerous products, please consider signing and promoting them.

Genetically modified organisms. GMOs are not chemicals, but I am including GM seeds and crops here because they are inextricably linked to, and dependant on, chemical herbicides like Roundup as well as the fact they are almost certainly causing similar long-term health outcomes for humans and other animals. The first commercial GM crops were produced in the mid-1990s and mass public exposure started in the US around 2006. Other countries like Brazil, Argentina, Australia and Canada soon joined the GM bandwagon and other countries followed. There was a 100-fold increase in GM crop production between 1996 and 2012. Thankfully, Europe has, so far, mainly avoided their use at least for human consumption. This is primarily because EU citizens have fought against GM crops with incredible determination, this despite the fact most EU regulators and other officials support GM use and declare there is no evidence they cause any harm. The European Commission has argued that the US has been using GM crops for two decades and there is no obvious evidence of any harm. The reality, however, is that the US has one of the highest rates of chronic, degenerative and inflammatory diseases in the developed world, as well as very high rates of allergy and declining fertility. The fact is no direct studies have ever been carried out on humans, but animal studies have in fact shown links between GM crops and these types of disease.

Why has the use of GM crops grown exponentially? The manufacturers' claimed benefits include: increased crop yields, reduced herbicide and pesticide use, and claim it is the only way in which the world can reduce hunger and feed the estimated 9 billion population predicted by 2050. The reality is, however, rather different. A 2009 report titled "Failure to Yield" by the Union of Concerned Scientists in the US says that genetic engineering has failed to consistently increase crop yields. By 2014 a number of US farmers were reducing their use of GM crops because they had realised that some actually had lower yields than conventional crops and, given that the GM seed costs were higher as well, it meant they could increase their profits by nearly 15% by changing back to natural seeds. The use of herbicides and pesticides has not reduced as claimed, instead it has increased. Weeds and pests are also developing increasing resistance to products like Roundup and the superweeds that result (there are now over 250 of them) require ever more herbicides and ever more powerful ones. Some weeds have become so resistant that farmers have no option but to try to remove them by hand. Finally, the claim that world hunger can only be solved by GM crops is incorrect because it misses the key points. A majority of GM crops are actually used for animal feeds and biofuels and not for human consumption and that's before we remember they do not produce any overall increase in crops yields.

A United Nations five-year project completed in 2008 by 400 scientists from 60 counties concluded that GM technology had no place in the alleviation of poverty and hunger. The main cause of hunger is a lack of access to food and not a lack of food itself. Around one-third of all world food is wasted. So, the reality is nearly all the claims for GM crops do not stand up to real scrutiny. There are, however, other factors that significantly exacerbate the problem of hunger especially in Africa. Consider the EU Common Agricultural Policy. The EU subsidises its farmers with about €30 billion each year. This allows it to literally "dump" thousands of tonnes of excess heavily subsidised food into Africa and many local farmers simply cannot compete. A typical example is thousands of tonnes of surplus powdered milk dumped in West African countries like Mali at a cheaper price than local cattle owners can sell at, thus devastating the economy, driving them out of business and significantly raising unemployment.

A second problem is that these farmers cannot immediately return to production if the EU then has a reduced crop yield a year later which can then lead to food shortages and hunger. The EU may appear to many people to be very philanthropic when it sends huge amounts of food to Africa, but in fact, just like many other apparently philanthropic "gifts", there can be unexpected and devastating consequences. At the same time, the EU imposes tariffs on most African food exports. All this means that Africa imports a significant proportion of its food but 20% of its entire population are still undernourished, making them vulnerable to disease, deficiencies and development stunting.

The real solution to this devastating tragedy of hunger lies in initiatives such as Africa Improved Foods (AIF). It took place three years ago in Rwanda and helped 2 million people avert malnutrition and hunger after just one year. Local small holder farmers were guaranteed set prices for their organic crops which were then processed in a factory in Kigali. The cost was $70 million. If this initiative was reproduced across Africa the total cost would be as little as $5 billion. To put this in context, official aid to Africa was $29 billion in 2017, yet hunger is still rising, millions remain in poverty and because the food from rich countries, like the EU, comprises calorie rich but nutrient light carbohydrates such as maize meal, it doesn't prevent stunting or other serious health issues such as anaemia. It can even make countries poorer because ill people cannot work and need more health care, and children who don't get the right nutrients and vitamins early in the first 1,000 days of life suffer impaired brain development and learning difficulties as well as all the physical deficiencies. The title of a Guardian newspaper article by Feike Sijbesma sums it all up: "Wiping out hunger in Africa could cost just $5 billion. What are we waiting for?" Sadly, and tragically, global business and political interests in the developed world will be a major hurdle in achieving this life-saving and life-changing outcome.

So, let's now consider the real motives behind GMO development. Natural open-pollinated seed varieties have always been universally available and could be saved for future crops and exchanged with other growers. But every GM seed is covered by a patent (just like drugs). It means the companies alone control the product and no one else can produce or use them without their consent. New seeds for planting have to be purchased each year and any farmer who tries to reuse them during subsequent years is sued. GM crop sales have increased 100-fold mainly due to the false promises made about yields and reduced use of herbicides and insecticides, as well as the claims that it would eliminate hunger in developing countries. All this has led to a situation where just three companies control over 60% of world seed production and around 75% of world herbicides and insecticides. These are Bayer 31%, Corteva 22% and ChemChina 8%. Four years ago, there were six such companies, but then Bayer took over Monsanto, ChemChina took over Syngenta, and Dow and DuPont merged to form Corteva. These three giant corporations are effectively taking control of the world's food supply by restricting the options available to farmers. All this has been magnified by the exponential growth in industrialised large-scale agriculture which has decimated smaller farmers who traditionally used natural seeds. The result? In the last century, nearly 75% of the genetic diversity of agricultural crops and over 90% of unique seed varieties have simply disappeared. We are now at a point where it is becoming difficult in many countries to revert back to conventional seed production even if this is what their farmers and governments want to do. There are now so many superweeds that can only be killed by new, more powerful and more costly chemical herbicides and, of course, these can only be used on GM seeds that were gene edited to resist them.

The real motives behind GM crop development were never altruistic; their only purpose was to generate patented products and gain total control of world seed production. As Henry Kissinger said, "Control oil and you control nations, control food and you control the people." This was exactly the plan of these global cartels and they are well on the way to achieving it given they are backed by most regulators and even governments in key developed countries.

However, there are some rays of hope. In some counties like India, anti-GMO activists like Vandana Shiva have done an extraordinary job in blocking GM crops (with the exception of cotton). In Europe grassroots public campaigns have so far kept out most GM food crops for human consumption, but even here the battle for animal feed has already been lost, with 85% of all animal feed now coming from GM seeds. If the cartels win this war, the future for mankind could be devastating. Just look at the predictions for antibiotic resistance in humans – key experts are predicting that 10 million deaths will occur each year and most medical operations will have to cease unless a solution can be found. It is quite possible that weed and insect resistance will continue and eventually no new herbicides and insecticides will work. At this point food decimation could threaten much of humanity. It is almost too frightening to contemplate. Please consider trying to support public campaigns that promote natural seed and food production as well as those that are attempting to get GM crops and foods banned or restricted and trying to get them adequately labelled to clearly stipulate their serious and lethal outcomes.

I'll finally outline a few key facts from the very latest 2021 peer-reviewed paper by Jonathan Latham PhD, "The Myth of a Food Crisis". This paper challenges the claims made by Big Ag and its regulatory, philanthropic and academic supporters that only GM crops and chemical intensive and industrial-scale agriculture can provide enough food for mankind. It explains how local organic food grown on small farms can offer tremendous benefits. It regenerates rural communities, it doesn't pollute rivers and groundwater or create dead zones, it can save coral reefs, it doesn't encroach on rainforests, it preserves soil, and it can restore the climate. Most importantly, it can do all of this while still satisfying all food needs for mankind. The fact is almost wherever one looks in global agriculture, food prices are low because products are in surplus. Farmers in many countries are going out of business because prices are falling and have been, with just a few exceptional periods, for over 100 years. In fact, the development of biofuel was done, in part, to minimise the amount of excess foods that had to be scrapped, and all this in spite of a rising global population. Big Ag made false claims that food shortages were imminent many years ago which have been proven to be wrong.

Now they are once again making the same claims that the current surpluses will eventually turn into significant shortages, and organisations like the Food and Agriculture Organization (FAO) use mathematical projections and models to calculate the supposed shortfall in world food. By 2050 they calculate that 60% more food will be needed and that conventional agriculture cannot meet this increase. The 2021 paper, however, clearly rebuts these claims and shows exactly what the false assumptions are that the FAO have made to manipulate the data. In fact, it shows that conventional agriculture could (if needed) produce enough food to feed another 12.5 billion people. None of this will change Big Ag's unscientific claims. Their multi-billion-dollar businesses would be finished if the truth ever became known to everyone. Powerful organisations who have invested tens of billions of dollars in Big Ag will also add their weight in promoting their false claims to protect these investments, and governments are also overly influenced by these organisations.

This 2021 paper concentrated specifically on food supply, but remember the key issue with chemical-laden GM crops is that they are causing devastating health conditions and deaths. As already stated, the future of humanity depends in part on who wins this unforgiveable battle led by global cartels whose only motive is money. Finally, it is worth mentioning that Bayer, the company that controls around a third of world seeds, herbicides and pesticides, is also one of the world's largest pharmaceutical companies. So, its agricultural products are causing serious diseases, but it then gets extra profit from the sale of its drugs that are used (often with minimal benefit) to try to treat the very diseases that it caused. What a sickening scandal.

Plastics. These now exist virtually everywhere. Approximately 370 million tonnes are produced annually. Once released into the environment, plastic waste leaches toxic chemicals which kill wildlife and contaminate the ecosystem. Around 150 million tonnes of plastics already contaminate the oceans and an additional 8 million tonnes from things like plastic carrier bags, food containers and drink bottles are dumped in them each year. Huge numbers of fish, marine animals and sea birds are killed by plastic pollution – either by consumption or entanglement. There are many types of plastics like PVC, phthalates, polycarbonates with bisphenol A and polyethylene. They are ubiquitous and nearly all of them can affect human health. However, one of the key dangers comes from plastics used in food-related items like containers, packaging, drink bottles and cling film. They can contaminate the food we eat and they have been linked to serious potential health conditions like infertility, cancer, immune system suppression, cognitive decline and developmental problems in children. It really is impossible to escape some level of contamination but there are some key things you can do to minimise the risks. Most importantly, don't use plastic for cooking or microwaving. At high temperatures the plastic can breakdown and leach into the food very rapidly. Also, try wherever possible to use glass bottles for drinks, other liquids and foods. Plastics can affect everyone but sadly, amongst those most seriously affected are young children either from food contamination during their development phase, or from contamination of their mothers during pregnancy. Fortunately, some governments have started to ban the use of certain plastics like baby bottles made from bisphenol A, but whilst very welcome, it is only one small step in reducing plastic risk.

Heavy metals. Lead and mercury are particularly dangerous and are known to contribute to conditions like Alzheimer's, poor brain development, mental retardation in children, miscarriage, kidney function, nervous system function and death. As far as lead is concerned, the good news is many governments, particularly in developed countries, are introducing well-needed tougher restrictions to limit people's environmental exposure. Lead mining and processing are key contributors to lead poisoning for those workers involved, but for the average citizen, the three main potential sources are leaded petrol, leaded paint and leaded aviation fuel. Leaded petrol has been eliminated in most developed countries and leaded paint is also on the way out, but in some developing countries they are still being used and are causing around 500,000 deaths per year as well as 10% of all intellectual disability.

Mercury is potentially an even more deadly metal and again, exposure in mining and industrial processes can cause serious outcomes. But, for most people, there are three main potential sources. These are dental amalgam fillings, certain vaccines and certain types of fish and seafood. Official bodies throughout the world declare that those vaccines that contain mercury are completely safe, but some independent scientists disagree, so this is a highly debatable issue especially when you consider what has recently happened with amalgam fillings. The official regulatory response to mercury in amalgam fillings used to be exactly the same as that for vaccines. In other words, the mercury released from these fillings was deemed to be completely safe. This message was endlessly repeated over many decades, but over the last few years there has been increasing official acceptance that it really can cause harm. In 2020 the Federal Drug Agency in the US recommended that certain groups of people should avoid dental amalgam fillings. These include young children, pregnant women, women intending to become pregnant, women who breastfeed, people with multiple sclerosis, Alzheimer's and Parkinson's, and those with impaired kidney function. Similar restrictions or recommendations have been made in the EU and counties like Sweden, Norway, Denmark and 30 others have in fact banned their use completely. In most other countries, however, including the UK, amalgam fillings are still used and even recommended for most other adults. The idea that children can suffer truly serious outcomes from dental mercury exposure but that for adults it has no detrimental effects whatsoever is, to say the least, impossible to believe. Part of the problem may be that amalgam fillings are cheaper to carry out than ceramic fillings. I am convinced that at some future date the UK will have to ban them, but until this happens people will continue to develop diseases and will never know they were caused by mercury "poisoning" from their fillings.

Certain types of fish can also be a major source of mercury. Predator fish and marine mammals that have long lives and eat other fish tend to have significantly higher levels of mercury because it bioaccumulates up the food chain over time. Mercury levels are thus higher in fish like king mackerel, shark, swordfish, barracuda and large tuna, as well as in seals and toothed whales. Countries that consume large quantities of these types of fish, like Greenland, Japan, Canada, China, the Faroe Islands and Brazil, generally have higher levels of mercury in the bodies and more detrimental health outcomes. Fortunately, for many countries, like the UK, the majority of the types of fish eaten have much lower levels of mercury and do not pose the same level of risk, Finally, here are some of the key side effects that mercury can cause. For adults, these include impairment of cognitive thinking, memory, language, and fine motor and visual skills, and for children, brain and nervous system development can be affected.

Processed foods. These contain a wide range of chemical additives. These include artificial colourings, preservatives, chemical flavourings, glazing agents, artificial sweeteners and thickeners. Ultra-processed foods made by Big Food are one of the key causes of many chronic diseases like obesity, heart disease, diabetes and cancer, and some of the chemical additives play a part in their development. However, there is a huge list of other factors involved. These include facts like they have few natural ingredients left after the intense processing they undergo, they contain low levels of essential vitamins, minerals and other natural compounds, they contain many chemically altered foods like hydrogenated vegetable oils, they contain significant amounts of sugar and other similarly dangerous foods, and they are intensely calorie rich. The ideal solution to this is simply to stop eating them or significantly reduce them and eat an all-natural diet as already explained in detail.

Finally, a great deal of evidence exists on the dangers of chemicals and heavy metals and how we can, and should, minimise our exposure to them. But no matter how hard we try, no one can escape some exposure such is their ubiquitous nature. Lifestyle medicine, however, has found a number of safe and simple ways in which we can help to minimise many of them. These include substances like spirulina (blue-green algae) which binds to toxic metals like mercury and plastics like and causes them to be excreted, although detoxification can take several months. Key vitamins and minerals like vitamin A, the B vitamin family, vitamins C, D and E, selenium and compounds like glutathione also help minimise chemical pollution exposure. Another successful option is the use of saunas which helps reduce our toxic burden by sweating out a range of chemicals and heavy metals. The key weapon, however, is still to minimise chemical exposure from all the other potential sources in the first place, by using cleaning products, toiletries and cosmetics made from natural ingredients rather than those made by large global corporations which invariably contain a range of hazardous chemicals. Let me give you one sickening example of this, which also illustrates just how far global corporations will go to maximise profits regardless of human harm.

The drug company Johnson and Johnson has been fined $2.1 billion – a fine that has just been upheld by the US Supreme Court in June 2021. Twenty-two women had sued the company claiming that Johnson's baby powder had caused their ovarian cancer because it contained asbestos. The courts upheld the claim and the lawyer acting for the women made the following court briefings. He said that J&J "had known for decades that their talc powders contained asbestos, a highly carcinogenic substance with no known safe exposure levels. They could have protected customers by switching from talc to cornstarch, as their own scientists proposed as early as 1973. But talc was cheaper and they were unwilling to sacrifice profits for a safer product."

Amazingly, there are another 21,800 more identical lawsuits against the company still pending. Despite the guilty verdict, the company still maintains that its baby powder is safe and does not contain asbestos or cause cancer, even though it stopped all sales in the US in 2020. The company is, in effect, implying that the Supreme Court judgement is wrong, which is a hugely controversial stance, especially when you consider it had previously been found guilty in another five separate lawsuits and fined $3 billion for a range of other illegal practices. I know who I believe, and it is certainly not J&J.

Sleep

Too little sleep is harmful for our health, but so is too much. There is a reasonable consensus that six to eight hours – depending on the individual needs – is about right for an average healthy adult. Babies and children, of course, need much more. Sleeping pills rarely solve sleep problems and they come with a range of very unwelcome side effects such as dizziness, dry mouth, confusion and diarrhoea. There are many ways in which lifestyle solutions can help you get an optimum level of sleep without any of the downsides of drugs. In fact, the other six key lifestyle factors already examined in detail really can provide the basis for good sleep. However, if you still have a problem then there are specific things you can do. Avoid drinking coffee within six hours of going to bed and try to avoid eating any food within a few hours. Really cut back on sugar and refined carbohydrates and use as many low GL foods as possible. Stick to a regular sleep pattern and keep your bedroom cool, dark and quiet. If poor sleep still persists, read the section on insomnia in Patrick Holford's book *Good Medicine* which contains some very specific solutions.

Other important factors that affect health

We have examined in some detail the seven key factors that profoundly and synergistically affect our health and life expectancy and that provide the basis for lifestyle medicine. Of course, some of the claims, particularly for vitamins and minerals, are still disputed by medicine even though the evidence is compelling. There are, however, many other aspects of our lifestyle and environment which contribute to our wellbeing. I have selected just six more random factors in headline form that will give you an idea of the diversity of lifestyle approaches to health. Some are important while others are simple things that individually give small benefits, but which collectively make a difference.

Teeth and gums

Looking after your teeth and gums is important for obvious reasons but did you know that poor oral hygiene is also implicated in heart disease? The bad bacteria responsible for gum disease can find their way into the bloodstream where they cause havoc – an extra reason to really look after them.

Mobile phones

Well over 200 studies have linked excessive mobile phone use to brain tumours and infertility. Children are particularly badly affected. The telecoms industry, of course, denies any link, and finding *definitive* proof is always very difficult. It took decades before scientists could finally prove beyond any doubt that smoking caused lung cancer. One day, however, the dangers of mobile phones will, despite the best efforts of the telecom industry and regulators, be proven. Until then try to limit their use and try to keep the mobile phone away from your body, because there is strong evidence, for example, that they are a key cause of the decline in sperm counts. The imminent expansion of 5G networks will significantly increase these risks and will also affect nearly every other form of animal life.

Keep moving

The human body evolved for, and is designed for, activity. Inactivity is really bad for us. Remember the young people who, before the Apollo moon landing, were kept in a state of almost complete rest to see what would happen. Within a few weeks their heart function had deteriorated so dramatically that the trial was stopped because of fears for their health. This trial led medicine to abandon its use of bed rest after heart attacks – and instead to replace it with exercise. Of course, we have already explored exercise in detail, but while exercise is truly beneficial, what you do for the rest of the time is also important. I'm sure you must have seen the warnings about sitting down for extended periods and its detrimental effect on health. Because of this, some people have recommended we stand instead of sit, but recent research suggests that even standing in one position, at a work station for example, could also have detrimental outcomes. The key is simply to try to move regularly. When you have been sitting down or even standing still for a while, try to move around even if it's only for a minute. The other good option is to keep changing position. In other words, for want of a better description, you should fidget quite frequently. I am very lucky because I actually do find it difficult to sit down for more than an hour and even then, I really do feel the need to move. So, I will change my sitting position, stretch my legs and stretch my arms regularly.

Eating window

Going without food for 12 to 14 hours can be beneficial in several ways. It helps keep blood sugar levels under control and improves insulin resistance. It helps control blood pressure and there are indications it may help in the prevention of diseases like Alzheimer's as well as increasing life expectancy. Most people prefer to do this by having nothing else to eat after their evening meal. Intermittent fasting for periods up to 24 hours can bring even more benefits but you should not contemplate this unless you have thoroughly researched the subject, and this applies particularly to people with diabetes. Regularly eating snacks between main meals is also something you really should try to avoid. These can lead to blood sugar levels staying constantly high and significantly increasing the risk of developing type 2 diabetes as well as the risk of serious side effects for those who already have the disease.

Innovative supplements

There are a number of innovative supplements that may be particularly beneficial for our health.

- Coenzyme Q10 is a vitamin-like substance present in virtually all cells and has proven benefits for heart function and blood pressure. When it was tested on fruit flies, it doubled their lifespan. Don't expect the same for humans, but nevertheless the evolving evidence is hugely encouraging for a number of other diseases. Incidentally, statin drugs destroy CoQ10, so anybody who takes them really should supplement with CoQ10 supplements. There is also a much more absorbent form called ubiquinol which is even more effective.
- Resveratrol is a red wine/grape extract and it has been shown to improve heart function. It has also increased the lifespan of fruit flies and other small mammals. It shows promise as a cancer treatment and for Alzheimer's, amongst others.
- Curcumin is a turmeric extract. It reduces inflammation and is used in the treatment of arthritis. Animal studies also show potential benefits in cancer treatment, Alzheimer's and diabetes.

Breathing

If you ever feel really stressed or unhappy about something, close your eyes and take a few very long, slow, deep breaths, both in and out. You may be surprised how you feel.

There are many studies which show how a healthy lifestyle really can increase life expectancy, and here are two specific examples. The Nurses' Health Study and the Health Professionals Follow-up Study which were carried out over 30 years showed significant increases in life expectancy by simply adopting just five healthy behaviours. These are: not smoking, BMI in the normal range, a high-quality diet score, taking regular exercise, and maintaining alcohol intake within sensible limits. Those who adopted all five had an average life expectancy of 13 years more than those who adopted none of them. I must add these are very high-profile studies but they analysed just these five specific lifestyle factors. If a study was done that analysed all the other key lifestyle factors that have been explored, the difference in life expectancy would, without doubt, have been at least around 20 years.

Further reading

Here are some key recommendations for learning more and keeping up with the latest developments and information on lifestyle medicine and its incredible benefits.

Sign up for a free weekly newsletter from the Alliance for Natural Health International (ANH). Simply press the "subscribe" button at the top of its website. You could also become a Pathfinder member for more benefits and to help support what is perhaps the most amazing, independent organisation of just half a dozen incredible people who help to protect, defend and promote lifestyle medicine. You will see shortly that around 20 years ago, the EU really was about to ban nearly all vitamin and mineral supplements and it was Robert Verkerk, the founder of ANH who made a legal challenge against it. Without this, most supplements really would have disappeared but thankfully he prevented it from happening and has helped millions of people to stay healthy. I have already recommended a really key book called *Reset Eating*, which is written by Robert Verkerk and Meleni Aldridge. I will recommend it once again.

In terms of other books relating to lifestyle and especially nutrition, Patrick Holford is also a real superstar. He has published over 30, often in conjunction with other experts. Throughout the book I will recommend several of them. Here are some of my top suggestions:

- *The 10 Secrets of Healthy Ageing*
- *The 10 Secrets of 100% Health People*

- *Food Is Better Medicine than Drugs*
- *The Hybrid Diet*

He has also written important books on individual diseases like heart disease, cancer, Alzheimer's, diabetes and arthritis to name just a few.

You could also consider signing up for the magazine What Doctors Don't Tell You, or simply have online access to it.

Lifestyle medicine - my own journey

The 12 hours that changed my life

Twenty-five years ago, my life changed forever in just 12 hours. One evening, I opened a letter containing the results of a blood test that showed I had very high cholesterol. This came as a complete shock and I remember telling a friend about it early the next morning. This friend suggested I read a book called *The 8-Week Cholesterol Cure* because her brother had cured his high cholesterol by following the dietary guidelines in the book. So, I bought the book and, at that time, test kits were also available from chemists that accurately measured cholesterol levels. This meant I was able to make the dietary changes and monitor my own progress, and literally eight weeks later, my cholesterol came down from 7.3 to 5.2.

Luck or chance, whichever you believe in, was on my side in an unbelievable way. All this came about because the company I worked for decided to offer its managers a comprehensive two-hour medical check-up. Like many other colleagues, I decided not to bother due to a busy work schedule, but on a whim, and at the last minute, I made an appointment. I still can't remember exactly why I changed my mind, but on such whims, lives are changed forever. The results of the blood test came through a week later. The doctor in his letter said I should try to eat more fruit and vegetables and that in 12 months' time we would discuss the options for treatment. Remember, although my cholesterol was very high, there was not the same hysteria at that time as there would be now, and statin drugs were nowhere near as widely prescribed. I was looking forward to telling him of my success, but this didn't happen because the company then went through a difficult time and the medicals had to be curtailed.

The second piece of luck came when I mentioned my cholesterol diagnosis to the "one in a million" friend who knew about this life-changing book. If I had mentioned it to anyone else instead, I would never have found out about the book and my health would have been on a downwards spiral. Had this unlikely series of events not taken place, my high cholesterol would eventually have been diagnosed by my GP who, without doubt, would have started me on statins. I would never have learnt anything about lifestyle medicine and would now be taking a cocktail of drugs. I would be on the drug merry-go-round not realising that each new condition was very likely caused by the previous drug(s) I was taking, and not realising how the right lifestyle could prevent me ever needing to get on the drug merry-go-round in the first place.

So, what happened after I had read *The 8-Week Cholesterol Cure* and reversed the high cholesterol simply by changing my diet and taking a few supplements? Well, something in my subconscious drew me back to the bookshop and the section on health. I started to look at the titles and saw a book called *Stop Ageing Now* which, not unsurprisingly, caught my eye. I read the synopsis and was immediately intrigued. The book was all about the latest research indicating that a good diet and ten key vitamins and minerals together with fish oils and foods like garlic could slow the ageing process significantly and add healthy years to your life. Normally, it takes me a few weeks to read a book, but I read this one in just a few hours. The logic and evidence seemed compelling and I decided there and then that I would follow the advice. Would I have been similarly swayed if I had not had first-hand experience of how powerful lifestyle changes could be? Probably not, but, of course, I did have that knowledge and so the decision was much easier. I had just one concern. Was it safe to take all these supplements? So, I found another book that gave the "safe level" of every vitamin and mineral. I was pleasantly surprised to see that the safe limits for nearly all of them were many times greater than the recommended doses in the book. So, with my safety concerns fully addressed, I started to follow the supplement and dietary advice. Before I explain what happened next, I need to briefly outline some of the health problems I was experiencing at the time.

If I tell you that every cold over the previous 20 years lasted 14 or 15 days, you would probably imagine it was a gross exaggeration, especially when I add that the symptoms were so bad that life was essentially on hold for two weeks. But this really is the truth. I vividly remember a ten-day holiday in Gran Canaria where I spent almost the entire time ill in bed, apart from occasional tiring trips to the supermarket for some food. There were several others including Greece and Croatia, where the holiday was similarly ruined. When that first tell-tale sign of a new cold – the sore throat – occurred, my heart sank. Anything I had planned for the next two weeks was not going to happen. The severe sore throat would, after two or three days, give way to the cold proper, when I would use up several boxes of tissues with alternating bouts of incredible sweating and shivering thrown in for good measure. To round everything off, the last week was dominated by a truly painful hacking cough when I would use three or four bottles of cough medicine to help minimise the lung pain. Since I had at least three colds each year, then at least six weeks, or 12% of my life, was spent literally in abject misery. I was, of course, the ideal patient for Big Pharma, consuming copious quantities of "cold remedies" and cough medicines. But I now realise that, apart from reducing the symptoms, none of these "remedies" affected the cold in any way whatsoever. It was my immune system, and only my immune system, that eventually defeated the cold virus. The incredibly long duration of the colds clearly indicated that my immune response was severely compromised, although I didn't realise any of this at the time.

The second problem was my finger joints. These had been slowly getting worse for about five years. They weren't too painful but the joints were stiff and had started to "click" whenever I flexed my fingers. The symptoms were particularly bad early in the morning and slowly reduced as the day progressed. I worried that eventually it would affect my piano playing which I had planned to be a major part of my retirement. I didn't visit my doctor because I thought that joint problems were just a normal and unavoidable part of ageing. But I now realise I had the classic symptoms of rheumatoid arthritis.

The third problem I suffered from was energy slumps. These usually occurred about an hour after lunch. If I was at home, I wouldn't try to fight it and would often just fall asleep. The tiredness only lasted for about 15 minutes. After that I felt absolutely normal as if nothing had happened. Of course, if they happened at work, I couldn't just fall asleep, so I would immediately force myself to walk around the factory until the tiredness had passed. The most terrifying thing that has ever happened to me occurred during the most severe energy slump I had ever experienced. It was unprecedented in its severity and something I would never have expected could happen. I was driving in the middle lane of the M6 motorway when I could feel the tiredness start. It was February and the outside temperature was below zero. I opened both windows and an icy gale came in but this barely helped. I even started to slap my face very hard to try to stay conscious but to no avail. What must have been no more than a second or two later I woke up shaking and terrified but luckily still in the correct lane.

I could have killed not just myself but countless others. At that time, I had a very stressful job, often working twelve hours a day, six, and sometimes seven, days each week. I simply put my tiredness down to these factors. But I now know that I was suffering from reactive hypoglycaemia which was caused by a high glycaemic diet.

My diet really was atrocious, although I didn't realise any of this at the time. I was simply following government and medical advice to cut down on fat and increase carbohydrates and I really believed I was doing the right thing for my health. While I did eat some vegetables, the other parts of my diet, like plain white baguettes, cakes, processed breakfast cereals and Coca Cola, particularly at lunch time, were slowly killing me. Reactive hypoglycaemia occurs when the body is overwhelmed by severe spikes in blood sugar caused by high glycaemic foods. Insulin is then released in large quantities to rapidly reduce this dangerously high blood glucose. But when blood sugar is so high it is difficult to bring it down quickly without "overshooting", and this means that for a short time, the level falls too low. It is this low blood sugar – hypoglycaemia – that causes the energy slumps and, in extreme cases, even complete black-outs, as I finally found out. During 7 million years of evolution, mankind has never eaten such highly processed glycaemic foods. This disastrous change in diets is one of the key factors in the escalation of many serious diseases of which reactive hypoglycaemia is just one example.

The fourth problem I had was regular attacks of hives that lasted about five days. Hives occur when the body's own immune system attacks something like a specific food or food additive that it starts to recognise as harmful. This battle between the immune system and the offending food causes the tell-tale rash that is incredibly itchy. This time I did see my doctor who prescribed antihistamines. These really did reduce the symptoms, but whilst the rash was subdued and only slightly itchy, my skin did not look or feel normal. They also made me drowsy and, of course, the drugs didn't stop the hives returning every few weeks.

The fifth problem was leg cramps that affected my calf muscles. These were excruciatingly painful. They always occurred in the middle of the night and I would wake up in agony. One night I got up after the initial pain had subsided but unusually, the cramp started again. This time the pain was so bad I passed out. I must have dropped like a stone because I woke up on the bathroom floor with a sore hip and eventually a huge bruise. I must have been incredibly lucky that I did not seriously damage my head. As well as the immediate savage pain, the damaged muscles caused further bouts of milder, but still unpleasant pain, for about another day particularly when walking.

So, what happened when I started on my regime of high dose supplements and a much-improved diet? One day, after about twelve months, I suddenly realised I hadn't had a 14-day cold that I was used to. I had had two "normal" colds that lasted around five days. This was a completely unexpected outcome. However, as I continued to learn how to keep improving my lifestyle and diet, colds became even shorter and less severe. In the last ten years I have had an average of two each year – nothing can stop you catching the cold viruses – but most of them are so mild I am able to carry on life exactly as normal, including going for a run. The symptoms, incredibly mild as they are, last just one or two days. In this same period I have had just three colds that lasted three or four days. I should add that I have also seen exactly the same sort of reduction in symptoms with flu although it occurs less frequently than colds.

Of all the benefits lifestyle medicine has given me, regaining over 12% of my life from the misery of severe colds and flu is, perhaps, the most tangible and impressive, but it is actually not the most important. The supplements, such as chromium which help regulate blood sugar, and my improved diet made a huge difference to my energy slumps. Gone were the white baguettes, cakes and Coca Cola and in came nuts, salad and fruit for lunch. The afternoon energy slumps disappeared almost immediately and are now a thing of the past, which is quite amazing when you think that just over 25 years ago, they nearly killed me.

I would like to tell you that my finger joints also improved, but they didn't – at least not immediately. But over the next five years there was a slow, but increasingly noticeable change. At that point only my little fingers were affected and even then, not all the time. Today my finger joints are perfect – no stiffness, pain or clicking. I can now look forward to many years of piano playing, without the constant worry that it will all be snatched away from me. The attacks of hives slowly became much less frequent, although they also took several years to disappear completely. The last attack I had was almost 20 years ago. It lasted no more than two hours and I didn't even take an antihistamine.

My muscle cramps also significantly reduced in frequency but did not completely disappear. It was only about 15 years ago that I found the final solution. I knew muscle cramps are often caused by a lack of magnesium, and at that time I was already taking a magnesium supplement. But then I read about how different types of magnesium are absorbed in significantly differing amounts by the body. I changed the supplement to one containing magnesium citrate and magnesium malate which are two of the most highly absorbable types. This really has worked. I have not had one episode of cramp since. Incidentally, if you look at the NHS web entry on muscle cramps, the main cause is stated as idiopathic – which means it is unknown. Medicine also has no drugs or other treatments for it, so most people just have to accept it and suffer from it. It's impossible to know whether the key decision makers in medicine really don't know about the benefits of magnesium (although I doubt that) or they are just keeping quiet about it. This is all very sad because muscle cramps really can be seriously painful and they affect a great many people. So, there is a truly effective natural solution that can prevent most of them but very few people know about it, and medicine seems intent on ensuring they never do.

What would have happened if I had not learnt about lifestyle medicine and just seen a doctor for all five of these medical conditions? Well, as far as muscle cramps are concerned, medicine has no treatments so I would still be having regular agonisingly painful episodes. Antihistamine drugs certainly do reduce the symptoms of hives but they never stop it from happening and, of course, they have very unpleasant side effects. There are drugs for rheumatoid arthritis but they don't cure it and only minimise the symptoms; the disease still slowly deteriorates and there are some very serious potential drug side effects. It really would be highly likely that I would now not be able to play my beloved piano. There are no medical treatments that can turn serious 14-day colds into superficial one- or two-day colds, so I would still be effectively "losing" 12% of my active life. If I had seen my doctor about the energy slumps, he probably would have diagnosed the reactive hypoglycaemia and advised me to reduce carbohydrate intakes. This would have helped, but it would definitely not have been as effective as the other major dietary changes that I made, as recommended by lifestyle practitioners.

By comparison, I have completely cured all of these diseases and conditions using simple lifestyle changes. But these are only one part of the benefits. I am enjoying life like never before. Of course, part of this is probably because I am now retired with fewer stressful situations, but I am working just as hard on a wide range of other things. I am significantly healthier now than I was 30 years ago even though medicine really does believe this is impossible. I'm also enjoying food like never before despite the fact that close to 50% of it consists of vegetables, and now I only rarely eat any of the "impossible not to eat foods" that I used to adore, like cakes, sweets, conventional chocolates and processed foods. Instead, I've found foods that taste wonderful but are far healthier like 85% dark chocolate, extra virgin olive oil, red grapefruit, pistachio nuts and pomegranates, and I'm eating really tasty foods like cheese and butter again that I had previously avoided. I'm also sleeping better in the last few years than I can ever remember. I am now within one kilo of my lowest ever weight as an adult, and this is seven kilos less than my highest weight. I've also never needed to see a doctor or take any drugs in the last 25 years. With the possible exception of antibiotics, I can say it is highly unlikely I would ever take any drug, because I know, quite simply, that lifestyle changes simply achieve better outcomes and have no side effects.

I'll now outline just a few of the other key things that have helped transform my health. Over the last five years, I started to try a number of fermented foods that can contain up to 100 different types of friendly bacteria. These included things like goat's milk kefir, sauerkraut and kimchi. There were also prebiotics like inulin that provide perfect foods for these incredible bacteria. I am convinced that most of the additional improvements in my health that I have seen over this time can be attributed to these foods that support and improve microbiome health and diversity. They have improved my natural immune system which has resulted in even further reductions in cold and flu symptoms and also my improvements in sleep. Incredibly, I also feel much more relaxed and have even more energy. When I tried all of these, I discovered something that went straight into my top ten favourite foods. Its name? Sauerkraut, which is basically fermented cabbage. I have one suggestion if you ever decide to try it – buy it from a UK company that specialises in it and not from a supermarket. If you don't like the taste, remember there are a range of other incredibly beneficial fermented foods and drinks like goat's milk kefir, kimchi and kombucha that are also available.

You have also seen that not far off 50% of my diet involves vegetables. I have to admit that many of them are not exactly exciting or tasty foods on their own, but I have found a way to actually make that happen. For my main meal, I usually have up to ten of the most beneficial vegetables which are steamed, like broccoli, kale, cauliflower, cavolo nero, cabbage, sprouts, carrots, spinach and asparagus together with fish. But I widely add other natural and incredibly tasty things that I love, like black peppercorn, extra virgin olive oil, mint sauce, red onion and herb sea salt, so that every forkful literally contains a taste of all of them. This simply makes these vegetables one of my favourite foods. Given the wide variety of taste preferences, most people would certainly not like what I add to vegetables, so my key suggestion is simply to find your own and try to use them so you too can really enjoy vegetables which are one of the absolute key foods for good health. There are, of course, also a wide range of homemade recipes containing vegetables in the books I recommend, like *Reset Eating*.

Let me add that herb sea salt is my favourite food additive. Most people, however, really do think this is something that should be seriously restricted because of the many negative claims made about it, but let me explain that salt is one of those vital ingredients for human life. It's true that if you really eat too much, it can be harmful, but if you had zero salt it would also harm you and you would eventually die from it. Eating too much or too little are both harmful. An important fact is that the processed foods many people eat nearly all contain salt. However, I rarely eat any of them, and many of the natural foods I do eat, like vegetables and fruits, contain zero amounts. So, apart from my cheese and butter which do have salt, then I really do need to add my incredibly tasty herb sea salt or my health really would be affected. If you love salt and want to know the real truth about it and the ideal amounts to eat, then read this book written by Dr James DiNicolantonio *The Salt Fix: Why the Experts Got it All Wrong and How Eating More Might Save Your Life*. There are in fact a wide range of different official recommendations, but many of them involve significantly restrictive salt use and this really can affect your health.

Before I started to learn about lifestyle medicine, I almost religiously followed the medical and government dietary guidelines involving low fat diets. From the mid-1970s, everyone, including the media, portrayed fat as the ultimate killer. TV regularly showed obese people and made sure that everyone "knew" they were obese simply because they ate too much saturated fat, and that this was also the main cause of heart disease and the huge numbers of deaths associated with it. If I tell you that two of my favourite foods are butter and cheese, you might understand why this was a devastating blow for me. However, the relentless warnings meant I did almost give them up at that time. I say almost, because just once a fortnight I would indulge in one meal with both of them and it was like going to heaven. However, I still vividly remember feeling incredibly guilty about doing it and almost praying it wouldn't cause me any harm. Even when I started to learn about lifestyle medicine and started to change my diet in the ways already explained, the two decades of incessant anti-fat propaganda were so engrained within my psyche that it took several more years before I had the courage to start to ramp up my fat intake. Now I know these guidelines were wrong and I can really enjoy these two wonderful foods without a hint of worry. In fact, I know with certainty that they are a major contributor to my current level of good health. The key point is if you cut out most fat you have to eat something else which usually means many more carbohydrates and it was these, often very refined, carbohydrates that were the main cause of nearly all my major health problems.

Over the last 25 years I have continued to learn about effective lifestyle solutions to most health conditions. Each year more information becomes available. If I had known all of this at the beginning, it wouldn't have taken me about five years to finally conquer my rheumatoid arthritis and hives, and ten years to finally conquer my muscle cramps. It could still perhaps have taken months or even one or two years because lifestyle changes don't always provide instant results, but ultimately, they can provide real and lasting cures. And, of course, they will now prevent these devastating conditions from reoccurring. For anyone now wanting to try lifestyle solutions for health, disease prevention or cure, much more information is available. However, please be very careful about trying to find information from the web. As already explained, those in power are making great efforts to censor lifestyle information and to divert everyone to the use of drugs and things like industrialised foods. Books are the very best way to learn about lifestyle medicine because they are not censored (at least at present). This is why I keep making certain key recommendations.

When researchers, medicine, regulators and governments embraced the saturated fat and cholesterol hypothesis for heart disease and obesity and all the other dietary recommendations, I was a model citizen. I believed everything I was told, and followed the guidelines almost religiously. Of course, I know now that this was ruining my health and had I not had my "lucky breaks" that led me to lifestyle medicine, I would today almost certainly be suffering from some chronic and probably life-threatening diseases like heart disease, diabetes and cancer. But now I also know the research that led to the dietary guidelines I so assiduously followed was biased and not based on science. I am angry at all those involved. Angry at Ancel Keys whose biased research was a key promoter of low fat diets, angry at those who should have checked his work but didn't, angry at the researchers who concluded that fat was the cause of heart disease when even their own data showed it wasn't, angry at the global food companies who poured huge sums of money into "proving" that saturated fat was bad just to protect sales of their own truly dangerous hydrogenated vegetable oils, angry at medicine's elite committees who suppressed powerful contradictory evidence, angry at medicine for allowing dogma to set in and refusing to reanalyse the data at any stage over the next 30 years, and angry at official organisations who even today advocate a low fat, high carbohydrate diet. I have been very lucky. Over the course of 25 years I learnt the awful truth and, as I learnt, I was able to ignore the advice given by all these "experts" and so-called guardians of our health and in doing so regained and even improved my health. But I am angry, more than anything, that hundreds of millions of people are still unwittingly following this advice and living shorter, unhealthier lives and succumbing to serious chronic diseases as a result. It really is almost unimaginable how this sort of health disaster occurs with such regularity, and how the experts get it wrong time after time. I will explore all of this in much more detail in Part 5.

I'll finish this section by explaining how two friends have also benefited from lifestyle medicine. Six years ago, one of them developed non-diabetic small fibre neuropathy the symptoms of which got progressively worse. Neuropathy is a condition where the nerves, usually in the legs and feet, are damaged. It results in intense pain and can cause the affected limbs to feel "on fire" or totally numb, and it can significantly affect physical movement and balancing. The condition got so bad he would not even see members of his own family for days and even weeks. His doctor offered a drug called gabapentin, but he didn't take it because there were risks of severe side effects, which I'll come back to. He was then sent to see a consultant neurologist who referred him to a hospital that applied electrical stimulation procedures. He described it like this: "Think jump leads attached to my legs and feet and electrical shocks sent through me. Awful, and no benefits seen." He was eventually given cognitive therapy and pain management courses where you simply have to try to learn how to live with the pain.

Previously, he had looked at other solutions for neuropathy like vitamins, but had dismissed them because it seemed improbable that they could work for such a serious disease. Eventually, however, he did try them. These included highly absorbable forms of vitamin B12 (methylcobalamin) and B1 (Benfotiamine) and vitamin D. It took around two months before he felt any changes, but then slowly, the pain started to ease. During the worst phase of the neuropathy, he was only sleeping an average of just one hour each night, but after taking the vitamins for several months he was back to sleeping between seven and eight hours. He was also able to start going for walks again, which had been almost completely off the agenda. The pain hasn't totally disappeared, but he is back to living almost a normal life.

It was a very good decision he made not to take the drug gabapentin. Why? Cast your mind back to the section on "fraud" within medical research and the drug Neurontin. I should explain that most drugs have two names and Neurontin is just another name for gabapentin. This was the drug that was fraudulently promoted without any clinical evidence for a range of off-label uses for which the manufacturer – Pfizer – was eventually fined $430 million. No trials were carried out on non-diabetic small fibre neuropathy so there is no proof that it has any benefits. I should add that gabapentin is officially used to treat diabetic neuropathy but this is a different disease and even for this, its benefits are minimal with just 15% of patients seeing some partial reduction in pain. The other key fact is the long list of alarming side effects. These include an increased risk of suicide, aggressive behaviour, jaundice, inflamed pancreas, nausea, increased risk of infection, feeling dizzy, swollen arms and legs, blurred vision and weight gain, to name just a few.

There is, however, another twist to this story. If you look on the NHS website, you will see that they do say that one of the possible causes of neuropathy can be vitamin B12 deficiency, but they do not approve its use for doctors. They also claim that other vitamins like B1 and D have no proof that they work. This is why doctors do not, and cannot, prescribe them for patients with neuropathy. However, the British Medical Association (BMA) publishes a book called *The Complete Home Medical Guide* which clearly states that vitamins B12 and B1 together can be very effective in treating neuropathy and can even cure it completely if they are taken before the condition deteriorates too far. So, quite shockingly, the BMA says these vitamins are an effective cure, while the NHS will simply not use them. The NHS also states that around 1 in 10 people over the age of 55 have neuropathy, which means that over 2 million are suffering from it. It is just one more devastatingly sad example of how medicine's key decision makers ignore simple, cheap and effective natural solutions to disease. How can they allow 2 million people to suffer unnecessarily from a curable devastating disease like neuropathy?

Another friend developed type 2 diabetes six years ago. Her initial blood sugar level was 14.8 which is very high and if left untreated would have led to serious complications. She told her doctor she wanted to try changing her diet first as she had started to read about the benefits of certain low carb foods. After about a month, the level had come down significantly to 9.5, but her doctor said it was still too high and prescribed two tablets a day of the drug metformin and a few weeks later increased this to four tablets a day. At the same time, she was still trying to improve her diet and taking several supplements like chromium. Her blood sugar eventually fell to around 7.5 and her diabetic nurse and doctor seemed reasonably satisfied with this progress. It stayed around this level for the next two years, but then she came across information about another supplement and a herbal product that seemed to have a significant effect on blood sugar. She decided to try them and the results were staggering. Her blood sugar fell by a further three points to around 4.5. In fact, this reduction was too much because very low blood sugar can cause dizziness and even result in passing out. She immediately reduced the amounts so that the blood sugar was at a more normal range of around 5.5 to 6. She then also decided to see what would happen if she stopped taking the metformin drug. Over a few weeks she slowly reduced the level to zero. What happened was that her blood sugar went up by an average of 1.1. What all this means is that, in total, she had been able to reduce her blood sugar from 14.8 to 4.5 which is a 70% reduction. The lifestyle changes she had made and the various supplements delivered a 63% reduction and the drug's contribution was just 7%. However, she then decided to go back to taking half the dose of metformin because I think she was worried her doctor and nurse would not be happy about what she had done. The key fact from all of this is it was the lifestyle changes that caused 90% of her blood sugar reduction. Without this, and just using the drugs, she would probably now be suffering from serious outcomes like amputations and heart disease.

The key message from these two friends' outcomes, as well as my own five original conditions, is that simple lifestyle changes can achieve staggering health outcomes that can beat drugs by many orders of magnitude and, of course, there are no side effects. The three of us are not unique. For the last 25 years I have read hundreds of articles about people (some on their own, and others helped by integrative medical doctors) who have used lifestyle solutions to cure conditions and transform their lives, including life-threatening diseases like cancer.

I want to outline now one other potentially life-threatening condition I developed. The reason I have left it until the end of this section is that, although my attempts to solve it have recently been encouraging, they are still in progress. Around 12 years ago, I started to notice my very short-term memory was occasionally failing. As an example, before I clean my teeth, I floss them. After doing this and when opening the toothpaste, I would sometimes suddenly think, "Have I flossed my teeth?" I simply couldn't remember. I would then have to check the place where I put the used floss and, on most occasions, it was there. So, I had in fact used it. All this meant that, on certain occasions, I was unable to remember something I had done less than a minute earlier. There were, of course, other examples of this short-term memory loss, but none of them caused any practical or significant problems and my life was, in all other respects, absolutely normal. However, almost immediately I realised this was one of the earliest signs of Alzheimer's disease, so I was truly concerned. I should add that both my mother and aunt had also developed the disease and had their remaining life destroyed. Most cases of Alzheimer's usually start to occur in people over the age of 70 and, in these cases, it is rarely hereditary. But if it develops well before that age, which it did in my case, then there is a significantly increased possibility of such a hereditary link. There is a special section on Alzheimer's disease in Part 5, but I will outline just a few key facts now and explain what I have been doing to treat it.

One key fact is there are no meaningful medical treatments for Alzheimer's, so there really was no point in seeing a doctor. In my mission to learn everything I could about lifestyle medicine, I had already read a great deal of information about ways in which it could influence the disease. My main option was to take a range of B vitamins, which had been analysed in a number of studies and trials. The studies showed they reduced the level of homocysteine, a compound that had been linked to Alzheimer's. As the disease progresses, the brain starts to shrink in size and the trials had shown that the vitamins and the lower homocysteine had significantly curtailed this shrinkage. So, I started to take extra key vitamins which included B12, B6 and folic acid and had a test done to check my homocysteine level before I started to take them and then six months later. The figure fell from 13 to 11, and while this was an improvement, I knew that a figure of seven or below was the sort of target I should be aiming for. Eventually, I started to learn about special, highly absorbable types of these vitamins and started to take methylcobalamin (a form of B12) and methylfolate (a safe natural form of folic acid). Six months later the homocysteine level had fallen to seven which was very encouraging. For the next few years, however, little changed. I still had similar levels of short-term memory loss, but encouragingly, it was definitely not getting any worse. Then six months ago I read about benfotiamine, a fat-based, highly absorbable form of vitamin B1 and its significant benefits for diseases like Alzheimer's and Parkinson's. It was the first time I had ever seen this type of information and decided immediately to try it because the evidence looked compelling as well as the fact it is one of the safest vitamins ever. Over the last few weeks, I began to realise that the incidence of memory problems had reduced. The recurrent and obvious problem when flossing my teeth used to occur three or four times a week but now it is around once. I will not get carried away yet, but I am becoming increasingly optimistic that I have certainly stopped any decline in memory loss and possibly that I have even started to reverse it even if only marginally. Only time will tell.

Incidentally, I have literally also just read about another form of vitamin B1 called allithiamine which is a naturally occurring compound in garlic and which is possibly even more effective than benfotiamine, at least for Alzheimer's. I am going to try it although it will probably take a number of months to see if it leads to any further improvement.

To end this section, however, there is one ominous cloud on the horizon. I will explain in detail in the next section that there are plans afoot – led by the pharmaceutical industry – to ban the sale of virtually all vitamin supplements with the exception of low dose multivitamins which have little therapeutic effects and certainly would have no effect on Alzheimer's. The problem for the industry is that vitamins work far better than drugs for many serious diseases and they are determined to stop this threat by taking them off the market. If this ever does happen, I fear I really will develop full blown Alzheimer's. This is my greatest fear in life. This plan would not just literally kill me in a slow and appalling way, but would affect millions of other lives in similar ways. It is why I can never forgive this evil industry which simply puts profit before human life.

The all-out war against lifestyle medicine

Lifestyle medicine has many enemies. The reasons are obvious. Healthy people do not need drugs, doctors, medical equipment, diagnostic tests or even much in the way of medical research. About $9 trillion is at stake annually and millions of jobs are involved. Many more jobs are similarly at risk in charities, regulators, universities and patient groups around the world. Global processed food and drinks industries, genetically modified grain, seed and plant manufacturers and many related chemical companies are also threatened since their products are one of the main causes of the epidemic of modern disease. Even the finance industry that invests trillions of dollars in all these institutions, companies and global cartels has a significant incentive to destroy or marginalise lifestyle medicine. The media and global news organisations, as well as social media and other internet companies, have also been incentivised and pressurised to join the war against lifestyle medicine, as have virtually all governments around the world.

Lifestyle medicine has enemies because it is exposing what is happening in healthcare on all these fronts. It also offers much better health and disease solutions. Everyone else is simply intent on maintaining the lucrative status quo regardless of what is happening to people's health and lives. There is no money to be made from healthy people. So, instead, all these organisations (some intentionally and others unintentionally) have created a world where sickness reigns supreme. People have been led to believe that being sick is normal, and drugs are portrayed as the only option to all these modern diseases; diseases that are nearly all increasing exponentially and affecting and killing young people who have never before developed some of them in the entire history of mankind. Lifestyle medicine, which simply exposes the truth about all these industries, organisations and professions, thus allowing people to stay healthy, is under serious attack from all sides.

I'll start with a brief history of this all-out war and outline just a few of the key methods of attack that have been, and still are being, used. The war against lifestyle medicine has been raging for around two centuries. But as already outlined, the whole process was ramped up in the late 1800s and early 1900s when some of the most powerful industrialists like John D. Rockefeller and Edward Carnegie became interested in health. They were interested because they saw a huge opportunity to make money by introducing industrial techniques and processes into the developing field of medicine. They had built their vast business empires by ruthlessly creating monopoly positions in their oil and other industrial businesses. Their vision was to create a similar monopoly within healthcare. They achieved this by donating huge sums of money to conventional medical organisations to enable them to expand their remit and to extend their control over all fields of healthcare as well as attacking what was, at that time, a significant use of natural solutions like herbal products. The power of conventional medicine and the various industries that supplied it grew enormously. The original vision of John D. Rockefeller was to create a monopoly position for medicine and that meant destroying the competition. Lifestyle medicine was, of course, the prime target and with their new formed powers and finances, the war on natural treatments was ramped up considerably.

Since that time, the key players, including the pharmaceutical industry, medical organisations, regulators and the global elite, have sought by every means at their disposal to discredit and destroy all aspects of lifestyle medicine. The methods employed have been vicious, indiscriminate and incessant, and the full force of the "establishment", from governments, regulators, police, media and big business lobby groups, have all been used. The details can be found in two books by investigative journalist Martin J. Walker called *Dirty Medicine* and *Dirty Medicine: The Handbook*. In these books you will find examples of how lifestyle medicine practitioners and doctors have been raided by anti-terrorist teams, imprisoned, intimidated and subjected to vile and vicious personal attacks. All this may sound impossible to believe in our supposedly democratic societies, but it is nonetheless true. Here is just one example. In 1992, armed police together with FDA officials raided the offices of Dr Jonathan Wright in Seattle who was a nutritional pioneer. The police were wielding guns and seized more than $100,000 worth of computers, medical records and nutritional supplements. He was not charged with anything and no charges were ever made because he had never done anything illegal. It took him years to get his seized property back and it is a wonder he didn't go bankrupt. These types of "illegal" police raids are what you might expect in dictatorships, but the fact they occur in supposedly democratic societies is shocking. Since then, the FDA has in fact carried out more than 25 similarly brutal "vitamin raids". The scale of the attacks on lifestyle medicine is unprecedented. The methods used include:

- declaring it is unscientific and without proof
- labelling the advocates, which include many doctors, as charlatans promoting fake news
- claiming some lifestyle treatments are dangerous and even life-threatening
- trying to discredit and neutralise individual practitioners using intimidation and personal attacks
- censorship of those individuals involved which includes many doctors
- withdrawing medical licences of doctors who continue to promote natural treatments
- introducing laws which severely restrict or ban the use of natural products and treatments
- laws making it illegal to communicate the benefits of any treatment, food or vitamin
- carrying out rigged trials to try to prove that lifestyle treatments don't work or are dangerous
- mobilising the media and press to spread this poison at every conceivable opportunity

Here is a description of one such media attack that involved the BBC and a pharmaceutical lobby group called the Campaign Against Health Fraud (CAHF). It was waged against the Bristol Cancer Help Centre (BCHC) which was a privately run organisation providing additional support for patients who were receiving conventional treatment for cancer. It offered care, compassion and support in abundance. It didn't offer any medical treatment and the most contentious thing it did was to recommend a more vegetarian diet. It was incredibly well supported and its patients thought the world of it. In 1990 the BBC was preparing a programme to celebrate the tenth anniversary of the BCHC. However, when the drug lobby group CAHF found out about the programme they contacted a producer at the BBC who was one of their members so that the purpose of the programme was changed into a hatchet job, in which premature, flawed and incorrect research was presented which showed that survival rates at the BCHC were significantly lower than those for patients treated just by the NHS. These allegations were untrue. Soon after the programme was shown amidst a frenzy of lurid press headlines, such as "veggie diet kills cancer patients", the lies and flaws started to be exposed by independent researchers. Retractions and apologies were subsequently made by the researchers and medical people involved. Professor Tim McElwain who was one of the main proponents of the attack on the BCHC committed suicide, possibly from feelings of shame over the damage he had done and the reprehensible methods he and the CAHF had used. But the damage had been done. Unlike the original media frenzy, the retractions were not published and no grovelling apologies were made by any media group. The BCHC did survive but it never really recovered from this vicious onslaught. This sort of attack was commonplace at that time. ITV produced a similar programme attacking the Breakspear hospital – a privately run organisation that used many natural treatments for allergies. Thankfully, such attacks are now much less common. But as we will see, this is simply down to a change of tactic from the establishment rather than a change of heart.

The war against lifestyle medicine is so one-sided it should have been won long ago. Lifestyle medicine has no friends in high places. By any measure this is not a David versus Goliath contest. It is more like David versus a million Goliaths. And yet, after everything the establishment has thrown at it and every nasty trick it has used, David is still standing. Millions of people still use lifestyle solutions to promote health and treat disease and this simple fact speaks volumes. In its desire to destroy lifestyle medicine, the establishment has had one intractable problem it simply cannot overcome: lifestyle medicine works. It transforms people's health and when they try it, they can see it works and continue to use it. But even after 100 years of incessant attacks and so much failure, the establishment was not about to give up.

Twenty years ago, a new plan was hatched, which even John D. Rockefeller would have been proud of. This envisaged the introduction of the most comprehensive and draconian set of laws the world has ever seen in peacetime. It was time to set aside human rights and civil liberty, as well as scientific principles, in a final effort to destroy lifestyle medicine. The development of these laws takes place behind closed doors. The media rarely, if ever, report on it. It all started in 1961 when the Codex Alimentarius Commission (CAC) was set up by the United Nations, and then the World Health Organization joined it in 1963. Its original purpose was to create international standards relating to foods, food production and food safety. This all sounds rational and very sensible, but unfortunately the whole process has been effectively taken over by global cartels like Big Food, Big Pharma and Big Ag and supported by all those with vested interests in their success, like global finance institutes and the global elite who have most of their wealth invested in these companies. These cartels help to fund what appear to be independent, so-called science-based organisations that help develop the CAC guidelines and standards. The end result has been that dangerous pesticides and hundreds of dubious food chemicals are being approved, and highly processed foods that have serious health implications proliferate around the world. Meanwhile, vitamin and mineral supplements have been savagely targeted and the CAC has produced guidelines setting exceptionally low limits for all of them, such that they would have virtually no therapeutic value for anyone. The ultimate aim is to make all these guidelines legally binding on a worldwide basis. If this ever happens, these natural substances, vital for health, will be lost forever and there will be no going back. Of course, we are not there yet, but this is the ultimate plan of the global cartels and the global elite.

The truth, however, is vitamins, minerals and other supplements are some of the safest things that we can consume (as we will see later), despite being one of the prime targets of governments and regulators who are being "guided" in that direction by CAC guidelines and other industry-led organisations. The EU and US are the leading advocates of this draconian approach. The official argument put forward by the authorities for this type of legislation is "to protect the public". They argue that lifestyle treatments and solutions, such as vitamin supplements, have no proof they work and "could" be dangerous and that low and mandatory limits must be placed on all such things. But this is not correct because it is important to remember one key fact. Regulators are mandated by law to protect the public and remove from use anything that seriously threatens human health and life. If harmful evidence against vitamins existed, then they would have been banned decades ago, especially given that the destruction of lifestyle medicine is one of the absolute priorities of the establishment.

For many years in the US, public pressure thwarted most of these tighter regulations because people were less likely to be taken in by these bogus arguments. Many of them intuitively understood that governments and regulators side remorselessly with big businesses rather than worry about civil liberties, the rights of individual citizens and even their ability to control their own health and lives. Indeed, after several particularly brutal raids by fully armed SWAT teams on supplement producers, during which employees were held at gun point while stock and records were seized, a spoof advert was filmed starring the actor Mel Gibson which caricatured the scene. He exclaimed to the SWAT team, "Hey, guys, it's just vitamin C. You know, like in oranges." When this advert came on national TV it struck a chord and helped create massive support for what ultimately became the Dietary Supplement Health and Education Act of 1994. This Act protects Americans' access to dietary supplements. However, despite such setbacks, the establishment never give up. They simply regroup and form new strategies as they have done for over 100 years.

At this point the main onslaught on lifestyle medicine passed to the EU. Here citizens are more likely to believe these fabricated claims particularly in countries like Sweden where draconian laws were introduced and shelves were emptied of many natural products with barely a whimper, simply because the people trust their politicians and regulators much more implicitly. At the time, regulators in the US looked enviously at such successes. I should add that the Swedish Supreme Court eventually overturned the decision three years later and the supplements were reinstated. This was because Swedish regulators had made the original decision without any legal framework either under Swedish or EU law.

A similar attack in Norway also failed spectacularly. Norwegians order most of their supplements online or by mail order from other countries. But in 2015 the Norwegian government passed and implemented overnight a law making the importation of all higher dose vitamin supplements illegal. People could, of course, have considered ignoring the law, but the government had provided additional resources to Norwegian customs to find and destroy these "illegal" supplements. If you then persisted in trying to buy them, you could ultimately be prosecuted and receive a criminal record. So, instead, thousands of people demonstrated outside parliament and many made it clear that if the law was not revoked, they would sell up and leave the country. The government eventually gave way and rescinded the law. This shows two things. People power will be essential in stopping this worldwide plan to destroy lifestyle medicine. It also shows just how passionately some people must believe in the benefits of supplements and how they value their health above everything else. If you are prepared to uproot your entire family and leave friends and loved ones and move to a foreign country, you must be pretty confident it is all worthwhile. How has society ever reached a stage where law abiding citizens in a free and democratic country like Norway could ever have been faced with the full force of the law for ordering vitamin supplements? Just how far will governments and regulators go to protect the interests of their friends in Big Business? Well, in fact the EU has already gone much further by introducing draconian regulations as we will now find out.

So, what exactly are these draconian EU regulations?

The EU has issued 12 directives relating to food. Five of the key directives will now be outlined together with their savage outcomes.

EU Food Supplement Directive 2002. This directive controls which vitamin and mineral supplements can be produced, the form of those supplements, and aims to specify the maximum levels which any supplement can contain. Only a limited range of vitamin and mineral forms were originally approved. Many others, including all forms of silver and vanadium, cannot be sold legally. The maximum levels for the other vitamins and minerals, however, have still not been finalised 18 years after the legislation was introduced, because this is probably the most contentious directive ever issued by the EU. Many countries disagree on the limits that should be imposed and opposition is strong since all the indications are that the relevant committees favour the exceptionally low levels as proposed by the CAC. This means they would have almost no therapeutic benefits and would literally take away overnight one of the most important ways in which people can maintain good health and minimise the risk of serious diseases. But, as well as all of this, a legal challenge was made against the directive at the European Court of Justice in 2005. Much more on this shortly.

EU Human Medicinal Products Directive 2001. This directive provides a legal framework for pharmaceutical drugs. The problem lies with the definition of what can be classified as a drug. Currently, the scope and definitions are so broad that every substance that has a therapeutic effect on the human body – and that really does mean every individual natural food, herb, vitamin, mineral and even water – could fall foul of this directive. What this means is a natural food, like garlic, which is known to thin the blood (much like the drug warfarin) – and hence it has a therapeutic effect – could in theory be labelled as a drug. But anything classed as a drug cannot be sold unless it is tested as a drug. This, of course, means expensive clinical trials costing over $2 billion which no supplier of natural foods could ever afford. So, without the clinical trials, garlic could – according to the directive – be banned from sale. Of course, no one, not even the mighty EU, would dare to ban a hugely popular food like garlic. It would spark public outrage and this would also apply to many other popular foods like carrots, cauliflowers, strawberries and blackberries. The problem is there are many other less well-known but very therapeutic foods that already have and will continue to fall foul of this insidious and evil directive (the herbal tea Essiac is one example). It is then likely that they will be "given" to the drug industry who will either just decide not to produce and sell them so they don't threaten existing drugs, or they will turn them into new "drugs" and charge thousands of dollars for them. If you doubt this could be true, here is one outrageous example. This occurred in the US and I will outline it here because it is the most outrageous example of this type of medicinal product law that I have yet seen.

Cannabidiol (CBD) is a natural hemp-derived product that has a significant benefit for pain reduction and has been used for many years. Even though people have to pay for it themselves, this natural supplement is widely used in western countries because it works better and has no side effects compared to most pharmaceutical drugs prescribed for pain. But the Federal Drug Agency approved a CBD drug called Epidolex in 2018 for the treatment of epilepsy and granted a patent to the drug company GW Pharmaceuticals. The company now charges around $32,500 for a year's supply. The patent means the company could, at any time it chooses, ask the FDA to remove the widely available and cheap CBD supplements off the market. This has not yet happened but if it does, most people will then be forced to revert back to inferior painkilling drugs because clearly very few could afford $32,500 each year.

The EU is also in the process of trying to ban the sale of CBD supplements and thus allow the pharmaceutical industry to take over full control of this incredible natural product. They are, however, using a different approach based on the Novel Food Regulation which will be explained shortly. The UK regulator seems determined not to be left out of this assault on natural foods. They have also classed other supplements like the herb milk thistle (which has a positive effect on liver function) as a drug.

EU Traditional Herbal Medicinal Products Directive 2004. This 2004 directive controls the supply of herbal products. Simple herbs that have been used for over 30 years can still be obtained but only those used for minor ailments such as coughs, colds and sore throats can be promoted. Herbs that were traditionally used to help treat other conditions such as heart disease and cancer are already banned. New herbs or herbal products from countries outside the EU are also banned. The new directive also requires expensive laboratory tests and the use of standardised extracts, extracted using alcohol, and stabilised in a pharmaceutical matrix of polymers. The cost of all the extra processing has meant that for the relatively few herbal products that remain available, prices rose significantly, typically by 300%. The potency of the products is in many cases also reduced, making them less beneficial. Given all these factors, sales of the relatively few remaining herbal products have also fallen significantly and many people have just had to accept this destruction of their human rights to use safe natural products that previous generations took for granted and benefited from for thousands of years. Some are using the internet to try to find alternative sources from outside the EU but this has its own problems and risks.

EU Nutrition and Health Claims Regulation 2006. This regulation controls what can be said about the benefits of any food, vitamin, mineral, herb and other botanical substances. Any health claim must be approved by the relevant EU committee. The only way to gain a health claim is, yet again, to carry out prohibitively expensive trials. There are nine essential amino acids without which every human would die but, unbelievably, none of these has been granted a health claim. There are over 2,000 other natural substances with plausible evidence of health benefit, but because they are not substantiated by these specific trials, such claims are also banned. A further 1,600 claims for botanical substances are still in limbo awaiting evaluation but these will almost certainly suffer the same fate. Many natural foods do, however, have substantial scientific evidence that support their benefits. Consider the example of walnuts.

In the US National Library of Medicine Database there are no fewer than 35 peer-reviewed published papers supporting the claim that walnuts improve vascular health. Yet this is simply dismissed by regulators like the FDA and EFSA. But Big Food is able to make positive health claims for unhealthy, highly processed fried foods and regulators seemingly turn a blind eye. Frito-Lay, a subsidiary of PepsiCo, makes products like Lays potato chips and Doritos. It makes the claim that they can "support a healthy heart" even though scientific evidence says exactly the opposite. This illustrates the power of these industries and how regulators simply protect their interests and at the same time help to destroy any competitors. This is what Bill Faloon, co-founder of the Life Extension Foundation, said about this devastating situation: "For the FDA to allow Frito-Lay to pretend there are heart benefits to ingesting their high calorie snack products, while censoring the ability of walnut companies to make scientifically substantiated claims, is tantamount to treason against the health of the public."

It is very clear that there will never be any fully approved health claims for any natural foods like cauliflowers, blackberries and flax seeds that could help to transform human health. Here is yet more proof. The manufacturers of glucosamine did fund an official trial as required by the EU to prove it worked which would then have enabled them to officially make the relevant health claim. Glucosamine is by far the top selling supplement for joint health. It has a great body of evidence to demonstrate it works and the new trial also produced significant benefits. What happened? The European Food Safety Authority still rejected it. Why? The manufacturer had sensibly and logically tested it on people with arthritis. In other words, the very people who would benefit from it. The EFSA said they should have tested it on young people whose joint health was fine, just like the pharmaceutical industry does. There couldn't be clearer evidence that regulators are determined to find any reason to reject every health claim for every natural product. They allow the drug industry to use young healthy people in clinical trials because older people usually take other drugs that could significantly stop the new drug from working. This in itself is appallingly unscientific. So, despite the fact that the manufacturers of glucosamine proved it worked well for people with impaired joints most of whom were also taking other drugs (something the drug industry can't do), the regulator still rejected the evidence because of this bizarre, unscientific technicality. This means that despite providing better scientific evidence about their product than the drug industry, the companies involved still cannot put any information about what glucosamine can achieve on the supplement package or make any other claims of what its benefits are. In fact, they are still in the same position as all other producers of any natural plant, fruit, vitamin, mineral or other similar product. They cannot tell people about their health benefits without being warned to stop, and if they persist, being fined and eventually imprisoned. It is a true health scandal. But this legislation is so scandalous that I want to provide one final example.

This involves fructose which is one of the two compounds that make up sugar (the other being glucose). The EFSA endorsed the following health claim: "Fructose has a beneficial impact on blood glucose when it is used to substitute sucrose or glucose in the finished product." This claim gives the misguided impression that fructose is good for people's health. It is true that blood glucose is lower in someone who eats fructose compared to the same amount of glucose, but what it doesn't make clear is that by definition, blood fructose will, of course, then be much higher. Why does this matter? Because blood fructose causes more serious outcomes overall than blood glucose. Robert Lustig is professor emeritus in paediatrics at California University in San Francisco specialising in obesity. This is what he said about it: "The scientific data on fructose shows it is one of the most egregious components of the western diet, directly contributing to heart disease and diabetes, and associated with cancer and dementia. Fructose causes seven times as much cell damage as does glucose."

The simple fact is sugar, glucose and fructose, causes severe health problems and everyone should be encouraged to reduce their intake of all of them – there should never be an approved "health claim" for any of them. Professor Lustig concluded his article with the following comment: "The EFSA has boosted the position of the sugar industry, either by incompetence or collusion. But it is clear that this recommendation is scientifically bogus. Nutrition policy should be based on science – not pseudoscience."

Many other obesity experts were also appalled by the EU move to approve a health claim for fructose, but the fructose industry was, unsurprisingly, delighted by the ruling. One manufacturer said it expected a surge in sales – a surge brought on by a regulator whose mandate is to protect public health but whose decision will lead to a significant increase in serious diseases like obesity and heart disease. If you ever doubted that global cartels (who don't care about human health and life) effectively control regulators, then look no further than this appalling Nutrition and Health Claims Regulation for the proof.

EU Novel Food Regulation 2015. Any food that was consumed in the EU prior to 15 May 1997 can continue to be sold legally. Any new food introduced after that date has to go through an expensive registration process. The regulation was originally intended to protect consumers from genetically and technologically altered foods but it has been extended to include any natural food grown in the EU or produced outside of the EU. But proving that a food was used before 1997 is difficult because the EU requires original records and invoices; they are the only proof it will accept. How many companies retain hard copies of original paper invoices for more than 20 years when financial and industrial law dictates they only need to be retained for eight years? Virtually none. Of course, the new EU registration process could be used, but again, with the exception of global food cartels, it is simply too expensive for most companies and this means that many "relatively" new foods that have been eaten safely for several decades could now face a ban.

Goji berries were a high-profile example that the EU was planning to ban but due to public outrage some "fudge" was used to allow them to continue to be sold. But most foods are not so high profile and are just banned because they are "under the radar". Of course, the EU claims the Novel Food Regulation was approved to protect the public like all the other food directives, but it is just one more insidious law designed to protect the interests of global cartels to the detriment of people's health and their choice of what they can eat. This regulation is being used by the EU to try to ban CBD supplements as already outlined and it is being increasingly used for many other foods because the law is so simple and unchallengeable. If a producer cannot produce an original paper invoice from before 1997 then the case is lost and the product is removed from sale with no recourse to any legal challenge. Of course, the regulators wrote this rule in full knowledge of this fact knowing it would give them the absolute power to take any food they want off the market.

EU Food Supplement Directive 2002 (part 2). I now want to return to the EU Food Supplement Directive. I outlined the fact that a legal challenge was made to the European Court of Justice shortly after it was approved. Had this legal challenge not taken place then virtually every vitamin and mineral supplement (except low dose multivitamins) would have been banned throughout the EU. Today, 18 years later, almost all of those supplements are still available. Let me outline the incredible story of how all this happened.

It involves someone you have probably never heard of, but he is one of the world's greatest unsung heroes. Just after the start of the new millennium, Dr Robert Verkerk, with a PhD in sustainable farming who worked at Imperial College London, discovered that the EU was planning to finalise and approve the Food Supplement Directive. His considerable knowledge about how our soils are dangerously depleted in essential nutrients meant he knew this regulation was a clear threat to human health. So, initially, he created an organisation called the Alliance for Natural Health International and then spent many months in Brussels, attempting to educate European ministers about the serious nutrient decline in foods and the safety of vitamin and mineral supplements that would help to offset this decline. He was also a member of the Health Freedom Movement which aimed to alert as many members of the public as possible, because virtually no one knew anything about these new insidious laws, mainly because the press and media were, as usual, remaining silent about them and the first time most people would have known was when supplements were physically taken off the shelves and banned forever.

Along with other colleagues he assembled masses of evidence to show the directive was based on poor science. But despite all their efforts, the EU Food Supplement Directive was approved in 2003. At this stage Rob and his colleagues then filed a legal challenge in the European Court of Justice. Any case that comes before the ECJ is first examined by the advocate general who gives his opinion before it then moves on to the ECJ itself. In April 2005, after reviewing the evidence, he concluded that "the Food Supplement Directive infringes the principle of proportionality because basic principles of community law, such as the requirements of legal protection, of legal certainty and of sound administration have not properly been taken into account. It is, therefore, invalid under EU law." In other words, the directive is illegal, too restrictive and based on flawed science. He declared the procedures to be "as transparent as a black box". The advocate general's opinion is not legally binding but represents a strong recommendation and, in the overwhelming majority of cases, the justices in the ECJ follow it.

However, in July 2005, in a surprise reversal, the ECJ upheld the directive's legality. It did, however, make two crucial amendments that were still a slap on the face for those who developed the directive. The first was that every natural vitamin and mineral would be regarded as safe and must be allowed on the directive's positive list, whereas the original directive planned to ban many of them. In other words, rather than supplement manufactures having to prove that natural safe foods were "safe", the regulators would have to prove they were unsafe before they could ban them, and even then, any proposed ban could be challenged in the courts. The original directive also stipulated that to get any ingredient back on the positive list in the future, a supplement company would have to go through a lengthy and costly process. Modern vitamin and mineral supplements can include up to 30 different ingredients. The cost of approving each one would be around £250,000 which meant that the cost for each supplement could be up to £7 million and, of course, there was still no guarantee that it would be approved.

The end result of all this is that virtually every natural supplement is still available and this actually proves quite conclusively that there is no scientific evidence they are unsafe, otherwise the regulators really would have banned them immediately in 2005. The ECJ also confirmed natural vitamins and minerals would continue to be classed as foods which would prevent them from being labelled as medicines. The quiet fortitude of Robert Verkerk, who mortgaged his house three times to provide financial support for this landmark legal challenge, is nothing less than heroic. Of course, because the ECJ approved the directive in principle, albeit with two significant changes, there was still another major hurdle in protecting people's access to supplements. This is because the EU could at any time impose strict upper limits on vitamins and minerals which would effectively have the same devastating consequences as the original directive's plan to ban them. I will now outline what has happened so far on this vital issue.

After the embarrassing 2005 ECJ judgement, the EU needed time to regroup before deciding how to carry on the fight against vitamins and minerals and impose strict limits on them. In 2009, however, UK organisations like the Alliance for Natural Health and Consumers for Health Choice and their "Save Our Supplements" campaign started alerting people to the fact the EU had made significant progress and was getting close to finalising very low vitamin limits. They asked all their supporters to write letters, asking that restrictive limits were not imposed, to the president of the European Commission, Jose Manuel Barroso – and to Commissioner John Dalli – as well as to UK MEPs and key UK politicians. I remember sending around 40 letters in total. Sending letters rather than emails was important since emails could be sorted electronically and then just deleted and senior officials may not have been aware of all of them, whereas letters had to be physically opened and given that hundreds of thousands were sent from around Europe, staff were often overwhelmed and President Barroso and Commissioner Dalli could physically see the opposition to these imminent laws.

Petitions were also launched in many EU countries and organisations like the Alliance for Natural Health continued to challenge them and produced peer-reviewed papers demonstrating the inappropriate science being used. All this paid off and eventually the whole process went on to the backburner. In 2014 there appeared to be a renewed push by Big Business to pressurise the European Commission to make decisive progress, but it had clearly started to understand that this directive was so controversial across the whole of Europe as well as the 28 individual governments that it was probably unsolvable on an EU-wide basis, so it continued to put it on hold. At this point, individual governments in countries like Germany, France and Sweden decided to take the law into their own hands. Not unsurprisingly, these countries have huge pharmaceutical industries and they all imposed slightly different but incredibly low maximum levels – the sort of levels the drug industry had wanted for 60 years. But these low levels can also lead to devastating health outcomes. We have already seen that medicine recently recommended that people take 10mcg of vitamin D because it had been scientifically proven to reduce muscle weakness and frail bones. But France and Germany had set the maximum vitamin D level at 5mcg. This meant that many people in these two countries who followed these devastating, unscientific limits would have suffered significant health problems that could in fact have been prevented. The whole thing is unforgiveable, but this is what happens when global cartels effectively control regulators and governments. In many of these countries, legal cases have been brought against national regulators and we have already seen the outcome of the one in Sweden where the Supreme Court overturned the supplement ban. But these trials can take years to conclude and many of them are still in progress. This means that even if the governments eventually lose the case, vitamins will still have been banned for years. The ECJ has actually intervened on several occasions to prevent overly low doses being adopted since this interferes with the free movement of goods throughout the EU. But the fact is individual governments are so determined to impose strict national vitamin limits that they are prepared to break their EU treaty obligation of adhering to the single EU market principles.

Regardless of the individual outcomes of these legal cases, it is clear that the ultimate goal of most national regulators and governments remains resolute. Even after 20 years of embarrassing setbacks they are determined to eventually severely restrict all vitamins and minerals except low dose multivitamins. That is unless public pressure and organisations like the Alliance for Natural Health International can continue to thwart them. Of course, it is simply the drug industry that is behind all of this and yet it still wants multivitamins to remain available. Why? Well, believe it or not, most low dose multivitamin supplements are actually made by Big Pharma and their EU-wide annual sales revenues alone are a significant €3 billion. These multivitamins contain very low doses and many of the individual vitamins and minerals are synthetic and chemically produced versions and are in a form that is poorly absorbed by the body. The levels are just high enough to prevent diseases like scurvy, rickets and beriberi, but are so low they will have virtually no effect on any of the other major life-taking diseases like heart disease, diabetes, cancer, dementia, mental illness and infectious diseases and this means they cannot threaten the use of drugs which is the industry's key priority. So, quite simply, they don't want to lose their annual €3 billion of sales because money always has been, and always will be, their only priority.

I have a very logical suggestion to you. Don't buy any supplements from pharmacies or supermarkets because most of them are made by Big Pharma, like Sanatogen made by Bayer, Multibionta by Merck, and Centrum by Pfizer. Please don't support a devastatingly corrupt industry which is determined to stop everyone from staying healthy so that drug sales can be maximised.

Finally, here is just one more example of the industry's incessant corruption. In 2001 eight drug companies were found guilty and given the largest fine at that time of €865 million for operating a multivitamin price fixing cartel in Europe. No doubt they would try this again if they were ever allowed to gain full control of multivitamins, which is, of course, the establishment plan.

But what about the UK? Unlike the vitamin clampdowns in countries like France and Germany, no serious additional restrictions have been placed on supplement levels here, but this may be partly due to the fact that Brexit almost completely dominated the entire political agenda for around four years. Even though this is now complete, it is important to remember that all the EU food directives and regulations are still legally in place in the UK. So, what is likely to happen in the future? Some people suggested it may be a chance to relax some of these draconian directives but that really is unlikely and while no restrictions have happened so far, I believe UK regulators with close ties to the drug industry will try to persuade the government to impose similar restrictions at some point. In fact, when individual EU governments voted on whether to implement the Food Supplement Directive in 2002, the then Labour government actually voted for it. Had they voted against it, then it would not have been passed into law and supplements would have been safe for many decades. We will have to hope that enough of the population are prepared to fight hard to resist this again, just as people did in 2010 when we were probably the key country that helped "persuade" President Manuel Barroso to put the whole process into the long grass. Organisations like the Alliance for Natural Health International will also be key players because of their expert knowledge of the science involved in the complex regulations as well as their understanding of how to prepare the best type of legal challenges if we ever get to that stage.

Finally, I want to give one more, rather different, insight into the unscientific nature and industry domination of these unforgiveable food directives. In 2011 I wrote to every UK MEP about the Food Supplement Directive asking them to oppose it. Most of those who replied used the standard response that it was being done to protect public health and that the expert committees would base all their decisions on robust science. This is the letter I sent back to them. When you have read it, you may understand why I did not get a single reply. I have removed the recipient's names because I think it would be unfair to list them at this stage.

18 May 2011

Dear **** MEP

THE EU FOOD SUPPLEMENT DIRECTIVE

Imagine a world where politicians let experts decide everything and then give them instructions to look only at the harm that everything can do, to look for even the flimsiest evidence of harm, and then to eliminate all known risks completely. What would happen? Quite simply, there would be no transport of any kind, no manufactured goods, no houses, no hospitals, no drugs, in fact no healthcare of any kind because all of them cause harm or death in varying degrees. In fact, we would have to revert to being hunter-gatherers again – without the spears, of course, as even these would be banned. Is this a supremely stupid suggestion? Of course, it is. But looked at objectively, "welcome to the world of the EU Food Supplement Directive."

I would like to thank you for replying to my letter of 9 March. I have written on several occasions to MPs and MEPs about this directive. In all cases the replies are very similar, reiterating the official EU mantra that this is simply a matter of public safety, that we should be reassured that vitamin levels will be set by a group of experts and be based on rigorous scientific assessment. None of the specific issues I raised have ever been answered directly. So, I want to issue you with a challenge to see if you have the courage to answer the specific questions I raise in this letter.

The Food Supplement Directive represents one of the greatest assaults on liberty and individual rights in the modern world. It is not based on good science as claimed and its aim is to eliminate all known risk, even though risk is a natural and even necessary part of life. Risk should always be balanced against benefits, but that is not allowed by this directive. Most politicians imply there is little or nothing they can do about the legislation, as "experts" will make the decisions. If this is the case, why do we need politicians? Politicians should listen to the views of experts, but they should then subject them to detailed scrutiny and then exercise their own judgement. That is what they are elected and paid for.

Experts are frequently wrong and they certainly are on this issue. Less than 50 years ago the same scientists who now advocate global warming were warning of global cooling. It's difficult to think of a more compelling example of the fallibility of science than this. There are thousands of other scientific failures that were originally developed or approved by experts. In terms of health, think of thalidomide, lobotomy and the drugs Avandia and Vioxx, all of which resulted in the deaths or serious injuries of tens of thousands of people and children. Every MP and MEP from every country in the EU should have to answer the questions I am now going to raise. If they had to do this, I wonder how many would start to question the experts and how many would vote for the directive with a clear conscience. I do hope that in your busy schedule that you can find time to read and respond to the following questions.

1) I am now going to break EU law by making a health claim: "Drinking water prevents dehydration and maintains bodily function." When I first read that the European Food Standards Agency (EFSA) had ruled against this nutritional health claim submitted by two German professors, I checked it wasn't 1 April. Then I got angry – really angry. If you doubt that the EFSA made this ruling (and thus made it illegal for anyone to say as much) then I suggest you check it out. That anyone could develop an official procedure that denies one of the most undeniable facts on the planet is simply unbelievable, but the fact that the ruling comes from the EU's top experts reveals that something far more sinister and shocking is happening. The reality, of course, is that this ruling will have no practical effect. No doctor confronted with dehydrated patients would let them die by not giving them water, whatever the EU experts officially rule. So, why am I incensed by all of this? Because the experts who made it are the people in whose hands rests the fate of the whole of natural medicine. The German professors who submitted this health claim did it deliberately to expose the EFSA in its true light. After this, can anyone say, hand on heart, that vitamins, minerals and herbal products could ever get a fair appraisal by these so-called experts? It is quite clear that the assessment processes being used are skewed in such a way that natural foods will never be able to gain official health claims. I normally consider myself a law abiding citizen, but breaking this disgraceful EU law makes me proud and unashamed.

Question 1 – Do you support this ruling by the EFSA that water does not prevent dehydration? If you don't, do you think that the committee members should retain their current jobs?

2) In setting safe upper limits (SULs) for vitamins and minerals, the various experts have been instructed to ignore completely the many benefits of nutritional supplements. I can't think of any single decision in the entire world where only one side of an issue or debate is examined – unless, of course, you happen to live in a dictatorship. There would not be a single approved drug in the world if regulators made decisions based on side effects alone. There simply cannot be a true scientific evaluation

of anything without evaluating both the pros and cons. So, any claim that the Food Supplement Directive is based on science is quite simply false at the first hurdle.

Question 2 – Do you support this one-sided, non-scientific approach?

3) The various experts are advocating radically different SULs. Perhaps you could ask an expert why, if the whole process is based on science as claimed, the experts disagree so radically. For vitamin C, for example, the range of SULs varies between 60 and 1000mg. A 17-fold difference.

Question 3 – Can you justify such an unscientific gulf? Let me help with one possible explanation. German experts are pressing strongly for extremely low SULs and, surprise, surprise, Germany just happens to be home to a multinational pharmaceutical company that is the largest manufacturer in the world of mass produced, synthetic low dose multivitamin supplements. If low levels become law, most high-quality natural vitamin manufacturers in the UK will be driven out of business, leaving the market open to this pharmaceutical giant, thus generating huge extra profits for the company and financial and employment benefits for Germany overall.

4) The example of vitamin C is very instructive in the way that the flimsiest of evidence is being used to justify draconian and totally unnecessary limits. (Note that vitamin C is normally sold in tablets with a maximum level of 1000mg.) The UK Food Standards Agency set up the Expert Group on Vitamins and Minerals (EVG) and they reported in 2003 and their conclusion on vitamin C is as follows: 1000mg may cause mild stomach upset in sensitive individuals. Probably only one in several hundred people would be affected, and unlike bacterial infections from contaminated food which can cause many days of sometimes serious bowel problems, the mild stomach upset from vitamin C disappears within a day of ceasing to take it. Note that there are absolutely no other side effects with vitamin C. Does this seem like a compelling reason why vitamin C should be subject to a draconian restriction that will almost certainly reduce the level to well under 100mg, especially when you consider that there are many hundreds of scientific studies and clinical trials that provide evidence of its beneficial effects on dozens of serious diseases? All that is needed is an appropriate label saying that anyone who experiences stomach upset should stop taking it and suggesting that the dose could be halved and taken twice daily when the mild upset will then never reoccur. Precautionary labelling is deemed acceptable for thousands of far more dangerous products that can even kill people, like prescription drugs, ladders and electrical equipment, so why not vitamin C? In the UK an estimated 5 million people suffer every day with upset stomachs and diarrhoea. How many of these are caused by vitamin C? Very few, probably no more than a few hundred. I'll hazard a guess that far more people get upset stomachs from eating apples than from vitamin C. Will the EU restrict apple sales? Of course not. The Food Supplement Directive is clearly just an attack on natural ways of staying healthy that threaten drug sales.

Question 4 – Why is precautionary labelling not the appropriate solution for vitamin C?

5) For most vitamins and minerals there is absolutely no evidence of harm to humans from taking supplements at the levels currently on sale. So, how do the

experts set a limit when there is no evidence of harm? The EVG used animal experiments where animals were given ever larger mega doses of a vitamin until some side effect eventually occurred. If you blatantly keep increasing levels indefinitely, then every substance and food will ultimately induce some effect. People have, for example, died from drinking huge amounts of water and I guarantee that if you were forced to eat 50 apples you would end up with an upset stomach at the very least. So, having eventually forced some side effect to occur in the animal, they then try to work out what the vitamin level might be that induces no side effects in a human. To do this they divide the original animal figure by various arbitrary factors. For vitamin B6, for example, they divided the figure by three, then by ten and then by ten again. But these are just arbitrary figures which produce some truly ridiculous outcomes. Applying the same logic for manganese, the maximum limit calculated would mean that every single human on the planet was eating more than this so-called safe amount just from their normal diets. Obviously, this is sheer nonsense and could not be legally adopted, so what did they do? They simply decided not to divide by the final figure of ten. The whole thing is laughable. It's just a shoddy attempt to try to justify low vitamin levels with phoney science, guesswork and inconsistent methodology. The experts already know which low level they want for each vitamin and then they "adjust the maths" to get to the figure they want. The "science" is so dubious that even a 15-year-old student could shoot holes through it. Some experts even seem to have given up all pretence of evaluating this matter scientifically. They are simply proposing that safe upper limits should be set at the recommended daily allowance without any logic whatsoever. It is hard to say which experts are the worst. Those that abandon science altogether, or those that use phoney science to get the result they want.

Question 5 - Can you justify the complete lack of a scientific approach to setting safe upper vitamin limits?

6) A significant percentage of all prescription drugs would not be on the market if the experts did not listen to and believe the people who take them in clinical trials. For conditions like pain and depression, experts can only know whether a drug works or not by asking individual people. Their collective views then determine whether a drug is approved and used. Why are experts so ready to accept the views of ordinary people when it suits them, but dismiss them completely when vitamins are involved. Millions of people take vitamins and minerals and report radically improved health. This is why we are all so angry, because we know our health will suffer if low limits are enforced and supplements banned from sale. Incidentally, a study in America shows that 82% of nurses and 78% of doctors take supplements and about half do so on a regular basis. The most common ones taken are vitamin C, vitamin D and fish oils. The slight possibility that a few of them might get a mild stomach upset clearly hasn't deterred any of them. Why do the experts think they know better than the millions of people and the doctors and nurses who take supplements, especially when they use flawed science, and cannot agree amongst themselves and are subject to vested interest group lobbying and national interests? EU commissioners may now be starting to understand the anger that the Food Supplement Directive is creating but they obviously don't understand why this anger exists.

Question 6 – Why are the views of millions of people being dismissed?

7) Everyone is freely able to smoke and drink themselves to serious illness and death. (Over 100,000 EU citizens die for this reason each year.) They take pharmaceutical drugs and engage in activities like driving cars and mountaineering, all of which can, and do, result in serious injury and death. It is their human right to do these things. But millions of people are about to be denied the right to take vitamin C at levels they have taken for decades because a few susceptible individuals may get a slight and temporary stomach upset. As far as all the other natural vitamins and minerals that will also be severely restricted are concerned, not one person has died from taking any of them.

Question 7 – Can you defend this on a human rights basis?

8) Tens of thousands of EU jobs in the supplement industry are about to be sacrificed as a result of this directive.

Question 8 – Do you consider that this is a price worth paying to avoid a few mild upset stomachs and claimed side effects of other vitamins that exist only in theory, based on animal experiments and their flawed human interpretation.?

Yours sincerely,

Anthony Armstrong

Corruption in the regulatory process

After everything you have already read, it may not surprise you to know that many of the "experts" who sit on the committees that produce these global industry biased regulations have conflicts of interest with pharmaceutical, agro-chemical and global food companies, and many have lucrative financial ties. Experts working for regulators move to these industry giants and vice-versa. These so-called revolving door arrangements are well documented and indisputable. The EU food laws give regulators the power to destroy the means by which people can look after their own health, and however unbelievable all this seems, they were based on the Codex Alimentarius plan hatched by Big Pharma and Big Food six decades ago. Similar plans are now being implemented in many other countries like Australia, South Africa and Canada. The US is also ramping up the war on lifestyle medicine and natural foods yet again using almost identical laws. Some parts of all this pre-planned legislation are not finalised and so can't yet be implemented fully. But even where they are, the regulators still tread carefully in certain areas like setting maximum levels for vitamins and minerals and classifying foods as drugs and banning them because public opposition could make this very difficult. We should also remember that many people already know how to ensure they stay healthy using lifestyle solutions and will, of course, ignore all the directives. Slowly but surely, however, the noose will tighten year by year, decade by decade. The Nutrition and Health Claims Regulation, for example, will not affect me. I already know which foods are healthy and which are unhealthy, so I can continue to consume the healthy ones and avoid the dangerous ones for the rest of my life, but what about the next generation? Unless those parents who do know continue to pass on such information to their children directly, it will eventually be lost to future generations because internet content and articles conveying such information will slowly and almost imperceptibly be censored and finally declared illegal. The plan is to roll out these draconian laws on a global scale. The EU, for example, has sent its experts to countries like South Africa to "help" regulators there to implement identical laws, guiding them through the processes and advising on how to minimise and overcome public opposition.

Let me now give you some proof about the corruption that pervades the EU health committees where these draconian laws were first brought into law and are now starting to be rolled out around the world. This is important because, despite Brexit, all of these laws and guidelines, as we have seen, still apply in the UK. In 2011 a remarkable event took place in the EU parliament. MEPs voted almost unanimously by 637 to 4 not to approve the annual accounts of the European Medicine's Agency (EMA). This should have been headline news throughout the EU. It should have started intensive investigative journalism and caused extreme public outrage, but it didn't. Let me explain why all these things should have happened. The EMA is the drug regulator for the whole of the EU. Its job is to approve new drugs and monitor existing drugs thereby protecting the health and lives of 500 million citizens. We have already seen many examples of how Big Pharma commits serial "fraud", kills people for profit and how its drugs are the third leading cause of death. If ever an industry needed a tough and honest regulator then this is it. Yet MEPs threw out its accounts. Why? They cited grave concerns - a phrase they used no less than five times - about the EMA's independence. They slammed the hiring practices, conflicts of interest and sources of funding and highlighted the "revolving doors" between the EMA and the pharmaceutical industry. With this report, the MEPs stated in black and white terms that the EMA is acting to promote the very industry it is meant to be regulating. The EU machine normally operates invisibly; it rarely shows its dirty linen in public in order to protect the external image of the institution. Everyone involved normally closes ranks to protect that image. So, such a public show of dissent and one that was so critical is a rare event. MEPs stuck their heads above the parapet and yet there was no critical media coverage. You might imagine that evidence of corruption in the EU would have been a godsend to the numerous anti-EU media groups. But even they wouldn't touch the story. Why? The problem for all concerned is that corruption is a two-way process. Also implicated is the mighty pharmaceutical industry and then, by extension, medicine itself. We have already seen many examples of media censorship to help protect the reputation of medicine and pharmaceuticals. Is this interpretation correct? It is impossible to say, but it is the only explanation I can think of that fits all the facts.

The EU ombudsman has also adjudicated on numerous occasions on the various EU health committees after numerous complaints on lack of transparency and conflicts of interest. His judgements are equally damning. One particularly revealing case was that of Dr Suzy Renckens who, after a five-year stint as head of the unit responsible for the risk assessment of genetically engineered plants, joined the biotechnology company Syngenta, which is a major manufacturer of such plants. She joined the company in a senior position advising on regulatory affairs just two months after leaving the EU committee. EU regulations require that staff are scrutinised for conflicts of interest both when entering or leaving their position. For two years after leaving, staff must inform the Commission of new jobs. If such jobs relate to the work they did as an official, and could lead to conflicts of interest, the Commission can forbid it or approve it subject to appropriate restrictions. The ombudsman was highly critical of this blatant example of "revolving doors" that was nodded through in clear breach of the relevant procedures.

The European Food Standards Agency (EFSA) is also mired in corruption and murky practices. Independent reports showed that, in 2011, two recently appointed members of the EFSA panel convened to assess food additives but failed to declare ongoing consultancy work for the International Life Sciences Institute. Hiding behind this innocuous name are nearly all of Big Food's global corporations, including Hershey, McDonalds, Nestle, Kraft Foods, Proctor & Gamble and Coca Cola. This revelation followed hot on the heels of another independent investigation that revealed that 55% of the same EFSA committee were conflicted by industry ties as defined by the OECD. Obviously, all of these companies have a clear vested interest in the EFSA maintaining its approval of all the food additives they use in their highly processed foods. One of the key additives is the artificial sweetener aspartame and all these conflicts of interest really matter because there is significant evidence that aspartame has been linked to a number of serious health outcomes ranging from premature births to cancer. Its continuing approval by EFSA is extremely concerning and controversial.

In 2013 one of the UK's leading experts on food policy, Erik Millstone, professor of science policy at Sussex University, challenged the biased and deeply flawed EFSA opinion that aspartame is safe. Professor Millstone highlighted 20 studies which have identified potentially dangerous outcomes. He explained that, of the 17 members of the EFSA panel, seven had direct commercial conflicts of interest and another five had institutional conflicts because their employers had already announced that aspartame was safe. In total, 70% of the panel had industry ties. He said that the EFSA should convene a new panel of experts with no conflicts of interest. This, of course, never happened.

John Dalli, former Commissioner for Health and Consumer Policy, who headed the EMA and all the other EU health committees, resigned ostensibly to "clear his name" after he was accused of corruption and taking bribes. The EMA also faced a separate fraud investigation by officers of the European Anti-Fraud Office relating to the drug Mediator which was responsible for the deaths of 2,000 people. The Nordic Cochrane Centre, part of the internationally renowned Cochrane Collaboration, accused the EMA of withholding clinical trial evidence in order not to jeopardise the profits of the drugs companies.

These examples demonstrate systemic corruption within the regulatory and health committees in the EU, and the seamless link between these and the pharmaceutical, food and agro-chemical industries; a truly disturbing situation. Of course, it isn't just the EU health committees where corruption and murky practices exist. It is widespread throughout the whole of the EU. Former commission president Manuel Barroso now works for Goldman Sachs who were instrumental in enabling Greece to join the euro. It is a poorly kept secret that this was a political decision, because Greece did not meet the conditions for entry and should never have been admitted. Greece employed Goldman Sachs to "prove" its finances were in order while the Brussels elite, with Barroso at its head, knowingly turned a blind eye to the deception. Goldman Sachs made hundreds of millions of euros and the appointment of Manuel Barroso is seen by many as their payback for this collusion. Such blatant abuses led to a huge public petition which called for "strong exemplary measures to be taken against what they considered to be the worst example of 'revolving door' practices that 'dishonour' the European Civil Service and the European Union as a whole."

Global corporations love large bureaucratic organisations and these don't come any bigger than the EU, which, before Brexit, controlled the laws and directives that governed 500 million people. Instead of negotiating with 28 different countries where their lobbying would be spread thinly and where 28 different sets of "revolving door" arrangements would be needed to enable them to achieve the lenient laws they want for their own products and the brutal laws needed to damage their lifestyle competitors, they can concentrate all their efforts on a few key individuals who control all the relevant regulations. It means the "financial incentives" that can be offered to them can be all the more lucrative and difficult to turn down.

Are vitamin and mineral supplements really dangerous?

The laws and directives the EU and many other countries are developing to limit the levels of vitamins and minerals in supplements are supposedly done to "protect the public" because they "might" be dangerous. At least that is the main excuse used by legislators and governments. So, are they really dangerous? Here are a few media headlines that suggest they are: "Vitamins are as dangerous as smoking", "Vitamins shorten life expectancy" and "Vitamins are a waste of money". Just three newspaper headlines that were meant to scare us into not taking them. I'll be surprised if you haven't seen at least one of them.

I will explain in detail why you can safely ignore these sensational, silly, totally misleading, unscientific and disgraceful headlines. I will also explain exactly who is behind them and what their motives are – although by now you should be able to hazard a guess.

So, what is the real truth? The first thing that needs to be made clear is that there are no dead bodies labelled "killed by vitamins". This statement is crucially important, but what do I mean by it? In the USA, for nearly four decades, the American Association of Poison Control Centers has issued detailed analyses on the causes of death. They have almost consistently reported each year that "there were no confirmed deaths from multiple vitamins or any single vitamin, no deaths from herbal medicine, no deaths from any amino acid or dietary mineral supplement, and no documented deaths from homeopathic medicines". In the few years where a death was reported, these were mainly linked to choking from taking a capsule and not from the vitamin or mineral itself. The Federal Drug Agency also did a study from 2006 to 2014 which found there were three such deaths which equates to one every three years. I should add that pharmaceutical drug capsules can also cause a small number of choking deaths, and to put the whole thing into perspective, in the US there are around 5,200 deaths every year caused by choking from food. The facts are pretty clear. Vitamins and minerals are incredibly safe. Consider that in the US over 40 people die each year from lightning strikes, and around 100 die from peanut allergy, meaning these two causes are around 120 and 300 times more lethal than vitamin supplements. All this should be compared with 187,750 official deaths in the FDA's adverse event database for 2021 caused by properly prescribed pharmaceutical drugs and even this figure is grossly understated as explored in detail in Part 3. One of the other exceptionally rare causes of supplement deaths is due to young children finding a bottle of their parents' iron sulphate tablets and eating them all. They think they are sweets but they have usually been prescribed by doctors for the treatment of anaemia.

So, is it possible to say that *natural* vitamins supplements are completely safe? Well, no one can say that. But what can be said is there is almost no evidence of serious harm. If someone really tried very hard and consumed incredibly huge quantities then some harm may occur. But remember, people have died from drinking too much water – nothing can be guaranteed as being completely safe. But if you take natural vitamin supplements at the recommended levels, your risk really is vanishingly small and probably zero. This comment, however, excludes the dangerous synthetic vitamins produced by Big Pharma that will be explored in more detail shortly.

There are no equivalent reports or statistics on vitamins in the UK. But it is clear there are identical outcomes. I wrote to the MHRA – the UK's own regulator – and asked them this question: how many people have been killed by vitamin and mineral supplements in the UK in the last ten years, and how many have needed medical attention due to a side effect from taking supplements? The answer from the MHRA was short and to the point: "It is not possible for the MHRA to provide a definitive answer to your question as we do not collect the type of data you have requested." Given that the MHRA is vigorously implementing and endorsing the draconian EU laws that are justified on the basis that they are protecting the public from dangerous supplements, you might imagine they would have at least some tangible proof they were indeed dangerous. In fact, the reply is just a cover for the fact that, once again, there really is no significant evidence, not just of any deaths, but even the absence of significant side effects from taking natural supplements. So, unlike pharmaceuticals where the drug itself can be shown to be the direct cause of death in tens of thousands of people, there is no such proof for vitamins and minerals.

Surely then, there must be some other type of proof to justify the sensational news headlines? Well, yes, there is, but before I explore this in detail and then rebut it, there is one more important point. All the key vitamins and minerals are essential for human life. If any of them were excluded completely from your diet, you would die. So, what we are really talking about is the level at which absolutely essential vitamins are claimed to become dangerous. The "proof" that some vitamins and minerals are dangerous at high levels relies on a few clinical trials most of which were done in the 1990s. The key vitamins implicated are: vitamin E, betacarotene and folic acid. So, I will now address each one of these in turn.

Vitamin E. Several studies show that taking high dose vitamin E increases the risk of cancer; a damning indictment indeed. I need to start the analysis by giving an analogy that illustrates the main problem with these trials. Please bear with me – it is absolutely relevant. Imagine you are a young javelin thrower and I am a new coach who promises to make you a star. My method involves exclusively developing and exercising your throwing arm for eight hours each day until it is the most powerful throwing arm in the world. After six months, you are ready and I ask you to throw the javelin for the first time as hard as you can. What happens? You immediately pull a muscle in your back or leg because these other muscles have not been developed to the same extent as your throwing arm – your body is out of balance. You are incapacitated for weeks.

Let's now turn back to vitamin E. What most people don't know, including many doctors, is that vitamin E is not a single compound. It is the collective name for eight different but closely related compounds. These are alpha, beta, delta and gamma tocopherols and alpha, beta, delta and gamma tocotrienols. These eight compounds occur naturally in food, so the average person will consume all eight in roughly the correct ratio for optimum health. All the trials claiming harm used what was erroneously called "vitamin E", when in fact only a synthetic version of alpha tocopherol was used and this was administered in very large doses. Perhaps you can see where this is leading. The huge dose of just one of the eight compounds destroys the delicate balance in the body; the synthetic alpha tocopherol swamps the body's receptors sites, crowding out the other seven compounds that make up vitamin E thus reducing their uptake. This includes the most abundant and most important natural form – gamma tocopherol. Just as in the javelin analogy, the body is not prepared for this disastrous imbalance and in this case the end result is an increase in cancer risk for some of the participants in the trial. The explanation for these negative trial results really is that simple.

You must be thinking that surely the researchers and other experts must have known about all of this from the start. Well, there are two possibilities. The first is they did know but this was used deliberately as part of the war against lifestyle medicine. In other words, they knowingly used it to produce evidence against vitamins to frighten people from using them. The other possibility is the researchers really didn't know because they are used to thinking in terms of a single magic bullet – a drug – to treat every disease. They are conditioned to think this way. The problem is the human body simply doesn't work like this. Vitamins, minerals and many other compounds in food work synergistically and using a synthetic one, especially in huge doses, can have harmful effects. The synthetic alpha tocopherol is manufactured by Big Pharma. It is this form that is used in most multivitamin tablets. In multivitamins the level of this so-called vitamin E is so low it does not cause any significant imbalance or damage to the body, so anyone taking a multivitamin need not be unduly concerned about the dangerous side effects uncovered in these trials. Incidentally, I take a moderately high dose vitamin E supplement, but this contains all eight of the naturally occurring tocopherols and tocotrienols. As you may guess, it isn't made by Big Pharma and when this balanced formula is used there is no evidence of any harm. So, what do these trials really prove? They prove that it is the isolated, high dose, synthetic versions of alpha tocopherol produced by Big Pharma that are actually dangerous. There is no evidence that natural vitamin E is dangerous in any way.

Betacarotene. "Taking more than the recommended dosage of betacarotene was found to increase the risk of developing lung cancer by up to 20%." This headline was from the Guardian newspaper in 2015. The original study was published in 1996 but was "resurrected" in 2015 by Professor Tim Byers who has made a career out of attacking vitamin supplements. He regurgitates the same old trials time and time again to put the knife into lifestyle medicine. The original 1996 study was carried out to see if high dose synthetic betacarotene supplements could reduce the risk of developing lung cancer in long-term heavy smokers with significant lung damage. But what was not mentioned in the Guardian or by Professor Byers was that some of the patients quit smoking during the trial. For these people their risk of developing cancer actually fell by 20%. What was also not mentioned is that a second study showed the increased risk for smokers was also confined to women only – men were unaffected.

I'm now going to make up a hypothetical clinical trial. You'll think I have gone mad when you read it, but please bear with me because once again it is very relevant. A clinical trial has shown that eating one kilo of pebbles leads to rapid death for all participants. Shock horror – surely the government should issue warnings to everyone about the dangers of consuming pebbles. Maybe restrictions should be placed on their availability to avoid this life-threatening outcome.

So, here we have something that will rapidly and completely kill everyone. But does any action need to be taken by governments? That would indeed be silly because no one in the history of the world has consumed a kilo of pebbles and no one is ever likely to do so. We have a potentially deadly scenario but it has no practical relevance. So, what has all this got to do with betacarotene? Well, I'll hazard a guess that before the 1996 trial was carried out, and even after it, not one single female heavy smoker would have taken exceptionally high doses of synthetic betacarotene supplements in isolation and for protracted periods. Why would they? The 1996 clinical trial clearly showed that taking high dose synthetic beta carotene if you are a female heavy smoker leads to an increased risk of cancer, but I would argue that it has little or no practical relevance. So, these shocking headlines were completely unnecessary and completely misleading. All that needs to happen is that the labels on betacarotene supplements should state that they should not be consumed by women who smoke. This is exactly what happens with most pharmaceutical drugs and foods, like peanuts, which cause harm to a percentage of the population.

Instead, we have banner headlines portraying betacarotene as a major killer (together with the implication that everyone who takes it is at risk) when in fact the research that led to them was a completely artificial medical trial that applied only to female heavy smokers. In fact, during the trial, those who gave up smoking achieved a 20% reduced cancer risk. Why was this information not shouted from the rooftops? Why was it actually suppressed?

Why did the researchers not carry out another trial on non-smokers given that betacarotene would almost certainly reduce their risk of cancer as well? All this brings into question the real motives behind the trial but, of course, this could only ever be speculation.

Folic acid. Folic acid is manufactured by Big Pharma and is a synthetic version of natural folate which is found in natural foods like green leafy vegetables. Some studies suggest a link between folic acid supplements and bowel cancer. However, others show no link and a study in the Lancet in 2013 which looked at 50,000 people concluded: "Folic acid supplements are not linked to an increased cancer risk when taken for up to five years." A few studies have even shown a reduction in risk. So, the case against folic acid really is unclear, but none of this evidence stopped Professor Byers from selectively quoting only the studies that showed an increased risk and thereby tarring vitamins yet again. The press, of course, never thought to check if there were trials that contradicted Professor Byers' claims and simply published his highly biased views.

So, what conclusions can we draw on folic acid supplements and bowel cancer? The evidence is simply inconclusive. It is quite possible synthetic folic acid in high doses is implicated in some bowel cancers although this is not definitively proven. But what we also know is that natural folate is actually protective against cancer because it enables the body to copy DNA accurately. Supplements of natural folate are available and there is no evidence of harm from these. So, once again we have a synthetic form of a natural product, manufactured by Big Pharma, that is possibly implicated in harm when taken in high doses. The message is simple. Do not take high doses of synthetic folic acid.

So, how can we sum up the evidence against vitamins? There is little rigorous evidence that they are dangerous, and the evidence for vitamin E, betacarotene and folic acid constitutes a significant part of this, so these are the "star witnesses for the prosecution" as far as the anti-vitamin lobby are concerned. The first thing is naturally occurring forms of these substances are safe. No one has ever suggested it is unsafe to consume large quantities of green leafy and orange-coloured vegetables that in turn contain large quantities of both natural folate and betacarotene. Nor has anyone suggested it is unsafe to consume nuts, seeds, fish, spinach, olive oil and berries which all contain vitamin E. Supplements derived from natural vitamins are also not implicated in harm. The evidence for harm involves the synthetic versions manufactured by Big Pharma and can be summed up in one sentence: don't touch the so-called vitamins produced by Big Pharma with a bargepole.

But this is not the worst part of this whole wretched attack on lifestyle medicine. Researchers like Professor Byers take all the negative study results from vitamin E, betacarotene and folic acid and then use them to discredit *all* vitamins and minerals. They do this by carrying out a meta-analysis of the negative studies. A meta-analysis, if you remember, combines the results from a number of different studies to arrive at an average outcome using complex statistical techniques. They then report that their meta-analysis shows that vitamins are harmful and shorten life. They deliberately misrepresent the facts. The wording implies that *all* vitamins are now dangerous even though there is no similar evidence against the others. It is a neat and nasty little trick of the sort made possible by statistics-based research. The media and press, of course, swallow this message hook, line and sinker that virtually *all* vitamin and mineral supplements are harmful and gleefully generate the misleading and sensational headlines we have seen. No one in the media would seek to challenge an "expert" like Professor Byers, so when you see sensational headlines like "vitamins are as dangerous as smoking", you now know the disgraceful and disturbing process by which they are generated.

But Professor Byers is not alone in this vitamin bashing game. If you see any negative reports on vitamins by any of the following "experts", beware because they all operate in the same way and with the same motives. Dr Paul Offit has written a book about vitamins called *Killing Us Softly*, but his day job is at the Children's Hospital of Philadelphia where he holds a $1.5 million research chair funded by the drug giant Merck. Edzard Ernst, Simon Singh, Dr Giles Yeo and Professor Sir Rory Collins are other notable vitamin bashers.

How do researchers "prove" that vitamins and minerals have no benefits?

There are other tricks, scams and junk science that researchers and people like Professor Byers use to dissuade people from taking vitamin supplements (as well as many other natural health solutions). These involve "proving" they do not have any effect in preventing or treating disease. I'll give four examples of the different types of tricks that are used.

Trials are carried out using doses of vitamins or other supplements that are too low to have a therapeutic effect. (A little bit like giving someone who is seriously dehydrated a spoonful of water and then seeing no improvement in symptoms.) The Physicians' Health Study ll, published in JAMA in 2008, is a classic example. Its aim was to see whether vitamin C and vitamin E could reduce the risk of heart disease. The level of vitamin C used in the trial was 500mg day, but natural medicine practitioners would say that at least 3000mg taken in divided doses would be the minimum level needed to start having any effect on the heart. The trial also gave "vitamin E" at a level of 250mg on alternate days. Once again this is insufficient to have a significant effect, but in addition, the type of supplement used was not vitamin E but the synthetic version of alpha tocopherol made by the drug industry that has just been examined in detail. This means it does not work like the natural vitamin and is even likely to block the beneficial effects of natural vitamin E available from the diet. Unsurprisingly, the trial showed no benefits from taking the vitamins. These types of trials are what scientist Steve Hickey PhD, calls "trials designed to fail".

Despite all of this, the reality is those trials where the appropriate high doses of vitamins are used really do show their true benefits. One such trial gave high dose vitamin C to students who developed colds and flu. They were given 1000mg every hour for the first six hours and then the same amount three times per day until the symptoms disappeared. Those given vitamin C showed an 85% decrease in symptoms compared to those who just took decongestants.

Another trick is to use a specific type of vitamin that cannot work on its own for the disease being studied. A second one is to stop using the vitamin before the end of the trial. A classic example of both of these occurred in 1975 when Dr Linus Pauling and Dr Ewan Cameron, who was a Scottish cancer specialist, carried out a study in which high dose vitamin C was given to terminal cancer patients. It was given intravenously as well as orally, and for the full duration of the trial. They gave it to 100 patients and compared their outcomes with patients given conventional cancer therapy. The results showed that vitamin C doubled life expectancy. After the trial was published, it was dismissed or attacked by most medical experts. The Mayo Clinic then carried out a new study that was supposed to exactly replicate the original trial – as per normal scientific protocols. This found no benefit from vitamin C. However, rather than replicate it, Mayo made two major changes. They only gave the vitamin orally (which simply cannot work without the intravenous dose) and stopped its use prematurely before the trial was completed. Despite this deliberate and blatant cheating that caused the trial's failure, medicine unsurprisingly just accepted it and vitamin C was simply discredited. I should add that Dr Linus Pauling was one of the most brilliant scientists ever. He was the only person to ever win two individual Nobel Prizes, he had 48 PhDs and almost certainly made more radical scientific discoveries than anyone else in the history of medicine. But if you dare to promote a nutritional solution for any disease, your reputation is effectively finished.

Other studies use patients who cannot benefit from the vitamin being tested and these will also, therefore, guarantee it "doesn't work". This is epitomised by a trial carried out in New Zealand in which a group of young adults were given either a placebo or vitamin D to see whether it was effective against the common cold. The trials showed vitamin D had no statistically significant effect when compared to the placebo. The results were disseminated to the press and media who dutifully reported the findings. It even made headlines on the BBC radio news. I was so incensed by this that I was moved to complain to the BBC for their gullibility and lack of investigative rigour. Why was I so angry? Well, another trial involving children from the US had demonstrated clearly that vitamin D did indeed have a profound effect on colds. But in this case the children all had low levels of vitamin D. Those who were given the supplements saw their incidence of colds fall by a staggering 50% compared to the placebo group. Remember that between 25% and 90% of the UK population are deficient in vitamin D particularly in winter, depending on their age, ethnicity and sun exposure? So, this is a really important study which conveys a vital health benefit. How does this relate to the New Zealand trial? Well, the sun has, of course, been mankind's major source of vitamin D for millions of years. New Zealand is a sunny country and its population are sporty outdoor folk, particularly the healthy young people who were the subject of this clinical trial. Because of their high levels of sun exposure which produces very high levels of natural vitamin D, giving them extra supplements would have had almost no additional effect. It is no surprise, therefore, that the study was able to claim there was no statistical difference between the supplement and placebo groups and, therefore, that vitamin D "didn't work". But researchers are clever people. They would surely know all these facts. This was almost certainly nothing more than a clever version of a "trial designed to fail"; a trial that could be used to discredit vitamins yet again.

I was angry that the BBC had allowed itself to be misled in this way, and that its medical correspondents had failed to uncover the US trial which proved just how effective and powerful vitamin D supplements can be. I found details of this trial after a one-minute search on the web. I argued that the BBC was effectively acting as an industry shill and that its shoddy journalism was preventing people from learning about the incredible benefits vitamin D could bring. The BBC's response was that "they had not broken any guidelines". Well, maybe not, but that still doesn't excuse what they did.

There are many examples of this type of scam. A large-scale clinical trial at Harvard University analysed the effect of omega 3 fish oils on memory loss. It found no difference between the control group and those taking the supplements. There were several major flaws in the trial protocol but the key one was that the trial participants had no significant memory problems. They were generally healthy people and their only medical problem was macular degeneration which was what the main part of the trial had been designed to assess. People without memory loss simply cannot benefit from a supplement that reduces memory loss. So, unsurprisingly, the researchers found no difference in patient outcomes and then used this to say that omega 3 fish oils didn't work. Of course, because this was a large clinical trial carried out at Harvard, no one would question the results and the press as usual said this was yet more "unchallengeable proof" that supplements didn't work and were a waste of millions of dollars.

So, you can see a clear methodology. Researchers devise bogus trials and use junk science to show vitamins don't work, while others make unscientific claims that they are dangerous. Experts like Professor Byers then use inappropriate statistical techniques and spin to summarise the various findings, and then use their status to widely disseminate the results to media groups. The media then blindly accept every single word without challenge and generate sensational and negative headlines aimed at deterring people from taking vitamins. Do all these appalling, unscientific or fraudulent claims actually work and deter people from taking them? Sadly, for many people, the answer is yes. Let me give you one example.

Two special friends were taking vitamin D supplements, but then read an article in a major newspaper about the dangers of a number of supplements. The article claimed it was unsafe to take more than 10mcg of vitamin D. They clearly accepted it and stopped taking them because they (and many other readers) understandably believed this newspaper was so respected it simply wouldn't report any lies. This claim on vitamin D, however, really is a lie. Here are the true facts. All vitamins are essential for life, so the Federal Drug Agency in the US lists the minimum levels that people need to take on a daily basis – called the Reference Daily Intake. For vitamin D, this *minimum* level is 20mcg. The NHS also accepts on its website that anything up to 100mcg is safe. These two facts alone tell you this article is simply a lie. There is, however, additional evidence that provides even more graphic proof of the vitamin's safety even at much higher doses.

There have been many hundreds of official scientific trials and studies over the last half century to assess vitamin D's benefits for a wide range of diseases. Most of them have used levels between 100 and 250mcg and yet no side effects have ever occurred. A recent major study involved 17,000 adults in a preventative health programme. They were given a daily range of the vitamin up to 500mcg and none of them experienced any toxicity. In 2015 the Mayo Clinic also completed a study on over 20,000 people over an incredible ten-year period to assess the possible toxicity of vitamin D. Just one patient experienced toxicity. However, this woman had been taking an unbelievable and totally unnecessary 1,250mcg for over three months. Even then she did recover once she stopped taking it. The Mayo Clinic report concluded that vitamin D toxicity is one of the rarest medical conditions and occurs only in people who take 1,250–2,500mcg per day. The simple fact is that no one needs to take supplements remotely close to this level. To help prevent or treat any disease (including cancer), very few would need to take more than 250mcg, and around 100mcg would be a reasonable average for many. Quite simply, ignore all the lies that are told and seriously consider taking vitamin D supplements so you can improve your health, help prevent serious diseases and increase your life expectancy by around two years.

Newspapers that publish this sort of data should be ashamed of themselves, and their investigative journalists really could, and really should, have explored all the factual data just outlined and slammed the false claims. What about those so-called experts who initially promoted these lies? I'd better not say what I really think about them because the language would not be acceptable in this book.

Here is one final amazing fact. The human body, of course, produces its own vitamin D from sun exposure but the amount can be staggering. White skinned Europeans with around 80% of their body uncovered in just 20 minutes of midday summer sun increase their vitamin D levels by the equivalent of that from 500mcg of supplements. The body after 7 million years of evolution would simply not produce this level if it caused any danger and it does this simply because it really helps to prevent many diseases and is essential for bodily functions. Of course, some people do not go out in the sun and others use sunscreen, so these people, and everyone else particularly in winter, really should take the supplements.

I will now finally explain perhaps the most shocking and unforgivable examples of "trials designed to fail" I have ever seen. These involve vitamin C which was used in conjunction with vitamin B1 to treat sepsis which is the main cause of death from infections around the world. The latest figures just released show there are an incredible 11 million deaths each year which means that sepsis causes 20% of all deaths worldwide. The annual UK deaths are around 50,000. Sepsis and its consequences are so important I need to explain everything in detail.

Sepsis is the body's extreme response to an infection. The main causes are various bacterial infections but other sources include viral infections like pneumonia and influenza. Many of the infections occur in hospitals through things like surgical wounds, intravenous drips, urinary catheters and bed sores. The patients most at risk are those with chronic illnesses, those with impaired immune systems, the very young and the very old. Antibiotics successfully treat well over half of all cases, but for those patients who end up in intensive care and are given conventional treatments, the mortality rate is up to 40% in developed countries, and 60% in developing countries. But some doctors have used a treatment involving intravenous vitamins and the results are staggering. Dr Paul Marik from the Eastern Virginia Medical School added high dose vitamin C, vitamin B1 and a steroid to the normal antibiotic protocol for patients with sepsis in his intensive care unit. The mortality rate fell by around 75%. Dr Marik and his team published results from this treatment in the CHEST journal in 2017. Those given conventional treatments had a mortality rate of 40.4% while for those in the vitamin C treatment group it was just 8.5%. These results led hundreds of other doctors in intensive care units around the world to use the same protocol. A totally separate trial involving patients with sepsis who required a special treatment for very low blood pressure showed that after 28 days the mortality was significantly lower in the vitamin C group at 14% compared to 64% in the placebo group.

Of course, once again, these are not large-scale medically endorsed clinical trials and so, according to medicine, they do not provide definitive proof. Normally, medicine dismisses such studies just for this reason. But in this case, probably because sepsis is such a serious and high-profile disease, it would have been difficult to just ignore the Marik study. So, another officially endorsed trial called the CITRIS-ALI trial was carried out with the results published in 2019. This concluded that the vitamin therapy did not work. The results, however, were very controversial and caused much debate amongst those doctors and scientists who examined the trial data in detail. Why? When a study like Dr Marik's has produced such spectacular results and you carry out a second trial to confirm whether it was correct or not, then you should reproduce the original trial protocols exactly. If you change them, then by definition, you will get different results and you cannot then say that the initial trial was either wrong or right. The purpose of these trials should be to see if the vitamins save the lives of sepsis patients. It was the primary outcome Dr Marik measured in his study and it is, without any doubt, the only outcome that matters for the 11 million patients who die from it every single year. Surely it should have been the primary end point of the new trial. But incredibly, the CITRIS-ALI trial instead measured certain complex chemicals that are associated with changes in organ function which are linked to the progression of sepsis and this was defined as the primary end point. The second main difference in the CITRIS-ALI trial was that the vitamins were only administered for four days whereas in Dr Marik's protocol, vitamin C was given until the patients had recovered and were transferred out of the intensive care unit. Dr Marik makes it clear that stopping the vitamins early can result in a rebound effect in the disease.

So, what did the results of the trial show? They showed there were no significant differences in organ function which was the official primary outcome. However, during the four days the vitamins were given there was a significant difference in deaths which was one of the secondary outcomes that was assessed. Those given the placebo had a mortality rate of 23% while for those given the vitamins the rate was just 5%. After day four, when vitamin administration was stopped, the mortality rates in that group started to rise again.

Dr Marik's clear statement that the disease is likely to regain toxicity and result in increasing mortality if the vitamin C is stopped too early means this outcome was to be expected.

What is the official medical interpretation of the results? The primary end point showed no difference in organ function between the placebo group and the vitamin group, and the primary end point is the only data that is considered in an official clinical trial. So, the official conclusion is simple: vitamins don't work at all for sepsis. Full stop. But what about the reduction in deaths when using vitamins? It is totally ignored because deaths were only classed as a secondary end point and these have no official validity. Think about this carefully because it is simply unbelievable. Some people have described the trial protocols and outcomes as nothing less than criminal. As already outlined, behind the scenes there was also much unrest in parts of the medical community about this contentious trial and its unbelievable conclusions.

Then, in 2020, the results of another trial were published. The VITAMIN trial again compared the vitamin C and vitamin B1 treatment against conventional treatments for sepsis. But once again there were major differences in the trial protocols. The primary end point was "time alive and off vasopressors after seven days". The trial found no difference between the two treatments in relation to this specific end point, so once again it stated that the vitamins don't work. However, just like the CITRIS-ALI trial there were very contentious changes to Dr Marik's protocol. Some of these are very complex so I won't even try to explain them, but the key change was the time taken from a diagnosis of sepsis to the time the first treatment was given. Sepsis is such a serious disease that death can occur within a few hours in many patients. This is recognised not just by Dr Marik but in conventional medical circles where the aim is to start treatments within one hour of a patient arriving in the emergency department. But in the VITAMIN trial, the average time to first treatment was around 30 hours. Please let this incredible time lag sink in. Dr Marik was incensed by it and said the study was rendered void by the futile administration of his protocol. He said, "It's like giving it to a patient who's dead. It's of no benefit". He also said, "I am very disappointed and saddened by the results of the VITAMIN study. There is no question in my mind that this intervention saves lives. This has been the experience of hundreds of clinicians around the world, who have used this intervention early in the course of severe sepsis and septic shock when combined with high-quality supportive care." He also said in a 2020 Critical Care Review Meeting, "I contend that doing a study that is designed to fail is ethically and morally unacceptable."

Another trial is also underway called VICTAS. This trial is still in progress as I write this section and yet it is possible to predict the outcome now. It will again conclude that vitamins don't work just like the CITRIS-ALI and the VITAMIN trials. Why? Because yet again, the primary end point does not involve deaths despite the fact this is the only thing that matters for every patient. This time it measures "days free of vasopressors and ventilators". Reductions in deaths are again a secondary outcome which means they have no validity as far as the trial's final conclusions are concerned. This is clearly another "trial designed to fail". Quite simply, no researcher would dare to do a trial that measured deaths as the primary outcome because it would prove that vitamin C and vitamin B1 work. What will happen when the VICTAS trial is concluded? Almost certainly someone will then carry out a meta-analysis of all the three trials. The final conclusion will obviously be that vitamins do not work for sepsis. Given that a meta-analysis is the ultimate "medical proof", then it will spell the end of this treatment that could save millions of lives each year. No new hospitals will be allowed to use it because of the "proof" it doesn't work. I suspect that even the doctors and intensive care units that currently use it and save 75% of their patients' lives will, at some point, be pressured to stop using it. Eventually, the whole thing will just be forgotten. But sepsis is not the only disease where "trials designed to fail" have been used to "disprove" the incredible life-saving benefits of vitamins. In Part 5, I will outline how this has also been done for vitamin treatments for cancer and Alzheimer's.

Yet, despite this devastatingly sad, tragic and unforgivable situation, a new study published in 2020 in the American Journal of Respiratory and Critical Care Medicine provides more evidence for Dr Marik's protocol. Sepsis is one of the leading causes of death in critically ill children and the Lurie Children's Hospital of Chicago, which is ranked as one of the nation's top children's hospitals, carried out the first paediatric study involving the use of vitamins to treat septic shock in children. It closely followed nearly all of Dr Marik's protocols. The 43 children given the vitamin treatment were compared to 43 others who received standard care. The mortality rate after 28 days for children given standard care was 28%, while for those given the vitamins it was just 9%. Similar results were found after 90 days when the standard care mortality was 35% and vitamin mortality 13%. The lead researcher Dr Wald said, "We were surprised and excited to see a substantial reduction in mortality after treating septic shock in children with a high dose vitamin C, vitamin B1 and cortisone. While based on a retrospective analysis, our results are especially compelling in that they are very similar to the positive outcomes found in a recent study for septic shock in adults." Dr Wald also said, "We hope to encourage larger, multi-centre studies in children with septic shock to confirm our data." However, if any studies are carried out, I guarantee they will not measure mortality and will continue to look only at what are really almost irrelevant outcomes, like time on ventilators, and that means they can again be claimed to fail and thus discredit Dr Ward's findings.

So, 11 million people will continue to die each year even though there is still convincing evidence that well over half of these deaths could be prevented by using the Marik vitamin protocol. I should add that there is also reasonable certainty that if people adopted the sort of really healthy lifestyle that has been explored in some detail, they would develop a strong natural immune system, and many more of them would simply defeat the infections that lead to sepsis naturally in the first place and avoid the need for intensive care altogether.

It is almost impossible to believe that researchers and key officials would allow around 6 million unnecessary deaths to occur each year. How can they live with themselves?

Who is really behind this all-out war against lifestyle medicine?

We have seen most of the reasons why lifestyle medicine finds itself on the wrong end of this vicious and unforgiveable war. But who are the real power brokers? Who are the real villains? The pharmaceutical industry is, of course, the key driving force behind the attack on lifestyle medicine and the draconian laws aimed at finally destroying it. Lifestyle medicine really does work better than drugs for most diseases and really can prevent many of them from happening in the first place, so it represents the ultimate threat to this trillion-dollar global industry. This leads it to provide much of the funding for the unscientific trials and studies that try to prove natural solutions do not work or may be dangerous. It also spends huge sums of money (more than any other industry) lobbying politicians, the media and every other organisation involved in healthcare with the message that lifestyle solutions do not work and that only drugs should be used to treat disease.

The finance industry is also a key player. We have already seen how investment banks like Goldman Sachs have made it clear they are unlikely to lend money to drug companies that want to find real and lasting cures for diseases, because it is a major threat to future profits. But lifestyle medicine provides an even greater threat to their investments because it can prevent significant numbers of diseases from happening, thus eliminating the need for many drugs. There are, however, other key financial players because nearly every drug company is publicly listed, and most individuals and organisations like pension funds that invest in stocks and shares do so via global investment companies. The two largest are Black Rock and Vanguard, which, between them, own $15 trillion worth of shares in nearly every major listed company including those in the pharmaceutical industry. They also have major investments in industries like processed foods, GMO agriculture and chemicals, which are responsible for much of the current epidemic of disease, and lifestyle medicine is helping to expose the truth about all of them. Given that the key priority for investment companies and banks is to maximise profits, they all have a huge vested interest in trying to eliminate the potential threat posed by lifestyle medicine. Much of this is probably done through what appear to be independent "scientific" organisations, as well as the global media and internet companies which they are also major shareholders of.

Many of the world's richest tycoons have major investments in Vanguard and so, the global elite have a significant level of influence particularly when you consider that just the top 50 wealthiest US entrepreneurs alone have a net wealth of over $2 trillion. But there is one billionaire who has gone much further by directly using much of his personal wealth to promote and develop drug and vaccine treatments and to discredit and destroy every lifestyle solution that threatens these investments. His name? Bill Gates. It is hard to believe that one man could be wielding so much power in the war against lifestyle medicine, but this really is happening. Evidence will be provided in Parts 5 and 6, which I guarantee will shock you to the core.

What about medicine? Once again, doctors, GPs and even consultants are not responsible for what is happening. They know very little about what is going on behind the scenes. Doctors simply have to follow medical guidelines and the guidelines relate almost exclusively to drugs. They are not allowed to promote non-medical solutions within official medical organisations like the NHS. The real medical villains who are attacking lifestyle medicine are relatively small in number. They comprise:

- a relatively small band of researchers who are prepared to develop and conduct biased, manipulated and unscientific research of the types already examined
- a very small group of "experts" who have made it their mission to destroy lifestyle solutions to health, like vitamins, by cherry picking trial data and spinning the results
- key medical decision makers who refuse to acknowledge the incredible level of evidence for lifestyle treatments
- experts who sit on health and regulatory committees who control the directives that aim to savagely restrict natural products

Most of these key individuals have links to all the industries involved and are handsomely rewarded for their efforts. They receive honoraria and well-funded research chairs, and can benefit from "revolving door" arrangements with the companies involved and can be paid huge sums of money to promote or positively endorse their products.

Regulators have several functions, but the key one is supposedly to protect the public. However, one only needs to look at the number of deaths and serious diseases caused by drugs and products like agricultural chemicals to realise there are serious flaws in how they operate. Regulators usually receive most of their funding directly from the industries involved, and this has led to lax regulations that enable the companies to prosper, regardless of serious public outcomes. It also means that anything else that threatens the industries will be attacked by the regulators who are the key players in developing the draconian legislation that aims to destroy every aspect of lifestyle medicine.

What about politicians? I have written many letters to MPs and MEPs and most of them simply repeat the party lines that the laws that are already curtailing lifestyle medicine are there to protect the public. Of course, occasionally something happens to spark them into rebellion – like the vote in the European Parliament that exposed widespread industry-based corruption in the EU health committees, and the Commons Health Select Committee report on the pharmaceutical industry which was lambasted for the way it unduly influences medicine and bribes virtually everyone. But these are rare events and even these heavyweight condemnations have never resulted in any significant changes to the laws involved. The real political power brokers who decide on the regulations that govern things like natural foods and vitamins are top politicians in health, finance and industry. However, they have no detailed knowledge in this field and most rely almost exclusively on their expert advisors and regulators. Of course, most of these experts have ties with the pharmaceutical and other industries involved, and they strongly promote the idea that only drugs are proven to work and vitamins and other lifestyle treatments have no scientific evidence and "could" even be dangerous. These senior experts have, of course, been hugely incentivised by Big Business to promote their interests. The top echelons of the UK's health regulator, the MHRA, are littered with former Big Pharma employees. For example, the directors Ian Hudson and Gerald Heddell previously held senior roles at GlaxoSmithKline. Senior politicians will, of course, know about some of the corruption and bias that takes place, but they are busy people and won't know the full extent. They rely on their expert advisors who simply keep repeating the anti-lifestyle message. But politicians are also keen to protect "vital and strategic" industries like pharmaceuticals, Big Food and agro-chemicals. Concerns about civil liberties and allowing people to control their own health seem to come a distant second.

The whole thing is so corrupt it really does beggar belief.

PART 5

How Do Medicine and Lifestyle Medicine Treat Diseases?

Now we can start to examine individual diseases in more detail. Detailed books have been written about these diseases, so I can only outline the key facts. I will, however, also give recommendations for further reading. Also, I can only examine a relatively small number of them, but they do include most of the serious life-taking and life-destroying ones like heart disease, strokes, type 2 diabetes, obesity, depression, Alzheimer's and cancer. I'll start, once again, with the biggest killer: heart disease. (*Note – For each disease, the key medical approaches will be evaluated first, followed by lifestyle solutions.)*

Heart disease

Chronic heart disease (CHD) is one of the few diseases that medicine claims it is trying to prevent, by using drugs like statins and blood pressure treatments. However, given that heart disease is still the leading cause of death around the world (with 135,000 deaths in the UK in 2019) then clearly these drugs are not the panacea they are claimed to be. It is true that over the last 60 years, deaths have fallen by around a half. However, the two main reasons are the 70% decline in cigarette smoking and incredible improvements in emergency medical treatments for those people who do have heart attacks and other life-threatening types of heart disease but reach hospital in time.

Heart disease – the medical approach

Medicine lists a number of factors it believes can lead to heart disease. These include smoking and lack of exercise, which have already been covered, and high blood pressure, high cholesterol, high saturated fat intake, obesity and type 2 diabetes. The last two will be covered separately, and I will also provide a brief section on blood pressure, but most of this section will be devoted to cholesterol, statin drugs and saturated fats. Why? Because over the last 30 years, they have all been endlessly promoted and statins are the most widely prescribed drugs ever produced. Virtually everyone knows about statins and cholesterol. They have been prescribed to hundreds of millions of people around the world and sales have recently reached $1 trillion. The real facts, however, will surprise and shock you.

History and development of statins

Before undertaking a detailed analysis of statin drugs and heart disease, it is essential to understand how the cholesterol theory started, and this means we need to go back to the 1950s. We have already seen how heart attacks were much rarer 100 years ago. The numbers increased modestly up to about 1930 but then accelerated significantly over the next 20 years. Once World War II was over and normality resumed, medicine and governments in the west realised a disaster was unfolding. Heart attacks had gone up in those 20 years by around 1000% (a ten-fold increase), and had become *the* major killer. In the USA there were 500,000 deaths annually which was a third of the total. At that point researchers and academics started to grapple with this new threat and to investigate what the cause of such an "epidemic" could be.

Investigators were drawn to the idea that changes in diet were likely to be the main culprit. Some scientists suggested the epidemic was caused by the rise of hydrogenated vegetable oils and their offsprings, such as margarine and shortenings, since the consumption of these products had grown steadily over the previous two decades, roughly in line with the increase in heart disease. Others suggested that the use of sugar, which was also increasing rapidly and in tandem with heart attacks, was the main cause. Other researchers including David Kritchevsky demonstrated that cholesterol fed to rabbits caused arthrosclerosis. He also showed that vegetable oils could reduce cholesterol levels. It was already known that the blockages that caused heart attacks were made up of plaques containing fat and cholesterol. So, this seemed a neat and logical solution to the problem. Saturated fats, like butter and eggs, which also contained cholesterol, would enter the bloodstream after digestion where they could eventually form the plaques that ultimately led to blockages in the arteries. Within a few years this lipid hypothesis had gained momentum.

There were, however, a number of influential scientists who did not endorse this new theory. They pointed to the fact that rabbits were vegetarian and couldn't metabolise cholesterol, and that they should not be used to predict what happens in humans. There were also a number of studies that indicated that high fat diets did not correlate with heart disease. A long and acrimonious debate ensued. Trials and counter trials were carried out, papers and counter papers produced, but the lipid hypothesis had already gained much traction. The global processed food companies, such as Kraft Foods and Proctor & Gamble who produced the hydrogenated vegetable oils and margarines, played a major role. If they ever lost this debate, it would be nothing short of a disaster for their businesses. So, they lobbied politicians hard to support the theory that saturated fats were the real culprit and they provided huge funds to allow research to be carried out to try to support this theory.

One of the key players in the saturated fat–lipid hypothesis was a researcher called Ancel Keys. He used a different approach by comparing heart disease rates in various countries where accurate data existed on the consumption of fats in the diet. In 1958 Keys launched the hugely influential "Seven Countries Study" which gave a huge boost to the lipid theory. Keys analysed the results of seven countries: Italy, Greece, former Yugoslavia, Netherlands, Finland, the USA and Japan. He found an almost perfect straight-line correlation between the amount of fat consumed and the number of heart attacks. this was nearly a knockout blow in favour of the lipid theory, but some vociferous dissent nevertheless remained. Eventually, however, several dietary intervention trials were carried out and researchers claimed they provided the final proof for the lipid hypothesis.

In 1984 in the USA, and 1987 in the UK, this majority consensus led to the publication of official and definitive dietary guidelines which recommended a significant reduction in saturated fat consumption of all types, including butter, eggs, animal fats and high fat milk. In their place people were advised to substitute vegetable oils, margarine, low fat milk and lean meats, such as chicken, and were also advised to increase their carbohydrate consumption with foods such as grains and cereals to make up for the "lost calories" from fats. Western governments also applied immense pressure to the global food manufacturers to reduce the levels of fat in the processed foods they produced. This was a real challenge because people like the taste of fat and it took several years and billions of dollars in research to reformulate the huge range of processed foods they made so people would still enjoy them and buy them. Indeed, changes were introduced slowly over a few years to allow people's palates to gradually adjust to the changes in taste, but eventually, the job was done and low fat foods are now ubiquitous and a huge money spinner for an initially reluctant industry.

The pharmaceutical industry was also waiting in the wings. Now that the lipid theory of heart disease was almost universally accepted, the industry set out to develop a new generation of drugs that would lower cholesterol, with the knowledge that if they succeeded, then governments and medicine would fund them. The first statin drug came onto the market in 1987, but several others followed over the course of the next decade. Huge advertising campaigns were subsequently initiated by Big Pharma so that everyone would get to know about these new "wonder drugs" and their dramatic effect on heart disease. The whole marketing process has been a true object lesson for any business on how to sell a product. Today, there can't be a single adult in the west who doesn't know about statins, cholesterol and heart disease, and who doesn't know that "bad cholesterol" is really bad for us and must be lowered at any cost. The saturated fat and high cholesterol theory of heart disease was indeed one of the most dramatic and influential theories ever developed by medical researchers. In time, statins would turn out to be the most profitable drugs ever invented. So much for the big build up. But do you sense a big "reality check" coming? You'll have to wait a little longer to find out. So, now we can start to examine statins and saturated fat in more detail.

Statins and cholesterol – a few facts

- Statins are the world's most prescribed drugs of all time (antidepressants are closing in rapidly).
- There are currently seven different statin drugs as well as several combination drugs using statins.
- Lipitor (atorvastatin) is the bestselling drug of all time; its total sales up to 2014 were $147 billion.
- Worldwide sales of all statin drugs has recently reached $1 trillion.
- Cholesterol in food such as eggs does not increase blood serum levels. This is proven conclusively.
- Cholesterol is produced by the liver and by each cell in the body. It is essential for human life.
- It is essential for maintaining cell function, brain synapses, hormones, plus many other key roles.
- If it was possible to reduce someone's "bad cholesterol" to zero they would die immediately.
- Fats make up the biggest component of the brain – around 60%.
- The brain produces and contains 25% of the body's entire cholesterol. It is essential for cell function.
- Most statin drugs have now lost their patent protection, meaning that profits have fallen by around 90%.

What proof is there that statins work?

Statins reduce cholesterol and this is a scientific fact. But high cholesterol is not a disease in itself; there are no symptoms of any kind with high cholesterol. Statins are given to protect against heart disease and nothing else. So, you might realistically expect that when the original clinical trials were carried out, they would have demonstrated that they did indeed reduce the number of heart attacks. But you would be wrong. In fact, Pfizer, the manufacturer of the bestselling drug of all time, the statin drug Lipitor, was forced to put this insert into its advertisements by the FDA: "Lipitor has not been shown to prevent heart disease or heart attacks." Not bad going for a drug whose only purpose is to prevent heart disease.

So, how did Lipitor and the other statin drugs gain approval? Well, if you remember the section on "surrogate end points" it will all fall into place. In the case of statins, cholesterol is a surrogate end point. The drug manufacturer simply has to prove that its drug lowers cholesterol and it will be automatically approved for preventing heart disease even though it has not been proven to do so directly. This they can do in a few weeks at little cost. It's much harder proving your drug actually prevents heart disease; it's so much easier just to assume it does. Of course, experts will say that the lipid hypothesis of heart disease proves this must be the case, but this also was never proven by clinical trials, only by other indirect methods. When drugs are going to be given to hundreds of millions of people, definitive clinical trials are the least the public should be able to expect, or at least that is the view of medicine, except, of course, when it suits them not to, as in the case of statins. Of course, this doesn't mean statins don't work. It just means you've unleashed a drug that doesn't have any scientific proof. Not bad for a profession that prides itself on being "evidence-based". Many years later, trials were carried out that claim to show statins save lives, but as we will see later the results of these trials are not what they seem.

When statins were first developed, they were given only to people who were thought to be at high risk of heart disease. But over the last 30 years the number of people taking them has increased significantly. People judged at moderate risk were next in the firing line, and the level of cholesterol which was deemed "safe" was also reduced. Then, in 2014, even people at low risk of heart disease were recommended for statin treatment by NICE. Overnight the numbers of people eligible for statins went up from 6 million to 12 million in the UK alone. Worldwide, around 300 million people are taking statins making them the most prescribed drug class of all time and the number is set to rise inexorably as developing countries that currently barely use them also join the statin bandwagon. Everyone knows about cholesterol and saturated fats and "knows" they cause heart disease. Except, I'm going to provide evidence that they don't. Even if you've been convinced by most of my arguments so far, I can imagine you're thinking this a step too far, that this simply couldn't be true. All I can say is defer your judgement until you have seen all the evidence. Incidentally, have you noticed the way in which statins are being reported has changed? Even as little as seven years ago all press reports on statins regularly contained the phrase "these wonder drugs". Now, you will often see headlines like "these controversial drugs".

Several senior medical figures like the queen's former physician Sir Richard Thompson, who was also a former president of the Royal College of Physicians, demanded that statin use was re-evaluated after a review into key trials concluded the pills were not effective at protecting against heart disease. He said, "The statin data needs to be urgently scrutinised. We are very worried about it and particularly side effect data which seems to have been swept under the carpet. If we are wrong about widespread prescribing of this drug we have to stand up and say sorry."

Of course, many other leading doctors say these reports are misleading and that people should continue with their statin treatment. But the fact this acrimonious battle is taking place openly within medicine is to say the least intriguing and unusual. The British Medical Journal has also waded into the debate with claims that side effects are far higher than are being acknowledged and that statins are less effective than claimed. Several studies have also been released in quick succession about "previously unknown side effects" of statin drugs. Given what we know about the power of the pharmaceutical industry and the iron grip it exerts on medicine and the press, just what is going on? All will be revealed shortly.

The truth about saturated fats

Medicine's theory of what causes heart disease has rested for decades on the assumption that saturated fat and cholesterol are two of the main culprits. I'll start with saturated fat. Let's start by going back to Ancel Keys. He is the researcher who in 1958 published the "Seven Countries Study". It was this study that proved so decisive in persuading most researchers, politicians and academics that saturated fat and cholesterol were the primary causes of heart disease. But a few years earlier Keys had floated his saturated fat theory at a meeting of leading cardiologists who tore his ideas to pieces. Keys apparently left the meeting humiliated. Of course, after he produced his seven-country study, he had the last laugh when his theory became widely accepted. The problem was no one considered it worthwhile to check his work. It was only many years later that some researchers did just that, and what they found was a bombshell.

In 1958 there were 22 countries that accurately monitored the consumption of fats. Keys had the data on all of them, but chose just seven for his study. The analysis of all 22 countries in fact showed there was no relationship whatsoever between saturated fat and heart disease. Put quite simply, the cause of heart disease is not saturated fat. In fact, if Keys had selectively chosen seven other countries, he could have even shown the exact opposite of his theory – that high fat actually reduces heart disease. So, why did Keys "cherry pick" the seven countries that "proved" his theory, and ignore the other 15 countries that would have totally derailed it? Was he a corrupt researcher? Was he driven to avenge his previous humiliation? We may never know the exact truth, but the fact is Keys really did believe that saturated fat caused heart disease and like many researchers, politicians and academics before and after him, when you "know" that something is true, it is natural to accept information that supports your ideas and reject information that doesn't. The people who do this don't see themselves as corrupt, because rejecting information that doesn't support your ideas is natural when you "know" beyond doubt you are right. It is simply a classic case of blind dogma. But whatever his motives, the fact remains that one of the key pieces of evidence that supported the saturated fat theory of heart disease, which led to widespread dietary changes, was simply wrong. There is an incredible amount of evidence that totally disproves the saturated fat theory and I will give you just a few more key examples.

There was never any real proof about saturated fats even when governments started issuing guidelines to reduce fat consumption. At that time there were six separate trials that had compared low fat diets to standard diets. But we now know, after a recent reappraisal of their findings, there was no significant difference in heart disease between the two groups. So, how do theories like the saturated fat theory gain acceptance when there is seemingly no hard evidence? This is Dr Malcolm Kendrick's view. It could be an idea that was simply put forward in a medical journal or at a conference and it may be impossible to find the source. Despite the lack of any scientific evidence, a strange thing then happens. Over time, the concept is repeated and cross-referenced between different authors and journals. Eventually, it becomes a universal concept and simply becomes accepted. Can this really be the way that such a momentous decision was taken to redefine diets for more than half a billion people? It certainly seems so.

Perhaps realising they were on shaky ground, and 11 years after the US Senate Select Committee published its recommendations against dietary fat, the US surgeon general's office set about preparing a report that would definitively link saturated fats and heart disease. After a further 11 years, and research costing millions of dollars, the project was quietly abandoned after they could find no evidence of such a link. It was never published. This complete lack of any evidence made not the slightest difference to the dietary recommendations. After all, everyone "knew" by that time that saturated fat caused heart disease, so this new evidence could be safely ignored. Perhaps there was something wrong in the way it had been done. Perhaps the researchers had just had a bad day at the office – or should that be a bad 11 years. Perhaps... Or more likely it was simply that no one wanted to jeopardise their inflated egos and reputations, or put at risk the big "fat" industry profit streams that were being made. All we know is that one of the longest studies ever carried out anywhere in the world was simply ignored, even though the results were beyond doubt: saturated fat simply could not be linked to heart disease.

But even more bad news was to follow. Researchers pointed out that France, which has one of the highest consumptions of saturated fat in the world, also had one of the lowest rates of heart disease. France had, and still has, around one-third of the number of heart attacks of the UK. How was this possible? The accepted theory, of course, said it was impossible, so there *must*, of course, be another explanation. When experts are faced with something that contradicts their views, they describe it as a "paradox". So, this simply became known as the French paradox. Researchers soon realised that if they could find a plausible explanation for the "French paradox" they would become famous and they would have "saved the day" for the saturated fat theory. The drug industry would almost certainly offer generous donations for such work. Eventually, researchers came up with the idea that the French had low rates of heart disease because of all the red wine they drank, the garlic they consumed and the freshly cooked vegetables they ate. Sighs of relief all round then. But wait a minute. If this really was true, it would be one of the greatest medical discoveries of all time. It would mean that if people in the UK, for example, started consuming garlic, fresh vegetables and red wine in abundance, the numbers of heart attacks would plummet by two-thirds. Governments across the world would surely change dietary guidelines immediately to save millions of lives, wouldn't they? But, of course, they didn't. This time quite rightly, because there was not a shred of evidence to back it up. It was just an unlikely and unproven hypothesis. Of course, it is almost certain that garlic, vegetables and red wine in moderation are good for us, but to suggest they could reduce heart attacks by 65% is plain fantasy. But none of this mattered – the saturated fat theory "had been saved". Hallelujah. The press and media swallowed this garbage hook, line and sinker; not one health correspondent could see these claims were utter nonsense. No one dared to challenge them. They were simply reported verbatim as if they were the gospel truth.

As Dr Malcolm Kendrick said, "Once experts have decided that saturated fat causes heart disease then *nothing* will change their minds!" But the bad news just kept on coming. A major study in Malmo in 2005 followed 28,098 people for 6.6 years. The findings were: "Saturated fat showed no relationship with cardiovascular disease in men. Amongst women, cardiovascular mortality showed a downwards trend with increasing saturated fat intake, but these didn't reach statistical significance." In other words, there was no difference.

Another major randomised intervention trial in the USA involved 48,835 women. The control group ate a normal diet while the active group followed a low fat regime. The trial lasted for 8.1 years. The findings were: "Among the study population as a whole there were no significant differences in the numbers of heart attacks or strokes or in total mortality."

What was the medical reaction to this trial? "The results of this study do not change established recommendations on disease prevention. Women should continue to work with their doctors to reduce their risk of heart disease including following a diet low in saturated fat, trans-fat and cholesterol," said Dr Elizabeth Nabel of the National Heart, Lung and Blood Institute. So, no matter how overwhelming the evidence was becoming, Dr Kendrick was right. *Nothing* was going to change minds.

There really are many more high-quality trials I could quote that show no link between saturated fat and heart disease, but I'll give you just one more substantive piece of evidence.

Fifty years ago, the Japanese had the highest rate of strokes anywhere in the world but at the same time one of the lowest rates of heart attack. There are two types of stroke and there was evidence that for haemorrhagic stroke, a low level of cholesterol actually caused an increased risk, while for ischaemic stroke, low cholesterol decreased the risk. To cut a long story short, the Japanese government advised its entire population to eat more saturated fat in attempt to stop so many of them dying from haemorrhagic stroke. What happened? In the 40-year period between 1960 and 2000, fat consumption in Japan went up from 5% to 20% of total calories. An incredible four-fold increase. Cholesterol levels went up by 20%. Surely, they must have started to drop like flies from heart attacks? Well, actually, they didn't. The number of heart attacks – which were already low – actually fell by a further 20%, while the number of haemorrhagic strokes fell by a staggering 83%. Medicine would say this was an epidemiological study and it doesn't definitively prove that increased fat consumption was the cause of the reductions in both stroke and heart attack. But Japan has a population of 117 million and the dietary change has lasted over 40 years, making it the largest intervention trial involving an entire population that has been carried out in the history of medicine ever. You might imagine that the results just might cause western medicine to wonder whether their theory that saturated fat and cholesterol are the cause of heart disease might be wrong. But *you* would be wrong. By now I'm sure you can see a clear trend emerging to account for any, and every, piece of unwanted evidence against the saturated fat theory. So, unsurprisingly, this latest one became known as the Japanese paradox, but tellingly, even today, no one has been able to offer any other plausible theory to explain it. That's simply because there isn't one. There is no Japanese paradox. It is simply the saturated fat theory that is wrong.

Despite the fact many of medicine's elite can't, and won't, accept they are wrong, others are not so reticent. In 1984 Time magazine was a key player in promoting the saturated fat and cholesterol hypothesis. Its front cover read: "Cholesterol – and now the bad news". The article explored Ancel Keys' "proof" that saturated fat caused heart disease and the dangers of high cholesterol. In 2014 it published an apology for having got it so wrong. The headline this time said: "Eat butter. Scientists labelled fat the enemy. Why they were wrong". In the accompanying feature, the magazine admitted that the war on fat had been wrong all along and that the science supporting the theory had been "junk". The dangers of saturated fat had in fact started to be voiced as early as the 1960s, well before official dietary guidelines were changed. This is what Rodney Bilton, emeritus professor of biochemistry at Liverpool John Moore's University, had to say on the saturated fat debate: "The idea is deeply embedded in the public consciousness as a result of half a century of flawed information and propaganda. The 'fat is bad' idea has become so established that many experts refuse even to consider opposing evidence from impeccable sources." Dr James DiNicolantonio from Ithaca College, New York said, "We have been led down the wrong dietary road for decades." He is now calling for a public health campaign as pervasive and aggressive as the one enjoyed by the low fat theory, telling the public that medicine simply got it wrong and that carbohydrates and sugars are the true villains.

The real tragedy is that, in the developed world, around 1 billion people are following low fat diets. Natural fats contribute to our health and the demonising of fat has made people sicker. But the really insidious part of this whole dietary disaster is that people have been told to replace the "deadly fat" with extra carbohydrates and grains. Much of this is in a highly processed industrialised form, such as white bread, corn flakes and other highly processed breakfast cereals, sugar and other junk foods. These are the real deadly foods that are killing us slowly but inexorably. It is this huge increase in industrialised foods – a by-product of the reduction in fat – that has resulted in one of the greatest self-inflicted health disasters of all time. At some point in the future, when it is politically expedient to do so, researchers will calculate how many hundreds of millions of lives have been shortened and by how much, and how many extra cases of diabetes, cancer and a host of other diseases have occurred, all because of this single dietary catastrophe. Before this can happen, of course, medicine and politicians need to simply and honourably accept they were wrong. Clearly, they are not yet ready to do so.

Statins

Statins reduce cholesterol levels, but is this a good thing or a bad thing? Most people would say I must be mad asking such a silly question. But consider the following facts. Study after study has shown that people with low cholesterol levels have a higher risk of dying overall than those with a normal level. And the lower the cholesterol goes, the higher the risk. This is an extract from a paper published in the Journal of the American Medical Association in 1987 titled "Cholesterol and mortality: 30 years of follow-up from the Framingham study": "There is a direct association between falling cholesterol levels over the first 14 years of the study and mortality over the following 18 years (11% overall and 14% cardiovascular death rate increase per 1mg/dl per year drop in cholesterol levels." So, lowering cholesterol levels results in increased deaths from heart disease, strokes and overall mortality. The Framingham study is one of the most influential and respected studies ever conducted.

Next is an extract from a paper published in the Lancet in August 2001 whish examined cholesterol levels and mortality in older people. The Honolulu researchers concluded: "Our data accord with previous findings of increased mortality in elderly people with low serum cholesterol, and show that long-term persistence of low cholesterol concentration actually increases the risk of death. Thus, the earlier that patients start to lower cholesterol, the greater the risk of death. We have been unable to explain our results. These data cast doubt on the scientific justification for lowering cholesterol to very low levels."

How about a study from Austria which followed 150,000 men and women aged between 20 and 95 for a total of 15 years, one of the biggest studies of its kind: "In men across the entire age range and in women from the age of 50 upwards, low cholesterol was significantly associated with all-cause mortality, showing significant associations with death through cancer, liver diseases, and mental diseases."

This next one is from a Finnish study published in the American Journal of Epidemiology in 1992: "Men with high cholesterol levels had lower all-cause mortality, because of their low cancer mortality and residual mortality."

So, now we have a new "paradox", because the cholesterol theory is contradicted by the facts and low cholesterol levels result in increased mortality. Panic stations all round in those promoting low cholesterol then? Not really because, of course, the cholesterol theory "must" be right because all the experts say so. Not unexpectedly, researchers have come to the rescue of the cholesterol theory with yet another tortured hypothesis that seeks to explain this "paradox". We have a researcher called Carlos Iribarren to thank for this one. He hypothesised that those people with low cholesterol who are dying disproportionally have some other underlying disease even though it has not yet been diagnosed. This other disease causes cholesterol to fall and, therefore, it is this disease and not the low cholesterol itself that is causing the increased death rate. This is tortured logic in the extreme. Can there really be so many people who are suffering from diseases that no doctor has actually been able to diagnose and that remain undiagnosed for many years? It is true that some advanced cancers and chronic liver disease can cause cholesterol levels to fall, but the idea that tiny cancers that are so small they cannot even be detected can also cause cholesterol to fall precipitously is fanciful in the extreme.

I'll show you why this hypothesis is just that: a hypothesis that doesn't stand up to rigorous examination. It is no better than the garlic and red wine hypothesis that "saved" the saturated fat theory, but it has indeed saved the day for the cholesterol theory and is quoted widely by all the statin experts. The Framingham researchers who had recorded that high mortality was associated with low cholesterol levels, particularly in the over fifties, also wondered if there could be some other underlying illness. They concluded that "this was an unlikely explanation". The Austrian researchers also reached an identical conclusion after re-examining all their results in the light of the Iribarren hypothesis. The Honolulu researchers similarly re-examined their findings and reported: "Iribarren and colleagues suggested that a decline in serum cholesterol levels might occur over a decade before diagnosis of a disease. Our data suggest that those individuals with low serum cholesterol maintained over a 20-year period will have the worst outlook for all-cause mortality. Our present analysis suggests that the Iribarren hypothesis is implausible and is unlikely to account for the adverse events of low cholesterol levels over 20 years."

As Dr Kendrick so eloquently puts it: "This is as close as one set of researchers will ever come to telling another set of researchers that they are talking complete bollocks! At least in public, anyway." He sums up the whole cholesterol situation succinctly: "The simple fact is that a low cholesterol level increases the risk of death in men and women. This fact has never been contradicted by any study."

Next, I'll present a different type of proof. It has been recognised for many years that women generally suffer much less heart disease than men, especially younger women. In the UK the difference is around 300% while in New Zealand it is a staggering 1000%. This is despite the fact that women have higher average cholesterol levels. Women, therefore, present a special problem for the cholesterol hypothesis. Higher cholesterol levels than men but much lower rates of heart disease. This must mean... Yes, you've probably guessed. It can only be the "female paradox". But, of course, this is the biggest paradox ever seen in medicine, because females make up slightly more than half of the global population. Of course, researchers again came to the rescue with a new hypothesis that at least temporarily rescued the cholesterol hypothesis. This was that women's sex hormones protected them against high cholesterol, at least until the menopause, after which this protection disappeared. The only evidence in support of this hypothesis was a hugely flawed and biased observational study which was later totally discredited. In fact, a study from 1963 had already concluded there was no effect from ovarian function on heart disease, and that the difference in cardiovascular mortality between men and women had to be down to other factors. Another paper published in 1987 in the New England Journal of Medicine also concluded: "The normal menopause, which causes a gradual decrease in oestrogen production, was not associated with any increase in the risk of coronary heart disease."

In fact, there has never been a study that shows that female sex hormones protect against heart disease. But, despite all this evidence, the sex hormone hypothesis gained momentum and credence. Indeed, so powerful did it become that by the 1990s, millions of women were actively being given HRT therapy to reduce their risk of heart disease. So, what changed? Well, a clinical trial involving 17,000 women was conducted to examine the effect of HRT on heart disease. This was called the Women's Health Initiative (WHI) study. Doctors stood back and waited for the "inevitable" proof that would finally justify the millions of HRT prescriptions they were writing. But what the trial found was yet another body blow to the medical establishment. The trial's conclusion was that HRT actually increased the risk of coronary heart disease. Today the American Heart Association, a bastion of conventional medical thinking, recommends strongly against using HRT to protect against heart disease.

But, of course, even after this further setback, the cholesterol hypothesis still "had to be correct". All the experts agreed and, of course, so much money was at stake. So, you can probably guess that a new hypothesis was quickly waved in to keep the whole cholesterol charade going. This time it was that women generally have higher HDL cholesterol, and it is this that protects them from heart disease. Dr Kendrick has demolished this new hypothesis, but it is quite a long and technical process so I am not going to try to summarise it. If you want to find out how, I suggest you read his book *The Great Cholesterol Con*. Incidentally, even medicine now no longer promotes this idea as it is quite simply wrong. But it served a purpose until another hypothesis could be found.

Hopefully, you can see the utter futility of it all, and the desperation of the drug industry and medicine in trying to keep the whole cholesterol charade going. This can be summarised as follows. The cholesterol hypothesis must be correct – all the experts agree. (Experts who, of course, are hugely incentivised by Big Pharma.) So, when overwhelming evidence emerges that disproves this hypothesis, a *new* hypothesis must be invented to explain away this evidence. When that is demolished by the facts, a further new hypothesis is invented. This process has been going on for nearly three decades and will go on indefinitely because the cholesterol hypothesis "must be correct". I know this all sounds truly silly and almost impossible to believe, but the root cause is simple: money and greed. Just remember that statin sales have now reached $1 trillion. *Nothing* can, or will, be allowed to stand in the way of this profit bonanza because, as we have seen, Big Pharma effectively controls medical research and most of medicine itself.

I'm going to look at one final piece of evidence. Several randomised clinical trials were carried out on statin drugs after they had been on the market for several years. If you had read the press releases on these trials you could be forgiven for thinking that statins were indeed "wonder drugs". But I'm going to show you the distorted truth behind these sensational headlines. Before I can do this, I need to explain two new concepts that form part of the evidence. These are "overall mortality" and "saving lives". I'll start with "saving lives".

The results of one of the clinical trials on statins, the Heart Protection Study, included this statement: "If 10 million high-risk people worldwide go onto statin treatment, this would save about 50,000 lives each year". But you cannot "save a life" because everyone is going to die. So, a more sensible question is: how much longer would these 50,000 people live, compared to someone not taking a statin? You may think I'm being unnecessarily pedantic in trying to make this distinction, but consider two random examples. If a six-month-old girl develops meningitis and is immediately treated with penicillin, she will not die. In fact, she is likely to have a further 80 years of healthy life. On the other hand, if someone has a massive heart attack and they are defibrillated and resuscitated it is quite possible they could arrest and die half an hour later. It is true that both these interventions could be said to be "life-saving" in some form or another. However, one form of life-saving is clearly of much greater value than the other – 80 years compared to half an hour. This clearly shows that you cannot use "life-saving" as a remotely useful measure of the benefits of a treatment or drug. So, how much longer do people who take statins actually live? All will be revealed shortly and you will be surprised by the answer.

Next, I need to explain "overall mortality". When we briefly looked at the breast cancer drug Herceptin in Part 3, the clinical trials showed that Herceptin reduced cancer risk but increased heart attack risk. Cancer risk reduced by 3.0%, but the heart attack risk increased by 2.1 %. This means that if 100 people were given Herceptin, three would not die from cancer but two others could die from heart attacks. Heart attacks they otherwise wouldn't have had. The overall benefit of taking Herceptin – the overall mortality – is therefore 0.9%, meaning that about 1 in a 100 will benefit. Given that drugs are the third leading cause of death due to their side effects, the overall mortality figure is a critical one. It is *the* most important outcome of any clinical trial dealing with life-threatening diseases. Drug trials for conditions like heart disease, cancer, Alzheimer's and stroke really should include a figure for overall mortality. Just quoting the mortality benefits of a drug without quoting the mortality levels from its side effects is unscientific, as well as being effectively fraudulent.

Before I move on to the trials themselves, I want to introduce you to a major player, in fact, probably the most influential figure in the world in the promotion of statins and the cholesterol hypothesis. His name is Professor Sir Rory Collins. Professor Collins is based in Oxford University and runs an organisation called the Cholesterol Treatment Trialists Collaboration (CCT). As we have already seen, the pharmaceutical industry rarely promotes its own products. Instead, they enlist the services of respected clinical experts and academics to do the promotion for them. Enter Professor Collins. It should perhaps be pointed out that the CCT group is part of the Clinical Trials Service Unit (CTSU) also in Oxford which has been paid hundreds of millions of pounds to carry out research on behalf of pharmaceutical companies. The CCT is the only organisation in the world that has been given access to the full data on every single clinical trial and study ever carried out on statins. Many of these papers have never been seen by anyone else. So, the pharmaceutical industry must have complete faith in Professor Collins' ability to promote statins, as well as a willingness to overlook all the glaring defects in the cholesterol hypothesis, and to play down the side effects. As we will see, he hasn't let them down.

The CCT have promoted the ever-increasing use of statins so that the figure now stands at 300 million people worldwide and rising. They have declared that statins have few side effects except a small percentage of minor muscle problems and conducted clinical trials that proclaim the "life-saving" abilities of statins. Of course, they have been handsomely remunerated for all of this. I will reveal the actual sum later – it will shock you. So, now we can examine the clinical trials on statins. I'll start with one of the trials conducted by Professor Collins and the CCT, the Heart Protection Study. I'll repeat the key euphoric conclusion of his press release: "If 10 million high-risk people worldwide go onto statin treatment, this would save about 50,000 lives each year". Let's start by putting this information into a context that is easier to interpret. If you divide 10 million by 50,000, you get 200. So, what this study demonstrated is that you need to treat 200 high-risk people with statins for one year for one extra person to be alive at the end of that year. The other 199 people will gain no benefit at all. But how much longer would that one lucky person live? Almost incredibly, the average is just three months. Compare the real facts and the minimal benefits of statins with the euphoric press release which claimed that "50,000 lives could be saved".

There is one other key point that needs to be made clearly and unequivocally. These trial participants were high-risk patients because they had all previously suffered from a heart attack or other cardiovascular event, which means they were at a very much higher risk of a second serious heart event. They are the people who should benefit most from statins. People with a low risk of heart disease, however, would expect to see significantly lower benefits from statins, but if only 1 in 200 high-risk patients benefit, and that benefit is just three months extra life, then the benefit for people at low risk must be tiny. Indeed, it is vanishingly small. Two studies from 2011 found that around 1,000 otherwise healthy people need to take statins for just one of them to avoid "dying" from a heart attack. But the other key fact is that other studies have shown that the increased life expectancy is typically around three days.

To depress you even further we now come to the critical figure for overall mortality. But guess what? There is no mention of overall mortality in the Heart Protection Study. Not one word, no figures, nothing. What does this tell us? It tells us that, at the very best, there is no benefit in overall mortality. If there had been, it would have been included in the results. Could the overall mortality be negative? In other words, could more people have died in the statin group than the placebo group? Knowing what we already know about low cholesterol levels, this is possible. Of course, we will never know because the data from the clinical trials is not available to independent researchers. So, despite a small benefit for one high-risk person in 200 taking a statin this will likely be cancelled out by other significant side effects.

What this study really shows, despite all the hype and clever words as well as the huge numbers that were chosen by Professor Collins simply to magnify the tiny benefits, is that statins will almost certainly not save a single life overall. All the other trials that have been carried out showing similar benefits for statins suffer from the same flaw. They contain no data on overall mortality. The only conclusion from this is that there is no overall benefit. But overall mortality is the only thing that really matters to most people. If someone doesn't die from a heart attack but dies from cancer at around the same time, is there really any benefit? Incidentally, no trial has ever shown a reduction in overall mortality in women or in men who had no previous history of heart disease. These two categories account for over 90% of the entire population.

But then came the JUPITER trial, the only trial that apparently showed a fall in overall mortality with statins. So, is this the final proof that statins really do work? Well, actually, no. When independent experts started to delve into the details, a different picture emerged. The original researchers had used highly selective relative risk analyses and other dubious techniques to hype up the benefits. Dr Kendrick explains the whole story in his book *Doctoring Data*. It is a long and laborious process so if you want to see all the details you need to read the book. Finally, Professor Michael de Lorgeril wrote a damning article published in the Archives of Internal Medicine. This is his final conclusion on the JUPITER trial: "Although it is quite unusual that the burden of calculating cardiovascular mortality is placed on the readers, all methods used, however, lead to the same conclusion: there is no significant difference in cardiovascular mortality between the two groups in the JUPITER trial."

As explained, all the clinical trials ever carried out on statins have been given to Professor Collins and the CTT. Most of them have never been seen by anyone except the drug companies, the CTT and drug regulators. Given the clear disputes about the benefits and side effects of statins, there have been calls for many years for regulators to release all the trial data so other experts can carry out an independent analysis. This has never happened and probably never will because if it could ever be achieved, most independent experts believe the truth would devastate the drug industry and show just how they manipulate the data to achieve the results they want or just hide it if it cannot be manipulated. So, to summarise this section on the clinical trials carried out on statins: statins do not reduce overall mortality in women. Statins do not reduce overall mortality in men who do not already have heart disease. Around 1 in 200 men who are at high risk of heart disease live for around three months longer but have no decrease in overall mortality. So, there you have it. A meagre offering indeed. So small in fact it almost vanishes from sight.

So far, I have avoided any real discussion on the side effects of statins. But given that statins don't save lives overall, then any side effects are of great concern. So, what is the truth? The answer is that no one really knows. This sounds appalling and it is. On the one hand, we have Professor Collins claiming side effects are virtually non-existent – no more than 1 in 100 people suffering minor muscle problems. Then we have the British Medical Journal which claims the figure is around 1 in 5. The drug companies on their patient leaflets say some side effects affect 1 in 10 people. When patients themselves have been asked, the side effects have been reported at around 1 in 2 people. So, you can take your pick. However, if the drug companies themselves admit that around 1 in 10 people are affected, then we can be fairly sure Professor Collins is way off the mark. Even if we stick with the pharmaceutical company figure, it still means that with 7.5 million people taking statins in the UK, then 750,000 are suffering side effects from a drug that offers no "overall life-saving" benefit. The types of side effect are numerous and include not just muscle pain, but stomach pains, diarrhoea, vomiting, memory loss, headache, sleep disturbances, dizziness, type 2 diabetes, cataracts, acute kidney disease, cognitive impairment, depression and fatigue. This seems like a hell of a bad deal all round. Except, of course, for the pharmaceutical industry, which has made $1 trillion in sales worldwide, and its highly remunerated experts like Professor Collins.

As I was just about to finish writing this section, I uncovered an article concerning Professor Collins and the side effect saga. This almost defies any logic. Professor Collins confessed to the Express newspaper that he hasn't actually done any analysis on the true side effects of statins. This is unbelievable. Statins are the most widely prescribed drugs and have been given to hundreds of millions of people over the last 30 years. And only now do we find out that the key medical expert who has rigorously and incessantly promoted them for over two decades has never done a scientific study on their side effects. But balancing the benefits and risks of any treatment is the absolute bedrock of medicine. It is a scientific necessity. Professor Collins really should be put on trial for effectively ignoring the side effects of statins and only promoting their minimal benefits. But don't worry, because now Professor Collins intends to ride to the rescue. He put himself forward as the best person to head a new and belated analysis of the data on statin side effects. Words almost fail me. You simply couldn't make this sort of thing up. Despite all the evidence about numerous and serious side effects, I guarantee Professor Collins will downplay them all and carry on protecting pharmaceutical interests rather than statin patients.

After the last two paragraphs, this is the perfect moment to look at how statin side effects can seriously affect real people's lives and I am going to concentrate just on muscle problems, which, according to Professor Collins, are just minor problems affecting no more than 1 in 100 patients. Muscle problems and pain were in fact one of the earliest and most frequently reported side effects that patients encountered when taking statins. The reality, however, is that this supposed minor side effect is much more sinister. Dr James Le Fanu writes a weekly medical column in the Daily Telegraph and in 2007 wrote a short item on the experience of one of his readers who had had a successful operation to repair an aortic aneurysm five years earlier. However, things had not gone well over the following years. He was in pain and his movement so limited that when he went for a three-week break to his son's wedding in Hawaii, he even had to use wheelchairs during flight transfers. When he arrived, he realised he had not packed his statin drugs which he had been taking for several years. However, his health had improved so incredibly by the time he returned to the UK, that he was able to walk unassisted through Heathrow Airport. Stopping his statins resulted in a near miraculous restoration of his overall health and wellbeing, and this led to a deluge of similar stories from people who had read Dr Le Fanu's article. I'll outline just three of them.

A woman in her mid-sixties had been taking statins for several years and over time started suffering from insomnia, incessant tiredness, weakness in her leg muscles, unhealing rashes and memory loss. She thought these problems were just a result of increasing age, but after she read the article, she wanted to see what happened if she stopped taking the statins. She asked her doctor who agreed for a short time. She now sleeps perfectly, has regained an active lifestyle, her memory is improving and the rashes have also significantly improved. She will never take statins again.

A Scottish woman, who was a regular club cyclist, was given statins by her doctor. After a few months her stamina was disappearing and she had to give up her club sessions. She asked her doctor and a pharmacist whether her drug could be responsible and was told no. She then started to get severe cramps in her neck during the night, and in the morning had very little neck movement, although this eased slowly during the day. She eventually went on the web and found a list of simvastatin side effects which included muscle cramps. This was enlightening because she took her simvastatin drug at 11 p.m. each night and at around 1 a.m. her neck cramps started. She didn't take the statin that evening and had no cramps that night. Unsurprisingly, she has never taken them since and the neck cramps have simply disappeared. After a few months her stamina also started to return and she was able to rejoin the cycling club and she even expects to get back to her full level of performance.

A very energetic 58-year-old woman had two main hobbies: long distance horse riding and walking her dog for miles each day. Three years previously her doctor had effectively frightened her to start taking statins. She had asked him what the side effects might be, and he said, "You will live longer." The actual side effects, however, were lack of energy, insomnia and aching joints. Initially, she put these down to the ageing process and her life and activity deteriorated seriously. Then she decided to see what happened if she stopped taking them, and after two weeks saw a miraculous improvement. She threw them away and is now back to her normal, energetic life.

I have seen literally hundreds of similar individual stories of how lives have been seriously devasted not just from statins but from a wide range of other drugs – sometimes for many years – only to find that when they eventually stopped taking them, their life miraculously returned to near normal. However, the reality is the vast majority of people who take statins and suffer serious side effects do not stop taking them because they have no idea they could be the cause of their problems. They believe they are simply the consequences of natural ageing. Most of those people who replied to Dr Le Fanu and stopped taking their statins would not have done so had they not seen his newspaper article.

But there is an even more sinister long-term problem. We have seen that even the drug industry admits that around 10% of patients will experience side effects like muscle problems. This means that at least 750,000 people are currently affected, but these obvious and devastating statin side effects can also lead to even more serious potential outcomes. Consider that when an active person is unable to go out for walks or other forms of activity because of the drug-induced muscle problems or fatigue, then their risk of serious diseases like heart disease, cancer and dementia can all increase significantly because of their reducing levels of exercise. We have also seen that having positive thoughts and low stress can significantly increase life expectancy, but when people are unable to do the things they really enjoy as well as experiencing pain and movement restrictions, then positive thoughts can be lost and replaced by depression and anxiety. This really can then start to reduce life expectancy.

Additionally, some people experiencing side effects may eventually go back and report the problems to their doctor. Neither they nor the doctor will understand that statins are the cause, and the doctor is likely to prescribe additional drugs (which have their own side effects) to try to minimise these symptoms. The reality is that the so-called minimal side effects of statins claimed by Professor Collins are simply unforgiveable.

In 2017 even the deputy chairman of the British Medical Association, Dr Kailash Chand, openly admitted he had stopped taking statin drugs because the side effects were too debilitating – in particular muscle weakness, muscle pain and fatigue. I have also seen a number of similar statements and actions from doctors and pharmacists. Would Professor Collins simply dismiss even these high-profile medical people? Of course, he would.

Here is one more concerning piece of so-called statin evidence. It involves two of the very latest 2022 studies on statin side effects that have just been released and that I felt needed to be inserted here. An EU group of experts carried out a meta-analysis of 176 worldwide studies that involved over 4 million patients which put the average level of side effects at 9%. Another UK trial involving 150,000 patients put the figure at 1%. The media amazingly used this last study to declare that statins were effectively "safe". This is the Telegraph headline: "Statins do not cause common aches and pains – those taking them are just getting old". Really? What about the incredible study involving 4 million patients that had nine times more side effects? These two studies with a nine-fold difference in outcomes really does question the integrity of so-called scientific research. The study that found 9% is also almost identical to the drug companies' 10% figure. Surprisingly, the researchers who carried out this study also admitted that around 50% of all patients who have been prescribed them either stop taking the statins, cut the dose or take them irregularly due to muscle pain and other side effects. But, of course, even these researchers then claimed that most of these side effects are not due to the statins. We have seen that around half of all medical research is fraudulent and in terms of statins, I know who I trust. And that is the patients.

Here are two final facts for you to ponder. In 2014 the UK medical guidelines issued by NICE were changed such that even low risk patients were to be prescribed statins. It was a meta-analysis by Professor Collins' team that led directly to this change. (It was later revealed that eight out of the twelve NICE panel members that recommended the change also had ties with statin manufacturers.) At that time, around 6 million people were taking statins. The new guidelines would have doubled this to 12 million. Remember, medical guidelines almost carry the force of law. Any doctor ignoring them can face serious charges. But guess what has happened? The current figure is around 7.5 million, meaning that only one-quarter of the expected uptake of statins has occurred. It would appear that most doctors are not pushing their use for low risk patients. Why? Doctors must clearly be unconvinced (and quite rightly) of the case for doing so. In fact, when the medical magazine Pulse interviewed GPs in confidence in 2014 (after the new statin guidelines for low risk people were published by NICE), more than half of them said they wouldn't follow the guidelines themselves or apply it to their families and friends. Such a significant "rebellion" had never happened before.

The second incredible fact is that the official promotion of statins in the UK Quality Outcomes Framework (QOF) has been "silently removed". The QOF, which was covered in Part 3, listed a range of drugs that doctors were paid to prescribe to mainly healthy older patients supposedly to prevent the incidence of diseases like heart attacks and strokes and the deaths resulting from them. Blood pressure drugs and statins were two of these key drugs. Of course, as we saw, the significant increase in these drug prescriptions (polypharmacy) had no beneficial effect at all. There was no reduction in overall deaths and the UK wasted £30 billion on the whole "experiment", as well as causing significant and serious side effects for the patients involved. Removing statins from the QOF clearly suggests that some key decision makers realised their benefits are almost non-existent but the fact this decision has never been made public shows they are not officially going to admit that anything was wrong. Despite all of this, 7.5 million UK patients are still being prescribed statins, gaining virtually no benefits and suffering a range of debilitating and longer term side effects.

This concludes the evidence on statins. Of course, the overwhelming body of medical experts would officially simply dismiss every single word. In fact, they are very much on the offensive. Take the alarming comment that says by "claiming that statins have high levels of side effects will put people off taking them and could cause unnecessary deaths for which you would be responsible." This was uttered by Professor Collins in a radio interview and directed at Dr Fiona Godlee, editor of the British Medical Journal, over their disagreement on the level of side effects from statins. This attack is all the more outrageous after what we have learnt about Professor Collins' admission that he had never even carried out any analysis of their side effects at that time.

Earlier I mentioned that the CTSU and Professor Collins had been handsomely remunerated by Big Pharma for all their efforts in promoting statins. But by how much? Well, we have seen that doctors can receive free continuing medical education at medical conferences which are organised and funded by Big Pharma, while many leading academics and key opinion leaders can expect to receive a minimum six-figure-level of remuneration for their "cooperation" with Big Pharma. But Professor Collins and his team are in a different league altogether. Their total funding up to 2014 was... cue drum roll... £268 million. We would never have known about this incredible sum had it not been for one investigative researcher, Dr Zoe Harcombe, who stumbled on the evidence almost by accident. She said of the glowing newspaper headlines that always greet Professor Collins' studies: "A more discerning headline, therefore might have been: Team paid £268 million by statin makers finds statins are miracle drugs with miraculously negligible side effects."

Professor Collins had never declared this funding, even though it is normal practice for researchers to declare any conflicts of interest. What has happened to this money? Has Professor Collins used it for the good of mankind by carrying out useful scientific research? Is it invested in off-shore pension funds or other personal investments? We will never know because that sort of information is completely inaccessible. The only thing we do know with certainty is that the £268 million was received by the CTSU. You can draw your own conclusions as to whether – to misquote a well-known saying – "money corrupts, and absolutely loads of money, corrupts absolutely." However, please remember the name Professor Sir Rory Collins. We will come across him again later in the section on Alzheimer's disease, and if you have been disturbed by his involvement in statins, you will be truly shocked by his work on Alzheimer's.

I want to round off this section with some speculation on what could happen next. We have already seen that some influential medical heavyweights, such as Sir Richard Thompson and the British Medical Journal, have been involved in acrimonious debates regarding statins. In addition, press coverage became more sceptical and numerous new studies are revealing previously "unknown" side effects. I asked whether this could only happen with the blessing of Big Pharma and posed the question: could this have anything to do with the fact that profits from statins have plunged by 90% now they are all off patent? The pharmaceutical industry certainly wants to make up for this lost profit stream somehow. So, what can they do? Well, it may not surprise you to learn that already a new generation of cholesterol lowering drugs are being promoted and used. These are called PCSK9 inhibitors. These drugs really do lower cholesterol, and then some more. They can reduce LDL levels by around 60%. What does it all mean and how will it play out? I must add that this next section is partly based on speculation because the whole process is still underway.

The future of statins and the "son" of statins

Statins now cost health authorities across the world about $20 per patient per year now that they are off patent, whereas previously they used to cost over $200. Big Pharma and their lucratively funded experts have done such a good job in selling these drugs and hyping up the benefits that they now have a major problem. How can they persuade health authorities to switch to a new and considerably more expensive drug when they have convinced everyone that statins are already "wonder drugs?" Some industry watchers anticipated that the Big Pharma game plan might be as follows. The only way of getting the new drugs accepted was somehow to discredit statins. This, of course, could not involve attacking the cholesterol theory itself, since the new drugs also worked by lowering cholesterol. The only way was to demonstrate that statins had more side effects than had previously been thought. But how do you do that without everyone looking completely incompetent? Well, eight years ago, thanks mainly to the efforts of Professor Collins, the medical guidelines issued by NICE were changed so that statin usage would nearly double. With millions more people taking them worldwide, it was thought that the drug industry might claim that side effects that previously "could not be detected" had "suddenly appeared". Statins could then be discredited because they were more dangerous than previously thought. The new PCSK9 drugs would be hailed as the perfect solution because they would be promoted as having "no side effects" (just as statins were when they were initially prescribed) and Big Pharma's lucrative profit stream would be re-established. Of course, the flaws in this plan are there for all to see. If you really can't detect side effects when around 200 million people are already taking statins, are we really to believe that they somehow miraculously appear when another 100 million start to take them? Of course, this is almost pure farce, but the statin advocates had dug themselves into such a deep hole that they were only left with desperate and feeble solutions.

What evidence was there to support this "supposed plan"? A significant number of trials looking specifically at side effects had been carried out and published in a relatively short space of time. These showed that statins increased the risk of developing type 2 diabetes, and other studies linked them to conditions like liver damage, fatigue, impaired cognitive function, memory loss, muscle problems and depression. From their initial use around 1990, however, Big Pharma had skilfully promoted statins both within medicine and via the media and press, and with almost 100% success it had deceptively engineered positive trials and successfully hidden virtually all contradictory evidence and side effects through its hired guns such as Professor Collins. Given that Big Pharma exerts such an iron grip, the side effect studies and the increasingly bad publicity could probably only be occurring with their blessing. Think back to the beta blocker scandal in 2014 that caused 800,000 deaths and the total media blackout that ensued. This censorship continues to be successfully maintained with almost 100% success even today.

It is impossible to say whether this plan was real, but it did have real credibility behind it. However, a new approach is now taking place. One problem apparently was that there has been much more resistance than was originally thought in the move to discredit statins. Maybe too many high-level medical reputations are at stake. But whatever the reasons were, the plan involved using the PCSK9 drugs to treat (at least initially) just one specific group of high-risk people. These have, what medicine calls, familial hypercholesterolemia (FH) which puts them at extra risk of heart disease. The price of the drugs is around $7,000 per patient per year, and in the UK, there are around 130,000 people with this condition which should produce sales of $1 billion a year. The equivalent figure for the US would be around $9 billion and, in the EU, $5 billion.

Initially, PCSK9 drugs were approved for use by drug regulators, even though there were no clinical trials proving they effectively treated heart disease. Their only claim to fame was that they lowered cholesterol – exactly the same way that statins were initially approved and promoted. Nevertheless, the drug's incredible 60% reduction in LDL cholesterol levels also prompted immense support from many senior experts who unequivocally supported their use, and claimed they would significantly reduce the rate of heart disease and deaths. So, initially, everything seemed to be going in favour of the PCSK9 drug companies and it appeared they would soon be making at least $15 billion annual profit. But this hasn't happened. In 2017 global sales were just $543 million and even in 2021 they had risen only to $1 billion.

So, why has this incredibly low uptake occurred? One of the initial problems was that when the first clinical trial (FOURIER) was finally carried out, the results were quite devastating for the PCSK9 proponents. Whilst the numbers of people having either a heart attack or needing a specialised revascularisation treatment were 15% lower in the drug group, the key outcome – the number of deaths – was lower in the placebo group. In fact, 251 deaths occurred in the drug group compared to 240 in the placebo group. If you ever wanted additional proof that low cholesterol doesn't really save lives, then the FOURIER results do just that, especially when you consider that cholesterol levels were lowered by 60% and yet the drug group still had more deaths.

However, there was also another major problem with the trial. It was designed to run for four years and yet it was stopped after just two. Trial protocols are supposed to be set in stone and it is unscientific to change them once the trial has started. So, why was it stopped? Well, the drug company Pfizer had also developed its own PCSK9 drug but actually stopped its trials because it was found that the drug's effectiveness in reducing cholesterol diminished significantly as the trial progressed. Is this what happened in the FOURIER trial? Independent researchers have asked to see the trial data, but the company is clearly not going to make it available, so we may never know. However, this is almost certainly the case and it means that if the trial had continued for the full four years, this problem would have been openly revealed. Drug regulators really should not allow this sort of thing to happen and should force the company to divulge all the information, but, of course, they don't.

Another reason why PCSK9 sales have not taken off is that they have to be given as injections which takes extra time for a medical profession already under extreme pressure, and the final reason is, of course, their significant price. Despite all of this, sales are still increasing and it is impossible to predict how this story will end but at present, statins simply remain the key cholesterol lowering drug.

It is clear that lowering cholesterol (even though it has no meaningful benefit and promotes devastating side effects) is going to continue. The key concern is that, if the new PCSK9 drugs continue to be more widely used, there is the frightening possibility that driving cholesterol down by 60% could lead to serious life-threatening diseases like cancer, liver disease, dementia and mental illness. We have seen evidence that people with the lowest cholesterol have the highest overall mortality, but there is no knowing what might happen when cholesterol is driven down to levels never before seen in the entire history of mankind. The sad reality is it may take years before increases in diseases like cancer and dementia start to be uncovered. Remember it took 27 years before it was proven that statins were causing type 2 diabetes. No rigorous trials on safety have been done, nor will they be done on any of the new cholesterol lowering drugs.

So, how can we sum up this section? The cholesterol theory of heart disease is, for most people, simply one of the greatest scams in history. Only a tiny percentage of high-risk men gain a minimal benefit. Not for the first time has medicine allowed itself to be deceived by clever pharmaceutical tricks and the money grabbing actions of a few high-profile medical experts. Most people have gained no benefit at all from statins, while significant side effects (many only recently discovered) are leading to new conditions and many serious outcomes. The saturated fat part of the lipid theory of heart disease also led to the official low fat dietary guidelines that are also causing devastating health outcomes for millions of people involving diseases like type 2 diabetes, strokes, cancer and many others. It is quite likely that the official low fat diet is causing even more devastating outcomes than even statins themselves. The whole thing is shocking and almost unbelievable.

I have inserted this paragraph on the very latest (Jan 2023) information on statins, because it is almost unbelievable. The UK's National Institute for Health and Care Excellence

(NICE) says the scope for using statins should be widened dramatically and they should be an option for those with even a small risk of cardiovascular disease. This means they could be offered to up to 15 million additional people between the ages of 25 and 84. Given all the evidence that has been explored in detail about the long list of statin side effects and their truly minimal benefits particularly for low risk people, this is an unbelievable decision. When NICE increased the number of people eligible for statins in 2014 from 6 million to 12 million, many GPs really did not promote them. I would hope that GPs will do the same thing this time and thus help protect their patients. In 2014 two-thirds of NICE's key decision makers had ties with the drug industry. I wonder how many had ties this time. This has not yet been exposed.

This section has perhaps already taken up too much space, but because the saturated fat and cholesterol theories have been at the very heart of medicine's approach to cardiovascular disease, I needed to provide a great deal of evidence and data if I was ever to have any chance of convincing you they are simply wrong. Before I move on to the lifestyle medicine approach to heart disease, I just want to briefly mention blood pressure lowering drugs which, of course, are also used to treat heart disease.

Blood pressure drugs are now widely prescribed, but when they were initially developed in the 1960s, they were given only to people with very high blood pressure. The US Veterans study in 1967, which involved 140 people with severe hypertension (over 190/115) were treated with the new drugs. The trial demonstrated an incredible life-saving benefit. After 18 months, 27 out of 70 in the placebo group had suffered serious heart disease outcomes or deaths, while for those in the drug group it was just one. The trial was stopped at this point because the outcomes were so significant, and those in the placebo group were then also given the drugs. It is certain that without the drugs, the serious outcomes and deaths would have risen even more with some experts predicting that almost 100% of the patients would develop them over a ten-year period. For those people with severe hypertension, this was probably the most effective life-saving drug treatment ever invented.

But then, 18 years later, a new trial was carried out to determine what happened when people with lower blood pressure were given the drugs. The MRC trial involved people with blood pressures within the range 140/90 and 180/110. We have already seen that when a drug or treatment works really well, only a small number of people are needed for trials to provide robust scientific proof. In the US Veterans study only 140 people were required to reveal the significant benefits. However, the MRC trial had to recruit 17,000 patients. Even then, in terms of the numbers of heart attacks there was no significant difference between the drug and placebo groups, while for strokes, the drug reduced the incidence, but only by 1.2%. However, the key overall mortality was almost exactly the same in both groups.

Then, in 2012, a review of several clinical trials looking at benefits for patients with blood pressures between 140/90 and 160/100 in an editorial of the BMJ concluded there were no benefits at all for heart disease, stroke and overall mortality. Despite all of this evidence, the prescribing of blood pressure lowering drugs has simply escalated. Most countries currently have blood pressure limits of 140/90 and the drugs can be prescribed to anyone above this level. Even more incredible is that in the US the figure has already been lowered again to 130/85. Yet again, this is all part of the pharmaceutical industry's plan to simply increase profits.

In summary, blood pressure lowering drugs have miraculous benefits for those people with severe hypertension. There are, however, no overall mortality benefits for anyone with lower blood pressure, but if you look at the drug leaflets you will see an incredible list of side effects.

Heart disease – the lifestyle approach

Lifestyle medicine considers most heart disease to be preventable. We have examined the logic and proof for this in great detail. So, what are the key things we can do to lower our heart disease risk to very low levels? The lifestyle approach is simple and logical, and it has near universal benefit for most other diseases. In other words, there isn't one lifestyle and diet that benefits heart disease and a completely different one if you want to prevent cancer or diabetes. There are usually some specific extra things you can do for individual diseases, but the lifestyle that promotes good overall health also does the job of minimising the risk of developing nearly all chronic diseases. If you think about it, this makes simple evolutionary sense. Before I start, I should add that smoking, obesity and being seriously underweight are high risk factors for virtually every disease. They are universally bad for our health and I won't necessarily keep referring to them when looking at each individual disease. So, let's revisit briefly the seven key factors which have already been examined in some detail and which all play a part in preventing heart disease.

Emotional health and stress. Emotional health is crucial to our overall health and this applies particularly to heart disease. The evidence is very strong that our emotional health significantly affects heart disease risk. Very disturbed and damaged emotions and stress can increase someone's risk by about 50%. Conversely, positive emotions can completely reverse this risk. High stress and damaging emotions like anger and fear can also cause significant increases in blood pressure and pulse rates.

Exercise. We have seen, courtesy of the NHS website, that exercise can reduce heart disease risk by up to 35%.

Diet. The food we eat is vitally important and almost every expert would say a good diet should be our number one priority for heart disease (and indeed for all other diseases). There are two key parts: eating healthy natural foods, but also significantly reducing or eliminating unhealthy and even dangerous processed foods. There is a key phrase in lifestyle medicine: "you can't outrun a bad diet", meaning that whilst exercise really is one of the vital factors for health, it cannot counteract a really poor diet.

Overall, a low carb, low GL diet is one of the keys for a healthy heart. Certain foods can also provide specific benefits, and research has been done on many of them and on specific food groups. In addition, there are many long-term epidemiological studies that can give strong indications of the benefits and harms of certain foods. Two examples provide evidence of how vital our food really is for our health. We have already seen that just eating extra virgin olive oil, nuts and fish oils daily can cut our risk of heart disease by 30%. This is supported by compelling evidence from three high-quality randomised clinical trials. The World Health Organization also estimates that a simple dietary intervention such as eating more fruit and vegetables and reducing trans-fats could decrease the risk of heart disease by around 20%.

Here is just a small selection of other really healthy foods that help maintain a healthy heart: seeds, beans, oats, beetroot, lentils, fish, quinoa, mushrooms, onions, garlic, eggs, herbs, spices and peppers. A randomised controlled trial showed the amazing result that flaxseed taken for six months by people aged between 70 and 88 reduced blood pressure by around ten points and reduced the rate of strokes and heart attacks by 50%. A meta-analysis of studies involving dark chocolate showed a 20% reduction in heart attacks if taken most days over a five-year period. A good diet is the most important thing we can do for our cardiovascular system and our overall health.

Of course, the flip side of a healthy diet is an unhealthy diet. This consists of foods that actually do harm to the body and the cardiovascular system and here are just a few: sugar, high fructose corn syrup, white bread, cake, fast food and highly processed food of all kinds, trans-fats and hydrogenated vegetable oils. Highly processed foods deserve a special mention because they invariably contain hidden sugars and hidden trans-fats, as well as thousands of chemicals, colourings, emulsifiers and preservatives (most are undeclared). The extensive processing also destroys many of the beneficial natural elements in the food as well as many of the key vitamins and minerals. A devastating fact is that 80% of all processed foods have added sugar.

Vitamins and minerals. Vitamins, minerals and other natural compounds are essential for life, but as we have seen their availability in the food we eat has been in continuous decline for nearly a century. In terms of heart health, some of the key ones are: magnesium, zinc, selenium, B vitamins like folate, B12 and B6 which reduce homocysteine which is linked to heart disease and strokes, and vitamins A, C, D and E. Another key supplement is coenzyme Q10 (particular a very absorbable form called ubiquinol). A Swedish trial found that those elderly patients given CoQ10 and selenium supplements for five years reduced the death rate from cardiovascular disease by 50%. A recent US study showed that magnesium supplements reduced the rate of coronary disease by 5.3% and vitamin K2 by 15.7%.

Our gut biome. Our friendly bacteria don't just help with the obvious digestion and immune responses. They also help to synthesise vitamins which are essential for overall health and heart disease as well as aiding their absorption. They also can improve our emotional health which is an important factor in heart disease. So, whilst the microbiome may not have an obvious direct effect, indirectly it is still important.

Chemical exposure. Smoking is a major risk factor for heart disease. The reason for this is that the chemicals contained in the smoke put a strain on the heart by making it work faster and they also can damage the lining of the arteries. But as we have seen, we are exposed to around 100,000 other chemicals – very few of which have ever been tested for their safety. These come from the air we breathe, the water we drink, the food we eat, and the things we put on our skin. We are exposed to chemicals that are just as dangerous as cigarette smoke without even realising it. Minimising this exposure and using methods to reduce the chemicals we can't avoid is important not just for heart disease, but for most other disease.

Sleep. Many studies have linked poor sleep to an increased risk of heart disease, so good sleep really is another important factor in preventing it.

All the evidence demonstrates it is possible to significantly reduce our risk of heart disease and although I haven't specifically mentioned strokes, these too can see their risk reduced by exactly the same interventions. These seven key factors are also universally relevant as you will see in all the other diseases still to be examined. Of course, all the other things that impact our health, like having healthy teeth and gums and keeping active, are also still important.

Here is one final fact. You can only reduce your risk of developing heart (or any other) disease by up to 100% and if it was possible to reach this you would have zero possibility of developing the disease. But if we simply add up all the maximum risk reduction percentages for exercise, emotional health and diet, it is possible to reach a figure above 100%, which is not possible. The explanation works like this. Imagine you exercise vigorously and also eat nuts or oily fish. The risk reduction for each is 35% and 30% respectively, but you will not then see a 65% reduction in your overall risk of heart disease. You might, and this can only be a guess because no one has ever done it, see a 50% reduction. If you added a third factor, like truly positive emotions at 50%, the individual reductions add up to 115%, but you might only see a 70% overall reduction in heart disease risk. The reason for this is that some of the individual benefits can overlap the same biological pathways and you can't get the same benefit twice. But, as we do more healthier things, we can continue to reduce our risk of heart disease, and continue to approach the 100% rate of prevention.

Further recommended reading:

- *Say No to Heart Disease* by Patrick Holford

Type 2 diabetes

Sixty years ago, the number of cases in the UK was around 200,000; now it is over 4 million, and by 2035 it is projected to reach 6 million. Approximately 1 in 8 people between 20 and 80 years of age have their deaths attributed to diabetes and its life-threatening side effects. These include heart disease, amputations, blindness, strokes, breast and colon cancers, kidney failure and liver damage. Diabetes reduces average life expectancy by over ten years, and is the leading cause of blindness in people of working age and the single greatest cause (44%) of kidney failure. There are a staggering 5,000 hospitalisations each day in the UK. The World Health Organization puts the worldwide number of cases at 420 million, rising to over 600 million by 2035. The disease used to affect only people over about 60, but now even young children are developing it. A recent study showed that for those under the age of 20, the incidence rose by 53% in just 13 years.

Type 2 diabetes – the medical approach

For decades, the medical approach to type 2 diabetes has been simple and straightforward. By carrying out random blood sugar tests at periodic intervals on those people they think are most at risk, they can eventually find out which of them have developed the disease. In other words, doctors wait until patients develop diabetes or pre-diabetes before taking any action. These patients are then given diabetes drugs. Medicine has consistently maintained that diabetes can never be reversed, so even though they now give advice on diet and exercise once it has been diagnosed, by then it is already too late to offer disease prevention. What is truly bizarre is that if there is one quintessential lifestyle disease, it is type 2 diabetes. Medicine accepts that it is caused by lifestyle factors, but there has never been any attempt to prevent it. Some people have described this situation as wanton neglect and even criminal behaviour. Surely the Hippocratic oath should drive the whole of medicine to explain how the right diet, exercise and other key factors would halt most of this epidemic in its tracks. But this is not happening, so what's the problem? Well, whilst medicine would deny it, the low fat diet recommended by medicine and governments (which, by definition, necessitates a high carb diet) is quite simply the key cause of type 2 diabetes. This is the same low fat diet that – as we have seen in detail – has now been totally discredited by most truly independent scientists.

The power of Big Pharma and Big Food is, as always, never far away, and their "dark hand" is also implicated in the diabetes epidemic. Big Pharma does not want the low fat diet to die, because it underpins the lipid theory of heart disease. This in turn supports the statin industry which has produced $1 trillion in sales, and new generations of cholesterol drugs are also now being used. Nothing will be allowed to derail this profit bonanza. Big Food also makes billions of dollars from low fat foods, and the "medical experts" who developed and advocate the low fat diet are clearly not prepared to accept they were wrong and see their reputations destroyed.

So, if people follow only conventional medical practice, then by 2035, 6 million people in the UK will have type 2 diabetes. The total cost to the economy will then be around £40 billion per year with the NHS alone spending between £15 billion and £20 billion just to treat its symptoms. Those people with the disease will see their risk of heart disease increase by around 300%, 15,000 will have limbs amputated every year and many thousands will develop cancer and strokes, lose their eyesight, develop kidney and liver diseases and have their lives shortened by an average of ten years. The diabetes epidemic will also continue to unfold around the world and countless millions of lives will be shortened and devastated. This is one of the greatest preventable tragedies in the history of mankind.

However, I do need to explain that in 2017 the DIRECT trial was carried out. This was an official medical trial and its aim was to reverse diabetes using severe calorie restrictions to reduce weight and it was based on conventional dietary recommendations. The main treatment involved a patented liquidised food of just 820 calories per day that was used for three to five months and then slowly increased depending on how well it worked. Other treatments were also added as necessary. The trial really did achieve remission of diabetes in around half of its patients after 12 months and has since gained official medical endorsement. However, there are several reasons why this treatment will never be a significant solution to curing diabetes. How many people will be prepared to adopt a liquid diet and give up the taste and wonderful sensation of eating normal foods? Severe calorie restriction has significant side effects and can also lead to serious long-term outcomes as will be explained in the section on obesity. The drug orlistat, which has many serious side effects, is part of the treatment if the required weight loss is not achieved. Also, rest assured that the pharmaceutical companies making diabetes drugs will definitely not allow this treatment to decimate what is the third leading drug type with current annual worldwide sales of $49 billion which are projected to increase to $78 billion by 2026. Only cancer and immunology drugs have greater sales. The reality is that four years after the main trial was published, just 5,000 people in England are now, in 2021, just being enrolled to start a treatment. But most importantly of all, there is a much more effective natural treatment which is more palatable, has no side effects and has many additional benefits for other key diseases. This will be explained in detail in the next section and, more importantly, even the mighty drug industry can't stop individuals from choosing to use it and cure their diabetes.

It is essential to also examine just how effective diabetes drugs are, and what side effects they cause. Diabetes drugs do reduce blood sugar, but the reductions are relatively small. Many patients (even those given up to three different drugs) do not see their blood sugar fall below the level of 6.5 which defines type 2 diabetes. The best drug, metformin, would typically reduce the level by just over one point from say 8.5 to 7.4. The other problem is that, over time, the drugs lose their effectiveness. After a few years, blood sugar levels will start to rise again. Doctors then have to increase drug doses and keep doing so. At some point they will need to add a second and even a third drug, but eventually even these can stop working effectively. The other problem is the drugs themselves have severe side effects. Metformin, for example, which is the most prescribed diabetes drug, can cause severe bowel problems like diarrhoea and flatulence together with nausea and vomiting. Researchers at the University of Surrey discovered that these conditions led around a third of patients to stop taking the drug, often without telling their doctors. Metformin can also reduce the levels of the essential vitamin B12, and anyone taking the drug really should consider taking a B12 supplement. Other drugs like gliclazide and pioglitazone cause sudden drops in blood sugar that can cause fainting and dizziness as well as eye sight problems and bone pain, and around 20% of patients also stop taking them because of these side effects. These drugs are also known to cause significant weight gain.

Finally, there is one more important fact. Over recent years, other prescription drugs have also been proven to be causing diabetes, and these are some of the drugs that are linked to it: beta blockers. diuretics, antidepressants, antipsychotics and statins. Several recent studies have shown, for example, that statins can cause diabetes. The three most referenced studies show that the drugs increased the risk by 36%, 46%, and 28%, which gives an overall average of 37%, while a very recent study showed an increased risk of 100%. It is impossible to accurately calculate how many diabetes cases have been caused by statins over the last 30 years of use, but given the millions of people who have taken them in the UK alone, it could be in the hundreds of thousands. A devastating outcome for just one drug, especially one that has such minimal benefits. Although this has to be speculation, it is not unrealistic to imagine that statins and the other listed prescription drugs could be causing at least 10% of all cases of type 2 diabetes.

The first statin drug was prescribed in 1987, and it is also an incredible fact that it was only in 2014 (27 years later) that tangible evidence started to emerge that led drug regulators to acknowledge this link with diabetes. I have explored numerous, almost unbelievable, examples of how long it can take for serious drug side effects to emerge. At 27 years, statins are perhaps in the "top ten" and once again this shows that the so-called gold standard of clinical trials simply can't be trusted. The world only finds out what serious damage drugs can cause and how many lives they destroy years, and even decades, later when real-world data starts to emerge.

Type 2 diabetes – the lifestyle medicine approach

The lifestyle approach is simple. The disease really can be prevented because its main cause is a poor diet, compounded by a lack of exercise. One of the main causes of diabetes is the poor dietary advice given by medicine and governments. So, why is this official diet so unhealthy? There are three main food groups: fats, proteins and carbohydrates. When dietary guidelines were issued in the 1980s, they recommended a significant decrease in saturated fat. But people have to eat something, so the reduction in fat had to be compensated by an increase in carbohydrates. It is the double whammy of a reduction in healthy fats, combined with the commensurate increase in unhealthy carbohydrates that is one of the key factors causing the current epidemic of chronic diseases. Diabetes is the ultimate and quintessential example of this dietary disaster.

The science is simple. When we eat a food like sugar or a refined carbohydrate like white bread, our blood glucose spikes sharply and quickly. High blood sugar is dangerous and so the body seeks to regulate blood glucose levels by producing insulin. The insulin converts the glucose into fat which is deposited throughout the body and blood glucose levels then return to normal before they can cause serious damage. This is the natural process that evolution has given us to avoid harm to the body. What is new is the profound change in the types of food that are now available. By evolutionary standards, sugar is new, as are high fructose corn syrup, processed white flour and other grains, breakfast cereals containing both sugar and processed grains, and all manner of confectionary and sweets. We were not programmed to deal with what, in evolutionary terms, was a sudden massive onslaught of high glycaemic foods that the body had never encountered over the previous 7 million years. (High glycaemic foods are those that cause rapid high spikes in blood sugar.)

High glycaemic foods were already being consumed in the 1970s, of course, and were already causing increases in diabetes, but their consumption was given a huge boost by the new dietary guidelines which were introduced in the 1980s. When the body's self-regulating mechanism for blood sugar control is repeatedly overloaded with constant high glucose spikes, it can eventually be overwhelmed. Either the body simply can't produce enough insulin or the insulin becomes less effective. The end result is the same: type 2 diabetes. This occurs when blood sugar remains constantly high. Of course, the flip side to all of this is that fats – at least the healthy ones – improve our health. However, the dietary guidelines recommended not just a reduction in fat consumption, but also recommended replacing natural healthy saturated fats, like butter and animal fats, with industrially manufactured fats like margarine and hydrogenated vegetable oils. These industrial fats contain high levels of omega 6 fats which have already been examined, as well as trans-fats, which even medicine now agrees are highly dangerous.

The solution to the diabetes epidemic is clear. It requires a change of diet that significantly reduces carbohydrates and high glycaemic foods, as well as increasing beneficial natural fats while reducing dangerous industrially manufactured fats and trans-fats. Restricting carbohydrates actually forces the body to use its stored fats for energy. Exercise is also a necessary and important part of the solution. Lifestyle medicine has been helping people to reverse their diabetes for decades as well as trying to get this message out to as many people as possible. Predictably, it has faced intense opposition from mainstream medicine which continues even today. This is contemptible.

Dietary interventions work. There are many case histories of complete reversal of diabetes. Medicine as usual responds with its usual get out of jail card: "It hasn't been proven by clinical trials." But this simply won't wash. Medicine has maintained for decades that diabetes cannot be cured or reversed, so if patients do indeed see their symptoms completely reversed this is sufficient proof that dietary intervention works, particularly when there are so many verifiable case studies. Clinical trials are not necessary to prove this, just as they weren't necessary to prove that penicillin worked.

Channel 4's *The Food Hospital* and BBC's *Doctor in the House* series have both included case studies of how lifestyle changes can reverse even years of diabetes. Dr Rangan Chatterjee, an Oldham GP who practises lifestyle solutions, achieved spectacular results with Sandeep Mistry who had had diabetes for over ten years. Despite taking three separate diabetes drugs, his blood sugar was still dangerously high at 9 and he had already developed nerve damage which meant he could have faced amputation at some future point. Medicine had failed Sandeep, but Dr Chatterjee brought his blood sugar down to 7 after just a few weeks. This result is all the more impressive because he got Sandeep to stop taking two of the drugs because they were implicated in his weight gain. Dr Chatterjee's methods used just dietary change and exercise. This sort of incredible success has been repeated in many thousands of people around the world by nutritionists and doctors like Dr Chatterjee who practise lifestyle medicine solutions. Even more tangible evidence comes from the Southport surgery of Dr David Unwin which has already been outlined. The surgery has reversed diabetes in half of its patients, and significantly reduced blood sugar levels in the others. It is saving £50,000 on diabetes drugs alone each year, and eliminating or significantly reducing its patients' risk of developing serious diabetic complications.

Then there is the diabetes organisation called "Diabetes.co.uk". This is different from Diabetes UK, which is the official diabetes charity that simply promotes the official medical position, and has never promoted a low carb diet. Diabetes.co.uk, on the other hand, promotes low carb and an incredible 100,000 people with diabetes have been adopting its dietary advice, and most of them have seen significant reductions in blood sugar and many have achieved complete remission. They have also achieved an average reduction in weight of 8kg.

Returning to Dr Unwin – a remarkable development has occurred in the last two years. Dr Unwin first went on a low carb diet himself in 2012, and then began using it for his diabetes patients. When they started to achieve incredible outcomes, he began trying to promote it to other doctors and medical organisations. Even though he achieved much recognition from the Royal College of General Practitioners, as well as many individual medical colleagues and the All-Party Parliamentary Group on diabetes, little progress was made in actually implementing his dietary protocol other than in his own surgery. Then, early in 2020, over 1,000 GPs signed up to take the e-learning course he had designed which was endorsed by the Royal College, and by mid-2021, nearly 3,500 doctors were now prescribing the low carb diet for their patients. This means that 250,000 diabetes patients are now benefiting and around half will be achieving remission of the disease.

Dr Ruth Tapsell from Devon recently shared the outcomes of her diabetes patients with the Daily Mail. For years she had been troubled that her diabetes patients made virtually no progress despite the drugs and dietary advice they were given: "If anything, they put on more weight, were hungrier and needed more medication to control their condition. I was also becoming increasingly concerned about the number of drugs we were prescribing, the cost to the NHS and the side effects or potential complications the medications can cause later in life – including weight gain. None of it made sense."

All that changed when she learnt about Dr Unwin's protocol and her surgery adopted it: "Like many GPs we'd previously been offering standard NHS diet advice for diabetics – to lose weight by eating smaller portions and following a low fat diet that was high in carbs such as pasta and rice. And it wasn't working." After adopting the low carb diet, however, patient outcomes have been transformed. A survey of the 161 diabetes patients at her surgery showed that 32% had already reversed their condition and most had reduced their blood sugar and medication. Other doctors and diabetes nurses have achieved even more impressive results, with some surgeries achieving up to 65% complete remission.

Dr Vipan Bhardwaj who runs a Wokingham surgery was another medical pioneer of the low carb diet. In 2016 he carried out an initial study on 40 of his patients and two-thirds achieved complete remission as well as significant weight loss. The surgery has continued this success for its current diabetes patients, but Dr Bhardwaj has also examined the effects that the low carb diet is having on other conditions. He found that the patients also see reductions in blood pressure and some have even been able to stop using their blood pressure drugs. He has also seen amazing results of fatty liver disease being reversed in weeks by the diet, and these were subsequently confirmed by ultrasound scans. Dr Bhardwaj explained that the most rewarding aspect for doctors is to see how this approach transforms the lives of patients, with so many also able to reduce their medication or go drug free.

Dr Tapsell also confirms that her patients "have been evangelistic about their results, but this is mixed with frustration that they didn't know about it sooner and the years that were wasted with poor advice". (This is an amazing patient critique of the official NHS treatments that have led to years of unnecessary ill health.)

The fact that all these doctors are ignoring the conventional and disastrous medical guidelines and helping their patients overcome a serious disease is very encouraging. However, there are around 54,000 GPs in the UK, but only 3,500 of them are helping diabetic patients with the low carb diet. This means only 6% of patients are receiving this life-changing dietary treatment. It is a sad fact that the official medical position remains unchanged (despite all the evidence) and most doctors simply follow the official low fat guidelines which simply don't work and are in fact one of the main causes of diabetes. Medical students are not being taught about the low carb diet, and unless many more doctors decide to rebel against their official mandatory guidelines, then little more progress will be made. What is certain is that the pharmaceutical industry will be using all its power to try to stop more doctors adopting the low carb diet. The reason is obvious. Annual worldwide diabetes drug sales now stand at $70 billion and by 2028 this will increase to $100 billion. The industry could see its profits savaged and there is no telling how damaging this could turn out to be. If every doctor in the UK prescribed the diet, then three of the key factors (blood sugar, blood pressure and obesity), which are major causes of many chronic diseases, would also be significantly reduced. The reduction in diabetes drugs alone would result in a fall in annual industry sales of at least £800 million just in the UK. On a worldwide basis the figure could be as much as $50 billion. The industry would also see reductions in blood pressure and other drug sales. The other key fact is that the typical weight loss for the patients using the Dr Unwin diet is around 8kg, and this would also result in a reduction in other serious diseases like heart disease, strokes and major cancers, which would further reduce drug sales. The drug industry only cares about profit, so they will do everything they can to discredit and minimise the use of low carb diets regardless of their potential to prevent disease and human suffering. Key medical and academic decision makers and organisations like Diabetes UK who have promoted the low fat diet for decades will also be reluctant to endorse the low carb diet and see their reputations destroyed.

It would be wonderful if GPs could eventually force medicine's elite to change their disastrous entrenched medical dogma on diabetes, but only time will tell. I have given copious evidence on what can happen to doctors who go against official medical policy, ranging from simply telling them to stop, to eventually losing their medical licences. However, with 3,500 GPs now using the diet, it would be impossible to sack them all without destroying local medical services and the outrage that would then ensue. In this situation it is impossible to predict what will happen, but if, in a year or two, you have heard nothing more about it, then you will know that the drug industry has "won" (yet again), and hundreds of millions of lives will carry on being destroyed.

There is another amazing fact. Whilst I respect and admire Dr Unwin and the GPs who are using the low carb diet to treat their patients, this has only been taking place at a significant level over the last two years. Yet the low carb diet was actually developed more than half a century ago, and courageous doctors and lifestyle medicine advocates have been using it ever since to help patients reverse and even prevent diseases like diabetes. This despite the fact they were ridiculed and attacked by medicine. All this was happening 50 years before Dr Unwin even started using it. Dr Robert C. Atkins, author of the *Dr Atkins' Diet Revolution* in 1972, was one of the most famous early pioneers. He wrote 17 books relating to the "Atkins diet" which was based on low carb protocols.

So, please, never forget John Hughlings Jackson's quote of, "It takes 50 years to get a wrong idea out of medicine. And 100 years to get a right one into medicine." When you first read it, I would guess you probably thought it was ridiculous. But I have given many devastating factual examples to confirm it (with even more to come) and the low carb diet is just one more. The world should pray that it will not take another 50 years before medicine officially accepts and uses the low carb diet, otherwise the level of preventable human suffering and deaths will be incalculable. If I was ever able to meet key medical decision makers, I would simply ask them how they can sleep at night when so many lives are being destroyed and lost, and they are simply refusing to accept the real-world evidence from their own doctors.

Another important fact is that these original low carb diets also use vitamin and mineral supplements as well as exercise and other lifestyle changes. These are vitally important, because the GPs using Dr Unwin's protocol use only dietary changes, and this is the key reason why only about half of patients see a complete reversal of diabetes. Utilising all these additional factors can significantly increase the reversal rate, and a figure of over 90% really does then become possible. Chromium supplements are one of the vital minerals that help control blood sugar. In a 2014 meta-analysis of 25 clinical trials, the researchers concluded that chromium not only significantly improved blood sugar but also reduced triglycerides and had no side effects at the doses used. Many detailed books have been written about diabetes and anyone wanting to reverse or prevent it would be well advised to read one. However, choosing the right one can be difficult because some still promote the official and disastrous low fat diet. *Say No to Diabetes* by Patrick Holford is one of the key books I would recommend for anyone wishing to prevent or reverse the disease. It contains detailed information on the best foods to eat and those to avoid and provides detailed information on vitamins, minerals and other supplements. (Some of the key ones in addition to chromium are magnesium, vitamins C and D, and cinnamon). There are also chapters on sleep, stress and exercise which all play a part in diabetes.

It is vitally important to repeat yet again that GPs and doctors are not responsible for this diabetes epidemic, which by 2035 will affect over 600 million people. The culprits are the relatively small number of top medical "experts" who define what medical students and doctors are taught and the guidelines they must follow when treating any disease. And, whist these experts would deny it, they in turn are controlled (and most of them are highly remunerated) by the drug industry which needs a world full of sick people, without whom its sales would plummet to almost nothing. Of course, the final key fact – and perhaps the most important fact of all – is that if you live a healthy lifestyle and eat a healthy diet, you are very unlikely to develop type 2 diabetes in the first place.

Obesity

Anyone over the age of 60 will be able to remember their school days, when they were surrounded by thin, mostly healthy children. At the age of 11, in a school of 600, I vividly remember that there were only two children who would be described today as obese, and the panoramic school photographs confirm this memory. (I should add that the average official figure for that time was around 1 in a 100 – or 6 in a school of 600, so maybe my school was just lucky). Today, however, in a similar school, 120 children would be obese and another 85 would be overweight. As far as adults are concerned, 28% are obese and 36% are overweight, meaning that a disturbing 64% of the population do not have a healthy weight.

Obesity – the medical approach

This is what the NHS says about obesity: "Obesity is generally caused by eating too much and moving too little. If you consume high amounts of energy, particularly fat and sugars, but do not burn off the energy through exercise and physical activity, much of the surplus energy will be stored by the body as fat."

Medicine believes, quite simply, that too many calories are the cause of obesity, although physical activity can help to offset it. The NHS lists a range of foods you should eat and those you should restrict, but the critical message is to minimise saturated fats and eat significant levels of carbohydrates. Medicine lists just one other thing that can cause weight gain (and eventually obesity), and this involves drugs for epilepsy and diabetes as well as steroids and antidepressants. The NHS recommends that men wanting to lose weight should consume no more than 1,900 calories per day and women no more than 1,400 calories. The aim should be to lose up to 1kg per week. They may recommend very low 800 calorie diets in certain specific cases, although these need to be carefully monitored because of the serious risks involved in very low food consumption.

Medicine also has two other main treatments for obesity, and these are bariatric surgery and the drug orlistat. Bariatric surgery is normally only used for certain people with a

BMI of over 40 for whom all other non-surgical procedures have failed. The side effects can be severe and include death for 1 in 100 people. Orlistat is normally used only for people with a BMI of 30 and above, but its weight loss benefits are minimal. After two or three years the average weight loss is 5kg, but even this only happens if food is also significantly restricted. It certainly cannot cure obesity. It also has a long list of severe bowel-related side effects as well as conditions like liver disease and kidney stones. When the drug started to be prescribed in the US, the manufacturer GlaxoSmithKline even said that users should "wear dark trousers and/or carry a change of clothes just in case they experienced the embarrassment of pooping their pants". I kid you not.

Nearly every other weight loss drug that has ever been approved and used has subsequently been taken off the market because of serious side effects. Amphetamines were the first weight loss drug, but were eventually withdrawn because they became addictive with harmful side effects. In the 1990s, Meridia and fen-phen were banned due to increased risks of serious heart disease. Fen-phen, almost unbelievably, caused around one-third of patients to develop heart valve defects and the drug firms had to pay out $13 billion in compensation. Another drug called Belviq was also withdrawn in 2020 because of cancer concerns. Drugs for weight loss have been one of the most dangerous and least effective types ever made over the last 100 years. Despite all of this, there is now more research taking place into the "next generation" of these drugs. The drug Wegovy produced by Novo Nordisk is already being used in the US and Denmark and is likely to be approved for the UK and EU in 2023. It is claimed to reduce weight by 15% but still has significant side effects, and those who have to stop taking it put their weight back on. Several other pharmaceutical companies like Pfizer and AstraZeneca are also developing their own similar drugs.

Here is a final key fact. In 2021 weight reducing drugs had worldwide sales of $2.4 billion. What do you think the projected sales are for 2030? An incredible $54 billion. You can bet with certainty that Big Pharma will fight like hell to ensure they are not taken off the market no matter how dangerous they are found to be.

There is one crucial and understandable fact regarding obesity. Most obese people really do, desperately, want to reduce their weight to normal levels and, in 1991, the University of Florida carried out a study by asking obese people how far they would be prepared to go to achieve a normal weight. They were asked whether they would rather be morbidly obese for life, or have a normal weight but have to suffer from one of the following serious condition: being deaf, having bad acne, having heart disease, being unable to read, having diabetes, being blind, or having one leg amputated. Every single person said they would be prepared to have any of the first five conditions, and over 90% said they would even be prepared to be blind or have a leg amputated if it meant that they really could maintain a normal weight for the rest of their lives. This study devastatingly encapsulates obese people's sheer desperation. Meanwhile, medicine and governments around the world have been promoting excess calories as the cause of weight gain and obesity for many decades. Most obese people, as we have just seen, would do almost anything to achieve a normal weight, and they really have meticulously tried the official calorie restricted diet. There is just one problem. It simply doesn't work in the long term. No country has ever succeeded in reducing obesity levels. In fact, the number of obese people worldwide simply continues to increase each year. So, something is devastatingly wrong.

So, what happens when people go on a low calorie diet like the one recommended by the NHS? Initially, nearly everyone loses weight and this can continue for several months, although the rate of decline also starts to fall over this period. After six months or so, the weight loss simply stops and then actually starts to increase again. During this period, people also report unpleasant side effects like feeling miserable, feeling cold and always feeling desperately hungry. Whilst some people can achieve significant initial weight loss, the overall average after six months is 7kg, but this then reduces back to just 4.5kg. Given that an average obese person would need to lose around 30kg in weight overall to reach a healthy BMI of 25, it is little surprise that most people eventually just give up with their low calorie diets especially when they realise its effect is minimal, that they are still obese, and have to face all the difficult side effects. When they go back to a "normal" diet, their weight increases to at least its original level but in many cases, it ends up even higher. This in turn can lead people to try to lose weight for a second or third time, and even more. Similar outcomes then reoccur, but the weight loss can become even more difficult to achieve and then when it fails again, and people revert back to a normal diet, their weight may go up even more. This type of yo-yo dieting is one of the worst things people can do for their overall health and can lead to hypertension, insulin resistance and dyslipidaemia resulting in increased mortality risk and, worse, cardiovascular outcomes.

So, why does the official low calorie diet not work other than in the short term? Let's first consider our 7 million years of evolution. Hunter-gatherers would normally eat a healthy varied diet but at times they could also face a lack of food from things like local droughts or having to move long distances through barren areas because of seasonal changes. In such circumstances, the body initially works as normal, and uses stored body fat as its source of energy. If the lack of food continues, however, and people lose more weight and their energy stores continue to diminish, the body will eventually respond by slowing down many of its key functions, thus reducing the overall energy needed, and helping to reduce the increasing risk of serious organ malfunction and even death that would eventually occur. Here are just a few examples of how the body can be "forced" to save energy in such circumstances. Bowel movements reduce to allow every single piece of food to be absorbed. For women, their periods stop since this is a "non-essential" bodily function. The skeletal repair system can also be compromised which could result in longer term bone density problems, as could the circulatory system which could lead to feeling constantly cold. The nervous system, endocrine system and other body systems would also slow down with other potential long-term problems and consequences.

When people use a low calorie diet to lose weight, this also forces the body to react in exactly the same way and eventually it slows down many key functions. The diet invariably fails and when they try it a second and third time, the body tries to minimise the damage by reducing bodily functions at even earlier times. This makes weight loss even more difficult unless food consumption continues to be drastically reduced which could lead to even more serious outcomes. The reality is simple: calorie-controlled weight loss does not work for most obese people except for a relatively short initial period. It simply does not cure obesity and several dietary studies have also confirmed this. One study in the US showed that between 1980 and 1990, Americans ate 4% fewer calories and 11% less fat than in the previous decade, yet obesity increased by a staggering 31%.

As well as having a devastating effect on the lives of those affected, obesity imposes a major financial cost for society as a whole and especially for the NHS. But the real tragedy is many of those who analyse and debate what should be done about it, just blame the people with obesity for "simply eating too much". Here is a short extract from a financial magazine article expressing the view of some of them about what policy makers should be doing about obesity: "Nothing, argue some; obese people should be allowed to get on with it. The argument is that, although this may be the biggest drain on the NHS while alive, the obese tend to die young and (arguably) cost less overall."

Michael Buerk the TV broadcaster has also said that the obese should be allowed to die an early death in order to save the NHS money. In the Radio Times he said, "The obese will die a decade earlier than the rest of us. See it as a selfless sacrifice in the fight against demographic imbalance, overpopulation and climate change." These are shocking and sad views and I have seen a number of other very similar ones. Essentially, they are saying that obese people have only themselves to blame, and they should be allowed to die young and save the country and the NHS money overall. Of course, medicine and governments would not dare endorse these very sad views, but after decades of incessant failure it is almost unbelievable that they seem impervious to the fact that it is the low calorie, low fat diet they promote that is the cause of the obesity epidemic, and that they are the ones to blame for much of this human catastrophe. I wonder what would happen if those making such views were ever to learn the truth that simply eating too much food (too many calories) is not the main cause of obesity.

The obesity crisis used to be just a western phenomenon, but now it is spreading throughout most of the world, with South and Central America, much of Asia and even parts of Africa currently affected. So far, the poorest nations have escaped its clutches, but they too will soon succumb as they become more affluent and start to adopt the "western lifestyle and diet". This incessant spread of obesity is yet more proof of just how disastrous our current lifestyle and diet really is. Anti-obesity strategies are also now commonplace around the world, but there hasn't been a single success story anywhere. Not one country has reversed the trend of rising obesity over the past 50 years. You might imagine that governments and medicine would take stock and consider whether they are doing the right thing, but the policy is always the same: simply tell people to reduce fat levels and total calories. Doing the same thing time and time again but expecting a different result is one definition of insanity.

In 2016 the National Obesity Forum and the Public Health Collaboration called for a major overhaul of dietary guidelines and accused public health bodies of colluding with the food industry and that food science has been corrupted by commercial interests that represent "a significant threat to public health". Dr Aseem Malhotra, consultant cardiologist and founding member of the Public Health Collaboration, said that dietary promotion of low fat foods "is perhaps the biggest mistake in modern medical history, resulting in devastating consequences for public health". Unsurprisingly, the report drew strong condemnation from senior medical professionals and the low fat, low calorie diet remains the official "solution" for obesity. It is unlikely that it will change in the foreseeable future and the obesity epidemic will continue around the world. Devastatingly sad.

Obesity – the lifestyle medicine approach

Food is the key cause of obesity, but it is the types of food we eat and when we eat them – not the calories – that are the critical factors. Let's briefly look at the foods the NHS recommends to treat obesity. Some of its key suggestions like eating plenty of vegetables and fruit while minimising sugar and processed and fast foods are, of course, correct and very important. The key problem is the recommendation to eat plenty of foods like potatoes, bread, rice, pasta and other starchy foods, and just small amounts of foods that are high in fat. Carbohydrates account for 55–60% of the diet and this is the official low fat diet that has already been examined in detail. There never was any proof that this diet prevented or cured heart disease which is why it was initially developed. It is also a major cause of type 2 diabetes (as seen in the last section) and is implicated in many other serious diseases. So, is it any surprise that it is also a major cause of obesity?

The optimum diet for weight loss consists of low carb, low GL foods. These are based on natural foods and healthy natural fats. So, what is the science behind it? When people are overweight or obese, the excess weight is stored mainly as fat. To lose weight, we need to "burn" this fat to provide our energy needs. The problem is when people eat a high carb diet, this results in high levels of glucose in the body. Glucose is the easiest way for the body to produce the energy it needs and it will always prioritise this as long as it is available in sufficient quantities. The body, however, can and will burn fat to provide energy, but only when glucose levels are low. There are two key things needed to achieve this. The first is the low carb natural diet, but the second is to restrict food intake to no more than three times a day. Current official dietary guidelines advise three main meals with three intermediate snacks. In other words, eating little and often. The problem is that this constantly keeps the body's glucose levels elevated and will ensure that very little stored fat is ever used to provide energy. Another key fact (examined in the section on diabetes) is that eating this official high carb diet causes blood glucose levels to rise rapidly and to high levels which then have to be quickly reduced by insulin. These rapid reductions can then make people feel hungry again, and this can often "force" them to eat even more snacks.

Natural weight loss works, but it is important to note it doesn't work in an exactly linear way. It is possible to lose a few kilos fairly quickly, but then it can become more erratic – a pound then nothing for days before restarting again at different rates. Nevertheless, the weight loss really will continue over time, and most people will achieve their healthy desired weight and, most importantly of all, maintain it. When you eat a natural low carb, low GL healthy diet, you will not just lose weight but start to feel great. You will probably see many health improvements like sleeping better, having more energy and reduced IBS symptoms. Most importantly, you will never feel hungry. Of course, all the other key aspects of lifestyle medicine like a positive mind, vitamins and minerals and exercise all play a part. Also, as already outlined, recent research has shown that our microbiome can play a key part in our weight. A healthy diet will, of course, also result in a healthier microbiome, but adding fermented foods will almost certainly provide extra help and add impetus to weight loss plans.

Of course, the official medical and government response to all of this is that they reject the low carb diet and continue to advocate the low fat diet which they advise everyone to adopt. It is rather strange then that the former Health Secretary Matt Hancock admitted in 2018 that he had lost two stone in weight by cutting out carbs like bread, potatoes and pasta. In other words, he had adopted the exact opposite of his own government's dietary guidelines that they relentlessly tell everyone to adopt and, of course, it really worked despite the fact the official position is it doesn't. Does he not realise this is truly shocking and almost criminal? He lost significant weight while the rest of the country that followed his official dietary advice continued to gain weight.

One final point. The key fact is if people eat a healthy low carb diet, they will almost certainly never become obese in the first place.

Top recommendations for further reading:

- *Reset Eating* by Robert Verkerk and Meleni Aldridge
- *The Low-GL Diet Bible* by Patrick Holford
- *The Diet Fix: How to Lose Weight and Keep It Off* by Dr Zoe Harcombe

Depression

Like nearly every other disease, the number of people with depression and other mental illnesses has increased over the last 60 years. It is, however, impossible to do a direct comparison of cases because the definitions of mental illness have also changed markedly in this period. For example, anxiety was the main type of mental diagnosis in the 1960s. Then, over the next few decades, depression became the main diagnosis, but part of this was due simply to changes in the official definitions of the two illnesses. However, just to give one specific example, Professor David Healy notes that in the 1980s about 1 in 10,000 patients in Britain were diagnosed with depression, while the current figure is more than 1 in 5 over their lifetime.

Depression – the medical approach

In 2004 NICE changed its official treatment plans for depression which aimed to increase the use of treatments like talking therapies and thereby reduce the use of drugs. The NHS now lists several ways of treating depression and these depend on whether it is judged mild, moderate or severe. With mild depression, some people will be advised to "wait and see" for a week or two, or to take exercise and self-help. If the depression persists, it would likely be classed as moderate which could lead to talking therapy. If it still persists or if the depression was initially much more serious, then it would be classed as severe. The two main treatments for this are antidepressant drugs like Prozac, Seroxat and Cipramil, and various forms of counselling and behavioural therapy. Despite the fact the NHS now recommends that drugs are not used initially for cases of depression unless it is severe, the reality is that drug prescriptions continue to soar. Around 25% of UK adults develop some form of mental illness each year and around two-thirds of them are given drugs. Now, at the end of 2021, NICE has once again issued recommendations for a range of non-pharmaceutical treatments for mild depression. Given that previous attempts have never worked, it will be interesting to see if this has any success or whether the drug industry will prevail yet again.

So, it is clear that at present antidepressants are still the main treatment for depression, and one of the reasons is doctors are so busy and have such a limited time with each patient (around ten minutes) that just prescribing a drug is simple and sometimes the only practical option. The other reason is antidepressants are very profitable drugs and they are endlessly promoted by the pharmaceutical industry and its highly remunerated advocates, both at medical conferences and in medical journals. But are these drugs really the best solution? What follows is a brief history of some of the key pieces of evidence relating to depression and antidepressants.

If asked what causes depression, most people would say it was due to a chemical imbalance in the brain. This is the message that has been carefully and skilfully implanted into the minds of doctors, politicians and the general public over many years by the pharmaceutical industry, which claimed the imbalance was caused by a lack of serotonin. In fact, the name of the most widely used psychiatric drugs – selective serotonin reuptake inhibitors (SSRIs) – summarises the claim that they increase serotonin and thus treat depression. There is just one problem. This theory is wrong. The chemical imbalance theory was originally proposed in the mid-1960s, but incredibly there has still never been any scientific proof to back it up. But could antidepressants still work for patients even though the theory has never been proven?

Let me outline one of the key studies that demonstrated that antidepressants really do not work directly for depression. Professor Irving Kirsch was a psychologist who regularly referred his patients to psychiatrists so they could be prescribed antidepressants. He unequivocally believed all their claims and that they really worked. He also carried out research and became particularly interested in the placebo effect. So, it was logical for him to carry out this research on placebos by comparing them to antidepressants. He confidently expected that antidepressants would work well for depression and his main aim was actually to see how placebos performed by comparison.

What he found was a profound shock, not just to him but to the whole of medicine. He found that placebos improved the symptoms of depression by 20% and the current antidepressant drugs by 25%. He was shocked at how little extra benefit the drugs actually gave.

When he compared the results of trials using the older generation of tricyclic antidepressants with the newer drugs, like Prozac, he found that both produced the same 25% benefit which he thought was strange. He soon uncovered other studies in which unusual drugs had been tested for depression. One was a sedative, one a sleeping aid and one a thyroid hormone. Incredibly, all three still produced around a 25% improvement in symptoms. This was now becoming faintly ridiculous. How could all these disparate drugs produce almost exactly the same benefits for depression? Did it mean that any active drug could function as an antidepressant? Well, apparently not. In 1998 Merck announced the discovery of a novel antidepressant called Emend, which had a completely different mode of action. But four months later it pulled the plug on any further development. The reason? It couldn't find any benefit over placebos in subsequent trials. We'll return to this drug in a moment.

What did all this mean? How could it all be explained? Professor Kirsch and his colleagues eventually realised and concluded that the only thing those drugs which improved depression had in common was that they all produced easily noticeable side effects. Did that fit in with the failure of Merck's new drug? Well, yes it did. Emend was initially announced as a breakthrough drug because it had virtually no side effects. Was this the reason it failed to work? It certainly seemed so.

We have already seen that when a patient in a (double blind) clinical trial finds out they are taking the real drug rather than the placebo (when the blinding is broken), they then invariably report that the drug works better than the placebo simply because they expect it to. Everything pointed to the fact that the small extra benefit seen from taking antidepressants compared to placebos might be explained simply because the obvious side effects of the drugs, such as a dry mouth, meant virtually everyone in the clinical trials who was taking them knew they were taking them. But this was still conjecture. Could it be proven beyond reasonable doubt?

Professor Kirsch then tracked down some trials that had compared antidepressants to active placebos. An active placebo is a substance that induces similar side effects to the real drug but, in all other respects, can have no therapeutic value for depression. These trials showed there was no significant difference between the drug and active placebo. Both produced a 25% improvement in symptoms. This is pretty strong evidence that the drug has no therapeutic effect itself, and works only because of the "active placebo" effect.

When Professor Kirsch published his work, it was greeted by many experts with scepticism. After all, everyone "knew" that antidepressants worked well, so surely there must be something wrong with his research. They also pointed out he had not included all the clinical trials that had been carried out on antidepressants. So, Professor Kirsch used the Freedom of Information Act to gain access to all the trials that had been submitted to the FDA by the drug companies. He then repeated his analysis. The findings were almost identical. In fact, the benefit of the drugs was even slightly less than in the original study. Professor Kirsch then asked nine leading scientists to independently check his work and findings. So, when the study was finally published, it was much more difficult for the supporters of antidepressants to criticise the results. In fact, one group of researchers involved in mental illness wrote: "Many have long been unimpressed by the magnitude of the differences between treatments and controls, what some of our colleagues refer to as the 'dirty little secret' in the pharmaceutical literature." The drug companies knew about the minimal benefits of the drugs, so did the regulators and many researchers. But most of the doctors who prescribed them didn't, let alone their patients.

The study made headline news in many countries. It did, however, split opinions in medicine, almost down the middle. Some doctors accepted they had been duped by the spin and marketing of the drug companies. Others maintained the view that, notwithstanding the negative study findings, they "knew" antidepressants worked in clinical practice. If you think about it, this is a strange position for doctors to take. On the one hand, they have an almost fervent religious belief that clinical trials are the ultimate and only type of proof acceptable within medicine, and yet, they are willing to ignore such proof in the case of antidepressants. This is just one more example that "evidence-based medicine" clearly isn't evidence based at all. With medicine split down the middle, prescriptions and, therefore, sales of antidepressants duly fell by around half.

But antidepressants were a major profit earner for the drug companies who were not about to take this disaster lying down. They marshalled their hired guns in academia and psychiatric practice to start the fight back. Lots of stage IV trials (that produced no scientific proof) were carried out to "demonstrate" the benefits of antidepressants and their highly remunerated experts went to town publishing papers and giving talks at conferences to promote them. Although the whole rehabilitation process took time, it worked frighteningly well.

Today antidepressants are the second most widely prescribed drugs of all time. Approximately 10% of the entire population take them at some point in a given year. It is as if all the detailed scientific analysis and findings by Professor Kirsch had never existed. It is just one more example of how the power and money of the drug companies can triumph over scientific fact, and demonstrates how medicine can be so easily duped. In the case of antidepressants, they were duped not just once, but twice. Quite mind-boggling when you think about it.

But what makes the whole thing so chilling is the side effects of the drugs. If there were no side effects, the fact that antidepressants don't work any better than active placebos wouldn't be an issue – apart from the financial cost, of course. But they do have side effects, and they are numerous, significant and even life-threatening. Antidepressants have been linked with suicide, homicide, obesity, type 2 diabetes, sexual dysfunction, dementia, gastrointestinal problems, rashes, severe personality changes and sleep disruption, to name just a few. Many people take them for years even though the official guidelines recommend they are normally only taken for a maximum of a few months. One of the reasons is that the withdrawal symptoms are so severe that many people simply dare not stop taking them. A recent review in the Journal of Addictive Behaviors found that more than half of users will experience withdrawal symptoms. That's 4 million people in England alone and for a quarter of them the symptoms are severe. They can also be incredibly addictive and it has been estimated that in the US around 7 million people have long-term addiction. The Federal Drug Agency has issued more "black box warnings" for antidepressants than almost any other family of drugs. The bestselling drug Prozac officially lists an incredibly shocking 242 different side effects. I'm not sure whether this is a world record, but it must surely be close to one. A child taking antidepressants is 15 times more likely to commit suicide than children who are drug free. In one review of drug reactions, it was found that "during a ten-year period, Prozac was associated with more hospitalisations, deaths and other serious adverse events reported to the FDA than any other drug in America".

Around 10% of the population of the developed world are now taking a class of drugs that have virtually no clinical benefits (no better than active placebos), they can be seriously addictive and come with hundreds of serious and even life-threatening side effects. This is so bizarre that I have to keep pinching myself to make sure I'm not just having a nightmare. I have asked this question before, but it needs asking again. How could mankind ever have reached such a situation?

Next, I want to look at one of the key reasons for the increase in mental illness. The number of people experiencing depression really has increased over the last 60 years, but something very sinister is also happening. To understand what is going on we need to explore the DSM (Diagnostic and Statistical Manual of Mental Disorders). The DSM includes a list of every official psychiatric disorder. Psychiatrists then select what they think is the appropriate one for each patient. It is produced in the US, but, crucially, it influences psychiatric practice throughout the world. The first edition was produced in 1952 and we are now on the fifth volume.

The first thing to say is psychiatric diagnoses are not an exact science. There are no biological markers that define mental illness – everything is subjective. There was frequently no consensus in the committees of the DSM as to what disorders should be included and even on the definition of their symptoms. Such things were often decided on a majority vote. This is hardly a scientific way to deal with one of the twenty-first century's most prevalent diseases. In addition, the various types of mental disorder usually overlap and the psychiatrist has to rely on the patient's description of their symptoms and try to match it with the symptoms described in the DSM manual. Different psychiatrists will frequently arrive at different diagnoses for exactly the same symptoms. Despite attempts to improve the definition of symptoms with each new edition of the DSM, things are no better than they were 60 years ago. Psychiatrists still disagree on diagnosis in around 40% of cases. If the psychiatric disorders and their symptoms are not universally agreed and if the symptoms can be so easily misinterpreted by experienced psychiatrists, then we have a deeply disturbing situation. In the midst of all this confusion and wrong diagnoses, how reliable can the treatments be?

All this reveals a deep flaw in psychiatry, but there is an even more disturbing problem. Around 100 years ago, psychiatrists recognised just seven mental disorders. When the original DSM manual was published in 1952, it listed 106 psychiatric disorders, DSM-II listed 182, DSM-III listed 265, DSM-IV listed 374, and the current version DSM-V lists 387. (Incidentally, 72% of the people on the DSM-V committee had financial ties to the drug industry – perish the thought, of course, that this could in any way influence their judgements and decisions.) Why is this so disturbing? Well, you will notice a clear trend. Each new edition lists more disorders than the previous one. It means more and more people will fall into one of the "arbitrary" boxes that psychiatry has conjured out of thin air; and more and more people will end up on drugs, since they are prescribed to a majority of those with a psychiatric diagnosis.

Today, between 25 and 30% of the adult population of the US will suffer from at least one DSM "disorder" in any given year according to the National Institute of Mental Health. The UK is not far behind. Psychiatry explains that this huge increase in diagnoses is due to the pressures of modern life and also because of the fact psychiatry is now better at recognising mental disorders which once would have "slipped below the radar". But is modern life really more stressful than decades ago? Many sociological studies suggest stress has actually decreased, while the idea that psychiatry is better at diagnosis is pretty fanciful given there are no objective tests that can confirm the validity of any psychiatric diagnosis and psychiatrists disagree in 40% of cases. Psychiatry has simply kept lowering the bar for what counts as mental illness, and has rebranded many natural responses to some of the inevitable problems of life as mental disorders, thus requiring psychiatric treatment. Here is a devastating example of these false diagnoses and over-medicalisation.

In March 2011 scientists undertook a comprehensive study on 1 million Canadian school children between the ages of six and twelve which looked specifically at how many had been diagnosed with ADHD in one year. The scientists were baffled by the results. These showed that there was a clear relationship between ADHD diagnoses and the month in which the child was born. As odd as this may seem, in each school year the youngest children consistently had the highest diagnoses of ADHD. Remember that in any class, children can have an age difference of up to a year. The youngest boys had a 30% increased ADHD diagnosis level compared to the oldest boys in the class, while the girls fared significantly worse at 70% more. The oldest children had a full 11-month developmental advantage compared to the youngest and at that age this represents an enormous difference in terms of mental and emotional maturity. The youngest children were being diagnosed with ADHD simply because their relative immaturity was being mistaken for the symptoms of ADHD. The relative immaturity of the youngest children was simply diagnosed as a psychiatric disease. This is not just happening in Canada. Similar studies have been carried out in several countries, such as the US and Sweden, and they all show the same type of results. Had these "youngest" children started school 11 months later, most of them would not have been diagnosed with ADHD. There was in fact nothing wrong with them in the first place. But now they have been labelled with a serious mental disease and many of them will be receiving drugs to "correct" this non-existent disease; drugs with huge numbers of side effects, including the risk of suicide.

This one example sums up the appalling and horrific consequences of a psychiatric profession that is out of control; a profession that should quite logically be labelled as "in need of psychiatric treatment" itself. Countless millions of people and children are being diagnosed with a mental disease that is just normal human behaviour. They are being medicalised and given dangerous drugs. Lives are quite literally being ripped apart and destroyed. On reading this section in the prequel to this book, a friend said, "If this is true, this is a profession whose advocates should be locked up and the keys thrown away." It is hard to disagree.

Let me give you a few examples of official "psychiatric disorders" listed in DSM:

- Stuttering
- Sexual aversion disorder (absence of desire for sex)
- Social phobia (shyness)
- Expressive language disorder (below average language skills)
- Reading disorder (falling substantially below the reading standard for your age)
- Female orgasmic disorder (persistent delay in, or absence of, orgasm)
- Caffeine-related disorders (caffeine withdrawal and dependency)
- Oppositional defiant disorder (for children with irritable mood swings and who defy authority)

As a child I remember I was often described as "shy", which is almost always just a temporary and natural part of growing up. This didn't last long and by the age of 16, I was playing drums in a local rock group. Had I been a child now, however, it is quite possible that I would be diagnosed as mentally ill (social phobia) and prescribed antidepressants and then be at risk of the hundreds of their known side effects including suicide. Truly shocking and frightening and, I believe, unforgiveable.

Some of the latest additions to DSM-V include:

- Generalised anxiety disorder – which threatens to turn the routine problems and disappointments of everyday life into a mental illness
- Disruptive mood dysregulation disorder – which will see children's temper tantrums become symptoms of mental disorder

But the most chilling example concerns the inclusion of grief due to bereavement. This means that feelings of deep sadness, sleeplessness, crying, inability to concentrate and low appetite, if they continue for more than just two weeks after the death of a loved one, could warrant the diagnosis of depression. This despite the simple fact these reactions are the natural human response to these sad losses. This is also simply unforgivable.

In 2012, before DSM-V was finally published, hundreds of articles, papers and editorials were written, including many in the leading medical journals, which strongly criticised the classification of bereavement grief as a mental illness. An online petition also went live protesting against most of the new mental "disorders" proposed by DSM-V. It was endorsed by over 50 organisations related to mental health, including the British and Danish Psychological Societies. They argued that by lowering diagnostic thresholds, many more people would be branded mentally ill and by including so many new disorders that lacked scientific justification, there would be more inappropriate medical treatment of vulnerable populations. All this was to no avail. DSM-V was published later in 2012 without any amendments. So, if you have ever grieved for the loss of a loved one for more than two weeks, or you have a child or grandchild who has temper tantrums, or you just feel the disappointments of everyday life, you can now at least be consoled that – according to the "experts" – you are all just mentally ill. Terribly reassuring, don't you think?

Incidentally, when DSM-VI is finally unleashed on the public, I too would officially be classed as mentally ill. Why? Well, many psychiatrists are desperately unhappy that the condition orthorexia did not make it into the DSM-V handbook. They are determined that it will be included in DSM-VI. Orthorexia describes a "condition" whereby people are determined to eat healthily and live healthily and where meals, for example, are prepared according to these principles on a regular basis. So, people who are determined to look after their health and regularly eat healthy foods will soon be officially classed as mentally ill. Don't laugh. I assure you this is factual; I did not write it on 1 April.

So far, I have outlined key facts about depression, psychiatry, and antidepressant drugs and their side effects. As shocking as all this is, the stories of individuals whose lives have been seriously affected and even destroyed are vital in understanding the true devastation of antidepressant drugs. These stories (and there are countless thousands of them) are often so devastating they are almost unbearable to read. I want to outline just two of them.

The first involves Katinka Blackford Newman who was a successful film maker with a raft of award-winning documentaries. In 2013, after 13 happy years, her marriage fell apart. She grew anxious and unhappy and went to see a psychiatrist who concluded that she was depressed and prescribed the drug Lexapro. After taking just a few pills she began hallucinating and was unable to stop moving. The whole thing was so devastating that at one point she thought she had killed both her children. In reality, she had simply slashed her own arm with a knife. Her two children called their aunt and uncle. Because Katinka had private health insurance, they took her to a leading private hospital in London where she was diagnosed with psychotic depression and over the next three weeks was prescribed a cascade of powerful drugs to try to treat her symptoms. She spent the next year in a near-catatonic state, in and out of hospital and needing to be cared for at home. She started smoking up to 70 cigarettes and drinking a bottle of vodka each day, never washed herself and couldn't speak a full sentence. She effectively lost her children who could not bear to see her. One day she told the community health worker, "I'm going to kill myself today." She meant it.

Luckily, she was transferred to a different hospital where the psychiatrist took the unusual step of stopping all her drugs with the plan of then restarting them at a later date to see which ones worked best. But, after three weeks of agonising withdrawals, she woke up one morning feeling almost normal. Amazingly, just a short time later, she rented a new home and was joined by her overjoyed children, she started a new job and after four months ran a half marathon. But this terrifying year-long ordeal led her to investigate the facts about antidepressants and their potential links with suicide and violence and to help spread the word in what she says is now her life's work. She wrote a book called *The Pill That Steals Lives* and her research led to a BBC Panorama programme called *A Prescription for Murder?* She has since been called as an expert witness in a number of cases in British courts related to homicide and suicide where antidepressants had potentially been involved. Katinka was one of the lucky people and after a year of hell, she returned to normal health. This, however, does not happen for everyone as we will now see.

The second involves Geraldine Burns from Boston. She was the life and soul of every party, held down a good job and loved life, loved working and loved her family. All this changed in 1988 when she gave birth to a daughter. She felt physically unwell and her doctor thought she had anxiety and prescribed the drug Ativan. A few months later she saw a psychiatrist who confirmed she should keep taking the drug (which she was told was harmless and non-addictive) for the rest of her life. Soon after, the psychiatrist added an antidepressant drug. As the months wore on, she became seriously anxious and found it impossible to leave the house. Eventually, the federal authorities classed her as "disabled by anxiety" and she was given disability payments. For eight years she was prescribed a wide range of psychiatric drugs, none of which worked. In fact, she developed many other conditions like rashes, weight gain, tachycardia, panic attacks and excessive menstrual bleeding which then led to a hysterectomy. She knew a number of women who were also taking Ativan and every one of them eventually had to have a hysterectomy. Then, in 1996, she had a new physician who, after examining her medical history, identified the drug that he said was the most likely cause of her conditions. Because the drug was incredibly addictive, it took her two years of hell before she could finally stop taking Ativan and all the other psychiatric drugs she had been prescribed. At one point she couldn't even sleep for weeks. It then took several more years before she felt physically better. Stopping the drugs resulted in really vital improvements in many aspects of her life, but the happy, socially at ease person she was before 1988 has never returned. "Am I back to my old self? No," she whispers, "I mourn who I used to be."

The book *Anatomy of an Epidemic* by Robert Whitaker explores in detail the incredible deceptions about psychiatric drug treatments and also includes stories of over 20 individuals whose lives have been devastated by them. These show the significant differences in the side effects of a range of antidepressants and other drugs used to treat depression. This helps to explain why some people can effectively recover if they stop taking them like Katinka, whereas others, like Geraldine, never fully recover. Incredibly, some of the leading psychiatrists consistently maintain there is nothing in the literature to back up the claims made about people like Katinka and Geraldine that it was the antidepressant drugs that were the cause of their devastating conditions. This, of course, is exactly what the tobacco industry said about cigarettes. The idea that the suffering of these women had nothing to do with the drugs they were taking would be laughable if it wasn't so appalling.

Quite amazingly, despite all the negative and dangerous evidence for antidepressants, and despite even the guidelines of both NICE and the NHS to minimise the use of drugs by promoting other effective treatments like exercise and talking and counselling therapies, the use of these drugs has soared. The number of prescribed antidepressants in the UK has doubled since 2010 and quadrupled since 2000. In 2011 a Channel 4 TV survey also showed they had been prescribed to over 15,000 UK children. As terrible as this is, here are two even more truly frightening facts. There are over a quarter of a million children in the US under the age of one who are being given antidepressant and other psychotropic drugs, as well as another 8 million children under the age of 18. Given how devastating these drugs can be for healthy adults, there is no knowing how deadly they might be for babies and young children and we should pray that such incredible figures do not spread to the UK. It is almost certainly one of the reasons why the US has the highest childhood mortality rate in the developed world and the highest levels of disease. The fact that the drug industry, drug regulators and some doctors allow all this to happen to millions of young children is, I believe, so evil they are no different to Hitler and ISIS.

If ever you (or anyone you know) are ever prescribed antidepressant or antipsychotic drugs, please make your own decisions on whether to take them after considering everything you have just read.

Depression – the lifestyle medicine approach

Well, other than in really serious and exceptional circumstances, antidepressants and other drugs are the very last thing anyone associated with lifestyle medicine would use. Most cases of shyness, temper tantrums and bereavement grief, for example, will resolve naturally. The people involved are not mentally ill and need no treatment other than friendly faces to help with the perfectly normal ups and downs of life. Many experts believe that more than half of all current diagnoses of mental illness fall into this "none mentally ill" category. There are, of course, still many people with real, serious and desperate mental health problems relating to issues such as domestic violence, bullying, social media attacks, family problems and social isolation. Here, counselling and psychotherapy provide better outcomes than antidepressants with none of the side effects. The problem, of course, is that psychotherapy takes more time. It's much easier for a doctor to just write a prescription for an antidepressant drug. But, of course, if psychiatry hadn't needlessly labelled so many normal people as mentally ill, they would now have much more time to help resolve the problems of those people with real and genuine need. But the very best place to start as always is by prevention. We have already seen – courtesy of the NHS – that 30% of the cases of depression could be prevented just by exercise. In fact, most people just need to remember the seven key secrets of good health:

- positive emotional health
- a healthy low carb, low GL diet
- exercise
- vitamin and mineral supplements
- gut health
- minimising chemical exposure
- sleep

Most people who actively pursue a healthy lifestyle and take these seven issues seriously are very unlikely to become depressed. Some people will still be unable to avoid traumatic events, such as a family breakdown, but for these, counselling and psychotherapy are invariably the best solutions.

There are also some key specific factors that can provide help. Studies have shown that people who suffer from IBS or have food allergies have a greater incidence of depression, so improving gut health is vitally important in treating and preventing depression.

Oily fish or omega 3 fish oil supplements can ease or help prevent depression as can B vitamins including B12, B6 and folate. Anti-inflammatory compounds like curcumin and turmeric can also help. Avoiding or minimising wheat and gluten are also important.

Chemical exposure has been clearly implicated in mental health. Leaded petrol was clearly a factor in mental problems and today other heavy metals, such as mercury, are also implicated.

For those people with depression, the herb St John's wort has been shown in many clinical trials to be just as effective as any drug but with virtually no side effects or addiction. A recent meta-analysis of 27 studies involving 3,120 people concluded: "St John's wort extract was just as effective in improving symptoms, as prescribed antidepressant drugs, with no difference in clinical response, remission or reduction in depression scores. Importantly, however, St John's wort extract had a significantly lower rate of side effects than antidepressants and superior safety in treating mild to moderate depression." Despite all this evidence and a significantly better safety profile, not one single psychiatrist or doctor ever prescribes it. St John's wort is also just a fraction of the price of antidepressant drugs and its use would save the NHS a fortune. This illustrates again the power and control the drug industry wields, and is just one more example of why the NHS never has enough money and never will.

Finally, here is one other important fact. The digital era is without doubt a significant factor in the increase in cases of depression. Many people, and not just teenagers, spend incredible amounts of time on social media, and even though there is a supposed 13-year age limit, many young children are also finding ways of becoming involved. Instead of natural face to face contact, social media is, for many people, their main way of communicating. For teenagers and children, in particular, this can lead to devastating outcomes.

Alzheimer's disease

There are five types of dementia, but Alzheimer's is one of the most devastating and accounts for nearly two-thirds of all cases. In 1906 there was just one case of Alzheimer's – the very first case ever recorded. Today dementia affects 55 million people worldwide with 800,000 in the UK. By 2050 the WHO predicts the global figure will rise to 140 million with 1.6 million in the UK. The increase in cases is possibly the biggest percentage increase of any major disease in the last 100 years. Apart from the human catastrophe, the costs of treating and caring for those with the disease is staggering. By 2050, in the US, it is projected to cost $1.5 trillion each year, and this does not include other costs such as lost wages for other family caregivers. It will financially devastate most economies.

Alzheimer's – the medical approach

There are several medical hypotheses regarding the causes of Alzheimer's disease, but the predominant one is the build-up of beta-amyloid plaque deposits and tau proteins that form neurofibrillary tangles in the brain. Most of the research carried out by pharmaceutical companies has been based on this theory, and over $40 billion has been spent over the last 50 years. Despite this enormous sum and the endless research effort, the drugs that have been developed cannot cure or stop the disease progression in any way. An increasing number of experts now believe the amyloid plaque and tau protein theory is simply incorrect and they are a reaction to Alzheimer's and not a cause.

So, how does medicine treat Alzheimer's disease? Medicine, of course, relies almost exclusively on drugs for treating nearly every disease. Despite the fact the Alzheimer's drugs that do exist – like Aricept – have almost no benefits, they are all that medicine has, and so they are still the only thing that can be prescribed. They are in fact given to millions of patients around the world, even though their effect is so limited that most patients and their carers usually see no benefit. The drugs do not stop progression of the disease and at best, for about 30% of patients, they minimally improve certain memory functions like awareness of time and place and reasoning for just a few months, and even then, only at a specific stage of the disease. After this, the decline continues unabated so that after a few more months there is no meaningful difference between those given the drug and those without treatment. In addition, drug side effects are numerous and include nausea, vomiting, anorexia, insomnia and muscle cramps. In fact, the official Aricept side effect list runs to 104 in total. Given that medicine has no other treatments, all it can really do is detect and diagnose the disease and then prepare family and carers for the inevitable decline and death of their loved ones. There is really nothing more that can be said about medicine's approach to Alzheimer's disease.

There is, however, one other important and serious fact. It is now known that there are a range of drugs for treating other diseases that can increase cognitive impairment and the risk of developing Alzheimer's. These include benzodiazepine tranquilizers, antidepressants, proton pump inhibitors and anticholinergics. A 2019 study published in JAMA linked anticholinergic drugs to a nearly 50% increased risk of developing dementia if used for several years. A large study also published in JAMA Neurology found that regular use of proton pump inhibitor drugs increased the risk of dementia by up to 52%.

Alzheimer's – the lifestyle medicine approach

Lifestyle medicine views Alzheimer's as a largely preventable disease. I know exactly what you are thinking right now: this is impossible. But please wait until you have read all the evidence before passing final judgement. Before starting, there is one important point that needs to be emphasised. Alzheimer's in its later stages probably cannot be reversed. This is because the disease results in actual physical brain shrinkage due to some brain cells dying off. This makes it very different to other diseases like heart disease and type 2 diabetes which really can be reversed by lifestyle changes. However, in the earlier stages, its progression can be slowed considerably and probably even stopped, such that most people would be able to live almost a normal life. Even so, the very best solution, as always, is to prevent the disease from happening in the first place by adopting a really healthy lifestyle. Unlike type 2 diabetes, where a poor diet and lack of exercise are the key factors, Alzheimer's is a much more complex disease. There are probably hundreds of factors that play a part in its development and this is in line with the almost infinite complexity of the human body. This does not mean that prevention or its progression cannot be achieved, because it is likely that a few dozen factors play the key roles.

So, what are the key factors that can help improve your memory and prevent the development of Alzheimer's? Adopting the seven key healthy lifestyle changes we have already explored in detail will take you a long way towards preventing Alzheimer's:

- mental wellbeing
- low carb, low GI natural diet
- exercise
- vitamins and minerals
- healthy microbiome
- minimising chemical exposure
- sleeping well

Is there any evidence that these really can reduce the risk of developing Alzheimer's? Well, we have already seen – courtesy of the NHS – that 30% of dementia and Alzheimer's could be prevented just by exercise.

A 2007 French study of over 8,000 men and women showed that those who ate a diet rich in fish, omega 3 oils, fruits and vegetables reduced their risk of Alzheimer's by up to 60%.

In 2013 a group of leading doctors, including a former chairman of the Royal College of GPs and the chairman of the National Obesity Forum, sent an open letter to the Health Secretary saying that the battle against dementia should focus on a Mediterranean style diet containing fresh fruits and vegetables, nuts, fish and olive oil rather than "dubious" drugs. They said there were numerous high-quality studies backing up this approach and that prevention was the thing to focus on.

A meta-analysis of five studies in the Journal of Ageing showed a significant improvement in cognition in those given probiotics compared to those in the placebo.

In 2016 a Lancet article also focused on why we should get serious about Alzheimer's prevention. It listed the following proven lifestyle treatments and their risk reductions:

- taking exercise 32%
- stopping smoking 31%
- getting some adult education 24%
- supplementing B vitamins 22%
- eating more fatty fish or taking omega 3 supplements 22%

There is also significant scientific evidence that mental issues, like stress and anxiety, as well as pesticides and heavy metals, like lead, mercury and aluminium, can all increase the risk of Alzheimer's. A damaged microbiome and poor sleep (less than five hours a night) are also known to increase the risk. Improving all these damaging conditions will, therefore, result in a reduced risk of developing Alzheimer's.

There are also many other specific factors that really can help to reduce the risk for dementia and here are just a few of them.

Sugar. Sugar is, of course, a major cause of type 2 diabetes and it is now known that people who have the disease are more likely to develop Alzheimer's. However, sugar is also known to be a cause of Alzheimer's even in people without diabetes. The Alzheimer's Society highlights a 2018 study that shows that those people with the highest sugar consumption are at the highest risk of developing Alzheimer's, and many researchers now, unsurprisingly, refer to it as type 3 diabetes. Of course, as we have seen, highly refined carbohydrates, like white bread, as well as other forms of industrially created sweeteners, like high fructose corn syrup, have similar devastating effects, So, reducing all of them and the processed foods they are part of is a crucial part of preventing Alzheimer's.

Flavonoids. Berries like blueberries and raspberries contain high levels of flavonoids and there are several studies that show their benefits. The latest 2020 study – part of the prestigious Framingham Offspring Cohort – shows that long-term dietary flavonoid intake reduces the risk of developing Alzheimer's and related dementias.

Eliminating gum disease. Researchers from King's College London showed that people who had gum disease saw their memory decline more rapidly than those with healthy gums.

Curcumin. This is a compound in the spice turmeric. A 2018 UCLA trial involving memory tests showed that curcumin supplements improved memory by 28% compared to the placebo group.

Antioxidants. Several studies, including a WebMD article, showed that antioxidants reduce the risk of developing Alzheimer's. Some of the key sources are natural plant foods like vegetables and fruits. These contain a range of antioxidants like vitamins, minerals and other key compounds like quercetin, isoflavones, catechins and anthocyanidins.

Challenge the brain. Never stop learning. Mentally stimulating activities like reading, crossword puzzles, games, singing, playing musical instruments, dancing and learning languages really do significantly reduce mental decline and improve memory function.

There are literally thousands of research studies that show how these wide range of lifestyle factors really can reduce the risk of Alzheimer's and memory decline. So, what is the official medical position about all this evidence? And indeed, what do organisations like the charity Alzheimer's Research UK and WebMD say about it? For some of the evidence, like a healthy Mediterranean diet and the need to reduce heavy metals and pesticides, they do tacitly agree that there are some benefits. However, they never seriously promote them, and if asked why, they would usually just say things like "more research is needed" or "large-scale clinical trials are necessary before we can authorise their use". Such research will, of course, never happen especially when you consider that for every £100,000 the UK Research Council spends on Alzheimer's, just £1 is spent on disease prevention and £999,999 on trying to develop drugs. Effectively, lifestyle benefits are simply ignored and brushed under the carpet and they are rarely reported by the media. But what happens when a clinical trial is carried out and the press report it? Medicine has to respond in some way.

I am going to examine one of them in detail: the amino acid homocysteine. A link between homocysteine and Alzheimer's was discovered in 1998 when researchers found high levels in the brains of people who had died from the disease. Other researchers then carried out dozens of studies that measured levels of homocysteine in patients with mental decline, and most of them showed a clear association. Such an association, however, does not necessarily mean it causes Alzheimer's, so a study from Boston University Medical School set out to explore whether this was true. Over 1,000 patients who had had their homocysteine levels measured eight years earlier and who did not have dementia had their homocysteine levels checked again and were monitored over the following eight years. In the study, 83 of them developed Alzheimer's and those who had the highest homocysteine before any mental deterioration started to occur had the greatest risk of developing the disease. The researchers concluded that "an increased homocysteine level is a strong, independent risk factor for the development of dementia."

One other key fact is there is also definitive proof that the B vitamins (B12, B6 and folic acid) can reduce homocysteine levels. So, strong evidence that high homocysteine is a cause of Alzheimer's and that B vitamins can reduce it. The key final question, therefore, is can B vitamins actually prevent or slow down the progress of the disease? Professor David Smith and his team at Oxford University set about finding out. They conducted a randomised, double blind, placebo-controlled clinical trial on 270 people with mild cognitive impairment (MCI). This is the stage where mental faculty is declining, but before the full symptoms of Alzheimer's disease start to occur. The volunteers were divided into two groups: one of which got high dose B vitamins and the other a placebo. Brain scans were carried out at the start and end of the two-year trial. The B vitamins used were folic acid 800mg, B6 20mg, and B12 500mcg. The remarkable result was that those people with high homocysteine who received the B vitamins had a 90% reduction in brain shrinkage compared to those with high homocysteine in the placebo group and this occurred in precisely the same region of the brain that Alzheimer's normally affects.

Normally, when a clinical trial like Professor Smith's produces such impressive results – particularly for such a devastating disease – new funding would be put in place within months so that a new trial could be undertaken to corroborate the original findings. But ten years later, Professor Smith and his team are still waiting for this funding. Why? When the results of the trial were published in 2011, they made headline news in the media, but it was also clear from the start that Professor Smith's work was not going to receive the same positive reception from the scientific community. Responses ranged from hostility to indifference. One professor jeered that the "fraudulent supplement industry would be delighted". Alzheimer's Research UK warned that "it was important not to raise false hopes". Minds had apparently already been made up before anyone had even read, let alone evaluated, the findings. Remember, medicine has an almost religious belief in the randomised clinical trial. It supposedly sits at the pinnacle of their evidence base. Medicine's constant dismissal of lifestyle solutions for diseases is usually based on the fact there are no clinical trials to back up the claims. Well, Professor Smith provided that proof unequivocally. So, why was the trial simply brushed aside, dismissed or ignored?

In addition to all of this, even worse was to follow, because those involved could not continue to simply dismiss his trial. They needed "scientific" proof if they were determined to discredit it completely. Two details are crucial in understanding what happened next. All those recruited into Professor Smith's trial had been diagnosed with cognitive impairment. This had to be the case, of course, because if people in any trial don't have the disease being evaluated, the treatment simply won't work and the trial would be meaningless. It was also already clear that only those people with a high homocysteine could benefit from B vitamins, so it was vital to measure the homocysteine levels in all participants so that the results could be analysed correctly.

In the section on sepsis, I explored in detail some of the ways in which medical research could be unscientifically (effectively fraudulently) manipulated. These are known as "trials designed to fail", and their aim is to "prove" that natural solutions that really do work "do not work". I also explained that when a successful clinical trial has been completed with impressive benefits for a serious disease, a second trial is usually carried out to confirm the results. In such a situation it is absolutely essential from a scientific perspective to replicate exactly the original trial protocols. Making changes is unscientific and unethical as well as demonstrating bias. So, when the new trials were carried out, the two key protocols that should have been reproduced exactly were to recruit only patients with mild cognitive impairment and to measure their homocysteine levels and evaluate the benefits of the B vitamins only on those with high levels.

Several clinical trials were nevertheless carried out and they ignored both of these vital protocols. Almost beyond belief, most of the patients were healthy and had no cognitive impairment. The trials never even measured homocysteine levels and one trial even used just a multivitamin in which the level of B vitamins was around one-five-hundredth of the level used by Professor Smith and would have had zero benefit. Nevertheless, the trials' conclusions simply claimed there was no difference in outcomes between those taking the vitamins and those with the placebos and, therefore, that the vitamins did not work.

Then, in 2014, a meta-analysis was also carried out on 11 trials involving B vitamins. The lead author, Dr Robert Clarke, said, "Our study draws a line under the debate. B vitamins don't reduce cognitive decline as we age. Taking folic acid and vitamin B12 is sadly not going to prevent Alzheimer's." However, anyone who examined the study in detail would see that exactly the same tricks were used as in the first set of trials. None of the trials involved anyone with cognitive impairment. This trick would be like "proving" a cancer treatment doesn't work by using people who don't have cancer. Quite simply, if you don't have cognitive impairment, B vitamins cannot stop or reduce a decline that is not happening. Quite sadly, no official organisations, like the Department of Health or Alzheimer's Research UK, ever challenged these glaring, disgraceful and unscientific tricks.

I asked the question why was Professor Smith's work simply dismissed out of hand when it was first published? To this can now be added why have other academics carried out research that ignored his methodology – using unscientific trials set up and designed to fail – thus discrediting his work? Well, the answer is simple. There is too much at stake. If it was ever proven unequivocally that vitamins could help prevent and slow down the progression of the most feared disease in the world, it would be a disaster for medicine, the drug industry, regulators, charities, governments and the finance industry. For years they have sought to denigrate lifestyle solutions to health, branding them unproven and even trying to claim they were dangerous, as well as introducing draconian laws to help destroy them. Proof that vitamins could work, and work in such a spectacular way, would give them all a bloody nose, call into question their collective judgements and cause the public to examine their hidden motives. In addition, most of the organisations and the individuals involved receive huge sums of money from the drug industry and this would be at risk if vitamins were shown to work, thus removing the need for drugs. But additionally, it would also open the door to other ways in which vitamins and other lifestyle approaches could transform people's health, including the treatment of all the other major chronic diseases like heart disease, diabetes, obesity and cancer. Quite simply, it could destroy a large section of medicine and the powerful industries that supply it, as well as those financing them.

One further shocking fact is that one of the other key authors of the meta-analysis that claimed that B vitamins did not work for Alzheimer's was Professor Sir Rory Collins, the researcher who endlessly promoted statins until they became the bestselling drugs ever. All this, despite their almost non-existent benefits for most patients, and the fact that for over 20 years he had never examined their side effects, but still claimed virtually none existed. He and his team received £267 million from drug companies. It is perhaps not too surprising he is now moving on and using his fame and prestige to help promote useless Alzheimer's drugs and discredit the natural solutions that pose a threat to his paymasters in Big Pharma.

It saddens me to see so many people raise so much money for charities like Alzheimer's Research UK, believing they are really helping in the search for a cure. But then we see the same charity casually dismiss the impeccable clinical trial of Professor Smith and then seemingly ignore what can only be called "fraudulent" medical research that "proved" he was wrong. The sad reality is all the major charities, like the British Heart Foundation, Cancer Research, Diabetes UK, as well as Alzheimer's Research UK, are all part of the problem, perpetuating the accepted establishment view that drugs, and drugs alone, are the only thing that can provide an answer to Alzheimer's and all the other major life-taking diseases and, at the same time, being prepared to dismiss credible science on lifestyle solutions. This is why I never give money to any of these so-called charities. I do donate money, but it is directed to those independent organisations that are promoting the prevention of disease and trying to expose the sad and frightening truth about how solutions to devastating diseases, like Alzheimer's, are simply being suppressed and discredited.

My own personal belief is that people like Professor Sir Rory Collins and Dr Robert Clarke really should be on trial in The Hague and charged with crimes against humanity for what they have done. I do not understand how they can live with themselves, knowing they have discredited a treatment that could have helped millions of people with the most feared disease ever. They are clever people and they knew exactly what they were doing when they tested B vitamins only on people who couldn't possibly benefit from them, and then used this so-called evidence to declare they didn't work. The charities who nodded these trials through aren't any better. Tens of millions of people and their families are suffering from this most dreaded of diseases and will continue to do so and the number will continue to increase to 140 million by 2050. A significant proportion of these destroyed lives and deaths really could be prevented by simple lifestyle changes and treatments like B vitamins. Hopefully, at some point, the truth may emerge and future generations will look back in horror and disbelief at what is now unfolding. They might wonder how money and greed could wreak such misery and devastation.

Finally, I want to make a recommendation for further reading about Alzheimer's disease. The book is called *The Alzheimer's Prevention Plan* and the author is Patrick Holford. You may wonder why I keep recommending his books. Well, he has devoted nearly all his working life to researching scientific evidence on the real causes of disease. He spent time with some of the greatest medical experts that ever lived, He was a student with two of the leading pioneers of nutritional medicine – Dr Carl Pfeiffer and Dr Abram Hoffer. Then in 1984 he founded the Institute for Optimum Nutrition with his mentor, Dr Linus Pauling, the only doctor ever to win two individual Nobel Prizes. These are some of the accolades he has received:

> If there's one person who's done more than anyone to transform the perception of food in Britain, it's the visionary nutritionist Patrick Holford. – Independent

> He [Patrick Holford] is fastidious in conducting legitimate research to back his claims. – Times, Body and Soul

> Holford may be regarded as outside of the mainstream, but increasingly his approach is being fostered in conventional medicine. – Guardian

> Patrick Holford is one of the world's leading authorities on new approaches to health and nutrition. – Daily Mail

> Finally, here are some of the reviews of his book *The Alzheimer's Prevention Plan*:

> This is an outstandingly interesting book on a subject which is perforce of growing importance to all of us as the expectation of life increases. We need to achieve not only extra years, but years of extra enjoyment. This book explains in eminently readable form that mental deterioration with age is for the vast majority not inevitable, but we have to work at keeping both mentally and physically fit. It is true that there are genetic factors involved, but by sensible physical and mental exercise coupled with attention to an optimum diet which Patrick Holford explains, we can significantly reduce the mental deterioration of age. – Dr John Marks, life fellow and former director of medical studies, University of Cambridge

> It is time we woke up to the fact that Alzheimer's is a preventable disease, not an inevitable part of ageing. Just as there is nothing inevitable about heart disease, there is nothing inevitable about Alzheimer's disease. Patrick Holford's book takes up this theme with zest and is to be greatly welcomed. Each of us needs to know that Alzheimer's can be prevented and governments need to recognise this too. The lesson to be learnt from this book is that we can help ourselves and our loved ones by starting to modify the way we live so that our chance of developing diseases like heart disease and Alzheimer's disease is greatly reduced. But we need to begin now; the disease process begins early in life, and already in our thirties some of us have signs of Alzheimer's disease in the brain, just as we have atherosclerosis in our blood vessels. Get started! – Professor David Smith, Oxford University

> We are on the threshold of an exciting new era in preventative medicine, and Patrick Holford's comprehensive prevention plan for Alzheimer's is a sensible step forward.

– Dr Andrew McCaddon MD, GP and honorary research fellow of the University of Wales College of Medicine

I have quoted these reviews so you can see there are some real "medical heavy weights" who endorse Patrick Holford's Alzheimer's prevention plan. If it wasn't based on good science these people would never have written such supportive comments. Incidentally, some very recent studies have shown that using omega 3 supplements and combining them with B vitamins produced incredible outcomes by reducing brain shrinkage in the early stages of Alzheimer's. If I tell you that Patrick Holford was recommending omega 3 supplements over ten years ago and that they are a key part of his book, it will give you an insight into how incredible it really is and how it really can help people prevent Alzheimer's.

Cancer

In 2019 there were 18 million cancer cases in the world and 9.5 million deaths. In the UK the figures were 370,000 cases and 166,000 deaths. By 2040 worldwide cases are projected to rise to about 27.5 million with 16.4 million deaths. For the UK the numbers are estimated to be around 450,000 and 200,000 respectively. There are over 200 different types of cancer, but in the UK, the "big four" – breast, bowel, lung and prostate – account for 53% of all cases.

Cancer – the medical approach

Medicine has a three-pronged traditional treatment regime for cancer, comprising surgery, radiotherapy and chemotherapy, but newer options like immunotherapy and hormone therapy are also slowly gaining traction. It also has screening programmes for the earlier detection of certain key cancers like breast and bowel. As far as the causes of cancer are concerned, medicine simply says that most types "are not fully understood", and there are just a few well-known exceptions like lung cancer and smoking. It does, however, list a number of factors that can increase the risk. For bowel cancer, these include a diet low in fibre and high in red and processed meats, smoking, low levels of exercise, excessive alcohol and obesity; it is also age-related with possible inherited gene risks. Medicine does not seriously promote lifestyle changes for healthy people to help them avoid developing cancers. It simply relies just on disease treatment once the cancers occur.

So, how well do conventional cancer treatments work and are there cures? This is what WebMD has to say: "When you have cancer, cure may be the word you want to hear more than any other. It's also a word most doctors won't say. Unlike other diseases, cancer has its own language. There's no cure for it, but there are treatments that may be able to cure some people of some cancers." Cancer treatments are usually assessed only in terms of five- or ten-year survival rates. As an example, looking at five-year survival rates, a woman who dies five years and one day after she was first diagnosed with breast cancer would be classed as a success and would be included in the survival rate, while another woman surviving for 4 years and 364 days would not be included. On average, for all cancers, 50% of patients live beyond ten years. Survival, however, depends significantly on the type of cancer. Skin, testicular and thyroid cancers have low overall death rates, while others like pancreatic and brain cancers have a very high rate. However, even ten-year survival rates do not mean patients are in long-term remission. They may still die from cancer or some of the treatment side effects well before their normal life expectancy. Incredibly, there are no statistics that measure longer term and full-term survival rates which is what most patients want. So, there is no evidence whether cancer treatments work for this or whether they mainly extend shorter term lives.

Because medicine just treats cancers rather than trying to prevent them, it has also meant that the number of cases has continued to rise significantly. Fifty years ago, 1 in 4 people developed cancer at some point during their life, but now the number has almost doubled to 1 in 2. This increase is affecting all age groups, so clearly lifestyle and environmental factors must be playing a significant part. The increase is not just age-related.

Surgery usually provides most of the benefits of conventional cancer treatments even though it can also cause some of the fatal outcomes. The majority of the serious treatment side effects and deaths, however, are caused by chemotherapy and radiotherapy. I will concentrate just on chemotherapy, but should add that radiotherapy also produces a range of similar outcomes. A 2008 study showed that after cancer treatments were given to seriously ill patients, 27% of deaths were due to the side effects of the chemotherapy, and not because of the cancer itself. The National Confidential Enquiry into Patient Outcome and Death investigated more than 600 deaths within 30 days of receiving chemotherapy. The study also concluded that 19% of those who died should not even have been given chemotherapy and that doctors should take more care when using it. This is even more shocking, given the minimal benefits of many chemotherapy treatments that have already been examined in previous sections.

Chemotherapy works by using toxic chemicals that simply kill cancer cells. Unfortunately, these chemicals also kill normal healthy cells and because of this, chemotherapy has to be used for just a few weeks, then stopped to allow the body to partly recover from the damage before starting treatment again. Unfortunately, during this period, the remaining cancer cells can mutate which can then prevent the drugs from working – just like bacteria learn how to resist antibiotics. This doesn't happen all the time but it is one of the reasons why many chemotherapy treatments fail. They can also increase the spread of the cancer to other organs and different parts of the body as well as making it more destructive. So, as well as helping to save some patients, chemotherapy is also the cause of death in others. The drugs also cause devastating and well-known side effects like hair loss, nausea, fatigue and diarrhoea, as well as seriously disabling fertility.

There is, however, a significant and fatal side effect which is not widely publicised. This happens because chemotherapy also kill the body's immune cells, leaving patients vulnerable to potentially fatal infections like E. coli, MRSA, septicaemia, influenza, pneumonia and COVID-19. It has been estimated that about 10% of chemo patients die from such infections, meaning that in the UK the death toll is around 15,000 each year. Many patients are never told about this. One of the reasons is that it is the infection that is recorded as the official cause of death. The fact that the original cause was the chemotherapy drugs is never recorded on the death certificate. So, a drug treatment regime that, on average, achieves just over a 2% increase in five-year survival rates also causes this long list of other side effects and deaths. Do the benefits exceed the long list of serious side effects? The next paragraph gives an indication.

In 2012 a group of senior cancer specialists met in Switzerland to assess cancer treatments. The question they wanted to analyse and answer was "Are we winning the war on cancer?" This is their summary verdict: "The conclusion was, in general, no. Despite the introduction of hundreds of new anti-cancer drugs, including advanced therapies (so-called magic bullets) aimed at particular weapons in the enemy's armamentarium, the consensus was that, for most forms of cancer, enduring disease-free responses are rare, and cures even rarer. Notable exceptions include some forms of leukaemia and certain types of breast cancer, testicular cancer and particular tumours – e.g. colorectal – which are amenable in early stages to complete surgical removal." This is a sobering judgement by a group of cancer experts which – apart from a few real successes – shows the limited benefit of most cancer treatments.

One of the shocking reasons many drugs have such minimal outcomes is the way that many are now being assessed in clinical trials. Question: what are the only two outcomes that cancer patients really care about? Quite simply, will the drug provide a cure, or at least extend their life expectancy? However, over half of cancer drug trials don't measure either of these outcomes. Instead, they only measure a surrogate outcome, like a reduction in tumour size. You might believe that if a drug really does reduce the size of a tumour then surely it must save lives. But this is not necessarily correct. For example, many cancers spread to other parts of the body and it is frequently these that cause actual deaths and not the original tumour even though it can be made to reduce in size. The drug industry has "persuaded" regulators to approve drugs based on such surrogate end points and around two-thirds of all recent cancer drugs have been approved in this way. The drug industry only cares about maximising profits and if they had measured life expectancy in the trials rather than tumour size, the drugs would probably never have been approved. Many people would consider this to be fraud, but because the regulators really do allow it to happen legally, it can only be called "fraud". This is before taking in to account the devastating and life-taking side effects of the drugs. Even worse is the fact that around 45% of all the other drugs that have been recently approved for nearly every other disease are also based on some form of surrogate end point. This is just one more devastating example of the way Big Pharma effectively controls both regulators and medicine so it can simply continue to maximise profits.

I will return to survival rates shortly, but first I want to look at cancer screening programmes. The two main screening programmes are for breast and bowel cancer, and whilst prostate cancer doesn't have a specific programme, many men are given the PSA test which performs a similar screening function. Like most medical interventions, screening programmes were started with the very best of intentions. The logic seemed clear. The sooner a cancer was detected and treated, then surely the odds of a successful outcome would increase significantly. Unfortunately, things haven't turned out as expected. It was many years after screening was first introduced that researchers were able to look at actual patient outcomes and to compare those people undergoing screening against those in control groups who weren't screened. Taking bowel cancer as an example, there have been four large studies in the USA, Denmark, Sweden and the UK involving over 300,000 people. In the UK the claim for screening is that it reduces the risk of dying from the disease by 16% and the other studies show similar results. So, on the face of it, bowel cancer screening appears to have a significant benefit. But all is not what it seems to be. We have already looked in detail at how the benefits of drugs and medical procedures can be made to appear impressive by using the statistical "scam" of relative risk. So, let me tell you what the results of the studies really found.

They found that if 1,000 people are screened for bowel cancer, only one of them will benefit and see their cancer cured. I'll bet that doesn't impress you as much as the claim that screening reduces the risk of death by 16%. Let me explain. What the studies showed was that over a ten-year follow-up period, for every 1,000 people, eight died from bowel cancer in the group that were not screened, and seven died from it in the group that were screened. Thus, the overall benefit on cancer survival is just 1 in every 1,000. (The 16% figure quoted by the NHS is the percentage difference between the figures of eight and seven.)

Okay, so you may be thinking even though this is not as impressive as I may have imagined, saving 1 in 1,000 people is surely still worthwhile. But this is where the second part of the "deception" kicks in. The studies which led to bowel cancer screening being widely introduced in many countries quoted only the change in mortality from the cancer itself. But we have already explored in detail the concept of overall mortality in such studies. This means you look at how many people died *in total* in those screened against those not screened, not just at cancer deaths in isolation. Why is the figure for overall mortality so important in studies like this? Well, when other researchers subsequently looked at all the data, they found that almost exactly the same number of people died in each group. So, whilst more people died from cancer if they had not been screened, more people died from something else, if they had been screened. This means that as near as anyone can measure, not one life is saved by bowel cancer screening. The people screened or not screened may die of different things, but overall, the death rates are effectively the same. So, what could explain the extra deaths in those screened? Well, those screened who test positive on the initial screening are retested, and if this is still positive then a colonoscopy is invariably performed. But this procedure has its risks. Most gastroenterologists will have personal experience of patients who have developed serious medical conditions or who died as a result of the procedure, from complications such as hyponatraemia or cardiac arrhythmias. In addition, the stress, fear and anxiety of the whole process even when cancer is not found can profoundly affect the health of the patients involved in many ways – for example, it could contribute to triggering a heart attack.

Very similar results emerged for breast cancer screening which was first introduced in 1988. Once real patient data started to emerge and the clinical trials were completed, a meta-analysis showed there was little difference in overall mortality between those patients who were screened and those in the control group. It is true there were slightly fewer deaths from breast cancer for those patients screened, but the numbers were even smaller than in the bowel cancer trials. Only one extra patient in 2,000 survived. However, ten healthy women who would not have developed cancer were being treated unnecessarily with surgery and chemotherapy or radiotherapy, and a further 200 who tested false positively were also suffering from stress, anxiety and fear with potentially serious outcomes like heart disease and stroke. An article in the British Medical Journal in 2009, which endorsed the meta-analysis findings also made the following statement: "We believe that if policy makers had had the knowledge we now have when they decided to introduce screening 20 years ago, when nobody had published data on over-diagnosis or on the imbalance between numbers of prevented deaths and numbers of false positive screening results and the psychological consequences of the false alarms, we probably would not have had mammography screening."

Given all the negative evidence that is now available, and the logical claim that if this information had been available in 1988 screening programmes would probably not have been introduced, then why are the breast and bowel cancer screening programmes still in place? Let's go back to the beginning. These programmes were introduced with the best of intentions. Everyone believed they would work and save lives; the logic appeared compelling. The devastating figures and results only emerged years later when long-term study results started to filter through. By that stage the programmes were well established. Imagine the predicament of both medicine and governments around the world who had promoted these programmes so assiduously. Could they really admit they had got it so wrong, squandered so much money and resources, and subjected so many people to unnecessary and invasive medical interventions for no real overall benefit? Whatever the motives and rationale of those making such decisions, the official policy on breast and bowel cancer screening remains unchanged, and despite all the contradictory evidence, these programmes will undoubtedly continue unabated.

Incidentally, the screening programmes provide additional evidence that helps to expose a major flaw within much of medicine. Researchers and doctors seem fixated almost exclusively on the benefits of treatments, and this means they continually underestimate the damage their procedures and treatments can inflict on patients. It should have been possible to predict that bowel cancer screening, for example, would have caused many unnecessary and risky colonoscopies that may have negated the benefits of screening. But it appears no one even considered it before embarking on such a massive public programme.

Let's return to the subject of cancer survival rates for a moment and I'll let you in on a "little secret". Five- and ten-year survival rates are based on how long people survive from the date of their first official diagnosis of a cancer until the day they die from it. Most people who are screened have an earlier diagnosis than they otherwise would have had. Thus, a woman may live for six years after breast cancer detected during screening (even if the treatment she is given doesn't work). But if the cancer was only discovered two years later when the woman discovered a developing lump herself (and her treatment also didn't work), she would only live for four years from that date. In this example, the woman would die on exactly the same day. If she had been screened, however, her treatment would be judged successful; if she hadn't been screened, it would be judged a failure. So, even though early diagnosis in some cancers really can increase the possibility that treatments will work better and thus extend life expectancy, the other outcome (regardless of any treatment benefits) is that it will also automatically increase cancer survival times. But, of course, this part of the increase in survival is not real; it is just an illusion. Could this be one of the reasons why medicine and governments are so keen to continue with the screening programmes?

The sad fact is, with some specific exceptions, most conventional cancer treatments have minimal benefits and serious and often devastating side effects. This is why, in 2012, Lord Saatchi campaigned for, and introduced, his Medical Innovation Bill for its first reading in the House of Lords. Its aim was to allow doctors to try other treatments for rare and deadly diseases rather than use just the conventional treatments that were mandated, even though they were often of limited benefit. All this happened after he devastatingly saw his wife Josephine die a protracted and painful death from ovarian cancer. Ovarian is one of the most lethal cancers, and around 80% of patients will eventually die from it, although some of those diagnosed early can survive for five or more years, while cancers diagnosed at later stages are almost always fatal. He argued that the rigid and legally enforceable medical guidelines meant no doctor dared to risk trying any other treatment even though they knew their patients were going to die from the conventional treatment they had to use. He told his fellow peers: "All cancer deaths are wasted lives. Scientific knowledge has not advanced by one centimetre as a result of all these deaths, because the current law requires the deceased receive only the standard procedure – the endless repetition of a failed experiment." Initially, the UK government said it would oppose the bill, but eventually they decided to support it, as did the UK's chief medical officer and scientific advisor and Britain's top judges. However, it was opposed by other medical organisations and over 100 doctors, who wrote a damning letter to the Times ridiculing the bill and claiming that only those treatments and drugs approved by clinical trials should ever be used. They had obviously overlooked the view of the forefather of the randomised clinical trial, Sir Austin Bradford Hill who said, "Any belief that the controlled trial is the only way to study therapeutic efficacy, would mean not that the pendulum had swung too far, but that it had come right off its hook." Did these doctors not know or more likely had simply "forgotten" that huge swathes of medical treatments have never been subject to these types of trials?

Despite all of this, key Conservative ministers and leaders of the Labour party agreed that they would permit an open debate which would allow MPs to independently decide whether Lord Saatchi's bill should be approved by parliament. However, at the time, the Conservatives and Liberal Democrats had formed a coalition government and under the terms of their agreement, the Lib Dems could veto any proposed law. Incredibly, they did veto the open debate and Lord Saatchi's bill was effectively thrown into the long grass, never to be considered again. Let me explain why this decision was one of the greatest tragedies in medical history. We have seen that it really can take decades to get bad ideas out of medicine. Only when medical dogma is seriously challenged can major treatment improvements be made. Allowing doctors to try new treatments that otherwise would never be tested really would result in new life-changing developments. Even though some of them would undoubtedly fail, others really would improve treatments and life expectancy and even possible cures. The doctors who opposed the bill claimed that the "unproven treatments" would threaten patients' health and lives even though their so-called proven treatments simply resulted in death for virtually all late-stage ovarian cancers and 80% of its early detected cases. Shouldn't those patients with such cancers have a right to try alternative treatments if they wanted to, rather than just having to accept death?

Finally, most patients with terminal cancers are given treatments like chemotherapy and radiotherapy that are claimed to extend life expectancy. But, did you know that most doctors would not take any such medical treatments if they were given a terminal diagnosis. For many years, making this public knowledge has been taboo in the medical world, although there have been a few exceptions. In one 1996 poll, around half of German specialists admitted they would not undergo the treatments they recommended to their patients. Many other doctors have since confirmed that they and most of their colleagues would do the same. They would simply walk away and enjoy what is left of their lives. In 2012 Ken Murray, professor of family medicine at the University of Southern California, published an essay which argued that "most practising doctors would not put themselves through the 'life-saving' interventions that are big on promises, but small on success, and involve great pain and distress." Dr Martin Scurr who has written articles for the Daily Mail for many years also wrote a long article about his own views and that of nearly all his colleagues about terminal cancer treatments. He said, "Should I discover tomorrow that I have advanced life-threatening cancer, I won't go rushing to the doctors for a heavily invasive course of medical treatment. No, I will shut up my London surgery, head to my home in Norfolk, stock up on gin and tonic and have a jolly good time until I meet my end. Like most doctors, I understand that much of the care we offer patients who have serious, life-threatening illnesses is ultimately futile. Worse, it can involve many months of gruelling treatments that might possibly extend the length of one's life, but do nothing for its quality."

Another group of doctors wrote a similar article and were "attacked" by the General Medical Council. Why? Even if only half of all terminally ill patients were aware of all this information and decided not to take treatments, then a significant number of doctors who normally carry them out would effectively be out of work. Summarising this section, anyone taking terminal cancer treatments would go through months of devastating chemo-induced sickness and agony probably unable to do anything enjoyable with their family and friends. Those who decide not to can often live a relatively normal life for a good part of their remaining time. They can enjoy their favourite foods, go on holidays with family and friends and maybe make their greatest dreams a reality. Only towards the end do they need to take things like powerful painkillers.

But are these sorts of decisions the only thing that people with cancer can make? Are there no other options that can help with this devastating disease? Well, as you will now see, lifestyle medicine really can help to significantly reduce the risk of developing cancer in the first place and avoid having to make such sad decisions. It can also help those who have already developed cancer. Get ready to have your spirits lifted.

Cancer – the lifestyle medicine approach

When you look at the devastating facts and statistics surrounding cancer incidence and conventional medical treatments and outcomes, doesn't prevention sound a much more appealing option? But can cancer really be prevented? This is the million-dollar question.

You may, however, be surprised to learn that everyone has cancer cells, and even healthy adults have several millions of them in their bodies every moment of the day. These are caused by faulty DNA during cell reproduction or because a cell is damaged in some way. Faulty DNA can occur when cells reproduce, especially when you consider that each time a cell divides it has to copy the 3 billion DNA "letters" that make up its genetic code – a mammoth task to do error free. If the body is exposed to things like tobacco smoke and certain chemicals, this can significantly increase the risk of such faulty DNA. The body has nevertheless, over millions of years of evolution, developed various types of immune response that can help prevent this from happening. Even if it does, the immune system can help prevent it from developing into individual cancer cells and also prevent such cells from dividing which prevent cancer itself from developing. For example, antioxidants can help prevent some types of damage to DNA. Amazingly, each cell also has "proofreading machines" that scan the DNA code, looking for faults and calling on "molecular repair teams" to fix any damage that's found. If this doesn't work, then the cell can be forced to "commit suicide". Even if all these initial immunity options fail, the natural immune system can then simply kill the cancer cell by using its natural killer cells and T cells. The key factor for all this to work, however, is that our natural immune system needs to be operating very efficiently and some of the best ways this can be achieved will be explored shortly. If the immune system has been significantly compromised, then cancer can occur.

What do conventional research studies say about whether cancer can be prevented? A well-publicised study from 2015 by scientists at Johns Hopkins University stated that two-thirds of cancers were down solely to chance or bad luck; with only one-third down to lifestyle and genes. This, however, flies in the face of a great deal of evidence to the contrary. Even the conservative Cancer Research UK says that over 40% of cancers are preventable. Other experts confidently put the figure at around 50%, while a more recent high-profile study by researchers at Stony Brook University, New York, stated that up to 90% of cancers were due to environmental and lifestyle factors and thus preventable. A study involving 45,000 identical twins with completely different incidences of cancer concluded that at least 80% of cases were due to what you do in your life and not what you inherit genetically. Very recent information from the American Cancer Society (ACS) accepts that genes cause less than 5% of cancer risk and that 95% is caused by epigenetic factors like diet, smoking, environmental pollutants, drugs, stress, obesity and physical inactivity.

In trying to decide which of these are more likely to be correct, remember one key thing. Apart from a few very specific types of cancer, such as lung cancer associated with smoking, no one in medicine understands what the real causes are. So, if the causes are unknown, how can anyone make a claim that they can't be prevented? Lung cancer and smoking is a classic example. The link between them is obvious today, and experts can confidently label smoking as the main cause, but this wasn't always the case. In the 1930s and 1940s doctors actually recommended that people with anxiety should smoke because cigarettes really did help calm the nerves. Today it is quite shocking to think medicine was effectively prescribing cigarettes. However, doctors involved in lung cancer at that time simply did not know about the smoking connection and just like many other cancers today, the cause would simply have been put down to "chance". But, as knowledge progresses, what was decreed "unpreventable" before, suddenly becomes preventable today. If everyone gave up smoking, all these lung cancer cases and deaths would disappear.

The researchers at Stony Brook University and the American Cancer Society who claim that up to 90% and 95% respectively of cancers are caused by lifestyle and environmental factors have some sound evidence to back up their claims. For example, Stoney Brook concludes that cancer incidence is too high to be explained away by random and, therefore, unpreventable cell mutations: "The rates of mutation accumulation by intrinsic processes are not sufficient to account for the observed cancer risks." They also point to the large and consistent body of evidence that shows how immigrants moving from countries with low cancer incidence to countries with high cancer incidence soon develop the same higher tumour rate, strongly suggesting the causes are driven by environment and lifestyle, rather than biological or genetic factors. The fact that different countries and regions have different cancer rates is further tangible evidence.

The UK government set up the "100,000 Genomes Project" and provided significant funding in order to try to find the genetic causes of many rare diseases and cancers. But the Stony Brook research and ACS information shows the project is unlikely to help the majority of cancer sufferers, because genes are not the main cause. Trying to tackle cancer by focusing on eradicating gene mutations is, as Dr Ira Goodman puts it, "a multi-billion-dollar wild goose chase after the wrong target." Kate Allen from World Cancer Research Fund commenting on the project said, "It's not true that most cases of cancer 'just happen', and that there is nothing we can do to prevent them occurring. Our research has shown that many cancers are caused by external factors, and that there are changes that we can all make to our lifestyles to significantly reduce our risk of cancer."

Paul Pharoah, professor of cancer epidemiology, University of Cambridge, said of the Stony Brook research, "These findings do not have any implications for cancer treatment, but they do tell us that most cancers would be preventable if we knew all of the extrinsic risk factors." But here lies the problem. The risk factors and causes of most cancers are not actively prioritised for research for all the reasons previously examined. Most research is controlled and paid for by the drug industry, which is looking for treatments for cancer and not for the definitive causes. Quite simply, no money can be made from researching causes and these could also pose a real threat to the need for cancer drugs. Of all the treatments for the major diseases, cancer drugs are the most expensive and the most profitable. They represent 16% in monetary value of worldwide drug sales.

So, there is very strong evidence that a majority of cancers could be prevented – we can debate whether the figure is 50% or 95% or anywhere in between – but we are not likely to find out how to achieve this from conventional medicine. Medicine never acts unless there is the so-called definitive clinical proof, and so they will continue just to treat cancer rather than wholeheartedly recommend prevention. But you don't need to wait decades, hoping medicine might eventually come up with the answers to prevention, because this is where lifestyle medicine comes into its own. There are many genuine clues as to what is really causing cancer, even though the final "definitive proof" is not available. The real beauty of lifestyle medicine is that you are not going to be harmed by it. Minimising your exposure to toxic chemicals and pollution, and improving your diet, for example, pose no risk, and in fact are going to benefit your overall health and help prevent other diseases, as well as almost certainly reducing your risk of developing cancer.

I'll give just one example. Bisphenol A (BPA) is a chemical found in plastic bottles and food packaging. It has been implicated in several diseases including breast and prostate cancer, although I should add that this, unsurprisingly, is denied by the plastic manufacturers. The lack of definitive proof means governments can't or won't take action to ban it.

Nevertheless, concentrations of BPA have been found in cancer tumours and there is other evidence linking it to cancer. Limiting your exposure to BPA won't do you any harm and the odds are very good that it will reduce your risk of cancer – so why not do it? Why wait for 50 years before medicine and governments finally get their act together?

The seven key lifestyle factors that have been examined in detail all lie at the heart of the lifestyle approach to preventing cancer, so I won't reiterate them all again. Instead, here are just a few important examples of lifestyle factors that specifically help prevent cancer and radically improve the natural immune system.

Many studies show that cruciferous vegetables, like broccoli, Brussel sprouts, cauliflower, cabbage and kale, really can help to prevent cancer due to their special antioxidants and also because they can improve the microbiome which plays a significant part in our immune system.

Obesity increases the risk of many major cancers by an average of around 15 to 20%. These range from 80% for kidney, liver and stomach cancer, to 10% for breast and thyroid with many more in between. We have seen in detail how obesity can be prevented or reversed by a low carb, low GL diet. This lifestyle diet really can solve obesity and, therefore, significantly reduce cancer cases.

A recent French study showed that eating more organic foods reduced the risk of developing cancer by 25% because they have minimal levels of the dangerous pesticides and herbicides that are used in industrial agriculture. These can significantly increase the risk of faulty DNA as can many of the other chemicals already explored in detail.

Exercise can reduce the risk of many major cancers, like breast and colon, by an average of 20% as confirmed by the NHS. It can also increase survival times for those with cancer by up to 50% depending on the type. Key vitamins and minerals like vitamin C, vitamin D and selenium also play an important role in cancer prevention.

Sugar has been linked to cancer for many decades. But while the scientific evidence that it can cause cancer and also speed up tumour growth continues to grow, there are parts of medicine that still dispute such a link. All I can say is that lifestyle medicine absolutely lists sugar as a major cause and you would do well to restrict its use to lower your cancer risk as well as all the other diseases like diabetes and obesity where its link is indisputable. Some experts and organisations do recommend replacing sugar with artificial sweeteners, like aspartame, but unfortunately, as well as affecting many other diseases they also affect cancer. New French research published in PLOS Medicine confirms this risk and shows they can cause a 22% increase in breast cancer cases.

There are, of course, many more vital factors, but I can't cover all of them. There are, however, two books that contain detailed information on how to minimise your risk of cancer by adopting a healthy lifestyle. We have already seen some of the work of the nutritionist Patrick Holford; his book *Say No to Cancer* would be an excellent choice. For anyone who has been diagnosed with cancer and who wants to try lifestyle options, the book *The Cancer Revolution* is another option.

Finally, I want to give you just one example of how effective lifestyle medicine can be, not just in the prevention of cancer, but in its treatment. This involves the work of Dr Patrick Kingsley. Dr Kingsley qualified from St. Bartholomew's Hospital in London in 1965 after which he spent time in post-graduate training, working in the pharmaceutical industry and as a GP. In 1981 he started his own private practice in nutritional and environmental medicine. Dr Kingsley's main expertise was in the fields of cancer and multiple sclerosis, although he also developed lifestyle-based protocols for other diseases including diabetes, asthma and cardiovascular disease. Dr Kingsley described himself as different to most other doctors because of his obsession with understanding why people get disease. Even at medical school while his fellow students were simply learning by rote all about the symptoms of disease and which drugs could be used to treat them, he never stopped wondering why people got the diseases in the first place. Of course, he never learnt anything about this from his tutors; they had no interest in that sort of thing. When he became a GP, he started finding out what was known about the real causes of disease. With the agreement of some of his patients, he then started "prescribing" lifestyle changes alongside conventional medical treatments. The success of these surprised not just himself but his patients. After building up his knowledge over four years, he decided he would set up his own private practice, so he could devote himself entirely to using lifestyle changes to treat disease. From that day in 1981 he never used a single drug to treat any of his patients.

His results speak for themselves. While medicine claims around a 55% survival rate for cancer treatment, Dr Kingsley achieved a 90% success rate. He treated around 5,000 patients and 4,500 survived. What makes these figures even more truly remarkable is the fact many of his patients had been given terminal cancer diagnoses and others had undergone conventional cancer treatment which had either not worked, or the cancer had initially cleared only to return at a later date. So, essentially, many of his patients were beyond any conventional treatment and he was their last hope. So, how did Dr Kingsley achieve such remarkable, indeed near miraculous results? The first stage was to conduct a comprehensive medical history with his patient, often going back to childhood. This was designed to look for clues as to the causes of their cancer. He described this process as "medical detective work". He usually recommended other close family members be in attendance as quite often they would be able to add very relevant information that the patient themselves may not have realised was important. This might include some deep or subconscious emotional problem. Some of the questions he asked may seem bizarre but they all had a purpose. For example:

- Do you have metal fillings in your teeth and if so, how many? (Mercury is implicated in some cancers.)
- Do you have headaches? (Migraines can be caused by food intolerances and these may be subtly involved in cancer.)
- Do you suffer from indigestion? (Problems with gut health can lead to a compromised immune system.)

There were many dozens of such questions which helped Dr Kingsley build up a comprehensive picture of the patient and each and every issue which could possibly have contributed to their cancer. He usually ended up with several probable causes. It was impossible to tell which of these factors was the most important, of course, so he had to tackle and resolve all of them. But the one thing that was present in many patients was a serious emotional problem, like a dominating or coercive family member which he had to help resolve. His treatments involved most of the lifestyle factors that have already been examined, although his knowledge and detail of the key factors was incredible. This sums up his treatment regime that produced such remarkable results.

One key fact is that some of the vitamin treatments he used had to be done intravenously. This particularly applied to vitamin C which was one of his key treatments and the significant amounts needed could not be achieved just by taking supplements orally. He never used any conventional treatments or drugs. He did, however, use his conventional medical training to carry out some very sophisticated medical tests that showed the progress that was being made in treating the cancer. This was not just to reassure himself that he was doing the right things, but the results would also demonstrate to the patient that the treatment was working. This was vital because maintaining a positive emotional outlook throughout the treatment process was a vital part of its success.

When he retired, Dr Kingsley wrote a book and set up a website hoping to get the message out about his incredibly successful treatment regimes, not just for cancer but also for multiple sclerosis. He wrote to the General Medical Council and several medical schools inviting them to look at his results. Sadly, not one of them responded. Several years later he died. I have no doubt that he must have been saddened and devastated by the fact no one in medicine had any interest in his treatments, even though they could have helped millions of patients. I had been aware of his remarkable work and incredible success for some time, so it was doubly devastating to learn of his death and also to find out that the medical establishment had totally ignored his work. Over 9 million people die from cancer each year. The medical profession was simply not prepared to look at Dr Kingsley's evidence. It defies any logic.

Dr Kingsley's book is titled *The New Medicine*, but in reality, as he acknowledges, it is not really that new. It has been practised by many doctors all over the world, especially since the middle of the last century. In fact, Hippocrates was probably the first person to suggest this approach to medicine. It is he who said, "Let food be thy medicine, and medicine thy food." But as true as all this is, no one has ever achieved the same remarkable success as Patrick Kingsley. He was a true genius. Is it too much to hope that one day his work may be recognised for the medical breakthrough it represents and the millions of lives it could save?

Other diseases

Clearly, I cannot cover every disease in this book, but lifestyle medicine really can help with nearly all of them including prevention and cure. I would strongly advise another Patrick Holford book: *Good Medicine: Safe, Natural Ways to Solve Over 75 Common Health Problems*. This includes a wide range of diseases like Parkinson's, chronic fatigue, indigestion, asthma and Crohn's disease.

Here is a short summary of just two more alarming health issues. Infertility, affecting both men and women, has been escalating alarmingly over the last 50 years and is still continuing. It is projected to become a devastating crisis in most developed nations. A meta-analysis of data between 1973 and 2011 showed there had been a 59% decline in sperm counts in men in North America, Europe, Australia and New Zealand and if the rate of this increase does not change, then by around 2050 sperm counts would be zero thus imperilling the future of the human race.

Medicine's answer to infertility is IVF treatment. However, assisted reproductive therapy has several major problems (all the figures quoted are from 2012):

- About 80% of the eggs produced by the drug treatments have chromosomal defects.
- One in ten babies has birth defects.
- Women undergoing IVF have a subsequent 350% increase in ovarian cancer risk.
- The success rate for IVF is 20%.
- The miscarriage rate is 25%.

Yet, there is a natural method of treating infertility developed by the UK charity Foresight Preconception. It has:

- a 90% success rate
- a 3% miscarriage rate
- to date, a zero birth defect rate

These figures are all the more remarkable because many of the women had already undergone conventional IVF treatment without success. How does it work? It simply gives guidance on diet, allergy, environmental pollutants, supplements and other lifestyle issues that promote improved fertility and good health in both men and women and, as unlikely as all this might seem, the proof, as they say, is in the results. I won't lament about why most women will never get to know about this unique and highly successful natural treatment protocol and how they will be deprived of the one thing they most want in life – a baby. Just remember IVF treatment and research is a huge global business. It uses drugs and medical equipment galore, and employs tens, if not hundreds, of thousands of people. Need I say more? Foresight only treats, at most, a few hundred very lucky couples each year. If it tried to aggressively promote its success, then it would almost certainly be attacked and discredited.

Finally, I'll summarise the epidemic of childhood diseases. Sixty years ago, very few UK children were classed by medicine as having a "diagnosable health condition". Now the figure for children under the age of 16 in the UK is around 50%. No, it isn't a misprint: 50%, and this excludes those children who are "merely" overweight. When I was that age, I can't remember any childhood friend who had asthma, or behavioural problems like ADHD, or mental illness, or a peanut allergy, or autism, or indeed any of the other problems that would today probably come under the banner of special needs or even obesity. Everyone I knew was simply healthy. Something sinister and incredibly frightening has been occurring in the last 60 years. Approximately 21% of children aged 11 are now obese, 6% have ADHD, 4% are autistic, 10% have a diagnosable mental disease, 3% have an anxiety disorder, and 9% have asthma. Other diseases like type 2 diabetes, cancer and Crohn's disease are also part of this continuing disease explosion.

This epidemic of childhood diseases is quite simply a potential time bomb that has the capacity to destroy western civilisation. Sadly, nothing can change unless medicine, governments, regulators and charities unite and demand a change that puts disease prevention as the key, but as we have seen throughout the book, the pharmaceutical industry effectively controls all of them and so nothing will happen. There is one other thing that at some point might hopefully occur. How many of today's parents know that half of all children have at least one chronic disease that could affect their entire lives and that will almost certainly reduce their life expectancy? Very few. The real likelihood is that, as the epidemics continue, virtually every child will eventually develop these types of disease. If parents ever did understand and were prepared to act in unison, then governments would find it hard to oppose tens of millions of them. Would a major media organisation also expose the truth as this disaster continues to unfold? We can only hope and pray.

One final fact. The disastrous childhood obesity epidemic has led the government to recently announce the introduction of specialist obesity clinics for children as young as two. Some people will think this could be a good thing that will surely help. But every single worldwide attempt (and there have been many) to prevent obesity over the last 30 years has simply failed and this new initiative must also fail because it will not involve prevention. The epidemic will sadly continue.

Infectious diseases

In the nineteenth century, infectious diseases were the main cause of death in westernised countries. In the mid-1800s, deaths from all types of infection started to decline and by 1950 they had plummeted by around 90% to almost 100%.

Infectious diseases – the medical approach

Medicine uses two main treatments for infectious diseases: vaccines and antibiotics. Antiviral drugs are also used for some diseases, although these often have limited benefits as well as many side effects. For those people who develop serious symptoms, hospital critical care is also used. They do not use or recommend any lifestyle options. Vaccination and antibiotics are portrayed as the ultimate achievements of modern medicine. They are credited with eliminating smallpox and significantly reducing the death rates and case numbers for many other diseases. These "facts" are embedded into the psyche not just of medicine, but the vast majority of people on the planet. For anyone who is prepared to examine all the facts, however, a different story emerges.

Every medical student is taught about the history of these treatments which started in the 1800s with the smallpox vaccines. They are taught that at that time, for those diseases for which vaccines were available, the deaths of most children and adults were prevented. However, students are also taught that the diseases for which there were no vaccines or antibiotics at that time – like scarlet fever, typhus, measles, tuberculosis and whooping cough – most deaths were also prevented and that this was simply due to better social conditions. The key fact is that up until around 1950 only four vaccines were available and even two of these were only given to a small specific section of the population like the army. So, for most infectious diseases there were simply no vaccines. Antibiotics also only became more widely available in the late 1940s. So, now you can already see a chink in the armour of the idea that vaccination was the single most important health intervention that had ever been introduced. In terms of the one vital disease outcome – the number of deaths – most diseases had been effectively defeated by 1950 simply by better living conditions, without a single doctor or vaccine ever being involved. To explore this further, I need to explain the history of some of the key vaccines, but first, in graphic detail, I need to explain what life was really like in the 1800s. It is truly shocking and horrific.

We are used to seeing historical dramas that impart a nostalgic and romantic view of the 1800s. For a privileged few people at that time, these dramas may be close to reality, but film makers would not dare to show the reality of the squalid, miserable and shockingly short lives of all the other poor souls who inhabited the slums and tenements of urban conurbations found in most western countries at that time. I apologise in advance for what you are about to read. It may make you feel ill and the descriptions may live with you for a long time, but it is the only way to understand how infectious diseases killed so many people and the truth about how these deadly outcomes were eventually largely overcome simply by better lifestyles.

The Industrial Revolution brought with it an incredible urbanisation of the population. In 1750 about 15% lived in towns but by 1880 this had grown to 80%. The largest city in the western world, London, had 800,000 inhabitants in 1801, but by 1901 this had grown to 7 million. Housing could not accommodate this population explosion. Tenements were created often from old industrial buildings and whole families would live in one or two rooms, most without light, ventilation and any form of sanitary arrangements or water supply. The dwellings, such as they were, intermingled with slaughter houses and industrial factories spewing out dangerous chemicals and air borne pollution. Many tenements were overrun with vermin and even in a hospital, a baby was eaten alive by rats. Human and animal waste, along with industrial and chemical waste, would flow in the streets and ended up in the local streams, lakes and rivers which also happened to be the only source of drinking water. Rotting waste was everywhere. Food was limited, of poor quality and often contaminated. Diseased food was ever present. People were severely malnourished and they were overrun both internally and externally with dangerous bacteria and parasites.

The minimum working day was 12 hours. For most, the work was menial and hard labour. At the end of the working day, people simply fell asleep, exhausted. Children as young as eight were sent down mines. Girls had the job of carrying a tonne of coal to the surface each day via rows of ascending ladders. A creel filled with coal and weighing around 100 pounds was placed on the girls' backs. They carried over 20 such loads each day and were bent double due to the weight. Others worked in factories barely seeing the light of day and carrying out menial and dangerous tasks. There were no health and safety laws, no protective clothes. Factories with unguarded machinery claimed many lives. Cotton and asbestos workers inhaled fine fibres and asbestos dust; their lives shortened considerably by lung diseases. Medicine contributed with unhygienic practices.

The inhuman living conditions, exhaustion, malnourishment, contaminated food and water and dangerous working conditions took their toll. In many tenements, average life expectancy was just 15. This is not a misprint – 15 years. Think on that. One in five babies died within the first few months of life. Around 30% of women who gave birth were killed by puerperal fever due to doctors' contaminated hands. Huge numbers died from uncontrolled bacterial diarrhoea and dehydration. Industrial accidents and industrial diseases were rife. But it was the infectious diseases like cholera, typhoid and scarlet fever that also took many lives at all ages. Once an epidemic started, it spread like a wildfire through the tenement slums. The death rate was incredibly high because in its 7-million-year history, mankind had never faced such devastation and people's natural immune systems were so damaged that even normally mild diseases like measles also turned into killers. Here are a few graphic descriptions of life and death in the slums:

> As we passed along the reeking banks of the sewer the sun shone upon a narrow strip of the water. It appeared the colour of strong green tea, it was more like watery mud than muddy water; and yet we were assured that this was the only water the wretched inhabitants had to drink. As we gazed in horror at it, we saw drains and sewers emptying their filthy contents into it; we saw a whole tier of door less privies in the open road, common to men and women, built over it; we heard bucket after bucket of filth splash into it... – Henry Mayhew (1812–1887), September 1849

> The stenches from the horribly foul cellars with their infernal system of sewerage must needs poison the tenants all the way up to the fifth story... The well-worn rut of the dead wagon and the ambulance to the gate, for the tenants died there like flies in all seasons, and a tenth of its population was always in hospital. – The Tenement House Commission

> For millions, entire lives – albeit often very short ones – were passed in new industrial cities of dreadful night with an all too typical socio pathology; foul housing, often in flooded cellars, gross overcrowding, atmospheric and water supply pollution, overflowing cesspools, contaminated pumps, poverty, hunger, fatigue and abjection everywhere. Such conditions bred rampant sickness of every kind. Appalling neo-natal, infant and child mortality accompanied the abomination of child labour in mines and factories; life expectations were exceedingly low – often under twenty years among the working classes - and everywhere sickness precipitated family breakdown, pauperisation and social crisis. – Written by British historian Roy Porter noted for his work on the history of medicine

> The most deadly feature of the new towns was the close proximity of human beings to each other. The report of a health officer for Darlington in the 1850s found six children, aged between 2 and 17, suffering from smallpox in a one room dwelling shared by their parents and elder brother and uncle. They all slept together on rags on the floor, with no bed. Millions of similar cases could be cited, with conditions getting even worse as disease victims died and their corpses remained rotting among families in single- roomed accommodation for days as the family scraped together the pennies to bury them. – Written by Dorothy Porter from her book *Health, Civilisation and the State*

Of course, not everyone fared so badly. Inhabitants of the wealthier town suburbs led somewhat better lives and life expectancy was higher, as it was for those in rural areas. Nevertheless, average life expectancy for the working class as a whole was still only around 35 years in 1850. Of course, the wealthy could expect to live much longer. Queen Victoria lived to the age of 82, and many others also made it into their seventies and eighties. In fact, if you made it to 65 in 1850, you could expect, on average, to live to the age of 76. Today a 65-year-old could expect to live to 83 on average. This relatively small difference is quite enlightening.

By the mid-1800s there was increasing unease at the plight of the poor. In 1858 the stench from the sewage and other rot was so putrid that even the House of Commons was forced to suspend its sessions. Bold plans were put in place and eventually, over several decades, the great Victorian sewage and fresh water systems came into being along with better housing. Working conditions slowly improved, child labour was curtailed and food became less dangerous. Similar stories played out in other western countries. Quite simply, it was these basic but vitally important improvements in lifestyle and environment that led to the incredible reduction in deaths from infectious diseases.

Smallpox. Smallpox was the first viral disease to be treated with a vaccine, so it is important to briefly examine its history which may surprise and shock you. In the mid-1700s, the first crude vaccine which contained material from a real smallpox lesion was given to healthy people in an attempt to stop them catching the disease. Unfortunately, many of those vaccinated died of smallpox directly due to the vaccine itself, and these victims also acted as a source of new epidemics. It soon fell out of favour. It was Edward Jenner who, in 1796, claimed better success with a vaccine based on cowpox. His work was not universally accepted but like so many inventions it slowly gained traction. In fact, vaccination was made compulsory in England in 1853 with stricter laws passed in 1867. Other countries followed the same draconian route in trying to force most of their populations into vaccination. But after years of mixing different animal viruses and passing them through humans and back into cows again, no one actually knew what was in these so-called vaccines. The simple fact is the vaccines still didn't work well. They were also frequently contaminated and caused diseases such as foot and mouth, jaundice, tuberculosis and syphilis. Here are just four different examples of the vaccine's ineffectiveness.

Official German figures showed that between 1870 and 1885 1 million vaccinated people died from smallpox. An 1871 Lancet article showed that out of 9,300 smallpox patients in London hospitals, 6,800 had been vaccinated. Prussia had the strictest – almost 100% – vaccination levels in Europe, including mandatory revaccination for school children. Despite all of this, in the epidemic of 1871, its mortality from smallpox was higher than in any other northern state. Other countries like Italy and Japan also recorded unprecedented smallpox death rates after successful vaccination campaigns.

Despite the actions taken by the UK government that ensured high vaccination rates, a massive epidemic of smallpox also hit all of England in the early 1870s. The town of Leicester was to play a pivotal role in finding alternative ways to fight the disease. This extract from the Leicester Mercury reflected the feelings of those who had lost faith in vaccination:

> It must strike the reflective observer as rather singular that all the recent smallpox outbreaks have made their appearance among populations where the laws enforcing vaccination have been rigorously and systematically enforced. 96% of births in London are protected by vaccination. May I venture to ask whether medical men who have defended and fostered a medieval procedure which eighty years' experience has demonstrated a disastrous and humiliating failure ought not to feel honourably bound on public grounds to retrace their steps and confess that vaccination, like other once popular prescriptions of inoculation, bleeding and mercurization, is a serious and mischievous blunder.

Laws were initially passed after people refused the vaccine because they could see the negative complications and its poor effectiveness. Many submitted because of the increasingly stringent laws but still were stricken with deadly smallpox epidemics. Then even more people rebelled, but the government took steps to further increase the rate of vaccination by prosecuting parents who refused to have their children vaccinated. The penalties included imprisonment. The people of Leicester were finally motivated to revolt. In great numbers – around 100,000 – they took to the streets to protest. At the time of the demonstration, thousands of prosecutions had already been brought and were continuing to be brought against parents. Leicester's council, which had rigorously enforced the vaccination laws, was replaced by one that opposed compulsory vaccination. By 1887 vaccination rates plummeted to just 10%. What happened? This is an extract from a council report from 1895:

> The last decade has witnessed an extraordinary decrease in vaccination, but nevertheless, the town has enjoyed an almost entire immunity from smallpox, there never having been more than two or three cases at any one time. A new method for which great utility is claimed has been enforced by the sanitary committee of the corporation. As soon as smallpox breaks out, the medical man and the householder are compelled under penalty to at once report the outbreak to the corporation. The smallpox van is ordered and within a few hours the sufferer is safely in the hospital. The family are placed in quarantine in comfortable quarters and the house thoroughly disinfected. The result is that in every instance the disease has been promptly and completely stamped out at paltry expense. Under such a system, the corporation have expressed their opinion that vaccination is unnecessary, as they claim to deal with the disease in a more direct and much more efficacious manner. This, and the widespread belief that death and disease have resulted from the operation of vaccination, may be said to be the foundation upon which the existing opposition to the Acts rests.

Even though it was clear that the Leicester method was superior to vaccination, those who strongly endorsed vaccination believed that the immunity enjoyed by the town was temporary and that sooner or later it would suffer a large smallpox epidemic. They were convinced that a great tragedy was inevitable and that the whole experiment would result in a terrible massacre of unprotected children. Despite such prophesies of doom from the medical profession, the majority of the town's residents remained steadfast. The prophecy that the Leicester residents would eventually be plagued with disaster never did come to pass. In fact, Leicester continued to enjoy better success against smallpox than well-vaccinated towns. Birmingham had four times more deaths in proportion to its population than Leicester, while Mold in Flintshire had 32 times more deaths. Other towns lay between these two extremes.

In 1911 Dr J. W. Hodge published a paper on how smallpox was controlled in Leicester:

> The experience of unvaccinated Leicester is an eye-opener to the people and an eye-sore to the pro-vaccinists the world over. Here is a great manufacturing town having a population of nearly a quarter of a million, which has demonstrated by a crucial test of an experience of more than a quarter of a century, that an unvaccinated population has been far less susceptible to smallpox and far less afflicted by that disease since it abandoned vaccination than it was at a time when 95% of its births were vaccinated and its adult population revaccinated.

Many other towns eventually started to follow Leicester's example, and vaccination rates declined. Concurrent with these changes, mortality from smallpox also started to fall across the country. In the 14 years from 1933 to 1946 there were only 28 deaths in a population of 40 million. By this time only one-third of the population was vaccinated, and in 1948 "mandatory" vaccination was also abandoned in England. The reality is that smallpox, which killed so many in the early 1800s, was associated with the deadly way of life at that time. The atrocious social conditions were a key reason it took so many lives and spread in such devastating plagues. Once these improved and once the methods of isolation and monitoring used in Leicester were implemented, smallpox became a disease that few feared and indeed it was eventually eradicated in western societies.

Notwithstanding all of this evidence, the medical fraternity's blind faith, that it was the smallpox vaccine that resulted in the elimination of smallpox, maintains to this day. If you look at the Wikipedia entry for smallpox, which is written by learned medical experts, you will find no mention of how social conditions played a major role in the eradication of smallpox in western countries and no mention of how unvaccinated Leicester fared significantly better than the other vaccinated towns. You will read only that vaccination, and vaccination alone, led to the eradication of smallpox. The Wikipedia evidence would seem compelling to a casual observer: full of complex statistics and scientific terms and is unequivocal in its message. But how can it claim to be based on science when it leaves out whole swathes of historical evidence which contradict its claims? Vaccination eradicated smallpox, say learned doctors. Historical records tell us otherwise. As usual in these situations there will never be an open debate about the facts. Global leaders have made up their collective minds and are in no mood to consider any alternative.

How was smallpox eradicated worldwide? Believe it or not, when infections started to reduce around the world, just like it did in England and other western countries, some of the cases started to be treated in the same way that Leicester used. Those infected and their close families were isolated, quarantined and monitored. This helped to reduce further infections and as they continued to fall, incredible efforts were made to find every single infected person and continue this process. One other key fact is that all these people were also given the smallpox vaccines which meant that medicine simply claimed it was vaccines, and vaccines alone, that eventually eliminated smallpox as already explored. Really?

But it was not only smallpox that saw this amazing decline. Beginning in the mid-1800s, the mortality rates for all infectious diseases declined amazingly and in unison. By the

1950s, for example, the deaths from scarlet fever had declined to almost zero. The deaths from whooping cough and measles also declined by over 99% and almost 100% respectively before any vaccines were deployed, and from 1900 to 1943, deaths from diarrhoea also declined by 93.5%. before any antibiotics started to be used. So, if deaths for every infectious disease plummeted, can medicine really be correct in saying that for smallpox it was the vaccine, and the vaccine alone, that caused this decline, especially when they unequivocally agree that for the other infectious diseases the decline occurred simply because of improved social conditions? The deadly threats that were once so commonplace slowly faded into the past. Even by the end of the 1800s, it was clear that sanitation and improved living conditions were making a significant impact against all such diseases. So, what was the point of developing vaccines for diseases that virtually everyone recovered from? Was it to prevent a few days of mild illness? Was it because huge profits could be made from mass vaccination programmes? Was it so that medicine would be able to claim that it alone had cured these once dreaded diseases just as it was doing with smallpox? Whatever the motives, there is one thing for certain. If you are aiming to develop vaccines for most of these diseases and give them to virtually everyone, then you had better be sure there are no adverse reactions to the vaccine, or you could end up killing more people than the few you expect to save.

Whooping cough. Also known as pertussis, this vaccine was developed in the 1940s and large-scale vaccination began in the United States in 1949 and in England in 1957. Remember that at this time the deaths from whooping cough had already declined by more than 99% from their peak and were continuing to fall. But very early on there were indications of problems. A 1948 article in the journal Pediatrics discussed a number of cases of brain damage following vaccination. The article is hauntingly similar to the number of cases of autism that would escalate decades later. The children, mostly boys, had been developing normally and showed no problems prior to receiving the vaccine, but they developed acute cerebral symptoms within hours of injection which failed to reverse. At the time of this study, deaths form pertussis had become rare. Further cases and reports of harm followed. All this represented a warning for the future, but most medical experts continued to ignore such reports and insisted that the vaccine only rarely led to neurological problems. As had occurred with the smallpox vaccine over 100 years earlier, there was a medical bias against admitting that a heavily promoted medical procedure was actually harmful. The other thing you need to be sure of before starting a mass vaccination programme is that the vaccine is actually going to work effectively, but this also turned out not to be the case. As had been the promise with all vaccines at their inception, there was the expectation that vaccinated people would be protected for life against whooping cough. But just as the promise of life-long protection for other vaccines was never met, it was also unmet for whooping cough. Early studies showed that the susceptibility to infection was as high as 95% after just 12 years. Today the incidence of whooping cough is increasing significantly and most of the people affected have already been vaccinated. In the US the rate of pertussis has increased around ten-fold since 1980.

After vaccination, the body will react according to how it was programmed by the vaccine. In the case of the whooping cough vaccine, a crucial part of the bacteria is missing. So, when someone is subsequently infected with the real bacteria it can take hold without the body being properly prepared. It gives the bacteria a two-week advantage before the body finally realises it has been duped. But there are two more disturbing facts. The pertussis bacteria have evolved and strengthened under the pressure of the vaccine. This new strain of bacteria is more resistant to the vaccination and any immunity that may be gained is even shorter. In fact, a new additional inhaled vaccine was then developed and given to children to try to re-improve protection. The real tragedy is that whooping cough was a relatively mild infection that nearly everyone (except those with seriously compromised immune systems) recovered from, and crucially, when they did, they were immune for the rest of their lives. Now it is likely that vaccine effectiveness will continue to wane, requiring a never-ending need for new vaccines. There is, however, the possibility of an even more sinister outcome. Antibiotics, as already outlined, are now failing to work against a number of new resistant strains of bacteria and 700,000 (soon to be 10 million) people are now dying each year. At some point in the future, similar outcomes could possibly also occur with failing vaccines.

Measles. The development of the measles vaccine in the 1950s mirrored that of the whooping cough vaccine. So, the same questions need to be asked and answered. Throughout the 1800s, measles epidemics occurred about every two years. Hospital wards overflowed with children and up to 20% died. However, by 1960, deaths had dropped to extremely low numbers and in England the decline from its peak level reached an astonishing 99.96% and was still falling by the time the measles vaccine was introduced in 1968. Some people think antibiotics were responsible for a major part of the decline in mortality, but for measles, the mortality rate had already dropped to less than 1% of the peak level even by the late 1940s when antibiotics started to become available.

But what about the crucial question of safety? Given that it could save very few lives, then surely it must be completely safe. Well, the first vaccine which used complete but dead viruses, actually had some serious outcomes. A study from 1967 revealed it could cause pneumonia as well as encephalopathy (inflammation of the brain). Serious neurological illness occurred in some children 7 to 14 days after vaccination. The study concluded that such results were unanticipated and recommended that the dead measles virus vaccine should no longer be administered. In addition to being dangerous, the killed vaccines soon became very ineffective. Whatever vaccine immunity was present, it declined rapidly, and the recipients again became susceptible. They were later advised to be revaccinated with a new live vaccine in the hope of rectifying the problem. But those who encountered wild measles or the new live vaccine, after having been vaccinated with the old killed virus, had a tendency to develop a more severe measles because their immune systems had been "wrongly programmed", just as with the whooping cough vaccine. The killed vaccines were abandoned but there were also significant issues with the new live vaccines, which produced a modified measles rash in about half of those injected essentially similar to a case of real measles. About 48% had a rash and around 83% had fevers up to 106 degrees post-injection. To counter these problems, "attenuated" vaccines were subsequently introduced, with the aim of minimising such obvious flaws with the vaccine. But these too had problems which I won't go into because they need detailed and lengthy explanation. But you can see a simple pattern emerge. "If at first you don't succeed, try, try again." Except in this case, harm is being done to children with each try and all this for a disease that was killing very few of them.

Nevertheless, in western countries, and at the end of a long and painful road, the numbers of people catching measles declined significantly over proceeding years. Some of this decline is definitely due to the vaccines, the latest of which is the MMR vaccine, and some was happening naturally. For example, long before the vaccine was introduced, infection rates were already falling and continued to do so, possibly because the measles virus was slowly losing its potency. Outbreaks of measles still occur even now, of course, and these are often in people who have been fully vaccinated, but, as of today, the overall level of people who catch measles is very low. So, did the measles vaccines eventually fulfil their promises despite the harm they had caused? They are hailed by medicine as a great success story, of course, but are there any nagging doubts? Human beings have built up a natural resistance to wild measles over countless millennia. Healthy well-nourished children do not die from measles. I, and virtually all my friends, caught measles and recovered from it.

Although I didn't realise it at the time, "measles parties" were often held in those days so that all the local children caught the disease at the same time and we could then resume normal life together. It was clear that virtually everyone who was infected with measles recovered from it in a few days and would then have life-long immunity. This natural resistance is also passed from generation to generation. The very few that did die usually had other serious medical conditions and even if they did not die from measles, they might just as easily die from other infections like influenza and pneumonia because of their damaged immune response. Vaccines are simply not the same as real viruses or bacteria, and they illicit different immune responses as we have seen. They only provide temporary immunity, unlike the life-long immunity provided by real virus infections, meaning that frequent revaccinations are always going to be needed and each vaccination has a potential for harm. The numbers of people developing measles really has been radically reduced, but at what cost for future generations?

Influenza. Here are a few facts about flu vaccines. When a swine flu virus appeared in 1976 in New Jersey, the CDC convinced the US president to launch a mass vaccination programme to avoid a pandemic that was projected to cause an estimated 1 million deaths. A few months later 40 million people had been vaccinated, but then hundreds of them started to develop a strange form of paralysis, known as Guillain-Barre syndrome. Around 500 were permanently paralysed and dozens died. While all this was happening, the epidemic never actually took place. Incredibly, just 13 people contracted the virus and there was one death. When the second swine flu infection occurred in 2009, the World Health Organization quickly declared it was a phase-6 pandemic – the highest risk factor for an infectious disease. In the UK alone, the projected death toll was 750,000. A number of major developed countries, including the UK, at that time had agreements with drug companies to buy vaccines and antiviral drugs that would be triggered immediately when the WHO declared a phase-6 pandemic. Once triggered, there was no way of rescinding the agreement.

However, the virus which originated in Mexico was originally associated with 200 deaths, but shortly afterwards this was reduced to just seven. It soon became clear that this was not a worldwide pandemic. In fact, the total UK deaths from it between 2009 and 2010 were just 457, which is much less than normal annual flu deaths. While all this was happening, the vaccine was distributed for people considered at highest risk, including doctors because of their close contacts with infected people. However, while most people took the vaccine, 65% of doctors refused to have it. So, despite being compelled by medical guidelines to advise their patients to be vaccinated, the doctors themselves obviously knew better. What then happened was that a number of children developed narcolepsy which is a long-term brain condition that causes a number of serious sudden sleep problems. The UK government has since paid out over £60 million to families whose children were damaged by this vaccine.

A vital question is why the WHO declared a serious pandemic that wasn't? Unsurprisingly, the drug industry has close ties with the WHO and those scientists who advised the WHO about the "pandemic" also had lucrative financial pharmaceutical ties. This is just one more example of how the industry controls virtually everyone with the sole aim of simply maximising its profits. Most governments were angry they had effectively been duped by the whole saga, but there was little they could do about it. In 2005 the United Nations also warned that a new avian flu (H5N1) would cause up to 150 million deaths. Three years later the death toll was just 257.

What about the current annual flu vaccines? They provide modest short-term protection against seasonal flu, typically being around 33% effective initially, but then this starts to decline to even lower levels. In 2020 a 14-year study found that they can also cause adverse effects like high fever, seizures, narcolepsy and Guillain-Barre syndrome. The study involved only elderly men but these side effects caused more deaths than were saved by the vaccine – an 8.9% increase in overall mortality.

Vaccination has been a core medical tool for many years, and as each piece of evidence against vaccination unfolds, it is casually dismissed by the "vaccine establishment". You will, however, see even more frightening evidence in the next few sections.

Infectious diseases – the lifestyle medicine approach

The natural immune system is one of the most vital and amazing parts of the human body and plays the crucial role in protecting us from infectious diseases. The main aim of lifestyle medicine is simply to ensure it is able to function at maximum effectiveness. Without it we would have no way to fight the potentially harmful things that are constantly entering our body or those that develop within it. It has an incredible array of "weapons" to fight this endless invasion from pathogens like bacteria, viruses, other parasites and fungi, as well as being able to kill things like cancer cells that occur in everyone. These types of pathogens have been around since the creation of life. Humans and all other types of living creatures and their natural immune systems have simply evolved so that we can either live with them, control them or, if necessary, kill them.

There are two parts to the immune system: the innate (non-specific) immune system and the adaptive (specific) immune system. The innate system provides a general defence against every type of pathogen. It involves a wide range of special white blood cells, like phagocytes and monocytes, as well as number of neutrophils that include natural killer cells which either engulf or attack the invaders or the cells that they have already infected. These cells also release various proteins that act as cell signalling messengers and coordinate the attack on the invader. The innate system also alerts the adaptive immune system to prepare to enter the battle if needed. The adaptive system develops specific weapons for each individual disease and includes B cells, T cells and antibodies which swing into action if the innate system has not contained the infection within around 12 hours. These each have several key types. There are four types of T cells, for example. One directly kills infected cells, one spurs other T and B cells into action, one calms the immune system so that it recognises and avoids attacking friendly microbes, and the memory T cells retain all the information to rapidly destroy any subsequent infection by the same virus. For many viruses, like measles, this can mean life-long immunity. T cells and B cells also work together to form antibodies which surround the pathogen and tag it for destruction by other killer immune cells.

The natural immune system is not just incredibly complex but is amazingly powerful. Up until the late 1960s (other than for smallpox) most people and children had not received any vaccines, except for polio (from 1956) and diphtheria (from 1942). Most of them would at some point be infected by a wide range of other diseases like measles, chicken pox, whooping cough and mumps, as well as colds and influenza which have around 100 different strains each. There are also a huge range of other infectious diseases, but vaccines are available only for a tiny fraction of them, yet virtually everyone recovers from all of them. Most of the deaths occur in people and children who have a seriously compromised immune system caused by conditions like cancer and diabetes. The simple fact is there has been only one real pandemic in westernised countries in the last century: the 1918–1919 Spanish flu which took around 50 million lives.

There are, however, three key facts and causes. This occurred at the end of the First World War when living conditions had been severely affected which would have compromised natural immunity. Also, the natural immune system works optimally when it is tested by regular infections, but before the 1918 pandemic, it had been well over 20 years since a previous flu outbreak had occurred which would also have compromised the immune system. A final key fact is that we now know it was not just the flu virus that caused the epidemic. In 2008 the National Institute of Allergy and Infectious Disease carried out a detailed analysis of original autopsy reports and then re-examined the still available post-mortem samples and found a bacterial infection was also present. The researchers concluded that this bacterial infection was a major cause of the deaths especially for outcomes like acute pneumonia. In normal times the Spanish flu epidemic on its own would probably have caused much lower levels of deaths.

Many people, however, have been led to believe that vaccines are the key to beating infectious diseases, and that without them, people would struggle to recover from most of them. Vaccine proponents are in effect saying that people must artificially manipulate their immune system as the only way to stay safe from infectious diseases. This is not true. Without the natural immune system, no vaccine would have any effect whatsoever. Vaccines are simply designed to activate the immune system. But as we have just seen, for people with a healthy immune system, it simply activates itself and defeats the viruses without a vaccine. This means the wide range of side effects caused by vaccines can also be avoided. Unequivocal historic data provides definitive proof that this is true, and those with seriously compromised immune systems struggle to defeat it even with a vaccine.

So, what are the things you can do to maximise the effectiveness of your natural immune system? By now, you may not be surprised to learn that the seven key lifestyle factors that have been examined in detail, play the major role. The immune system can be seriously compromised by:

- mental issues like stress and fear
- a poor industrialised type diet
- lack of exercise
- dangerous chemicals
- a badly disturbed microbiome
- low levels of vitamins, minerals and a range of other natural compounds
- poor sleep

It can also be badly compromised by a range of drugs like antacids and proton pump inhibitors. There are, however, specific factors that can play a significant role in minimising the symptoms of infectious diseases, including certain vitamins, minerals and other natural compounds. These will be covered in much more detail in the next section on COVID-19, so I won't say any more here.

Anyone wanting to learn more about infectious diseases and vaccination should read the book *Dissolving Illusions: Disease, Vaccines and the Forgotten History* by Suzanne Humphries MD and Roman Bystrianyk.

COVID-19

The world is still in the midst of the global "pandemic" nearly three years after it started. A significant number of countries, like the UK, reached the end of the initial phase with virtually all restrictions lifted early in 2022. China, however, was still using savage lockdowns for many millions of people through most of the year although towards the end of December they have now started to significantly ease them. Because it is still not clear exactly how it will all progress, I will simply explain the key facts relating to COVID-19, and then at the end, bring them together to summarise what has happened, what could, and perhaps should, have happened, and what the future may hold.

There has been a single, official worldwide COVID-19 narrative which is unprecedented. It has been incessantly promoted and imposed globally by virtually every official organisation and government and it has simply taken over most people's lives. News and media organisations which historically earned their reputations by always searching for the truth, and challenging and helping to bring to justice, people, organisations and even presidents who lied and committed crimes, have simply kowtowed and obediently promoted this official global narrative. There is, however, one key problem. Much of what we have been told about COVID-19 is also simply not correct.

I do understand that many people really will want to dismiss everything that follows, but let me give you one crucial fact to consider. Most of the information you will see has been exposed and published by some of the world's most eminent doctors and scientists. If what they claim to be true really is a lie, then governments, regulators and medical organisations could, and should, charge them in a court of law so that they could legally be found guilty and thus completely discredited and convicted, as indeed they should be if they really are lying. This hasn't happened because it would simply allow the real truth to be exposed. Instead, the doctors and scientists have simply been censored. So, please be prepared to read these facts even though you will be truly shocked by most of them.

First, one piece of information. SARS-CoV-2 is the name of the virus that causes COVID-19 which in turn is simply the name given to the disease that then develops.

COVID-19 – the medical approach

Vaccination. Almost from the beginning of the Covid outbreak, medicine, regulators, Big Pharma and governments made one simple claim: vaccines were the only way to defeat the virus. They claimed there were no available treatments and no drugs and that the virus simply had to be curtailed with things like lockdowns, social distancing, travel restrictions and masks until the vaccines became available. Despite this claim, however, there is strong evidence that alternative treatments really do exist, and in fact they existed right from the start of the "pandemic".

Alternative treatments. In March 2020 an expert panel called the Front Line COVID-19 Critical Care Alliance (FLCCC) was created and led by Professor Paul Marik in the US. Most of these doctors had many years of experience treating seriously ill patients in hospitals and intensive care units particularly for severe infections. They had developed a number of highly successful treatments for various diseases and as soon as COVID-19 emerged they examined the basic science and using their previous experience, they developed a treatment protocol they called MATH+. This treatment was used in their two main hospitals and once it had been optimised, the death rate was 6.1%. This compared to an equivalent mortality rate of 23% in other equivalent hospitals using conventional medical treatments based on an average of 45 studies over the same period.

Ivermectin. Evidence then started to emerge about an old drug called ivermectin which showed that it could achieve remarkable reductions for all the key Covid outcomes like deaths, hospital admissions and intensive care admissions. FLCCC then developed two new treatment protocols based around ivermectin called I-MASK+ (for prevention) and IMATH+ (for hospital treatment). These also contained a number of supplements like vitamins D and C and zinc which have all shown significant benefits for Covid. Ivermectin is an old drug whose main use has been to treat parasitic infections in humans as well as animals.

Since the early 1990s, 3.7 billion people have been successfully treated with it, and the three scientists who proved its effectiveness were awarded the Nobel Prize. It is also on the World Health Organization's list of essential medicines. It originated from a bacterium unearthed from soil in Japan which was then developed into ivermectin. Its benefits for COVID-19 are also incredible. There have been over 50 individual trials around the world (28 of them the gold standard randomised clinical trial) and every one of them has shown a reduction in deaths as well as other benefits. Meta-analyses (some of them peer reviewed) have also been performed on many of the trials and the reduction in deaths range from 62% to 81% (with an average of around 70%). An important fact is that these trials used just ivermectin. When the FLCCC treatment protocols using ivermectin with several other compounds, like vitamin D, were used in their hospitals, the average reduction in deaths was around 85%.

You may also be surprised to learn that some countries have also used ivermectin with amazing success. These include Japan, Brazil, Mexico and Peru. In Japan, doctors were urged to use ivermectin by the head of the Tokyo Medical Association in August 2021 and individual people were then also able to buy it themselves. Case numbers and deaths then fell significantly. In Brazil, three regions distributed ivermectin to their residents while six others did not. The three that used it saw deaths decline by 36%, 75% and 42%, while the states that did not showed little change. A more recent study involved the city of Itatjai where 113,000 people took just four tablets per month and achieved a 68% reduction in deaths and 56% in hospitalisations. Mexico used ivermectin for those patients who had just tested positive and they were each given four tablets to be taken over two days. Studies showed a reduction in hospitalisations of around 60% just from these four tablets. In May 2020 Peru widely used ivermectin and achieved a 14-fold reduction in deaths.

There is also the incredible case of Africa which has nearly one-fifth of the world's population, but only a tiny fraction of its people has been vaccinated. It has nevertheless maintained one of the lowest Covid death rates at just 4% of world deaths up to mid-2021. One of the reasons for this is that Africa has relatively more younger people who, of course, are less likely to die from Covid. However, even though the following information cannot be proven conclusively, many independent experts think that ivermectin is almost certainly another key factor, because it is widely available in Africa and costs so little. It has been used to treat common parasitic infections for many decades and because doctors can see that it works for Covid, they are likely to be giving it to some of their local patients. This really is highly plausible because conventional medical experts have so far been unable to find any other explanations as to why Africa is faring so much better – with incredibly lower death rates – than even the richest developed nations that have high levels of vaccination and health services like the UK, Europe and America.

Given all this incredible evidence, why is there not a single western country using ivermectin as a treatment for COVID-19? Quite simply, the roll out of vaccines and the claims made early in 2020 by all the key organisations and governments that vaccines were the only solution to Covid has meant all other treatments (including those with impeccable proof) have simply had to be ignored, dismissed and even savagely attacked to protect the roll out of the vaccines. The key fact is Covid vaccines have been approved for emergency use only. Such emergency approval can only legally be made if there are no other effective treatments available. The vaccines were granted approval after just six months. Compare this to every other previous vaccine development timescale of over ten years. So, despite the huge number of clinical trials and studies on ivermectin, the WHO incredulously said, "More data needed." Really? The Federal Drug Agency said, "Currently, available data do not show ivermectin is effective against COVID-19." Really? For a regulator that approves new treatments based on just one or two clinical trials to then dismiss the 28 randomised clinical trials for ivermectin is simply unbelievable. This is even more appalling when you consider that the emergency trials for Covid were not even completed before they were approved and, therefore, could not guarantee their long-term effectiveness or safety.

Countless other approaches to try to discredit ivermectin are also being used. Fake news stories have been common. One classic example in the US that had nationwide press coverage was that gunshot victims were being turned away from an Oklahoma hospital because all the beds were filled with people who were dying from overdoses of ivermectin. This put millions of people off even considering ivermectin, even though it was soon exposed as a blatant lie. Incredibly, even now, the media continue to promote the official policy with similar false stories.

Dr Andrew Hill, who is a senior research fellow in pharmacology at Liverpool University, carried out one of the original meta-analyses on the clinical trials for ivermectin. His study of six randomised trials showed that ivermectin produced a reduction in deaths of 75%. Within a month, however, he was under extreme pressure from his sponsor Unitaid to revoke the study. Unitaid is a global health initiative funded by a number of countries and organisations including the UK, France and the Bill and Melinda Gates Foundation. Its main aim is to bring innovations in diagnoses and treatments for diseases like malaria and tuberculosis particularly in low-income countries. It is disturbing, therefore, that Unitaid pressurised Dr Hill to reverse his study on ivermectin. A new study which claimed the exact opposite – that ivermectin did not work for Covid – was then published. Dr Hill later admitted to a colleague that the results had been manipulated and that Unitaid (which has links to the vaccine industry) had in fact been involved in rewriting the new conclusions. This colleague was Dr Tess Lawrie who is a world-renowned and iconic global health scientist. She had found out that the manipulated results were about to be published and tried to persuade him not to release them, but such was the pressure he was facing that she did not succeed. Four days before the revised study was published, Dr Hill's sponsor Unitaid gave Liverpool University a $40 million donation, no doubt as a "thank you" for the study's reversal. Unitaid is meant to help the people in low-income countries, so why would it give $40 million to a major UK university other than to achieve this shocking data manipulation? As disturbing as all this is, I will give you more information in Part 6 on who the key player was behind all of this and you will be even more appalled that, while money was a key driver, there is an even more sinister reason.

A new study published in JAMA by Malaysian researchers concluded that ivermectin does not prevent severe Covid infection or hospitalisation. Professor Norman Fenton, however, called the study "scientific publishing fraud" because the ivermectin group had a 70% lower death rate. The control group had 10 deaths out of 249 patients, while the ivermectin group had just 3 out of 241 patients, yet the researchers claimed it had no benefit.

In the US, the FLCCC, which produced various protocols involving ivermectin for treating Covid, used them in their own hospitals. Dr Paul Marik is one of the key doctors who helped develop these treatments and used them in the Sentara hospital where he was director of ICU. They had been used since March 2020, but in November 2021, the hospital banned their use shortly after the FDA, CDC and NIH official bodies all warned that ivermectin and other natural treatments should not be used to treat Covid. Dr Marik said that many of his patients were now dying unnecessarily. It is clear that the all-out war to discredit ivermectin, and all those doctors who use it or promote it, is in full flow. This despite the fact that around 80% of all Covid deaths could have been prevented had it been used early in the pandemic.

Dr Tess Lawrie (who carried out one of the other key meta-analyses on ivermectin, and who had tried to persuade Dr Hill not to publish the manipulated data), together with other world medical experts, held a Covid conference and this is her closing address. It offers a searing insight into the whole problem:

> The story of ivermectin has highlighted that we are at a remarkable juncture in medical history. The tools that we use to heal and our connection with our patients are being systematically undermined by relentless disinformation stemming from corporate greed. The story of ivermectin shows that we as a public have misplaced our trust in the authorities and have underestimated the extent to which money and power corrupts. Had ivermectin been employed in 2020 when medical colleagues around the world first alerted the authorities to its efficacy, millions of lives could have been saved, and the pandemic with all its associated suffering and loss brought to a rapid and timely end. Since then, hundreds of millions of people have been involved in the largest medical experiment in human history. Mass vaccination was an unproven novel therapy. Hundreds of billions will be made by Big Pharma and paid for by the public. With politicians and other nonmedical individuals dictating to us what we are allowed to prescribe to the ill, we as doctors, have been put in a position such that our ability to uphold the Hippocratic oath is under attack. At this fateful juncture, we must therefore choose, will we continue to be held ransom by corrupt organisations, health authorities, Big Pharma and billionaire sociopaths, or will we do our moral and professional duty to do no harm and always do the best for those in our care? The latter includes urgently reaching out to colleagues around the world to discuss which of our tried and tested safe older medicines can be used against Covid.

All this is nothing short of a human tragedy, but ivermectin isn't the only incredible treatment undergoing this devastating form of attack. There is another successful old drug called hydroxychloroquine (HCQ) which was first approved for inflammatory conditions in 1955, as well as a range of vitamins, minerals and other supplements all of which have significant evidence including clinical trials. They are all facing exactly the same sort of attacks and their advocates are also being attacked and censored and some have lost their medical licences.

Hydroxychloroquine. From 2003 hydroxychloroquine (HCQ), and a similar compound called chloroquine, had been shown to be a valid treatment for a number of SARS-related infections like SARS-CoV in 2003, and MERS-CoV in 2012. CDC and Canadian scientists published an official paper confirming its benefits against SARS viruses in 2003 and European scientists did the same in 2004. The CDC paper concluded: "Chloroquine has strong antiviral effects on SARS-COV infection." Nine years later, in 2014, scientists at Dr Anthony Fauci's agency NIAID also published a study showing the same benefits as did two other separate groups of European scientists. Interestingly, hydroxychloroquine is an analogue of the quinine found in the bark of the cinchona tree that George Washington used to protect his troops from malaria. It has been used for many decades to protect against malaria particularly in Africa and India by hundreds of millions of residents and visitors, and its safety and effectiveness were well-established and unchallenged facts.

When COVID-19 emerged, US doctors were aware of these facts and a survey showed that two-thirds of them said they would prescribe HCQ as a treatment for family members as well as themselves. Incredibly, Dr Fauci also said in March 2020 that if he became ill with Covid, he would take it as his remedy. Even President Trump was given hydroxychloroquine by his doctors when he was infected with Covid as were many other world leaders as testified by the president of El Salvador who also took it. HCQ was even granted emergency use authorisation by the FDA as a COVID-19 therapy in March 2020 and millions of tablets were added to the Strategic National Stockpile. There were also over 60 studies showing how it could treat COVID-19 and that it was particularly effective in the early (five-day) phase of the disease. However, shortly after this, Dr Fauci started an aggressive campaign to deny HCQ and all other early treatments to the rest of humanity. In June 2020 the FDA, having initially approved it, then revoked its use. Key medical organisations like the Mayo Clinic also started claiming there were no COVID-19 medications that worked. Even worse was to follow.

The Lancet journal published a despicable study that had used fabricated data to show that HCQ did not work for Covid. Thirteen days later it was forced to retract it after 200 independent scientists exposed what was pure fraud. During the 13 days the study was "officially approved", however, many countries like France and Switzerland banned HCQ's use. This scandal later became known as #LancetGate. On the same day as the Lancet retraction, the New England Journal of Medicine retracted another similar study that had also used unverifiable and fabricated data. Shockingly, even when these retractions were made, the use of HCQ was not reinstated in most of the countries that had banned it. However, Switzerland did reapprove it and a study by Johns Hopkins University showed an amazing change in death rates. Hydroxychloroquine had been used in Switzerland from the early stage of the pandemic, but when its use was stopped for two weeks, deaths tripled but then reduced again by two-thirds when it was reinstated. Staggeringly, other countries simply ignored this incredible reduction in deaths. I must also add that some other doctors had not just used hydroxychloroquine on its own, but used it with two additional compounds: zinc sulphate and azithromycin. This treatment, given quickly after infection occurred, reduced death rates by more than 90%.

After the Lancet and New England studies were retracted and shown to be fraudulent, key medical and regulatory organisations simply had to find another way of discrediting hydroxychloroquine to help ensure the vaccines emergency use did not have to be stopped. Several large multicentre international trials were then carried out. If you are determined to "prove" a treatment doesn't work, then there are a number of fraudulent options you can use. These include using the wrong dose, giving it to people who can't benefit from it, and applying it at the wrong time. Despicably, all of them were used in these trials. We have already seen that HCQ works best when it is given within the first few days of infection, but these new trials selected inappropriate late stage patients some of whom were already near death and for which HCQ (as well as any other treatment) could have little or no benefit. A claim could then be made that it didn't work. Also, most drugs become lethal if given at high doses and these trials also used dangerously high levels of HCQ. Hydroxychloroquine is perfectly safe at conventional prescription levels that have been given to hundreds of millions of patients over many decades. However, these multicentre international trials used up to four times the maximum dosage that had been used safely since its approval in 1955. Independent researchers were shocked beyond belief that this was done, because it would have caused the deaths of some of the patients in the trials and they could only conclude that it was done deliberately to help "prove" that hydroxychloroquine did not work by using these deaths to offset the deaths it saved.

When I learnt about all of this, my first thought was that no one would believe it could possibly be true. So, I decided not to include it in the book, but eventually changed my mind because it really is factual and shows the appalling and despicable depths to which vaccine advocates were prepared to go in order to save the Covid vaccines. Just like the tobacco industry, they don't seem to care about human life.

Vitamins and minerals. The third group of treatments for COVID-19 that are being similarly attacked and discredited is a range of vitamins, minerals and other supplements. These also have lots of evidence that they work, but I will give more information about them in the lifestyle approach section. The simple fact is, despite the data manipulation, "fraud" and rigged trials that have been widely used to try to discredit all these incredibly successful treatments, the official medical organisations are so powerful and exert such influence over the press and media that they have succeeded in eliminating and discrediting every form of alternative Covid treatment that could have saved around 80–90% of all Covid deaths. Every doctor using or promoting them has simply been viciously attacked, censored and even sacked.

Here is a final crucial fact about ivermectin and hydroxychloroquine. Once a drug has been given official approval for one or more specific diseases by a regulator, doctors have always had a legally endorsed ability to prescribe it for off-label use for other conditions where they believe it can help. Both of these drugs have been approved to treat several diseases, but now, in most countries including the UK, a doctor cannot use either of them. Yet one more despicable example of how those in control of the Covid pandemic will not accept anything that threatens the vaccines.

Remdesivir. This is the ideal moment to examine a new drug called remdesivir that received an emergency use authorisation in May 2020 by Dr Anthony Fauci's National Institute of Allergy and Infectious Disease (NIAID). Dr Fauci euphorically claimed it was the "new standard of care" for COVID-19. I have explained how the emergency use of vaccines could not have been be approved if there had been any other successful treatment available and hence why the all-out attack on treatments like ivermectin, hydroxychloroquine and vitamin D was taking place. There is, however, another reason why these have been suppressed and why remdesivir has been approved. The Federal Drug Agency, and similar agencies around the world, now simply exist to protect the interests of the pharmaceutical industry rather than protecting the public, and numerous examples of this shocking situation have already been explored in great detail throughout the book. Ivermectin and hydroxychloroquine are old drugs that lost their patents decades ago. The companies that produce both ivermectin and HCQ make very little profit from them and the industry in unison does not want them promoted. A five-day course of either of them costs just a few dollars, whereas the same course of remdesivir costs over $3,000. Gilead, the company that makes it, will now make several billion dollars in profit each year and some of that will, of course, also filter back to the regulators who approved it. But how effective is remdesivir? A staggering fact is that the initial trial carried out by Gilead did not use proper inert placebos which are a vital part of the clinical trial procedure and instead used sulfobutyl. Why? Because Gilead knew remdesivir caused severe side effects and they also knew that sulfobutyl had similar effects which would make remdesivir appear no different to the placebo and thus safe. Despite this fraud, the researchers could not get remdesivir to show any improvement in Covid survival.

In addition to all of this, a number of other studies on remdesivir have also been carried out and one by the World Health Organization was exceptionally large involving 11,266 Covid patients in 405 hospitals and 30 countries compared to Gilead's trial with just 1,062 patients. The WHO study concluded that the drug had "little or no effect on mortality." Other studies showed similarly poor outcomes and a review by the European Union reported serious side effects, while one from Johns Hopkins showed it caused longer hospital stays. Given this disastrous data that it didn't actually save lives and in fact had adverse events, those involved in the drug's approval and promotion like Dr Fauci had to find another way of claiming its use was worthwhile as well as trying to protect their own reputations, So, they then looked at how long it took surviving patients to recover, and a study showed that those taking remdesivir recovered in ten days while those on the placebo took 15 days. They were then able to claim that the cost of five days extra hospitalisation was more than the $3,000 for the drug. So, relief all round then? But was this really a truthful get out of jail card? Well, according to Robert F. Kennedy Jr.'s bestselling book *The Real Anthony Fauci*, even this was fraudulent. Compared to those taking the placebo, almost twice as many patients taking remdesivir had to be readmitted to the hospital after their initial discharge, and this information was not included in the trial's conclusions. This was almost certainly due to the fact they were deliberately discharged too early to fraudulently make the drug look effective. You can be sure that all this is true. Why? If it wasn't, Robert F. Kennedy Jr. would have been sued out of existence by the US government and all the medical organisations involved, and quite simply he hasn't been and won't be. He is, of course, still attacked, vilified and censored like everyone else who simply has the courage to tell the truth about what is happening and the sort of fraud that those in charge are committing. However, even prestigious organisations like the British Medical Journal and the Scripps Research Translational Institute also made savage criticisms about Dr Fauci's remdesivir trial.

But here is another vital and distressing fact. Even though remdesivir does not save lives in relation to Covid, and achieves little else, it does in fact kill some of those patients that are prescribed it. Dr Fauci's National Institute of Allergy and Infectious Disease had previously carried out a clinical trial using remdesivir to treat Ebola, and within 28 days those patients given the drug developed diseases like kidney failure, septic shock and multiple organ failures and a staggering 54% of them died. Yet Dr Fauci gave it emergency authorisation use for Covid. This whole story about remdesivir is almost unbelievable and just one more example of the shocking things that are being done in the name of Covid. It really is all true.

Deaths and hospital admissions from Covid. What are the "facts" we have been given? Official figures showed that in the two years between early 2020 and the end of 2021, the total number of official deaths from COVID-19 in the UK was around 157,000. These official figures are defined as deaths within 28 days of a positive Covid test. The problem with this definition is that people who really do die from something else, like a car crash or a heart attack, but test positive are still classed as dying from Covid. It means quite simply that the numbers of official deaths and hospitalisations are incorrect and overstated. Even the previous UK Health Secretary Sajid Javid admitted that daily government figures were unreliable because people continue to die from conditions unrelated to COVID-19. He also admitted that about 40% of patients at that time who were classed as hospitalised Covid patients were not admitted due to Covid symptoms and simply tested positive at some point during their hospitalisation. In mid-2021, the Telegraph gained access to leaked NHS data which showed an even higher figure; 56% of admissions were not for Covid and the patients simply tested positive in hospital.

Ontario in Canada also confirmed that the true numbers are 46% less than its official figures. Many other countries like the US also admitted that hospitalisations had been overstated and the New York governor announced that almost half of patients were hospitalised for non-Covid reasons. Given that hospital admissions have been a key reason for the severe Covid restrictions that everyone has been forced to adopt, it is truly shocking and even unforgiveable that the real figures are significantly less than the official numbers. Almost none of those patients would have died from Covid. All of this adds extra solid evidence that the numbers of deaths have also been grossly overstated and are simply incorrect. But how incorrect? Official figures for 2020–2021 show that the number of UK deaths where Covid was the *only* cause listed are around 20,000. This means that these people who had no other diseases almost certainly died from Covid. But what about the other 137,000 people who died? All of them had other underlying serious health conditions and studies have shown that around 90% actually had two or more comorbidities or pre-existing health conditions, like heart disease and cancer, a wide range of other serious diseases as well as physical accidents. This means that these conditions would be the main cause of death in a significant number of cases and not Covid.

There is, however, no official data for this, so trying to estimate the real figure depends on how the deaths are assessed. As an example, for many patients who have serious diseases, Covid may play a part in the death but it wouldn't be the main cause and the death would almost certainly happen anyway. Also, given that the average age of death of those with a positive test was 82.5, then Covid could play a part, but its effect on life expectancy could be minimal for many patients given that the average UK life expectancy is even lower at around 81. For many people, the deaths are not caused by Covid. These include those who have heart attacks, strokes, terminal end cancers and car accidents We also now know from the CDC that PCR tests can give significant false positive results and they have recently told everyone to avoid a PCR test after they have been diagnosed with Covid. These false positives can last up to 12 weeks after someone has had, and recovered from, Covid. This is because PCR can detect even tiny traces or just fragments of the virus that can remain in the body for weeks. So, people really can have the disease, fully recover from it, but still test positive. It means that many people in hospital officially listed with Covid don't even have the disease and, therefore, couldn't possibly die from it.

Another PCR "scandal" involved duplicate tests. If someone tested positive and was then tested each week until they got a negative result, some of these tests were counted as a separate "case" – once again overstating real case numbers. Here is one more example of how this overstating has been done. The CDC has simply recategorised and shifted some influenza and pneumonia deaths to Covid deaths which was confirmed by law makers in Minnesota who audited death records. At the beginning of the pandemic in 2020, deaths were incorrectly overstated particularly in care homes. One son, whose mother had severe lung disease, was upset that when she died the death certificate incorrectly listed Covid as the cause and he complained to her doctor who explained that, at that time, care home residents who died could not always be seen and when that happened, doctors were actually encouraged to simply list Covid as the cause of death. Also, at the start of the pandemic, patients in hospital needing oxygen were invariably put on powerful mechanical ventilators, in part to help prevent the spread of their Covid virus. These, however, turned out to be dangerous for many patients. It has been estimated that up to 50% of them died from this rather than from Covid itself during the first phase of the pandemic in spring 2020.

So, given all this information, the true death rate is likely to be significantly less than the official figure. A true calculation, however, is impossible given such a wide range and variety of inaccurate, unprovable and conflicting data. Nevertheless, the likely range is somewhere between 40,000 and 80,000 for 2020 and 2021. I'll make what is probably an overestimate that the figure is 70,000 so that it can be compared to other diseases and thus expose another frightening reality. Using this estimate, it means that the average number of Covid deaths in the UK in each of the first two years of the pandemic was 35,000, even though in the first year there were no vaccines available. Of course, each death really does matter, but compare 35,000 to the average normal annual deaths from infections like pneumonia and flu of around 40,000 and those from sepsis of 50,000. Compare it to annual cancer deaths of 165,000, and a similar figure for cardiovascular disease. Given these figures, why has COVID-19 effectively shut down the UK and most of the world for nearly two years? Especially when it has resulted in other devastating outcomes like delayed and poor treatments for diseases like cancer and heart disease, increases in other conditions like mental health and obesity, as well as devastating effects on children's lives.

The pandemic has also cost the world an incredible $13.5 trillion, including £370 billion for the UK. This has been one of the major causes of the current high inflation and government debt. It will take decades to pay back and have a lingering effect on humanity. The key decision makers who caused all of this have seemingly indoctrinated the whole population with the idea that the only deaths that matter are those from Covid, even though they probably only accounted for around 5% of UK deaths in the first two years. I should add that the more recent Covid variants, like Omicron and BA.5, now have significantly lower mortality levels even though the existing vaccines have virtually no effectiveness for them. So, the current rate of Covid deaths is significantly lower. In fact, the Institute for Health Metrics and Evaluation estimates that the latest variants have a death rate of under 0.001% (1 in 100,000). This means that even if all 50 million adults in the UK had contracted Covid in 2022, just 500 deaths would have occurred. If you really want another shocking example of the overstating of deaths, then consider a recent article by the BBC which listed 38,000 official COVID-19 deaths in 2022. This is unbelievable given that these variants are no worse than colds for nearly everyone.

Finally, here is some other vital data. All the figures for Covid deaths that have so far been quoted are, of course, just the overall average for all age groups. However, the deaths vary incredibly with age. Older people are most at risk and the average age of death is just over 82. For the first two years of the pandemic, around 80% of all deaths occurred in those over 70 and nearly 60% for those over 80. Less than 3% occurred in those under 50. The younger you are, the lower your risk and for young children the rate is incredibly low at around 0.0001% (one per million), but even these rare deaths are usually related to other underlying health conditions.

Case numbers. In the first wave in 2020, there were very few tests available to determine who had the virus. The official figures were very low, mainly just those who entered hospitals. Recent estimates indicate that a realistic figure for this wave was around 4 million. Testing levels improved in the second wave but even then, they were still limited and the true number of cases would still be higher than the official figures. Testing then increased through 2021 when the lateral flow tests started to become available to an increasing number of people. Even then, however, the true numbers would still be higher because many people didn't take tests for various reasons. For example, it could mean they might have to self-isolate and risk losing wages or risk damaging their employment especially if they were self-employed. In addition, around 40% of infected people have little or no symptoms meaning they would not even know they had the disease and would be less likely to carry out tests. All this means that while the official number of cases at the end of January 2022 was 17.5 million, the real figure was likely to be higher. However, a further key problem, as already explained, is that PCR tests can do the opposite, and falsely increase the number of cases. All this means that many cases were underreported, but others were overreported and the true overall figure really is impossible to calculate.

However, we know with reasonable certainty that almost everyone has now been infected for the following reasons. The Omicron variant had soaring case numbers but was much less deadly, and when the other variants like BA.4 and BA.2.12.1 then emerged, the case numbers rose even faster but they too also had mild effects. The very latest BA.5 variant is a virus with the highest infectiousness and transmissibility known to man – very similar to measles – but also has symptoms no worse than a mild cold for most people. All this means that by the end of summer 2022, virtually everyone had been infected with at least one Covid variant. In fact, many people have now had two or even three Covid infections, even though around 85% of the UK population have had at least two jabs. This gives the ultimate proof that they do not prevent infection or transmission. New variants are regularly emerging and this will almost certainly continue. Covid will probably be with us forever, even though it will hopefully be no worse than colds and flu.

mRNA Covid "vaccines" are not vaccines. This is a key fact that most people do not know. Vaccines have been used for many decades and their two main aims have been to prevent infection and minimise transmission of the virus so herd immunity can be reached and cases kept to low levels. The official CDC definition of a vaccine in 2020 was: "A product that stimulates a person's immune system to produce immunity to a specific disease, protecting the person from that disease." It also defined immunity as "protection from an infectious disease" meaning that "if you are immune to a disease, you can be exposed to it without becoming infected". But then, on 1 September 2021, that definition was changed. It simply said, "A preparation that is used to stimulate the body's immune response against diseases." There is now no mention of protecting people from developing a disease or transmitting it, even though these were the key requirements that led to the development of every other individual vaccine throughout the entire history of medicine. So, why was this dramatic change made? Quite simply, the mRNA Covid "vaccines" are not vaccines. They are in fact a gene edited therapy that operates in a totally different way to conventional vaccines. They do not use killed or modified types of the real virus to naturally stimulate the immune system. Instead, the gene editing makes the immune system act in a completely unnatural way by forcing it to produce and then attack just one type of protein (the spike protein) on the virus, and this type of "vaccine" does not prevent infection or transmission. The key problem for the vaccine promoters was that most people have an aversion and concern about gene editing drugs because of their unknown and unpredictable risks and outcomes. Those promoting Covid vaccination knew the mRNA "vaccine" needed to be classed officially as a vaccine so they could avoid having to try to promote a gene edited therapy to a reticent public. This quite simply is why the vaccine definition had to be changed. Even now, most people still do not know that the mRNA jab is in fact simply a gene edited drug therapy.

The way the gene editing works means the vaccines started to lose their effectiveness even against the initial Alpha variant. But this loss of effectiveness increased with each new variant and it started to wane sooner when the Delta variant emerged in the UK in mid-2021 and replaced the Alpha variant. Then when the Omicron variant took hold in December, it quickly phased out Delta and vaccine effectiveness fell even more rapidly to almost zero. Of course, most of the media were playing down this decline and the official position was that they were still working effectively. They still claimed that vaccines and booster shots were the only way of defeating Covid. But this wasn't true, just like the number of deaths and hospitalisations weren't true. If you don't want to believe any of this then consider what some of the most prestigious official experts and organisations in the world have said. Dr Fauci is the most prolific official vaccine promoter in the world and the most influential scientist on infectious diseases not just in the US, but in the UK and much of the rest of the world. In a New York Times podcast in mid-November 2021, he said that the Covid vaccine's effectiveness against infection, hospitalisation and even death, for all age groups, is waning to the point where booster doses will become essential. He also told the Times that vaccines are waning such that you're seeing more and more people getting breakthrough infections and winding up in hospital. The CDC director, Dr Rochelle Walensky, admitted that Covid injections simply do not prevent transmission. Even the CEO of Pfizer said that the jabs do not provide robust protection against Omicron in terms of severity of illness, hospitalisation and death. He also said that the booster shots provide limited protection for only a short time. In December 2021 the European Medicines Agency which had been recommending booster shots then warned that repeated boosters could seriously damage the natural immune system. The World Health Organization also said, "A vaccination strategy based on repeated doses of the original vaccine composition is unlikely to be appropriate or sustainable." All these people and organisations are at the very pinnacle of conventional medicine and these admissions are, to say the least, unexpected, even though they are all true. The WHO also said that what was now needed were vaccines that can prevent infection and transmission as well as severe disease and deaths, and that they should produce an immune response that is broad, strong and long-lasting in order to reduce the need for successive boosters.

There have been the most intense and often undemocratic strategies to try to force everyone to get vaccinated, but these facts represent a staggering put down of the mRNA vaccines and their current minimal benefits. Shockingly, in virtually every country like the UK, the US and the EU, people are still being aggressively told to "get vaccinated" or "get booster jabs", even though key experts have openly admitted that their benefits, especially with Omicron, quickly fell to low levels and with the more recent BA.4 and BA.5 variants they have even less effectiveness. This whole situation is extremely concerning in itself, but is even more shocking when you consider jab side effects.

Vaccine side effects. Given all of this damning evidence, you might expect that the vaccines would at least be safe and this is exactly what official medical organisations like the NHS continue to say: "The Coronavirus (COVID-19) vaccines are safe and effective." But the emerging evidence shows that mRNA shots have more side effects and are far more dangerous than any other vaccine in medical history. In the US, the Vaccine Adverse Events Reporting System (VAERS) has been in use since 1990. In the years before Covid emerged, the total number of adverse events reported for every vaccine administered averaged 39,000 per year. What do you think the figure is for Covid? A staggering figure of around 790,000, meaning that it has caused more adverse events in one year than all the other vaccines added together over the last 20 years. The average annual deaths reported from every other vaccine was 155, while for Covid, the deaths are over 9,100, meaning that Covid vaccines, in just one year, have caused twice as many deaths than every other vaccine added together since VAERS started over 30 years ago. Quite amazingly, 21% of these deaths occurred within 48 hours of vaccination.

However, another vital fact is that the adverse events and deaths listed in VAERS are significantly under-reported. One reason for this is that many people think the conditions they suffer from occur just by "chance" and don't realise the vaccines could be the cause. Many people also don't even know there are official government reporting systems. It can also take many months from when an adverse event report is received to when it is officially accepted in the VAERS data set. There is also a very limited time slot for completing the form and many people cannot fill it in on time. It is then automatically deleted and they have to start again and many of them just give up when this happens. Independent scientists believe this is all done deliberately by regulators to minimise the truth about the real number of vaccine side effects. Also, consider how many doctors could afford to spend around half an hour to submit a single adverse event?

Given all of this, in 2010, the US government commissioned a study that showed that only 1 in 100 adverse events were ever officially reported. The CDC (which unsurprisingly promotes vaccines) claims the figure is "just" 1 in 6, while a new study by Steve Kirsch of the Vaccine Safety Research Foundation puts the figure at 1 in 41. This means the real number of US deaths caused by the mRNA vaccines in one year is almost certainly somewhere between 58,000 and 910,000 with a sensible estimate being around 300,000. I must add that officially, and almost unbelievably, the Federal Drug Agency denies there has been a single death from the Covid vaccines. This means it has simply dismissed all the Covid VAERS data, even though VAERS is the US's official monitoring system which has been used by the FDA to assess all other vaccines for over 30 years. This is all truly appalling, but perhaps unsurprising when you consider how they unscientifically categorised the number of deaths and hospitalisations that we now know were vastly overstated and incorrect. The fact is they are simply determined to deny anything that threatens the mRNA vaccines regardless of the lives they take.

If you find all this hard to believe, here are a few more examples of the incredible increase in Covid jab adverse events. Researchers at Germany's largest hospital estimated there were eight serious events per 1,000 vaccinated people compared to the official German figure of just 1 in 5,000. In other words, their figure was 40 times higher than the official figure. This is almost the same as that in the study by Steve Kirsch in the US. The UK's MHRA has also recorded significantly increased levels in reported adverse vaccine reactions with over 433,000 up to the end of August 2022. In Iceland, the reported Covid adverse events were calculated at 750 times higher than those from flu jabs. This despite the fact that even flu jabs themselves, before 2020, had the highest level of recorded adverse events compared to other vaccines. The Ministry of Health (MOH) in Israel commissioned a team of researchers to analyse the data from their own adverse events reporting system. The results showed many serious and long-term side effects from the Pfizer vaccine. The researchers were so concerned that they told the MOH officials: "You have to think very carefully about how you communicate this to the public, because you may open yourself to legal lawsuits and liability issues because what you reported is, in fact, not the reality in what we see in the reports." Perhaps unsurprisingly, the Israeli government has not released this devastating data and no media group has reported it.

Finally, here is one more very recently exposed example. The CDC has in fact been using another type of adverse event reporting system and not just VAERS. This is called the V-safe programme, which, I should add, does not include deaths. Its information, however, was only available to people within the CDC, even though such government data should be legally available to anyone requesting it. An organisation called the Informed Consent Action Network requested it but got nowhere. They simply had no choice but to sue the CDC. It took numerous legal appeals, two lawsuits, and over a year, but the CDC finally capitulated and did what they should have done from day one. Around 10 million people had used V-safe and between the start of 2021 and July 2022, they reported an incredible 71 million individual adverse symptoms including things like joint pain, swelling, chills and fatigue. Approximately 770,000 people had to seek medical care or hospitalisation and another 2.5 million had to miss work or school or other normal activities. Around 4 million suffered from pain with 400,000 classed as severe. Perhaps it is not surprising that, originally, the CDC had effectively decided to cover up this damning information even though doing so was quite simply illegal.

Here is another important fact. Soon after the Covid vaccines were given to young men, there was an alarming increase in cases of myocarditis which will be explained next. The key point here is that it is almost certain that this was caused by the vaccines because most of it developed within five days of vaccination and huge numbers of scientists were highlighting it. This meant that the FDA did not dare to try to suppress it like they were doing with all the other adverse events.

Myocarditis. The increase in the number of cases of myocarditis, which have skyrocketed to a new level particularly in younger people and especially males, is truly worrying. In

2017 research in the US showed that the average number of cases of myocarditis was around 240 per year. How many cases of myocarditis do you imagine might have been reported in VAERS after this age group was vaccinated in 2021? The figure is 14,400, meaning a staggering increase of 60-fold. Unsurprisingly, the FDA and CDC dispute these numbers but they do accept that the vaccines really have caused some cases. Another fact is that the data shows that the Moderna vaccine is more likely to cause myocarditis than Pfizer's, and a number of European countries, like France, Germany, Sweden, Finland, Norway and Denmark, have recently halted Moderna vaccination for young males.

Young people should not be given mRNA vaccines. There are serious concerns regarding vaccination of young people and especially children. Even the UK's Joint Committee on Vaccination and Immunisation advised against vaccination for 12- to 18-year-olds. Why? Because clearly it causes more deaths and side effects in this age group than it saves, and the outcomes are even worse for children under 12. Countries like Finland and Singapore have not reported any childhood deaths from Covid. As already examined, only around one in a million young children die from Covid and even these are often related to other serious underlying health conditions. The US Joint Committee on Vaccination and Immunization recently released data showing that for the Omicron variant, 2 million children have to be vaccinated to prevent just one intensive care admission. Despite all of this, most governments and drug authorities, including the UK, have approved vaccination for children over the age of five. One of the key reasons that was originally given was that it would help to reduce overall deaths, particularly for older people, by reducing transmission. An opinion piece in the BMJ by three vaccine experts said, "Should society really be considering vaccinating children, subjecting them to any risk, not for the purpose of benefitting them but in order to protect adults?" Robert F. Kennedy Jr. said, "Never before has a society demanded that children take risks that might sacrifice their health in order to protect the old." Many other people agree that young children should not be allowed to die and lose around 70 to 80 years of life, just to reduce the risk of perhaps 1 in a 100 old people from dying probably a few weeks or months earlier than normal. Of course, the shocking fact is it is now universally accepted that the vaccines don't even prevent infection or transmission, so giving them to children would in fact have no benefit at all for older people. Recently, 16,000 members of the Alliance of Physicians and Medical Scientists signed a declaration stating that, "Healthy children should not be subjected to forced vaccination as their clinical risk from SARS-CoV-2 infection is negligible."

These are just a few examples of the significant opposition to childhood Covid vaccination. Nevertheless, despite all of this, the determination of governments, key medical agencies and vaccine advocates to impose child vaccination and include it in the childhood vaccine schedule continues. It is one of the most despicable and unforgiveable parts of the pandemic, and those trying to enforce it are themselves despicable and should never be forgiven.

Finally, here is another appalling fact about childhood Covid vaccines. Pfizer's Covid vaccine trial enrolled 4,526 children aged between six months and four years. However, 3,000 of them were then excluded from the results without any explanation. Participants can individually drop out of a trial, and drug companies also exclude others because severe side effects occur and they just want to hide them to protect their approval. Normally, however, these dropouts represent a relatively small percentage of the total, but in the Pfizer trial, two-thirds were excluded without any explanation. This is almost unheard of, and Dr Clare Craig, a diagnostic pathologist, said that a 66% dropout should have been sufficient to deem the trial null and void. While it is impossible to prove, it is almost certain that the reason was to hide a wide range of side effects.

Other serious vaccine outcomes. Myocarditis is a major concern, but here are a number of other diseases, side effects and deaths that have significantly increased since the start of vaccination. These include a wide range of other heart-related diseases, like heart attacks, heart failure, blood clots and pericarditis. Other increasing diseases include strokes, menstrual changes and still births, shingles, certain cancers, Creutzfeldt-Jakob disease, Bell's palsy, embolisms, Guillain-Barre syndrome, multi-organ failure, paralysis, aneurysms, and neurological disfunction. Independent experts relate much of these increases to Covid vaccines, but unsurprisingly, key medical organisations and regulators dispute virtually all of this and say the reasons for the increases are not yet known. However, the truth will almost certainly emerge at some point, just as it has about their original bogus claims that vaccines alone would solve Covid, their overstating of Covid deaths and hospital admissions, and their claims that vaccines would prevent infection and transmission. But there is a further problem. What about long-term side effects from the mRNA vaccines? We have seen many examples of drug side effects that took years and even decades to uncover and that resulted in incredible numbers of deaths. Beta blocker drugs caused the deaths of 800,000 EU citizens, but it took five years before it was uncovered. It also took 27 years before it was finally confirmed that statins increase the risk of patients developing type 2 diabetes by an average of over 50%. A number of independent viral experts are predicting that within the next ten years, the current gene therapy Covid vaccines – because of the ways they seriously compromise natural immunity – will increase the risk of a wide range of other autoimmune diseases like Parkinson's and multiple sclerosis, neurodegenerative diseases, cancers and blood disorders like blood clots, haemorrhaging, stroke and heart failure, which are also likely to affect much younger age groups. Although it cannot yet be proven, the future could be devastating.

Recent data, however, has shown that sudden cardiac arrest in young adults has increased since vaccination was undertaken. Athletes in particular have seen deaths skyrocket, although why it is affecting them so severely is as yet unknown. Historically, the annual number of sudden worldwide cardiac deaths in athletes has been between 29 and 69 – averaging around 50. In the 19 months up to August 2022, however, the figure was 847, which is equivalent to 535 in a year. This is over ten times the average number in previous years. The average age of death is around 25 and around 80% have no family history of heart disease and no actual symptoms. Virtually all of them had been vaccinated. Unsurprisingly, the media have reported very few of these deaths and certainly won't expose the total devastating number and start demanding a serious investigation to uncover the real causes of it all.

The increase in all of these diseases, and their disabilities and deaths, appears to be linked in a significant way to the vaccines, although there are certainly other causes like the increases in waiting lists and waiting times for hospital treatments. It's also primarily affecting working age people between 18 and 64. It is now known that in 2022 there have been 50,000 excess deaths in the UK. Very few of these were due to Covid. However, every official body including regulators and governments as well as the press are simply saying that the reasons for these excess deaths are not yet fully known but would include increased hospital waiting times. The one thing they do "claim" is that they are not caused by the vaccines which they continue to claim are safe. Despite this claim, we have seen that everyone involved had been desperately trying to hide the true level of vaccine side effects and deaths and to censor or simply not report the studies by reputable scientists showing that all this is happening.

The increase in diseases and deaths particularly in younger people is truly concerning, and here are just three examples of doctors trying to get health authorities and governments to take action against the vaccines, despite their unwavering claim that they are safe.

In September 2022 top doctors in India and 34 other countries declared a medical crisis due to the number of people being harmed by Covid jabs. This medical crisis declaration calls on governments and medical organisations to stop the continued injections of Covid jabs. They also call for investigations into sudden deaths following Covid jabs in previously healthy people and those suffering from the huge range of adverse events. An organisation called New Zealand Doctors Speaking out with Science (NZDSOS) published an open letter calling for investigations to be undertaken into the disturbing number of injuries and deaths being reported following Covid jabs. In August 2022 413 German doctors published an open letter criticising the government's Covid policies and called for the immediate suspension of the Covid jab programme due to the serious adverse events being experienced by so many.

There is also a very specific and significant increase in deaths and infections within the two weeks after vaccination. One of the world's top pathologists, Peter Schirmacher, has calculated that around 35% of these deaths were caused by the vaccine. Professor Norman Fenton also asked the UK Office for National Statistics to withdraw its February 2022 report because he says they were seriously underreporting both Covid and non-Covid deaths that occurred within the two weeks after vaccination. The simple fact behind all of this is that Pfizer knew, from its vaccine trials, that for this post-vaccine period, people of all ages experienced a temporary weakening of their immune system. This is almost certainly one of the key causes of these excess deaths and infections. The key reason that this has effectively been hidden is that people are not classed as vaccinated until two weeks after the second jab. So, although the jab is almost certainly the main cause, it is falsely and unbelievably blamed on the unvaccinated. Did the vaccine decision makers deliberately introduce this two-week definition for vaccination, so they could simply cover up these serious events and deaths? Almost certainly, even though it is impossible to prove.

Inadequate testing of Covid vaccines. Before Covid appeared, every other vaccine had been tested and trialled for between 10 and 15 years before being approved. Why such lengthy research? Just like drugs, all vaccines cause side effects and some deaths, but the deaths caused by most infectious diseases like measles and chicken pox are also very low, and even when Covid appeared, it was clear that children and even adults under 50 also had extremely low levels of deaths. It is vital, therefore, that vaccines don't kill more people or children than the disease itself. It is why they are tested in detail on animals first and then slowly on humans. A key point is that even when all this happens and after ten or more years of detailed research, some vaccines are still found to be too dangerous and are not approved for use. Others are approved, but then when they are given to hundreds of thousands or millions of people and children, serious outcomes and deaths can also appear at that stage, and they are then either removed from use or severely restricted. Here are two examples. The dengue fever vaccine caused a scandal in the Philippines in 2017. It was given to 700,000 children but actually made dengue fever worse and more deadly for anyone who hadn't previously had the disease. The scandal engulfed the nation.

In 2017 a study was also carried out on the DTP vaccine in the West African nation of Guinea Bissau. The vaccine did help to protect children from diphtheria, tetanus and pertussis, but in fact it caused a five-fold increase in overall deaths because it increased their susceptibility to other infectious diseases by compromising their immune system. These two examples are deeply disturbing. After more than a decade of research, testing and final approval, they both were found to increase mortality rates in the children taking them. How do outcomes like these happen? The problem is, in most cases, vaccines are only tested in a way that measures their benefits. So, for DTP vaccines, their effect on outcomes for diphtheria, tetanus and pertussis were measured, but nothing else. We have already seen that all-cause mortality is also very rarely assessed in most clinical drug trials even though it should be. This really is unforgiveable, because, quite simply, if a vaccine or drug kills more people than it saves it should not be used. This is exactly the sort of thing that drug regulators should control but they don't. They simply allow the drug industry to get away with such devastating and unscientific scandals and deaths.

For Covid, however, the mRNA vaccines were approved for use in just a few months by granting them emergency use authorisation (EUA). Unlike conventional vaccines, this type of gene editing therapy had never been officially approved or used before on humans. Now, it has been approved without any animal testing, and at warp speed with the shortest vaccine trials in the history of medicine. No one can know what the long-term side effects might be, and the idea that claims are being made that they are completely safe now and in the future is one of the most unbelievable and unscientific statements ever made. In fact, mRNA trials had previously been carried out for other diseases on animals, but no vaccine had ever been approved, and even Moderna had carried out several of these mRNA trials but they too were never approved because of serious outcomes which is quite alarming. It is possible that this Covid vaccine EUA approval could turn out to be the greatest medical disaster ever.

The unvaccinated. What about the unvaccinated? You will have heard incessantly that this is a pandemic of the unvaxxed. Claims have been made that they make up most hospitalisations and deaths, usually 85% to 95%. Yet this is just one more example of false data. In mid-July 2021 the CDC director Dr Rochelle Walensky claimed in a White House briefing that over 95% of hospitalisations and deaths were unvaccinated. However, it was finally revealed three weeks later just how these figures had actually been obtained. The data analysis was done from January to June. In January, however, only 0.5% of the population had received just one shot, so in that month virtually everyone was unvaccinated meaning that almost 100% of hospitalisations would simply have to have been unvaccinated. Whilst vaccinations increased each month, reaching 43% in June, a significant majority of the population was unvaccinated during that six-month timeframe meaning that the figures were skewed and clearly biased. Remember also that people are only officially classed as vaccinated two weeks after the second dose, and this would also have significantly increased the number of so-called unvaccinated. In fact, given the typical gap between first and second doses of two months plus the extra 14 days, then virtually no one would have been classed as vaccinated until at least April. So, why did the CDC choose this savagely biased and unfair timeframe? They were clearly determined to promote vaccination by making the unvaccinated appear to be almost the sole cause of the pandemic, but if they had given the latest actual numbers for July, they would not have been able to make such an absurdly false claim.

Most other countries have also been accused of manipulating data regarding the unvaccinated. Sweden's health authorities were recently accused of misrecording jabbed versus unjabbed deaths to cover up the true number of vaccine-related deaths. Sweden, like other countries, has been counting partially jabbed people as unjabbed.

The vaccine industry and its media and web promoters have continued to make similar manipulated claims, but here are some real facts that contradict them and indicate the true reality. During the third Covid wave in July 2021, official data from Israel showed that 71% of critically ill cases were amongst those who were double jabbed even though the double vaccination rate was even less at 61%, meaning they were at higher risk than the unvaccinated. Data from Israel are accepted by many experts as one of the most reliable in the world. Official figures from England's Office for National Statistics showed that in the months up to October 2021 there were more per capita deaths amongst the fully vaccinated than the unvaccinated. Official figures from Scotland showed that 87% of those who died from Covid in October 2021 were vaccinated (which means the unvaccinated accounted for no more than 13%). A more recent Scottish analysis published in January 2022 showed that deaths with Covid were higher in those jabbed compared to the unvaccinated. For Wales, 87% of hospitalisations for October were also for the fully vaccinated. In March 2022 a reporter from the Expose noted that while the world has been distracted by Russia's invasion of Ukraine, the UK government quietly released a report that confirmed that 9 in every 10 deaths from COVID-19 were in people who were fully vaccinated. Please remember that all these are based on official unchallengeable data, even though the press and media never published any of it and simply kept repeating the official line that the unvaxxed were to blame.

In the US, the Covid data for the vaccinated are also manipulated in another different way to the unvaxxed. Those vaccinated are given a Covid test with a very low sensitivity so that most test "negative", while the unvaxxed have a highly sensitive test which picks up every single case as well as classing those who recovered from infection weeks and even months before as still being infected. This means case rates for the unvaxxed are apparently (but incorrectly) much higher. The determination to make the unvaccinated appear to be the main cause of the pandemic is almost unbelievable and the scams that are used are simply unforgiveable.

Incidentally, here is one almost unbelievable fact. In May 2021, during a US senate hearing, Senator Burr asked Dr Anthony Fauci how many NIH employees had received the Covid vaccine. He said a little more than half to 60% and Dr Peter Marks of the FDA confirmed a similar percentage. So, around 45% of NIH and FDA staff had refused the vaccine. Dr Walensky of the CDC managed to dodge the question but if their rates had been any higher, she would have said so. Quite simply, these are the three key medical organisations that are labelling the unvaxxed as the cause of the epidemic, yet they were clearly the least vaccinated in the whole of the US. Could it be because many of the employees saw all the real data on Covid? This would mean they would know the limited effectiveness of the vaccines as well as their serious side effects, rather than the manipulated and false data given to the public via a complicit media. Whatever the reason, this is shocking and further emphasises the sad truth about the vaccines.

The Omicron variant has led to even more evidence that the savagely biased claims made about the unvaccinated are not just untrue, but that the reverse is now the case. Official UK government data show infection rates are higher amongst the fully vaccinated in every age group. Hospitalisations are also higher. Here is an extract from the Herald: "Double-jabbed Scots are now more likely to be admitted to hospital with Covid than the unvaccinated amid an increase in elderly people falling ill due to waning immunity. It comes amid weird data showing that case rates have been lower in unvaccinated individuals than the single, double- or even triple-jabbed since Omicron became the dominant variant in Scotland."

Data from Australia also shows that the fully vaccinated are 2.2 times more likely to catch Omicron than the unvaccinated. Israel had given four doses of the jab in just 12 months but then had one of the highest rates of infection in the world. In March 2022 UK government data showed that double-vaccinated people were more likely to be diagnosed with Covid and more likely to be hospitalised compared to the unvaccinated. Those who were triple vaccinated had even worse infection rates. A large study at the Cleveland Clinic involving 51,011 of its employees showed that, compared to the unvaccinated, workers who had received one jab were 1.7 times more likely to get Covid. For those with two jabs the figure was 2.6 times, for triple jabbed it was 3.1 times, and those with four jabs were 3.8 times more likely to get infected. In August 2022 the Eurostat revealed that while Portugal is the highest Covid vaccinated country in the EU (around 97%), it has had the highest level of excess deaths since January 2021 which coincides with the vaccine roll out. The latest data from New South Wales in Australia in August 2022 showed that of the 789 Covid deaths in the last eight weeks, all but two were vaccinated. Why is all this happening? As already explained, the mRNA vaccines force the natural immune system to work in a devastatingly unnatural way. They force it to attack only the original spike protein but this has undergone radical changes in the Omicron variant, meaning the genetically modified immune system simply cannot attack it effectively. Quite simply, a natural immune system really does have an incredibly better response against Omicron than a genetically modified immune system.

From early in 2022 the absolutely incessant and savage attacks on the unvaccinated by most governments and all vaccine promoting organisations effectively stopped. We have just seen that the vaccinated now have higher infection rates and significantly worse outcomes than the unvaccinated, although with just a few exceptions, most news organisations failed to report it. However, once this information started to emerge, every major medical organisation like the CDC, as well as all governments, simply stopped carrying out official infection rate monitoring. The reason? Almost certainly so the real truth could not emerge, because if it does, they will be held responsible for probably the worst medical scandal in history. This has to be why the devastating attacks on the unvaccinated have now stopped.

Finally, given all this information, the crucial question is why were the unvaccinated attacked so ruthlessly? Quite simply, whilst the vaccines did provide some initial benefits (although not as much as claimed), it was soon clear they were failing to halt the pandemic despite the original claims that it would. Infections, hospitalisations and deaths were simply continuing at high levels. Trying to blame the unvaccinated for all of this was simply a ploy that helped to hide the real truth about the vaccines. However, there is another key fact. Imagine a country that offered Covid vaccines but simply left the choice to every individual, and then ended up with half its population fully vaccinated and the other half unvaccinated. This would then create a perfect situation in which the benefits of the vaccines together with their side effects could be accurately monitored by independent scientists and the outcomes of both groups compared, not just for a few months, but over their entire lifetimes. The fact is those in charge did not want to allow this to happen because it would quite simply expose the truth about the devastating effects of the vaccines on human life, together with their limited benefits which also decline rapidly. So, the plan was to try to "enforce" vaccination which would have made it impossible to ever do such vital scientific comparisons and research. Luckily, there have been enough non-vaccinated people who have allowed this essential comparison to still be made and the truth to emerge, even though it is now being censored and hidden from most people. Of course, another key reason was that mass vaccination would produce incredible profits for the drug industry and all those who invested in it.

Court case to enforce release of Pfizer trial data. In September 2021 a group called Public Health and Medical Professionals for Transparency (PHMPT) filed a Freedom of Information Act request with the FDA to obtain all the trial documentation they had used to approve the Pfizer Covid vaccine. The FDA initially did not respond and eventually the PHMPT had to sue them. The FDA then asked the judge to allow them to delay the full release of the documents (comprising 329,000 pages) until 2075 and said they could only release 500 pages per month because they didn't have enough staff to check all the data (even though they employ 18,000 staff). The FDA's request was suspicious because they claimed they had thoroughly examined all the data to approve the drug, and yet this took just 108 days to complete. To claim the re-examination and release would now take 55 years was unbelievable. Then, a short while later, the FDA claimed they had "found" another 59,000 pages of data, which meant they would need to add another 20 years to the release of all this information. How could they just forget about 59,000 pages when this was perhaps the most important trial for decades? Then, early in January 2022, Judge Mark Pittman came to a judgement on the FDA's request for a 75-year overall delay in releasing all the information. He rejected it and told them they must complete the full release within eight months even though he recognised the burden on their resources. He said, "There may not be a more important issue at the Food and Drug Administration than the pandemic, the Pfizer vaccine, getting every American vaccinated, and making sure that the American public is assured that this was not rushed."

Perhaps unsurprisingly, the FDA (this time together with Pfizer) appealed the judgement, but all they achieved was to simply delay the initial release and add another month to final completion. So, towards the end of 2022, most of the data will be released so that independent scientists can carry out a detailed analysis, although I should add that the FDA are allowed to redact certain information that, for example, contains confidential business and patient information. No doubt they will do whatever they can to legally hide as much data as possible, but the world could soon face an incredible level of damaging evidence. However, a key question is, will the press and media report it accurately or will they downplay it or not report any of it? They have after all simply reported the official medical and government line on virtually everything related to Covid, even though they would have known that many of the key "facts" like hospital admissions and deaths were incorrect. No one in authority will want the true facts to come out about the vaccine side effects and deaths, so only time will tell whether the media and press will continue with their suppression of the truth.

Bivalent booster jabs. It has already been shown that extra booster jabs with the original vaccines actually increases Covid infection rates and adverse events. But what about the new type of mRNA boosters? On 15 August 2022 the UK was the first country to approve Moderna's new bivalent Covid booster although it will also be approved in Europe and countries like Australia and Canada. This contains its initial vaccine for the original Wuhan virus together with one for the first Omicron (BA.1) variant. Moderna claims it is effective against both of these variants. There is just one incredible problem. Both of them now effectively don't exist and have simply been "outed" by new variants like BA.2, BA.4 and BA.5 and the latest one called XBB.1.5. The key problem is the SARS-CoV-2 viruses (as well as other Coronaviruses) mutate naturally. However, the surface-based spike protein is the most rapidly mutating part of the Covid virus, and because the vaccines unnaturally force the immune system to produce these spike proteins, they are in fact causing even faster mutations than would normally occur. In 2022 dozens of variants have evolved around the world. This means that, in many cases, new booster vaccines, which take months to develop and then produce, will be out of date and will simply be used against a new variant for which there will be no proof it works. Even if it does offer some protection, it will deteriorate rapidly like it has done for every other variant.

An even more shocking fact is that now new boosters undergo no clinical trials at all. Given these involve different types of gene editing, there is no knowing what adverse events these will cause or how they will react with the initial gene editing from the first vaccines. Given there are no clinical trials, the claim that these new boosters work is made on just one very unscientific claim. Moderna's claim is it increases the antibody levels for the spike protein. How was this claim made? It was tested on just a few mice which in itself is appallingly unscientific. However, there is also simply no proof that specific antibodies offer any benefits, and even the Pfizer vice president for viral vaccines, Kena Swanson, acknowledged that there is no established correlation between antibody levels and protection from disease. The simple fact is, while the natural human immune system does, of course, contain a wide range of antibodies, they are just one part of its incredibly complex system like T cells, B cells, killer cells and phagocytes which are involved in defeating viral infections. One part of the innate immune system – neutrophils – has killer cells that can directly kill viruses without the need for antibodies. Just continually producing one single spike protein antibody is not only unlikely to work, it is likely to cause more serious adverse events. The key fact is continuously inflated antibodies caused by repeated booster shots signal to your body you are always infected, and the resulting enforced and unnatural continuous immune responses really could prove detrimental, keeping your body in a dangerous state. Covid analyst Marc Girardot has stated it really could lead to autoimmune diseases like Parkinson's and multiple sclerosis.

The simple fact is the only way Moderna could prove this new booster jab could provide any meaningful benefit and was safe would involve a clinical trial. However, Moderna really will make billions of dollars of extra profit from these boosters, so you can be certain they will never risk a clinical trial that would almost certainly fail and stop this from happening. Of course, we also know the drug agencies will not force them to do it (which is what they should do), because they also own part of the patents, meaning they also will make hundreds of millions of dollars as well. I should finally add that Pfizer has also produced a new bivalent booster jab which will probably be used in the US. However, it has made exactly the same claims as Moderna relating to the antibodies. Pfizer also tested it on just eight mice to promote its use. The whole thing is almost too shocking to believe.

Other important Covid facts. The Covid pandemic involves an incredible number and complexity of issues. To explore them all in detail would need another book. It is also important to understand that most of the crucial information originates in the US and this is because Pfizer and Moderna are US companies meaning the crucial authorities controlling them are the FDA and CDC. Another key fact is the US has a wide range of respected individuals and organisations who are trying to ensure the truth about the vaccines is exposed. These include senior doctors, scientists and researchers, attorneys, senators, and organisations like the Children's Health Defense, many of which are now involved in legal challenges. So, here are more crucial facts briefly outlined.

Pfizer's clinical trial data for the mRNA vaccine revealed incredible outcomes. The trial lasted six months and involved 22,000 participants who were vaccinated and another 22,000 who were given a placebo jab. There are two key facts. The first is there was one death from Covid in the vaccine group and two deaths from Covid in the placebo group. So, the vaccine achieved one less death. In other words, it actually showed that 22,000 people had to be vaccinated to prevent one Covid death. If this trial data was released exactly as I have just explained, there is little doubt that very few people would risk taking the vaccine. So, what did Pfizer do? They used the well-established technique of quoting "relative risk" rather than the reality of "absolute risk". The difference between one death and two deaths meant Pfizer could claim the vaccine provides a 100% improvement over the placebo. The real improvement is, of course, 1 in 22,000 which is around 0.005% – 22,000 times less than the claim made by Pfizer. Of course, it is not illegal to quote a "relative risk", but it really is completely deceiving. Many people really would think Pfizer's claim that the vaccine provided a 100% improvement really means it prevents every death, which is exactly what Pfizer would be hoping for. I should add that the media really did obligingly report Pfizer's extraordinary 100% efficacy claim even though their science reporters would definitely have known the truth. Are you shocked by this trial data? You should be. But now prepare for something even more shocking in this second fact.

The trial results also showed that overall there were 20 deaths in the vaccine group but only 14 in the placebo group. Pfizer was apparently so alarmed by the fact vaccination caused more deaths that it omitted five of these deaths from its final summary and only disclosed them in a fine print buried deep in the body of the report, no doubt hoping most people would not see them. The real factual data, however, meant the vaccines caused a 42% increased risk of overall deaths. Perhaps by now, you may not be surprised that the FDA still gave its approval for the vaccines. There are other examples of drug regulators approving dangerous drugs that kill more people than they save, but Covid vaccines could eventually turn out to be one of the most dangerous. There is real-world data that shows that, just like the Pfizer trial, the vaccinated are now dying at higher numbers than the unvaccinated.

One final fact is that one key reason for the increased deaths in the vaccine group was cardiac arrests. Five people in the vaccine group died from this compared to just one in the control group. Cardiac type deaths really are now also increasing alarmingly around the globe.

Significant evidence relating to the side effects of the Covid mRNA vaccines has been examined in detail. So, what have the key regulators like the FDA and CDC been doing about it all? Here are a few examples:

- We have seen that the FDA wanted to avoid releasing the Pfizer clinical trial data for up to 75 years. Luckily, a judge overruled this plan to hide the truth, and independent scientists have now started to analyse and report some of the serious outcomes.
- The CDC also refused to release any of the information on the V-safe adverse events reporting system, but again after an 18-month legal fight, they were eventually forced to do so.
- The FDA has consistently maintained that the vaccines are safe and dismisses all the VAERS data. It said that the only evidence it would accept regarding possible vaccine deaths is if an autopsy confirmed this. Initially, few autopsies were ever carried out but now these are increasing and once again scientists want to see this data. But once again, the FDA is refusing to release the data saying simply it doesn't want to release private and personal information. Of course, this is just an excuse because patients' names could simply be redacted as they have been on many occasions for similar types of independent research. I suspect independent organisations will have to take the FDA to court yet again to get the data. Why is the FDA really refusing to release it? Almost certainly because the data show the vaccines are a significant cause of the deaths. Despite all of this, there is one positive piece of news in December 2022. The Florida governor Ron DeSantis is now implementing official autopsy surveillance of post-jab sudden deaths and has established an Independent Public Health Integrity Committee. The Florida surgeon general Dr Joseph Ladapo said, "Healthcare professionals should always communicate the risk of a medical intervention to their patients in a manner that is clinically appropriate and meets standards of ethical practice. President Biden and Big Pharma have completely prevented that from happening – it is wrong. With these new actions, we will shed light on the forces that have obscured truthful communication about the COVID-19 vaccines."
- In July 2021 the FDA quietly disclosed an increase in four types of serious adverse events in elderly people who had received the Pfizer jab. These were myocardial infarction, disseminated intravascular coagulation, immune thrombocytopenia and pulmonary embolism. No press release or other alert was sent to doctors or the public. The FDA promised it would "share further updates and information with the public as they became available" and agreed to do a more detailed follow-up study. Over a year later and the FDA has not published any information, despite the fact that now

there are a number of other studies, including one from the BMJ, that are exposing similar serious outcomes.

- There are a range of other studies showing various side effects where the FDA is seemingly burying the results. The CDC publishes a "Mortality and Morbidity Weekly Report" which analyses the causes of deaths. The Ethical Skeptic analysed this data to show how the CDC hides and even deletes excess jab-related deaths, particularly in categories like cancer, cardiac deaths and strokes. In June 2022 the CDC was supposedly doing a "system upgrade" and did not release any new data for two months. When it came back online, a large number of previous jab-related death categories had been moved into either the Covid death category or a "holding category" where the deaths were classed as undetermined. These two major recategorised changes make the deaths from cancer, heart attacks and strokes appear far lower than they actually are. Of course, the CDC would deny any wrongdoing, but independent experts are predicting this is simply manipulation of the data and it cannot continue forever. The "holding category" now has 70% more cases that supposedly have unknown causes. These are simply being left there in incredibly high numbers that have never been seen before and there is little doubt they are just trying to hide jab-related heart deaths. There are significantly increased cancer cases as well, but these are now being classed as Covid deaths. Currently, 20% of all weekly Covid deaths have cancer listed only as an "underlying cause", while Covid is classed as the main cause. This significant misalignment of data will surely reach the point where the false manipulation will become self-evident.
- Quite simply, the FDA and CDC are refusing to release vital data which they are officially mandated to do. They are either not carrying out, or not publishing, research they promised to do on dangerous jab side effects. They are not acting on vital evidence, and they are now manipulating databases to artificially hide excess jab deaths. Why would any of this have been done if the vaccines really were safe as claimed? This is what Dr Joseph Mercola has said about it: "All in all, it seems the wheels are coming off the Covid jab bus. Sparks are already flying. The FDA and CDC could have saved themselves by coming clean a few months into the Covid jab scam. At this point, there's no way to save face, let alone anyone's career. Both agencies are doomed, as are their leadership." The world should hope he is right, that the real truth finally emerges, and that the key decision makers are brought to justice.

We have seen that the vaccine industry, particularly in western countries, is exempt from any claims from vaccine adverse events. There are, however, a number of countries where vaccine-damaged people can still take the manufacturers to court. Did you know that in December 2021 the World Bank president, David Malpass, said Pfizer will not give mRNA shots to countries where they face legal liabilities for side effects? If Pfizer really knew its Covid jabs were safe, why would it not supply them? Quite simply, Pfizer does, of course, know the vaccines have serious outcomes, and it will not risk losing more money in the courts than it makes from vaccine sales.

A prestigious meta-analysis of 12 clinical trials was published in JAMA in 2022. Its aim was to evaluate the adverse events of Covid vaccines and was carried out by a team of some of the most highly respected doctors and researchers including Ted Kaptchuk from Harvard Medical School. It showed a clear and statistically significant increase in adverse events in those receiving the vaccines compared to those receiving controls, and the second dose caused the biggest increase. Another equally prestigious team also carried out a meticulous study of the Pfizer and Moderna trial data. They found a consistently higher risk of serious adverse events – between 1.36 and 1.57 times greater – for those vaccinated compared to those receiving controls. They even used criteria approved by the WHO. Has any official body accepted any of these studies? Absolutely not. To try to hide the adverse events of the Covid jabs, one of their recent claims is that "long Covid" is itself a cause, but while this may play a part in some outcomes, it is not the main cause and it certainly cannot contradict the data from these two meticulous studies.

Recent evidence has shown that vaccine batches are not all identical which is causing different levels of adverse events. In the US, How Bad Is My Batch is a website that compiles data on adverse events from VAERS. By separating each adverse event into its corresponding vaccine batch, it has shown there are differences in side effects and deaths and Dr Meryl Nass at the FLCCC has confirmed this is happening even though at this stage the reasons why are unclear. It could be due to certain impurities or the fact that some batches contain varying levels of the spike proteins. A separate analysis suggests that some batches are hyper concentrated because of the way they collect at the top of the large vats they are produced in, and even suggests that 5% of batches could be responsible for around 80% of the harm. Whatever the reasons are, the wide range of adverse events that people are suffering from could, in part, depend simply on bad luck or good luck in their individual vaccine jab.

Approximately 85% of Canadians have received at least two Covid shots and in June 2022 Dr Charles Hoffe analysed the official data which showed that 92% of all Covid deaths were in the fully jabbed. However, only 34% had received three or four doses, yet they accounted for 81% of all the deaths. While this does not provide absolute proof, it really does indicate that the more jabs you have, the more likely you will die of Covid.

Three countries are now restricting Covid jabs. Denmark has effectively banned the vaccines and booster jabs for anyone under the age of 50 unless they have evidence of a serious medical condition and a doctor's note. Norway has done the same for anyone under the age of 65. Why? Maybe they understand how ineffective and dangerous the jabs are. Maybe they read all the official data that shows the vaccinated are now much more likely to get Covid than the unvaccinated. Finland is not recommending the fourth Covid jab because continued revaccination could damage and weaken the immune system. Also, in the US, the surgeon general Dr Joseph Ladapo issued new vaccine guidance for his state of Florida, recommending men between the ages of 18 and 39 abstain from the Covid jab, as its own data shows an increase in heart-related death within 28 days of injection. Children aged 5 to 17 years and those under five are also not recommended for jabs. In January 2023, even the UK has just announced that healthy people under the age of 50 will no longer be able to get Covid vaccines or boosters.

In early October 2022, during a Covid hearing in the Dutch parliament, the member Rob Roos questioned Pfizer's president of international developed markets, Janine Small, about whether Pfizer had in fact tested and confirmed their mRNA jab would prevent transmission prior to its roll out. Small responded, "No, we had to really move at the speed of science... and we had to do everything at risk... We were building the airplane while we were trying to fly it". As noted by Roos, "This means the Covid passport was based on a big lie. The only purpose of the Covid passport: forcing people to get vaccinated." Roos added that he found this deception "shocking – even criminal".

Since the roll out of the Covid shots, health officials have adamantly claimed the jabs are safe for all pregnant women. There has nevertheless been an increase in miscarriage rates and many mothers and independent experts do believe the vaccines are dangerous particularly in the first trimester. A CDC study was carried out in 2021 that claimed to show the vaccines were safe during pregnancy and was published in the New England Journal of Medicine. The miscarriage rate was claimed to be 12.5% which they said was only slightly above the normal average of 10%. However, miscarriages are only officially measured in the first 20 weeks of pregnancy, but the numbers that were analysed in this study included vaccinated women in the third trimester (weeks 28–40). These should simply not have been included and when independent experts excluded them, the actual miscarriage rate was 82%. This is not a misprint. I should also add that birth rates are falling in most countries and this escalated around nine months after pregnant women started to be vaccinated. Here are a few examples. In the first quarter of 2022 birth rates fell by 10% in Germany, 14% in Sweden, 15% in Switzerland, 10% in the UK and 20% in Hungary. A July 2022 article by Mike Campbell reported that in the five countries with the highest Covid jab uptake, fertility has dropped by an average of 15.2%, whereas the five countries with the lowest jabs had an average reduction of just 4.7%. I must add that the official medical position remains unchanged and all women are still recommended to take the jabs.

When the FDA authorised the use of doses four and five of the original vaccine booster jabs, it reportedly based its decision on Israeli data from the Sheba Medical Center in February 2022. This is what the authors of this study reported: "Vaccine efficacy against infection was 30% and 11% for BNT162b2 (Pfizer) and mRNA1273 (Moderna) respectively. Local and systemic adverse reactions were reported in 80% and 40% respectively." Quite simply, the FDA authorised these boosters based on data showing the Moderna shot was only 11% effective, and caused side effects in 40% of recipients. The Pfizer shot was 30% effective and caused side effects in 80% of recipients. You must be shaking your head in disbelief.

Children and many adults are now seeing a significant increase in infectious diseases like flu and RSV and are having more serious outcomes. Why? In August 2021 a French group of paediatric infectious disease experts warned that "immunity debt" caused by a lack of exposure to common viruses and bacteria during Covid lockdowns and school closures could predispose children to suffer more infectious diseases in the future. Quite simply, the human immune system, and particularly that for children, needs regular exposure to a range of viruses and bacteria to help train and optimise it, as well as enabling it to regularly defeat them with relatively mild symptoms. Lockdowns simply stopped most infections for close to three years and much of mankind is now suffering alarmingly.

A 2022 study in the New England Journal of Medicine shows that natural Covid immunity is significantly better than that from Covid jabs. Natural infection offered better protection against the Omicron variant after one year than three shots of the Covid vaccines did after just one month. Here are the numbers. Natural immunity was 54.9% effective against Omicron after more than 12 months, while just one month after the third dose of the Pfizer vaccine it was only 44.7% effective. The figure for the Moderna vaccines was even worse with a one-month figure of just 41.2%. What we also now know is that well before 12 months, vaccine effectiveness had not just fallen to zero, but that it actually increases infection rates.

In June 2022 the US became the first country in the world to grant emergency use authorisation for Covid jabs for toddlers as young as six months and in December the FDA also authorised the new bivalent booster for this age group as well, even though no trials have been carried out showing whether it has any benefits or is safe. There has been wide-scale alarm about all of this given the serious side effects the vaccines create and the fact that even prestigious doctors and medical organisations confirm that young children really do have an incredibly low risk from Covid. So, how can we explain these irrational behaviours of the FDA and CDC? Now that the Covid jabs are part of the official US vaccine schedule, the drug industry is quite simply shielded from liability for injuries and deaths that occur in any age group. It also means schools can mandate child vaccination. Quite simply, it means drug company profits will escalate yet again, and that they can't lose any money by being sued for the serious outcomes and deaths their vaccines are creating. Amazingly, Pfizer also intends to raise the price of its Covid jab by 400% – from $30 to around $120. But here is one more staggering fact. In the US, the Covid jabs are all still used under emergency use authorisation (EUA). Here are the criteria that must be fulfilled before emergency use can be granted:

- There must be an emergency.
- A vaccine must be at least 30% to 50% effective.
- The known and potential benefits must outweigh the potential risks.
- There can be no other adequate, approved and available treatments.

Unless all four criteria are met, EUA cannot be granted or cannot be continued. By any reasonable measurement, Covid is no longer an emergency; life is effectively back to normal. For young children there is zero evidence on the vaccine's effectiveness. There is also incredible evidence that it causes more harm than benefit. The FDA and CDC are simply operating outside their own rules and regulations. This doesn't even include the fact there are effective alternative treatments. How do they continue to get away with all of this?

Data from the US show the despair and lack of purpose in children, caused by lockdowns and school closures, led to an increase in the use of drugs like fentanyl by high school-aged adolescents during 2020 and 2021. This caused an incredible 94% increase in deaths from these drugs over previous years. New research from a joint Australian and New Zealand study also showed that there was a worrying increase in self-harm in those aged 12–17 and hospital admissions increased by almost 60%. which the authors blamed simply on the devastating effects of Covid restrictions.

Those doctors and researchers who tried to expose all the failings and side effects of the vaccines and viral drugs were attacked, censored and discredited even though we now know they were right. Here is just one example. Even as early as 9 February 2021, Dr Joseph Mercola published an article that explained that the mRNA Covid vaccines did not meet the legal definition of a vaccine, in part because they don't prevent infections or spread, and were in fact experimental gene therapies. Shortly after, the New York Times published a hit piece on him saying his assertions were "easily disprovable" even though we now know he was telling the truth. Since then he has become the most censored and attacked doctor in the world even though I am not aware of a single thing he has said that has been shown to be incorrect.

We have seen that the Pfizer and Moderna Covid "vaccines" aren't vaccines but gene edited therapy and it is now indisputable that they don't prevent infection or transmission and any benefits quickly fall. All this, however, has enabled the promotion of multiple boosters which have minimal benefits and make those who take them more likely to develop serious outcomes. But there is, of course, one "positive" outcome, which is the incredible increase in industry profits. The Pfizer vaccine has become the most profitable drug in history at $37 billion in one year. Pfizer also has the antiviral drug Paxlovid. Amazingly, this causes a rebound in symptoms a few days later for a significant number of patients, thus necessitating more prescriptions and multiple additional doses. We also now know the Covid jabs are associated with increased rates of the respiratory syncytial virus (RSV) in children and this side effect was shown to occur even in Moderna's clinical trial. Now, both Pfizer and Moderna are developing RSV jabs which could become another profit bonanza. Quite simply, as they have done throughout recent history, the drug companies care only about profit. They are quite happy to develop drugs and vaccines that don't work well, that have serious side effects and that then need additional drugs or vaccine which will give them continually increasing profits.

Dr Peter Breggin's latest book *COVID-19 and the Global Predators: We Are the Prey* explains that while other mRNA vaccines have previously been developed and tested on other types of Coronaviruses, none ever made it to market. Other more conventional types of vaccines were also developed, but none of these have also ever worked effectively and been approved. For some reason, it seems clear that vaccines for all types of Coronavirus routinely cause severe illness when people are exposed to the wild virus – a phenomenon known as antibody dependant enhancement (ADE). Dr Breggin also cites a 2020 paper by independent researchers warning that all Covid vaccines – both mRNAs and natural killed viruses – are too dangerous to even try on humans. This paper gave an incredible warning that can be compared to the adverse events and deaths that are now occurring after the current mRNA Covid vaccines. Another analysis shows that the mRNA therapies that have been undergoing development and testing for 20 years were all previously tested on animals which is the long established vital first part of the clinical trial process. Almost unbelievably, all of them caused autoimmune diseases which meant the trials had to be stopped and no human trials were ever authorised. Given all this evidence, why did all the vaccine makers develop similar mRNA spike protein Covid vaccines and why did regulators then give them emergency use approval? Truly shocking. But even worse, a wide range of other mRNA vaccines are now being developed.

The "end" of the pandemic. In early 2022 many governments had started the lifting of lockdowns, mask wearing, working from home, Covid testing, social distancing and school restrictions. There was seemingly an acceptance that the pandemic was more or less over, and that we must now learn to live with a virus that has mainly mild symptoms and will probably be with us forever, just like the flu. Unsurprisingly, the official claim is that it was the vaccines that created this outcome. This despite the fact vaccines make infections and hospitalisations even worse for Omicron and the other newer variants. The truth is life is back to normal because the Omicron variant spread incredibly fast but had incredibly mild symptoms. Huge swathes of the population have had it and defeated it. If it had not appeared, some form of restrictions would probably have remained in place with the Delta variant. The world should be truly grateful for Omicron.

Maybe you have also noticed that from early in 2022 the media have held almost no serious discussions and programmes about Covid, and they now only very occasionally report data mainly on case numbers or new variants. This is part of what is clearly a coordinated worldwide plan that is happening in virtually every developed country. If asked why, they would say that the data are now more unreliable. Really? Why would it suddenly be so unreliable? A more likely reason is that by no longer carrying out Covid testing and almost removing it from the news, they do not need to reveal or report that vaccinated people are now more at risk of infection and hospitalisation. This means they can keep reiterating the "official" but untrue narrative that it is the vaccines that have "solved" the pandemic. It means they can continue to pressurise everyone to get vaccinated and to take every booster jab that becomes available even though they result in worse outcomes. When the global elite made the claim that vaccines were the only solution to Covid, when they had spent tens of billions of dollars worldwide in developing them, when they had deliberately stopped virtually everyone from using truly effective, simple, cheap and natural cures like ivermectin, hydroxychloroquine and vitamin D, and when the lockdowns and wide range of restrictions had cost $13.7 trillion across the globe, they couldn't now admit that the vaccines have in fact failed and are now causing devastating outcomes. If enough people knew the truth, the key vaccine advocates would have their reputations and careers destroyed and could face serious legal charges for what they have done or not done.

Please remember that the WHO said that what was needed were vaccines that could prevent infection and transmission as well as severe disease and deaths, and that they should produce an immune response that was broad, strong and long-lasting in order to reduce the need for successive boosters. Staggeringly, the current mRNA vaccines now achieve not one of these things, and there couldn't really be better evidence that they should stop being used particularly for younger people, given the side effects and deaths they are now causing.

The financial side of Covid vaccines. In 2019 before the SARS-CoV-2 virus emerged, the annual worldwide sales of every vaccine totalled just under $60 billion. What about the Pfizer and Moderna Covid vaccines? In 2021 sales of both of them were $54 billion, meaning their sales value is almost the same as every other vaccine in the entire world. It is important to remember that other countries like China, Russia and India also produced their own vaccines and there were many other versions like AstraZeneca and Janssen. Total worldwide sales were probably around $100 billion. Given that the pharmaceutical industry's total annual global sales of every drug and vaccine are just over $1,000 billion, then this one new virus has increased its sales by a staggering 10%, which is more than any other drug in history. Another interesting fact is that the drug Humira by AbbVie, which is currently the single bestselling drug in the world, reached sales of just under $20 billion in 2018. Incredibly, the Pfizer vaccine alone in 2021 had sales of $36 billion which makes it by far the bestselling drug of all time in terms of annual sales.

Incidentally, we have already seen that the drug industry has been charged with fraud and fined billions of dollars on numerous occasions. It may surprise you that Pfizer is in fact the number one culprit with 34 separate convictions up to 2017, with fines of $4.72 billion. Of course, this is dwarfed just by the mRNA vaccine sales of $36 billion in a single year. We may soon find out whether Pfizer committed any fraud on the Covid jab trials with the upcoming release of the trial data. The other fact is that, as far as the Moderna vaccine is concerned, the US National Institutes for Health own half of the patents, meaning they could collect half the royalties. Four NIH scientists have filed their own patent application for it, meaning they could become very rich individuals. Could any of these unbelievable financial profits have played any part in the way the mRNA vaccines have been incessantly promoted, how their serious adverse events have been hidden, and how far more effective Covid treatments like ivermectin have been falsely discredited?

COVID-19 origin. Finally, I want to provide some information on the origin of the SARS-CoV-2 virus. You may have been persuaded to accept that it developed naturally in wild bats and then transferred to humans in a wet market in Wuhan. There is, however, a huge body of evidence (although it cannot yet be proven conclusively) that it arose in the Wuhan Institute of Virology (WIV) which carries out wide-ranging research on viruses that also involves their genetic modification. This viral manipulation is called "gain-of-function" research and its aims are to produce new variants to explore their potential for infecting humans and the effects they might produce. This would in theory then help to develop new treatments like vaccines and antiviral drugs for such variants. All this may appear to make gain-of-function research seem logical and positive until you understand the mutated variants it produces can be much more dangerous, infectious and deadly than the original natural virus and once they are produced, there is always a risk they may escape from the laboratory and then cause serious infections in mankind that would otherwise never have happened. Many scientists have criticised gain-of-function research because it creates a real possibility of starting new pandemics from accidental (as well as intentional) viral release, and they believe we need to ban all such research worldwide in which pathogens are purposely manipulated to make them more dangerous.

In light of all of this, significant evidence really does exist that the Wuhan Institute really did develop the SARS-CoV-2 virus. On 1 August 2021 Michael McCaul, the ranking member of the House Foreign Affairs Committee, published an addendum to the investigation into its origins. The investigation concluded: "The preponderance of evidence suggests SARS-CoV-2 was accidentally released from a Wuhan Institute of Virology laboratory sometime prior to September 12, 2019. The virus, or viral sequence that was genetically manipulated, was likely collected in a cave in Yunnan province between 2012 and 2015." Multiple pieces of information led the committee to this conclusion and also to the fact the whole thing had been covered up. Another startling fact is that the US National Institute of Allergy and Infectious Diseases, led by Dr Anthony Fauci, had also funded some of the gain-of-function research at Wuhan between 2014 to 2019, and this occurred after the Obama administration had imposed a moratorium on such research in the US because of its lethal risk. This means that the US and Dr Fauci could also be partially implicated in the SARS-CoV-2 virus. I must add that President Biden later released a statement calling the intelligence report inconclusive, which is unsurprising given the ramifications that would occur if it was true and if it was exposed to the world.

Another crucial piece of evidence came from four very senior virologists led by Kristian G. Andersen of the Scripps Research Institute who examined the detailed structure of the virus. They showed there were small snippets of a genetic element that had never been seen in other natural Coronaviruses or any of their variants. They concluded it simply couldn't have happened naturally and had been mutated in a laboratory and they sent a copy of the research to Dr Fauci. Then almost unbelievably, just four days later, Anderson and several other virologists produced a new paper which claimed there was no evidence that the virus had been engineered. Whilst it is impossible to verify, some independent scientists believe Dr Fauci and other key officials had pressurised and effectively forced this reversal, probably by explaining that if the idea that the virus was produced and leaked from Wuhan was confirmed, then it could lead to major international ramifications. However, another incredible fact has also recently emerged after the release of Twitter files by Elon Musk. Robert F. Kennedy Jr. obtained key information and emails that showed how Jeremy Farrar who was director of the Wellcome Trust was also a major player in this reversal, and had directed all these virologists to say it didn't come from a lab. This is what Robert Kennedy said about him: "Because of the control he has over the funding of virology and infectious disease, and biomedical research globally, he was able to marshal these core groups of virologists who just lied to us openly. And then they all got payoffs from Fauci. Kristian Anderson PhD got $9 million after he lied to us. Eddie Holmes got $9 million… We now have their emails. And all those guys believed it was a lab leak, secretly, privately… but they were telling the public it wasn't. And they all got payoffs of millions and millions of dollars."

A key problem is governments are not banning gain-of-function research meaning future pandemics will almost certainly occur and could be far more dangerous than Covid. This is because viral lab leaks have occurred on multiple occasions around the world, although most without a serious pandemic type result so far. In China alone, for example, since 2003 there have been four different lab leaks of SARS viruses. It is, therefore, really only a matter of time before something far more deadly than Covid emerges which really could kill much of mankind. The world really needs to hope that enough people find out about the true origin of Covid and that they can help to force all governments to completely stop all gain-of-function research. Frighteningly, however, the Biden administration has just announced a new strategy involving $88 billion to start a new biodefence protocol, part of which appears to include gain-of-function research.

One final point. A new paper has just been published in October 2022. According to the researchers, the chance of SARS-CoV-2 having a natural origin is less than 1 in 100 million. The researchers have found a tell-tale signature of genetic engineering that had not been previously identified and that could only have been produced in a laboratory. Just one more piece of incredible evidence that the Covid pandemic really was man-made. The key question is whether it was released from the Wuhan lab accidentally (most likely) or deliberately (much less likely, but not impossible).

COVID-19 – the lifestyle medicine approach

Natural immunity. The natural human immune system is one of the greatest achievements our body has developed in our 7-million-year evolutionary history. Healthy people can, and do, naturally defeat hundreds of different infectious diseases ranging from colds and influenza, to measles and chicken pox, and Coronaviruses, including the current SARS-CoV-2 virus, as well as having the ability to kill things like cancer cells. The evidence is simple and indisputable. In the first year of the pandemic there were no vaccines and the original Wuhan strain was the deadliest of all the variants that have followed. There is no accurate ratio of the true number of people who died and the true number of cases, but various experts put the figure between 1 in 100 to 1 in 400. This means that somewhere between 99 out of 100 and 399 out of 400 people recovered from the infection and this was simply achieved by the natural immune system. Of course, some seriously ill patients were helped to recover in intensive care units, but that number really is very small compared to those who survived naturally. Another crucial fact is that without the natural immune system, no vaccines could ever work. They would have no effect whatsoever. Vaccines simply stimulate the immune system and it alone cures every disease. Incredibly, many people really have been led to believe it is the vaccines that cure Covid as well as other infectious diseases, which is simply a lie.

We now know that around 40% of those who defeated the virus naturally also had no obvious symptoms. Many more had minimal symptoms like a mild cold, while others had a range of increasingly serious symptoms and just a small percentage ended up in intensive care. The key question from all of this is why do some people recover so well they don't even know they've had the virus, while others have this wide range of increasing symptoms? This relates quite simply to the effectiveness of each individual's immune system. Given this indisputable fact, why are no official bodies looking at what causes this difference in immune response between individuals so that those with weakened immunity could then redevelop strong immunity that would allow them to also defeat Covid (and other viruses) with minimal symptoms. The problem is the immune system is mainly reliant on the lifestyle we all lead, and an unhealthy lifestyle really can lead to poor immunity. We have seen copious evidence that official medical organisations dismiss lifestyle solutions to most diseases and are simply committed to using just drugs and vaccines. This means that anyone wanting to improve their own immunity, so they really could naturally defeat virtually every infectious disease including COVID-19 without serious side effects, will need to do so themselves. The main factors will be outlined at the end of this section. Medicine's key decision makers should be ashamed of themselves for ignoring this.

Here is another key fact about the natural immune system. For decades, the official medical position for many infectious diseases has been that those people who have been naturally infected do not then need to receive a vaccine. Quite simply, natural immunity nearly always provides life-long protection from reinfection and medicine has never given vaccines to people who have had diseases like measles and chicken pox. Despite all of this evidence, the vaccine industry (as explained in the section on infectious diseases) has relentlessly tried to promote vaccines as the only solution to infections even though this is a clear lie, and they have also tried to marginalise natural immunity. But when COVID-19 emerged, this "attack" escalated incredibly and key organisations – quite unbelievably – are now seemingly attempting to "erase" natural immunity altogether as far as the public is concerned. Here are just four examples:

- In a September 2021 interview, Dr Anthony Fauci explained that natural immunity was not even being discussed at government health agencies.
- For decades it has been an unequivocally accepted medical fact that population herd immunity for a disease can be achieved by natural immune recovery as well as by vaccination. However, in December 2020, the WHO deleted the line "immunity developed through previous infection" from the very definition of herd immunity, implying it can only be achieved by vaccines.
- Even the media are involved. The Washington Post made this false claim: "There's a pervasive idea that your body and your immune system can be healthy enough to ward off COVID-19. No one's body can. No one's body is healthy enough to recognise and just totally ward this off without a vaccine." How do they think that more than 99% of people recovered from the virus in 2020 before any vaccine was available? This type of lie is simply despicable and almost unbelievable.
- Until recently, the Mayo Clinic's data source had shown that individuals who survived the 1918 influenza pandemic still had natural immunity to its H1N1 influenza virus. That the natural immune system still worked 90 years after being infected gives a graphic example of just how amazing it really is. But in the spring of 2021 this information was removed from its website.

It would seem the medical elite (no doubt "financially encouraged" by Big Pharma) have a plan to ensure future generations will never hear or learn about natural immunity, and the only thing they will ever be told is that infectious diseases can only be controlled by vaccines. Can they succeed? It seems impossible given that every doctor and scientist knows about the human immune system, but remember they censored the deaths of 800,000 EU citizens who were killed by a drug and even now, eight years later, virtually no one knows about it and probably never will. Without the natural human immune system, everyone would die from a viral infection and mankind would simply be extinct. The global elite and the vaccine industry know all of this, but are so determined to literally "force" everyone to take an ever-increasing number of vaccines (not just the Covid jab as will be explained in Part 6), they are simply trying to suppress the truth.

For COVID-19 in particular, a key question is why do people who have recovered naturally need to be vaccinated when they have much longer (possibly life-long) immunity for each variant compared to the rapidly declining immunity of those who have been vaccinated? The answer, of course, is they shouldn't be vaccinated, just like medicine accepts and agrees that people who had measles shouldn't be vaccinated and simply don't need it. A number of highly reputable medical experts who have been advisors to the CDC, WHO and NIH, and the editors of journals like MedPage Today have said that natural immunity should be given the same status as vaccinations. Marty Makary of the Johns Hopkins School of Medicine argues that the medical profession has hurt its credibility in pretending that natural immunity is virtually irrelevant to the Covid equation and the dogmatic "get vaccinated" position constitutes a lack of honesty about the data. But, of course, medicine's elite claimed vaccines were the only solution for COVID-19, so they simply won't accept any of this and will simply continue to pressurise everyone to get vaccinated regardless of the evidence.

Here is a final fact which explains why natural immunity beats vaccine immunity. The SARS-CoV-2 virus contains five proteins. The gene edited Covid vaccine forces the immune system to unnaturally produce antibodies against just one of them – the spike protein. So, when the Delta variant appeared which involved changes to the spike protein, the vaccine was compromised, and when the Omicron variant appeared with even more spike protein changes, the vaccine was even less successful and its effectiveness soon fell to zero. The natural immune system, on the other hand, develops antibodies against all parts of the virus as well as creating memory T cells. So, when the spike protein changed due to the Delta and Omicron variants, it offered continuing protection because it recognises and can continue to attack all the other different proteins. Of course, now the BA.5 variant has changed so much that even the natural immune system can't recognise it from previous infections but it still defeats it from scratch, just like it does for the hundreds of different types of flu and colds.

Just going back to how the vaccine was developed and the way it operates, an analysis by geneticist Alexandra Henrion-Caude PhD at the French Institute of Health showed an alarming possibility. She pointed out that if you wanted to create a vaccine, you would not target the part of the virus that is most prone to mutation, which for Covid is the spike protein. You would choose one of many other parts of the virus that are much less likely to mutate. By targeting the spike protein, however, there would be a need for repeated multiple vaccinations and boosters to keep up with all the mutations. So, choosing the spike protein might well have been driven simply by a desire for significant and continuing vaccine profits. Choosing the spike protein, however, also meant the body would be forced to produce the most toxic part of the virus which was known to be pathogenic and produce adverse events like blood clots and abnormal bleeding. It's just astounding that these shots were produced and rolled out to billions of people worldwide knowing they had such outcomes. We know this is now happening with the significant increase in cases of myocarditis and a range of other diseases and heart conditions. It's almost certainly another devastating example of the drug industry's priority of profit before human life.

Key factors for natural immunity. From a lifestyle perspective, the key question is how can people maximise their immune response so they can defeat COVID-19 naturally with relatively mild symptoms? The seven key lifestyle factors that are crucial for our health and that have been covered in detail are also essential for our natural immune system. Radically improving all these key factors really can achieve a strong immune response for Covid for most people. Even Tufts University has said that around 60% of serious cases of Covid could be avoided if people just ate a healthy diet. However, there are some very specific factors that can play a significant role in helping to minimise symptoms and prevent serious outcomes.

The first thing to say is that certain medical conditions play a major role in the severity of Covid. You may have seen media data that around 80% of hospitalisations involve patients who are obese. If there had been no obesity in the UK, then the hospitalisations and deaths would be only a fraction of what they are now. Other diseases like diabetes also increase the risk. A recent study showed that around 35% of all people who died from Covid had diabetes. Evidence on how to avoid, reverse or significantly decrease your risk of this and other diseases has also already been explained in detail, so again I won't repeat any of this information. You just need to understand how vital it all is. One other fact is that the immune system can be seriously compromised by a wide range of drugs like antacids, proton pump inhibitors and antibiotics.

Vitamins, minerals and other natural compounds, however, play a special role in the immune system and the evidence for their incredible effects on COVID-19 is significant. Of course, the official medical position always remains the same: "more data is needed" before they could be approved. This is just part of the all-out war on lifestyle medicine and simply needs to be ignored. I'll start with the most important vitamin.

Vitamin D. Optimising this vitamin is probably the easiest, least expensive, and most beneficial strategy the average person can do to minimise their risk from COVID-19. Vitamin D already had thousands of trials and studies showing its incredible effect on a wide range of other infectious diseases some of which have been covered in the previous section. Here are a few of the recent ones relating to Covid:

- A US study based on data from 191,779 patients showed that those with blood vitamin D levels above 55ng/ml had a 47% lower rate of Covid compared to those with levels below 20ng/ml.
- An Israeli study had similar results. Those with levels above 30ng/ml had a 58% lower risk of testing positive than those below 20ng/ml. This Israeli study also looked at how it affected hospitalisations. Those with low vitamin D levels below 30ng/ml had almost twice the risk of being hospitalised.
- A study published in the journal Nutrients found that patients with really low vitamin D levels – below 12ng/ml – had a six times higher risk of severe diseases that needed ventilation and a 14 times higher risk of death.
- An Italian study found similar outcomes. Those patients with very low vitamin D levels – below 10ng/ml – had a ten times higher risk of death.
- In September 2020 a trial in Córdoba gave hospital patients calcifediol – a highly absorbent vitamin D supplement. Fifty patients were given the vitamin and just one of them had to be admitted to intensive care but none of them died. The control group had 26 patients who received standard care. Thirteen of them had to be admitted to the ICU unit, and two of them died. Overall, 2% of those taking vitamin D were admitted to ICU while for those who didn't, the figure was 50%. This trial made headlines in several newspapers and so, unsurprisingly, a number of experts tried to discredit it. They claimed the number of patients was too small, that there was no information on the patients' normal vitamin D levels and that the study did not specify or make allowances for any other comorbidities. However, two researchers – Irwin Jungreis and Manolis Kellis – at the Broad Institute of MIT and Harvard, Cambridge, MA, carried out a detailed analysis of the results using rigorous and well-established techniques and concluded that the trial randomisation, the 25-fold reduction in ICU admissions and its high statistical significance addressed most of the concerns raised. They said the likelihood that this could have happened just by chance, or because of things like different comorbidities, was extremely unlikely. They gave a simple graphic example. If you flip a coin 50 times, the chance of getting five or fewer heads would only occur about twice in a billion attempts. The idea that the 25-fold reduction in ICU admissions could have occurred because of any of the claims made would require very similar odds. The title of their paper sums up the evidence: "Mathematical analysis of Córdoba calcifediol trial suggests strong role for Vitamin D in reducing ICU admissions of hospitalised COVID-19 patients." Despite all of this, the Córdoba trial is still simply ignored or dismissed, as indeed are all the others.
- But finally, here is a new study from Israel published in the journal PLOS One, which adds even greater evidence to the incredible benefits of vitamin D for Covid. The

> researchers included in this study virtually all of the protocols that the critics of the Córdoba trial said should have been used. For example, they assessed the blood levels of vitamin D in 253 adult patients for nearly a year before they were admitted with Covid. Of these, 52% were deficient in the vitamin with levels less than 20ng/ml, and these patients were 14 times more likely to fall severely ill than those with normal levels. Approximately 25.6% of them also died with the virus compared to just 2.3% for those with normal levels. The researchers said the association was so strong they could predict patient outcomes just by their age and vitamin D levels. This trial has also been covered in several newspapers and one title said, "Does vitamin D protect against Covid after all?" So, what will the medical elite do about it? Quite simply, they will find a way to attack or dismiss it regardless of its impeccable scientific evidence.

A vital fact about vitamin D is that it is a key element in both the innate and adaptive immune systems but to be really effective it has to be given early – just like ivermectin and hydroxychloroquine. The best way would be for everyone to be encouraged to take it long term so that whenever they are infected with viruses like SARS-CoV-2, influenza and colds, their blood levels would already be high and their risk of serious disease significantly reduced. For those people who still get serious symptoms, it is vitally important that they are given calcifediol as soon as they are admitted to hospital. If it is only used when patients enter ICU then it is too late and will have little effect.

Incidentally, one thing that the medical elite might do to try to finally "prove" that vitamin D doesn't work would be to arrange several very large clinical trials in which calcifediol was given just to late-stage ICU patients. It really wouldn't work and they would then claim it was useless. Giving natural treatments too late when the disease cannot be cured is the sort of scam they have used many times before. I can never understand how they can live with themselves and sleep at night when they clearly don't care about saving lives and only care about destroying the benefits of vitamins. It is quite simply just one more example of their all-out war on lifestyle medicine. The other key fact is that vitamin D is exceptionally safe. Not one of the thousands of studies for a range of viral infections, where it has been used even at high doses, has shown any side effects.

Vitamin C. This can work in the same two ways as vitamin D. People who have high levels in the body by eating vitamin rich foods and taking oral supplements can reduce their risk of serious infection. Those who do develop serious symptoms could still achieve significantly improved outcomes, but only if the vitamin is then given intravenously and in large doses. In reality, this means most people can't benefit from it because medicine does not officially endorse its use. So, unless you can find some of the rare doctors who are prepared to risk their careers by using it, you will not have access to this. There are nevertheless a number of trials showing vitamin C's effectiveness and the key ones were included in a study published by five doctors from the UK, USA and New Zealand, led by the nutritionist Patrick Holford who has assiduously promoted vitamin C for decades and witnessed its incredible effectiveness. The study, "Vitamin C – An Adjunctive Therapy for Respiratory Infection, Sepsis and COVID-19", was sent to those sections of the NHS responsible for monitoring research including the Rapid C-19 group. Investigative health journalist Jerome Burne exposed what happened, or more realistically what didn't happen, and here are just a few of the key facts.

Several other reviews on vitamin C had also been sent to the NHS, but there was no response to any of them. Nine months later, the Rapid C-19 group confirmed it had received all the studies but that it hadn't done any review. Given that rapid analysis of data that could benefit Covid outcomes was its primary role, then ignoring all this scientific data is nothing short of unbelievable and reprehensible. One of the randomised clinical trials that was submitted to Rapid C-19 showed that critically ill patients achieved a significant reduction in 28-day mortality when given vitamin C. At that time, the trial had not been peer-reviewed, but this has now been completed and the reduction in mortality is 80%. This is a truly amazing outcome but there is no doubt that it will simply continue to be ignored.

While all this effective "refusal" to examine the evidence was happening, an official medically approved trial called REDMAP-CAP had been set up to provide "final scientific proof" on whether intravenous vitamin C would be effective for treating patients in intensive care. Patients had even started to be recruited in November 2020, but shortly after, the trial had to be stopped. Why? Amazingly, it was claimed they couldn't get any vitamin C. Really? They had placed the order for it with a company called Phoenix, but then the company had a supply problem. Almost a year later and it has still not been resolved and the trial has apparently been abandoned, even though they could have bought it in a few days from multiple sources throughout the world. As explained many times, the problem is simply that no official medical organisation, not just in the UK, but around the world, will ever admit that vitamin C is effective in treating Covid or indeed any other disease. That they can get away with such blatant scams and continue to avoid looking at the scientific data would be incredibly hilarious if only it didn't involve so many lost lives.

The official medical line remains unchanged and will probably do so for the rest of eternity: there is insufficient evidence to justify the use of vitamin C. In 2020 there was, however, one hospital in the UK that gave low dose (2g) intravenous vitamin C in its ICU. This is a very low level compared to that recommended by other doctors who use it, but nevertheless its death rate was 32.7% while the national UK average at the time was 41%. So, even this low level of vitamin cut deaths by 20%. Unsurprisingly, it was totally ignored.

Other key vitamins and minerals and lifestyle solutions. Having given lots of evidence on vitamins D and C, I will just outline some of the other important vitamins, minerals and supplements that have very positive effects on Covid.

Zinc is an amazingly powerful mineral that has well-known antiviral effects when it enters the body's cells. For COVID-19, it destroys the capacity of the virus to replicate. The US National Institutes for Health currently lists 26 studies on zinc, and many of them show that those with very low zinc levels have considerably higher Covid mortality rates. A 2022 randomised clinical trial from the Bourguiba University Hospital in Tunisia showed that those taking the oral zinc had a 40% lower risk of death and admission to intensive care than those taking the placebo.

Quercetin is a plant flavonoid found in foods like cherries, onions and red wine, but is also available as a supplement. There are several studies that show it is related to significantly reduced severity of Covid symptoms. It works in several ways but one of the key ones is that it acts in a way that helps zinc to enter your cells. Zinc on its own will help, but quercetin significantly increases its cell absorption and thus its overall effectiveness. Ideally, take both together (plus vitamin C) because all three work synergistically together.

Selenium is another key mineral for many diseases like cancer, osteoporosis and male fertility, but it is also vital for viral diseases like Covid. Studies show it can help reduce serious outcomes and increase survival rates.

N-acetyl cysteine (NAC) has 17 trials that illustrate its benefits for Covid, as well as over 50 more for a variety of other conditions.

There have so far been no trials on B vitamins – particularly B3 (niacin) – but the evidence on other infectious diseases suggests they could also play a significant part in Covid.

Magnesium is an absolutely essential mineral with a vast range of benefits for the human body, including the natural immune system. It helps to activate vitamin D which plays a crucial role in rapidly defeating Covid.

A very recent South African study examined the beneficial effects of exercise on hospitalisations from Covid and also explained that lockdowns were counterproductive for immunity. It showed that those who met the official recommendations of 150 minutes of exercise per week had significantly fewer hospitalisations. Professor Jon Patricios said, "In terms of policy, retrospectively we can say those hard lockdowns were counterproductive from an immune point of view... We've always understood that physical activity has protective effect against non-communicable diseases, but now we know we can protect against viral infection." I should add that while all this is very welcome, those advocating lifestyle medicine have known for decades that exercise is one key part of the natural immune system.

The amazing fact is most people really could improve their immunity by adopting the seven key lifestyle factors and taking a few key supplements so they could naturally defeat Covid without serious side effects or the need for hospitalisation. Add the early use of old drugs like ivermectin and hydroxychloroquine and around 90% of all deaths could have been prevented. I should also add that long Covid occurs mainly in those who develop serious symptoms. The sicker someone is and the longer the symptoms persist, the higher the risk of long Covid. So, almost certainly, many cases of this really could also have been prevented.

Fighting the dangerous vaccine-induced spike proteins. Finally, I also want to provide some information on how to minimise the serious adverse side effects of the mRNA "vaccines" like myocarditis, heart attacks and infertility. As already explained, these are caused by the gene editing therapy which simply forces the immune system to unnaturally produce endless numbers of these dangerous spike proteins around the entire body. A key way to minimise these adverse events is to try to inhibit, neutralise and eliminate these proteins and anyone who wants to try this should look at the detailed information from key organisations that have developed such treatments. My top recommendation would be the World Health Council. On their website you will see around 50 mainly natural things you can take that have been shown to help minimise the damage caused by the spike proteins. You certainly don't need to take all of them and in fact the top ten detox essentials are separately listed. These are vitamin D, vitamin C, N-acetyl cysteine, ivermectin, nigella seed, quercetin, zinc, magnesium, curcumin and milk thistle extract. In the UK you cannot buy ivermectin. It may be possible to get it directly from the US, but even if you can't, or don't want to, all the other options really will achieve a great deal. Please read all the data carefully before you start. It will almost certainly minimise the severe side effects from the mRNA jabs. If you want to look at other options you could also go online to the Front Line COVID-19 Critical Care Alliance.

Summarising the pandemic

How can we sum up COVID-19? Yes, it has been a serious disease, at least in the first 20 months, but it has been deliberately made to appear much worse than it really was. Many untrue "facts" have been spread around the world in an attempt to make everyone believe vaccines were the only solution and that everyone should get vaccinated and boosted. This incessant propaganda has been identical in virtually every single country, which makes you wonder who was involved in setting this agenda and communicating it worldwide. This will be examined in detail in Part 6. Every official body as well as the press, media and internet have maintained, and still maintain, this official line, even when some of the lies that were being told started to be uncovered. The vaccines soon started to lose their effectiveness, they didn't prevent infection or transmission and they have an incredible level of serious adverse events which are being hidden. The official Covid deaths are simply not correct and are significantly overstated. There are no scientific studies proving that face masks actually work in preventing Covid. In fact, the studies that have been carried out show they don't work and also show that they produce certain side effects. Despite all of this, they were mandated in virtually every country and in some, they still are.

Most of the world went into several severe lockdowns that included social distancing and mask wearing for months. We were initially told that, because the virus killed mainly older people, once those aged over about 70 had been vaccinated the pandemic would essentially be over because hospitalisations and deaths would plummet by around 90% and nearly all younger people were recovering from the disease without vaccination. Of course, this didn't happen and severe restrictions were reintroduced well after vaccination had started. We were told that the vaccines would prevent transmission and infections and in July 2021, President Biden promised that "if you get vaccinated, you're not going to get Covid". Younger people who had very low risk from Covid were told to get vaccinated to help reduce transmissions and thus infections and deaths in older people. But slowly, the truth started to emerge. These claims now lie in tatters; the vaccines do not prevent infection or transmission. We were told (and still are) that the vaccines are 100% safe, but now VAERS (and data from other countries) show they have more side effects and deaths than all other vaccination adverse events added together over the last 20 years. The young people who got vaccinated now have a significantly increased risk of serious outcomes and deaths, but agencies like the FDA and CDC are simply trying to suppress information relating to these adverse events.

In 2021 unvaccinated people were claimed to be the main cause of deaths and hospitalisations, but most of the data used was simply false or fabricated. Early in 2022 official figures showed the vaccinated, and particularly those boosted, had higher infection rates, deaths and hospitalisations than the unvaccinated. This is one of the reasons why governments are no longer analysing Covid outcomes, meaning that all this devastating information isn't available and can simply be covered up.

Covid deaths and hospitalisations were initially reduced after the first two jabs, but remember that the official Covid deaths are grossly overstated so the official vaccine benefits are also less than claimed. The other key fact is vaccines started to lose their effectiveness after a few weeks and fell to very low levels after six to eight months. After each variant occurred, fewer deaths were saved and even these then fell more rapidly. When the Omicron variant emerged, there was effectively no benefit. In fact, those who are vaccinated now have higher levels of mortality and infection than the unvaccinated. So, even though the vaccines initially reduced Covid deaths, we now know they also cause others, and many independent scientists really do believe they will ultimately produce more deaths overall. Despite their claimed initial success, the mRNA vaccines are turning into an unmitigated disaster for mankind, but everything is being covered up and censored.

Dr Pierre Kory, the president and chief medical officer at the Front Line COVID-19 Critical Care Alliance made the following incredibly short summary in a Substack article about Covid vaccines during 2021. It is a tongue in cheek way of summarising how the claims made about vaccine protection rapidly disappeared. It is close to – but not exactly – correct time-wise. However, it really does, very simply, expose much of the reality.

- May – 90% protection
- June – 70% protection

- July – 50% protection
- August – No protection, but reduces the spread
- September – Doesn't reduce the spread, but reduces severity
- October – Doesn't reduce severity, but reduces hospitalisations
- November – Doesn't reduce hospitalisations, but you aren't going to die
- December – You die, but you go to heaven

A crucial question is what actually enabled most people in the UK and nearly every other country to get back to a normal life early in 2022? Was it due to vaccination as the official claims imply? Absolutely not. It was in fact the Omicron variant that effectively brought life back to normal. Omicron was so mild that for most people it was no worse than a cold. It also spread incredibly fast and by spring 2022 most people had been infected and had recovered. If the Delta variant had not been phased out by Omicron, restrictions would almost certainly have had to remain in place for a long time particularly as the vaccines were rapidly losing their effectiveness for it. As you will see in Part 6, Bill Gates is the biggest promoter of vaccines in the world, but even he admitted that Omicron proved to be better. This is his quote: "The virus itself, particularly the variant called Omicron, is a type of vaccine, in that it creates both T cell and B cell immunity, and it does a better job of getting out to the population than we have with vaccines." Surprisingly, in January 2023, Bill Gates also effectively trashed the effectiveness of the mRNA Covid vaccines with the following admission: "We also need to fix the three problems of COVID-19 vaccines. The current vaccines are not infection blocking. They're not broad, so when new variants come up you lose protection, and they have short duration, particularly in the people who matter, which are old people." This really is an incredible reversal from the man who once advertised the jabs as the cure to the Coronavirus. This is what he originally said: "Everyone who takes the vaccine is not just protecting themselves but reducing their transmission to other people and allowing society to get back to normal."

One very interesting development has been a significant change in vaccination rates. Over 90% of the eligible UK population have now had the first jab. The figure for the second jab is around 85% and for the third it is around 70%. For the fourth jab it is just 22% and this is the percentage for those it was recommended for over the age of 50. It has been interesting to see how friends and acquaintances have reacted to the vaccination roll out. Initially, they were nearly all convinced that vaccination was essential and that it would be safe because of the universal claims made by medicine and governments. I was aware of four people who didn't take any jabs. One of my friends also knew a young man who developed myocarditis after the first jab and unsurprisingly, he didn't take any more. All the others simply took the first two jabs and most, but not all of them, took the first booster. However, things then changed rapidly. Most didn't take the second booster. What happened? Many had had side effects even after the first and second jabs but had simply accepted them because they were told it was all normal, showed the vaccine was working, and would disappear quickly.

However, the first booster shot caused more serious and disturbing symptoms, some of which lasted for weeks, meaning some could not do normal activities and some were unable to work or even shop. Many started to discuss the adverse events with other people for the first time and found that they were more widespread than they could ever have imagined. This concern led most of them to refuse the second booster. Another fact that helped was the significant reduction in serious outcomes and deaths that was already happening with the Omicron variant. There is now increasing concern and scepticism about the jabs around the world.

One of the most disturbing and alarming facts is that with almost absolute certainty this pandemic only happened because a man-made, genetically modified virus was somehow leaked from a laboratory in Wuhan. Previous SARS type virus outbreaks had simply been defeated by the natural immune system with very few deaths. SARS-CoV-2, however, is simply more lethal almost certainly because of its deliberate genetic modification.

The UK and most of the world have been in some form of lockdown for much of the initial two years for a disease that is unlikely to have caused more than 5% of total deaths, most of which occurred in older people with an average age of 82. The impact of this has been catastrophic in terms of all other human health outcomes, devastating for children, and caused one of the most serious financial disasters in modern times. For nearly two years, these lockdowns were mandatory and classed as essential, and this was also literally enforced by every single news agency. Now, however, we know that even this is not true, and the evidence is now unassailable from many eminent scientists, like Professor Mark Goodman, who have shown that the lockdowns actually caused more harm than good, and even major media organisations like the Guardian newspaper have now reported this devastating fact. Additional data from the OECD and the UK's Office for National Statistics reveals staggering differences in overall mortality relating to various lockdown rules. Sweden, which had almost no type of lockdown, did initially have a higher Covid death rate than many other western countries including its neighbours Denmark, Netherlands and Finland. But now, all-cause excess mortality, which adds the deaths from imposed lockdowns, such as those from rising suicides and those from cancer caused by lack of early treatment, to those deaths from Covid itself, tells a different story. Sweden's excess mortality from March 2020 to October 2022 was 2.7%. But for Denmark it was 5.2%, Finland 7.1%, Netherlands 11.8%, the UK 10.6% and the US 20.9%. These are incredible differences and give an insight into what perhaps could have happened in these countries if they had adopted the Swedish approach. I am not aware that this has been reported by any news agency particularly in the UK and the US so very few people will know anything about it. A number of independent experts predicted that lockdowns would have serious implications in spring 2020 when the pandemic was declared by the WHO. Once again, they were simply attacked and censored and some had their careers destroyed, even though what they said is now indisputable.

In the early days of the pandemic, courts, particularly in the US, effectively fell into line with the official Covid policies and legal cases opposing them were invariably lost. Recently, however, there has been rising success for those brave people who have been determined to expose the truth about Covid. Organisations like the Public Health and Medical Professionals for Transparency were determined to get vital Covid data released from official bodies like the FDA and CDC so that independent scientists could analyse it and make it available to the public. In the end they had to take lawsuits against them in order to get Pfizer vaccine trial data and V-safe adverse events data released and these legal court cases were won. Other organisations have also started to take legal action to try to defeat official vaccine mandates. In 2022 the courts ruled against President Biden's draconian mandate for federal workers. They also ruled against the Washington, D.C. school district's plan to vaccinate kids as young as 11 without parental consent. Even Congress has just passed a bill that struck down the Covid vaccine mandate for members of the US Armed Forces. The Children's Health Defense also recently financed a lawsuit for a group of medical practitioners in the New York State Department of Health who were threatened with its vaccine mandate. The New York State Supreme Court ruled that the state's mandate was "arbitrary and capricious" on the basis that COVID-19 vaccines do not stop transmission of the virus, thereby eliminating any rational basis for such a policy. The lead attorney Sujata Gibson stated, "This is a huge win for New York healthcare workers, who have been deprived of their livelihoods for more than a year."

She also added, "The damage done to healthcare workers and to all New York residents is irreparable. Thousands of people lost their jobs. Countless had to cash out their retirement accounts to feed their families; many lost their homes. Far too many left the state. Meanwhile, thousands of patients were deprived of critical care due to the staffing shortages this mandate caused."

In January 2023 another crucial legal case has been launched. Robert F. Kennedy Jr. and the Children's Health Defense (CHD) together with a number of others like Dr Mercola, filed a first-of-its-kind landmark antitrust lawsuit in an effort to protect freedom of speech and stop the deliberate, concerted efforts made by the legacy media, colluding with Big Tech, Big Pharma and the government, to suppress critical information. The lawsuit is against members of a partnership group of media conglomerates called the Trusted News Initiative (TNI). Members of the TNI include the Washington Post, Reuters and the BBC, as well as the tech giants Twitter, Facebook, Microsoft and Google. The TNI made efforts to silence the CHD, Dr Mercola and all the other plaintiffs who had combined followers of over 11 million, reaching billions of people with their content. TNI suppressed truthful information on safe and effective treatments for Covid and the harms and risks of the Covid jabs which caused millions of people to suffer unnecessary injuries and deaths as well as the loss of jobs and livelihoods. This lawsuit will probably take many months, but it would be quite devastating for the BBC if they and all the other big tech and media giants were eventually found guilty. They would, however, deserve it for the incredible censorship of truth that they have committed. The BBC and all the others, for example, have simply promoted the official claim that "vaccines are safe", even though this is not true. In January 2023 thousands of UK vaccine-injured people, and relatives of those killed by them, gathered to share their experiences outside the BBC headquarters in London. Unsurprisingly, the BBC never made (and wouldn't dare to make) a single mention of it and they simply continue to attack all those who say the vaccines have caused many serious outcomes.

Finally, a California judge in January 2023 issued a preliminary injunction which is the first critical step aimed at stopping the state medical board from censoring their doctors who dare to say anything against the official medical consensus, even if what they say is correct. The judge has simply shown that this so-called official medical consensus has no genuine scientific backing and no established meaning. Something so flimsy should not be used to silence doctors. If this eventually becomes the law, it will be a vital victory over the censorship being imposed on anyone who challenges medicine.

The most important fact, however, that you will see in the next section, is that nearly all of the devastating outcomes that have been outlined in this section really could have been prevented.

How the pandemic could have, and should have, been defeated

Before COVID-19, it was well known that all the other SARS viruses were highly transmissible and able to mutate rapidly. Not a single vaccine trial had ever worked for any of them and they all caused significant adverse events. Here is another important fact as quoted by Dr Peter McCullough: "Once a highly transmissible virus like Covid has a beachhead in a population, it is inevitable that it will spread to every individual who lacks immunity. You can slow the spread, but you cannot prevent it." In other words, it was clear right from the start that everyone would eventually get the infection and that the vaccines would not stop this from happening. So, the key question is was there a better way of tackling the pandemic?

We have seen that, right from the start, some doctors and hospitals were using existing treatments that really did significantly reduce the severity and deaths of Covid. Dr McCullough maintains that an international network linking the world's 11 million frontline doctors should have been set up almost immediately when the pandemic started because of the many successful and safe early treatments that were reducing deaths by around 70%. Towards the end of 2020, before the first vaccine had even started to be used, the death rate had been reduced even further to almost 90% by improving the treatment protocols. As well as these amazing reductions in deaths, there was also incredible proof that giving people who were at risk of infection preventative treatments, like ivermectin, vitamin D and zinc, would also reduce the number of cases and serious outcomes. By distributing this information around the globe, every hospital would have been able to start using these successful treatments. Also, because many more trials to improve the treatments could then have been carried out, the 90% reduction in deaths may been achieved even sooner and even reduced further.

Of course, it would have been necessary to have some specific short-term restrictions while the procedures were trialled and then adopted around the world and to ramp up the supply of old drugs like hydroxychloroquine and vitamins and minerals like vitamins D and C and zinc. These would have been given mainly as preventative treatments to key people and those more at risk. Isolating the old and frail and some of those with serious underlying health conditions would still have been necessary. But everyone else would have been able to continue life mostly as normal and most would get the disease and defeat it.

After some short-term specific restrictions while everything was set up, children would have been allowed to remain at school while their teachers were given all the treatments that would have prevented most serious outcomes. Similarly, most workers could have been treated in a similar way and allowed to work almost as normal. Because the virus would then spread rapidly but have minimal symptoms in most people under the age of say 60 (the exact age needed to be accurately assessed), then the pandemic would have quickly subsided just as it did with the Omicron variant and its incredible number of cases. Once most people had been infected and recovered, they would all have natural immunity which would probably last a lifetime. Even if other variants occurred, and people were again infected, then they would still defeat it with just mild symptoms, just as those who had the Alpha or Delta variants and then got the Omicron variant also had very mild symptoms.

If all this had happened, the NHS would not have gone through the same devastation that has resulted in a lack of treatments and disastrous waiting times for people with serious diseases like cancer and heart disease and even longer ones for those with less fatal diseases. There would have been no need for "vaccines" and the serious adverse events they are now creating would also never have happened. Children's lives, mental health and education would not have been devastated like they really have been. They would not have become sad, angry, demotivated, isolated and confused with friendships curtailed and life opportunities taken away from them. Their obesity levels would not have increased by a further 25%. The latest indications are that they will now also live shorter and poorer lives which would also have been prevented. Tens of thousands of companies would not have gone bust. The £370 billion that the UK government had to spend on Covid would probably have been reduced by around 90% and we would now not be in the current financially catastrophic position. All these things would, of course, have occurred around the world which could have saved around $12 trillion.

In a sane and unbiased world, especially given that the treatments involved were incredibly safe, medical organisations in every country really should have tried them in a number of their own hospitals and then, when it was clear they were working, they should have quickly endorsed their widespread use. Why was this not even considered? The problem that has been explored throughout the book is simple. It is the drug industry that effectively controls medicine, governments and regulators, meaning that anything that threatens drug and vaccine profits is simply not allowed to happen.

What does the future hold?

Most people around the world have now had Covid and recovered from it and many have had it twice or even three times. Some countries like Australia had very long and severe lockdowns, but it became clear that regardless of the lockdowns, everyone was still going to get the virus at some point and that the devastating economic costs and the effects on human life simply could not continue indefinitely and again most people there have also now had the virus and recovered from it. Even China, which enforced the most draconian lockdowns the world has ever seen for almost three years, has also now given in because its economy has suffered a really serious downturn and people started to protest about the savage destruction of their lives. In just a few months, most people in China will also have had and recovered from the virus. So, what could the world face at that stage?

The most likely outcome is that Covid will simply remain a mild type of virus for most healthy people even though there will almost certainly be new variants occurring each year. It is also certain that vaccines simply cannot stop infection and transmission and people will just have to accept that Covid will continue to exist. It is not impossible that a more serious variant could occur, but most experts really do believe this is extremely unlikely. So, except for those people with other serious health conditions, Covid will almost certainly be a relatively mild but frequent viral infection just like colds and flu.

Does this mean that people can now relax and forget all about pandemics, especially since the last one occurred over 100 years ago? No. There is one crucial fact to always remember. The current Covid pandemic was almost certainly caused by a lab leak of a genetically engineered virus created by "gain-of-function" research and the disturbing possibility is that other similarly caused pandemics will occur and they really could be much more lethal than Covid. We have seen that gain-of-function research produces genetically engineered truly dangerous viruses with the supposed aim of creating new vaccines that could then help to prevent and treat them. The concept that this type of high-risk research is a good idea is quite simply shocking, and it is opposed by countless scientists and researchers around the world. Apart from the potential escape of deadly viruses from the labs involved (which really has happened regularly), the other risk is that the vaccines then don't work well. Covid vaccines provide clear evidence about this risk. They have been an unmitigated failure in preventing infection and transmission, benefits deteriorate rapidly and have even turned negative, and they also cause many serious and life-taking adverse events. Quite simply, this dangerous gain-of-function research should be banned worldwide but it is continuing unabated.

So, what is happening that could lead to a new lethal pandemic? Here are just two examples. Mad scientists at Boston University's biosafety level 4 laboratory have engineered an Alpha/Omicron hybrid strain of SARS-CoV-2. When mice were given the Omicron variant alone, they had mild symptoms and no deaths, but when given this new engineered variant they had an 80% mortality rate. By combining the more infectious spike protein from Omicron with the far more dangerous original Alpha virus, the scientists have created what can only be described as a biological superweapon. If this gene engineered virus ever escaped from the lab it would also likely kill around 80% of the US population and do so within a few weeks. It would also spread around the world. Creating such a dangerous virus that is far more lethal than even the original Alpha SARS-CoV-2 variant is so shocking that it seems almost impossible to believe. Some of the funding for Boston University was provided by NIH and Dr Fauci's NIAID although they are now trying to claim they didn't know what the money had been used for. But even if this is true, surely they should mandate that gain-of-function research should not be carried out. The Daily Caller published scathing rebukes like this one from Justin Goodman: "Fauci and other mad scientists need to be stopped before they cause another pandemic by recklessly supercharging deadly viruses in wasteful taxpayer-funded animal experiments… Stop the madness." Dr Shmuel Shapira, a leading scientist in the Israeli government, said, "This should be totally forbidden, it's playing with fire." Jeff Childers is an attorney and the president of the Childers Law firm. Here are parts of his own detailed review: "Try to imagine the dumbest thing the public health experts could do at this point… They know it's been illegal to conduct gain-of-function research in the US since the Obama administration… Why, oh why, are these criminals, I mean scientists, still allowed to tinker around with this kind of explosive material… Have we learned *nothing* from the Wuhan lab leak?… Thanks to our witless health agencies, we – taxpayers – are funding our own destruction."

The other example involves the Spanish flu virus which, in 1918, caused the most lethal pandemic in recent history. Scientists funded by the NIH and Dr Fauci's NIAID resurrected the virus through reverse genetics and tested it on the macaque species. Their aim was to create a more dangerous version of an already dangerous virus, supposedly to enable better vaccines to be produced against it. Why do this when the virus simply no longer exists in nature and, therefore, poses zero threat to mankind? Luckily, the recreated virus failed to kill any of the animals involved even at the highest doses and the scientists were apparently frustrated and upset that somehow they had failed. If they had succeeded, a more lethal Spanish flu virus would have posed another incredible threat to mankind. The worry is that they may try again to create a different but incredibly dangerous new variant. We can only hope they don't.

These two examples are just the tip of the serious risk of gain-of-function research which is taking place in a number of countries. The US has recently funded what it calls a goal to "detect emerging viruses". Independent experts say this will simply lead to gain-of-function research through the backdoor and is being used simply to hide the reality. Also, before Dr Fauci retired, he had given the EcoHealth Alliance five years of funding, which, if you remember, was the organisation involved in funding the Wuhan Institute of Virology for part of its gain-of-function research on the Covid virus. Other countries also carry out such research but unsurprisingly, it is usually kept well under wraps. Certain key people seem determined to carry on with this, even though at some point it really could destroy most or all human life on Earth. There is not much more that can be said, other than if enough people ever understood the risks involved, they could probably protest and force governments to commit to a worldwide ban on all such evil research.

Here is another pandemic possibility. We have seen that in October 2019 Bill Gates funded a simulation of a possible future pandemic called Event 201. This was a pandemic table top exercise that amazingly "predicted" what happened during the real-world Covid pandemic three months later. In October 2022 he then co-hosted another pandemic exercise called "Catastrophic Contagion". This involved a novel pathogen called "severe epidemic enterovirus respiratory syndrome 2025" (SEERS-25) that primarily kills children. Could this really happen? It seems difficult to believe because if it did it would give incredible proof that these two pandemics were deliberately planned. The chance that they just happen by chance would be perhaps one in a million. It's impossible to predict what will happen, but if it does, you will know who is responsible.

Another key point about the future is that sadly the mRNA Covid vaccine serious adverse events may last for a long time. These gene editing drugs literally force the immune system to act unnaturally and produce endless spike proteins which are now known to affect every crucial part of the body like the heart. This is a key reason why we are now seeing a huge increase in a range of heart diseases like myocarditis, heart attacks, blood clots and pericarditis as well as many others like infertility, miscarriage rates, cancers and strokes. Everything will depend on how long the vaccines continue to force the immune system to keep producing these devastating spike proteins and this is as yet unknown. There is an even more shocking fact. The drug industry is now planning to develop even more of these new gene editing therapies for a range of other diseases and these will once again be classed as "vaccines". Each of them will almost certainly lead to yet more serious outcomes just like the Covid jabs. Even more concerning is that once these different gene editing therapies start to be used together, there is a real risk that they will interact in ways that would cause even more serious damage to the natural immune system and all parts of the body.

Why is the industry planning to increase the development of these "vaccines"? They would claim that they will be more effective than drugs for many diseases. Really? Presumably they have just forgotten about the failed Covid jabs. The truth is there are four very different and truly shocking reasons, all of which are related to profit:

1) The pharmaceutical industry can be taken to court by patients if their drugs cause serious adverse events and deaths and it has had to pay tens of billions of dollars in such settlements over the last three decades. Before 1986 they were subject to the same court cases for vaccines, and because their adverse events were increasing and becoming widely recognised by patients, court cases and fines were also rising rapidly. The drug industry effectively told governments that unless this was stopped, they would stop producing vaccines. Governments then simply gave way. So now, when a vaccine is approved and added to the official vaccination schedule, the drug industry is completely exempt from all such legal cases. If the industry killed a million people with a vaccine, it would cost them nothing, whereas if it was caused by a drug, it would be fined tens of billions of dollars. Perhaps you can now understand why they prefer vaccines. A sad fact is that people now have to try to get compensation from governments which is incredibly difficult; most people fail and literally spend the rest of their lives with serious vaccine-related diseases and literally end up in poverty.
2) I should emphasise that, for all this to take place legally, the product must be classed as a vaccine. This meant that for the Covid jabs, the FDA simply had to change the definition of vaccines which enabled them to class a non-vaccine gene editing therapy as a "vaccine". Truly appalling.
3) The Covid vaccines were also approved for emergency use authorisation, meaning that instead of clinical trials that would officially have taken ten years, they were "completed" in just a few months. This saved the industry hundreds of millions of dollars for each single vaccine. Perhaps unsurprisingly, the FDA will now almost certainly authorise emergency use for virtually all of the new mRNA type "vaccines". The public will then suffer again because it is simply impossible to prove these are safe or even effective in such a short time. But, of course, industry profits will soar yet again.
4) The FDA has recently surpassed all these unbelievable, unscientific and disastrous changes. If matters weren't already beyond horrible, it is considering allowing manufacturers to reformulate their Covid injections in perpetuity without conducting any clinical trials. In other words, they'd allow drug companies to change the mRNA and all the other vaccine ingredients without any safety or efficacy testing whatsoever. They have, of course, already done this with the new bivalent Covid booster shots which were approved without even an emergency use trial. They were simply given to a few mice for a few days to show that their antibodies increased, even though

this provides no proof whatsoever of the vaccine's effectiveness or safety. Part 6 will examine some of the reasons why all these devastating actions are taking place.

It is unfortunate but true that everyone who has received a Covid jab has simply participated in an uncontrolled medical experiment and its failures and serious outcomes are systematically being uncovered by courageous independent doctors and scientists. We are living in unprecedented and precarious times. Logic, reason, science and sanity itself has been tossed aside by those who claim this right to make decisions for all of mankind. The incredible decisions that are now being taken by agencies like the FDA are beyond belief. They simply threaten most of mankind unless, of course, mankind fights back to stop it all. Throughout history, people have had the right to make their own decisions on any medical treatment. This is the moment when people in democratic societies need to defend this human right to autonomy and freedom. I can only suggest that all these new gene editing therapies – even though they will almost certainly be labelled as vaccines – should be looked at with extreme concern, and if people refuse them, the world would almost certainly be a safer place not just for us but for future generations.

Finally, COVID-19 was serious but it did not turn out to be the catastrophic event that was predicted and there are other diseases like cardiovascular disease and cancer that take far more lives and which have been unbelievably side-lined because of it. There is, however, another disease that could be infinitely worse than Covid, heart disease and cancer all added together. It is even now unfolding before our very eyes, despite the fact most people have absolutely no knowledge of what is happening. This book has exposed increases in virtually every disease that are already reducing or stalling average life expectancy in countries like the US and the UK. The next section, however, exposes what could turn out to be the ultimate medical catastrophe that really could effectively destroy much of mankind.

Autism

Autism now affects an average of around 1 in 35 children. (The organisations that measure autism cases often analyse the data and define it in different ways which can result in different rates. For example, Northern Ireland's latest official figure is 1 in 22 children, while that of the CDC in the US is 1 in 44. Most other organisations have figures in between them. This is why I have used an average figure of 1 in 35. I should, however, add that the CDC has been accused by one of its key investigators of manipulating the data to try to minimise cases and thus "hiding" the seriousness of the epidemic. The other key fact is that the Northern Ireland figure is for 2020 while the CDC's is for 2018 which also partly explains the difference. All this means that the real figure is much more likely to be 1 in 22.) In 1970 the cases were 1 in 10,000 and going back 100 years the disease did not exist. Cases have increased 280-fold since 1970 and the increase has literally been exponential since 1989. This is an autism epidemic that, unless something changes, could literally end up destroying mankind.

Autism – the medical approach

Medical experts and organisations are simply trying to claim that autism has always existed, that the number of cases has not really changed, and that in the past our knowledge was just insufficient to diagnose it. This is what the CDC says about autism spectrum disorder (ASD): "More people than ever are being diagnosed with ASD. It is unclear how much of this increase is due to a broader definition of ASD and to better efforts in diagnosis. However, a true increase in the number of people with ASD cannot be ruled out." The CDC is effectively saying there is no real increase in autism; it's all down to broader definitions and better diagnosis. They clearly don't believe that there is a true increase at present, and this is confirmed by the release of their latest autism rate of 1 in 44 children which was 23% higher than the previous figure. The CDC said this "reflects more awareness – rather than a true increase". If this wasn't a deadly serious issue then it would be laughable. Here is the most powerful body on the planet responsible for monitoring disease, and yet it can't, or more likely it doesn't, want to recognise a devastating epidemic that has seen a 28,000% increase in cases in the last 50 years – an epidemic that threatens mankind.

Could the idea that autism has always existed really be true? Could no medical experts have detected any form of autism or recorded what would have been many millions of cases over the last two centuries? Absolutely not. The great clinicians of the time were incredibly fastidious over their records of disease and they described in meticulous detail their symptoms, characteristics and progression. They did this so accurately that even today doctors would be able to read these records and come up with the correct answer for most diseases even if the names had been blanked out. Quite simply, if autism had existed 100 years ago, its serious and blatantly obvious types of cases really would have been identified and accurately documented, but they weren't. There is, however, an even more obvious type of proof. If it had always existed, then there would now be nearly 5 million adults over the age of 35 in the US and around 700,000 in the UK with autism. Where are these cases? Quite simply, they do not exist. Of course, there will be a few thousand cases in the US because the first case of autism was recorded in 1931 but these only increased slowly, and even by the 1970s they still affected just 1 in 10,000 children. Compare these few thousands to the 5 million cases that should exist – it is only a tiny fraction. So, autism really does have to be a new disease. Despite all this evidence, however, official medical organisations like the CDC will simply not admit or declare that we are in the midst of an autism epidemic, even though around 1.8 million US children now have autism. This means no action is being taken, there is no desperate search for a cause, no major government task forces, no WHO initiatives. The epidemic simply continues unabated.

Next, I'll outline some key facts about autism which can take various forms. It can affect sensory inputs and manifest as behavioural and coordination dysfunction. Children can lack interaction, can have impaired speech development, and frequently use repetitive behaviour. Over 80% have serious gastrointestinal disorders and many develop seizures and epilepsy. Robert F. Kennedy Jr. says that half of them will never speak or go on a toilet, and will need lifetime care, often 24 hours a day. But it can also be even more severe. Many children are seriously disabled with harrowing symptoms that will cause a lifetime of agony. They will live in pain but be unable to communicate that pain or indeed anything else. Many of them commit self-harm and have to wear crash helmets to help protect them; some people believe they are trying to kill themselves to escape the torment. Of course, there are also children with milder symptoms who can live a near normal life and those who have incredible but specific "genius-like" symptoms. But the simple fact is over 80% of autistic children will need some form of care for their entire lives and they really will not live a normal life. Autism does not just debilitate the affected child. The diagnosis destroys the personal, emotional, spiritual and financial energies of everyone involved, imposing ruinous financial costs, derailing careers, straining marriages and marginalising families.

There are two characteristic types of autism. Regressive autism describes the condition where a child is developing normally, and then sudden changes occur in their behaviour and the symptoms of autism emerge rapidly. Regressive autism is usually diagnosed in those aged one to three years. The other type, early onset autism, develops soon after birth. Some of these cases can be diagnosed by the age of six months while others take longer. But trying to establish how many cases of autism are regressive and how many are early onset is difficult because the figures from different sources usually put regressive autism in the range 20 to 40%. There are likely to be some cases where the distinction is unclear and categorisation is, therefore, difficult, but something else may be going on. Parents have reported that doctors are reluctant to classify cases of regressive autism especially those that occur soon after the MMR jab. The authorities are acutely aware that regressive autism and its association with MMR vaccines is something they need to play down. Whilst it can't be proven, it is possible that doctors are in effect, and maybe even subconsciously, doing just that.

The story of an American mother, Katie Wright, gives a classic example of what can happen. Her son developed severe regressive autism and when she took him to see various doctors and explained how it had suddenly happened, they all doubted her claim and said she had probably just missed the earlier autistic signs. Thankfully, she had a number of home movies. These showed her 18-month-old son speaking in complex sentences and cuddling his baby brother. Then they were shown videos a few months later when he was severely autistic, non-verbal, screaming and head banging. When the doctors and psychologists saw these videos, it was clear they were shocked and were trying to process what they didn't believe could be true. But for many parents who don't have this sort of evidence, the medical reluctance to accept regressive autism seems to be quite common.

There have been many organisations and websites around the world set up by devastated parents with autistic children. Ed Arranga and his wife Teri who had two autistic children set up AutismOne which is the most respected parental autism organisation in the US. Its annual conference attracts parents from around the globe and covers all aspects of autism, especially cutting-edge treatments and therapies. Parents explain in huge numbers how their children were developing normally but then changed dramatically, many of them soon after the MMR vaccination. The official line from the CDC, the NHS and other medical organisations, however, is that there is absolutely no connection between the MMR vaccine and autism and that any suggestion of a connection is scaremongering that has been totally disproved. Despicably, organisations like AutismOne are subject to fierce opposition by the medical cartel and its media allies, but Ed stood up to the bullies and continued to help thousands of families. Despite all of this, many cases of autism are still officially diagnosed soon after vaccination, but parents are told it is "just coincidence" and would have happened anyway. This is despite the fact there have been hundreds of thousands of such "coincidences" around the world.

The other fact we know is that autism predominantly affects boys. Various studies typically put the average ratio of boys to girls at between three to four boys to one girl. This means the latest average figure of 1 in 35 children is made up of around 1 in 22 boys, and 1 in 70 girls, while in Northern Ireland the official figures are 1 in 15 boys and 1 in 45 girls. Here are other sobering facts. In the US, school pass grades have been lowered twice over recent years to ensure the same overall pass rates. Around 13% of schoolchildren are in special education and 1 in 14 have problems with speech, language, hearing and communication. Why? These effects are more pronounced in boys than in girls. Could this reduction in educational abilities and IQ have any connection with autism? This, of course, can't be proven, but is it just a coincidence that the prevalence of autism in boys is increasing, and their educational attainments are declining, or is there a real connection? If this really is the case, and low educational attainment is just a mild form of autism, then autism would take on a whole new meaning, with even greater implications for the future of mankind.

But as disturbing as all this is, if the rising number of cases is simply extrapolated, it projects that for those born in 2032, 1 in 2 children will have autism. This is not a misprint. The projection is that half of American children born in 2032 will develop the disease. If this, or anything remotely close to it, occurs, the US as a country is finished – the half of the country that is well will simply be looking after the half that is autistic. (I keep referring to the US because this is where much of the hard and easily accessible data exists, but, of course, it would also be applicable in the UK and other parts of the world.)

Of course, the exponential rise in the cases of autism may suddenly stop, but given that the trend has been in place for over three decades, there is no logical reason why it should. Independent experts started to extrapolate the alarming increase in cases around two decades ago and their projected case numbers have continued to be eerily correct. You might argue that surely even if the rise in cases continues, then something will be done before it reaches that final cataclysmic stage. But autism is already at epidemic (and many experts would already say cataclysmic) levels, yet nothing is happening. It is as if no one dares to be the first to break ranks and say officially, "We have a potentially world destroying epidemic on our hands." Why? Because, whatever the causes of autism, they simply have to be "man-made".

Imagine for a moment that the MMR vaccine was to blame, or vaccines in general, or pesticides or other chemicals. If it was any of these or any combination and the truth came out, the consequences could destroy nations and society as we know it. Governments would be faced with claims for compensation that would be impossible to fund. The cost of lifetime care for a seriously vaccine-damaged child in the US is around $2 million, and the National Vaccine Injury Compensation Program has paid out such sums. But these are relatively small in number because legally proving that vaccines are the cause is currently very difficult. If it was ever officially confirmed that vaccines were the cause of autism, however, then for the 1.8 million children currently with the disease, this would cost $4.5 trillion. If the numbers ever reached 1 in 2, this would rise to more than $50 trillion in today's terms just for the US. This is more than half the GDP of the entire world. The overall ramifications would be cataclysmic. Maybe you can see why no one wants to push the starting button and why everything is seemingly brushed under the carpet. Of course, if autism does keep increasing and reaches the projected 1 in 2, then the world would still disintegrate, even if no compensation is ever paid out. With half the entire population needing the other half just to look after them, the entire fabric of society would collapse. Even when the autism rate in the EU was just 1 in 60 a few years ago, the European Commission calculated that society would not be able to bear the indirect cost of the disease when those autistic children reached the age of 50 given their lack of earnings and those of the families looking after them. Autism rates have doubled since this sombre analysis was done, and even if autism suddenly stopped (which, of course, it won't) then it will still become a worldwide financial disaster and not just a human catastrophe.

Of course, everyone in authority would ignore and dismiss all the facts that have so far been examined as the ramblings of a deranged and dangerous lunatic. But there is one thing that even the massed, coordinated and concerted efforts of all those in power cannot hide, and that is the sheer scale of the escalating numbers of children with autism. If you look at the facts dispassionately, it is clear that despite all their claims, a tragedy of incalculable proportions is unfolding before our very eyes. Please ask yourself whether you had any idea that the official current rate of autism for boys is already around 1 in 15. But when it reaches 1 in 10 and then 1 in 5 boys, can those in power simply continue to hide or dismiss it? It really is impossible to predict how all this will unfold. Will the public, or certain media groups, or more doctors, or even some governments, suddenly be prepared to rebel and tell the truth and then demand desperate action? Only time will tell.

Here are some more facts about vaccination and autism. In the 1960s and 1970s autism rates were low and early onset autism predominated. Regressive autism only emerged in the late 1980s and increased rapidly in the 1990s. Since the 1960s, the numbers of vaccines administered has increased significantly and the age at which they have been given has fallen. In 1968 the polio and DPT vaccines were administered at the ages of six and seven months. But this was changed in 1988 and vaccines were given at the ages of three, four and five months with the MMR vaccine following at 13 months. This coincided with the start of the exponential increase in autism. Today, the number of individual vaccinations administered before the age of one in the UK is 19 and some of these are given just after birth. Different countries have different vaccine schedules for children below one. The USA has 22 vaccinations while Sweden and Japan, for example, have the lowest number with 12. There is a clear trend; the countries with the most vaccines have the highest level of infant mortality. The level is, on average, double those with the lowest number of vaccines, meaning that the US has twice the level of infant mortality than Sweden and Japan.

Unvaccinated children don't appear to develop regressive autism. For example, the Amish community do not allow vaccinations and no cases of regressive autism have ever been reported. There was no evidence of regressive autism when single vaccines were used and when vaccinations were spread out over time and were given later in the child's life. Early onset autism might be related to vaccines administered just after birth or at two or three months, before a child has developed any sort of natural immunity. This, of course, would be dismissed out of hand by medicine. But something has to explain the exponential rise in early onset autism as well as the exponential rise in regressive autism.

Despite the claims that vaccines, in general, are completely safe, the US government has paid out over 4 billion dollars in compensation to the families of vaccine-damaged children. The UK government has also paid out millions of pounds. Surprisingly, the drug companies making the vaccines seem to be more transparent than politicians or doctors. Merck admits its MMR vaccine can cause any one of 39 serious reactions including learning difficulties, blindness, diabetes, autism and death. This information is included in the vaccine package insert sent to doctors, but this is almost never shown to patients. Of course, the drug industry can afford to be honest, because once a vaccine has been added to the official childhood vaccination schedule, it is indemnified by governments against any parental claims for vaccine damage. This means that if any link was ever found, governments, and governments alone, would pick up the bill for compensation. The pharmaceutical industry insisted on this indemnity. Why were they so insistent if vaccines are completely safe? Well, it may surprise you to learn that an older version of the DTP vaccine was causing severe brain damage in many children. The manufacturers were facing increasing parental lawsuits and there was concern amongst US politicians that the vaccine makers might stop much of their vaccine production to avoid these huge legal fines. This is why, in 1986, a new law indemnifying them against any claims was introduced leaving the government to pick up the bill. Of course, the reality is that it is the general public who really pay for it all via taxes. Before this bill was introduced, vaccine manufacturers were producing only limited new vaccines to avoid the risk that serious side effects could result in huge fines and serious financial losses. But, once the bill had been introduced and they were free from any prosecution, then vaccine research and development increased exponentially. In 1983 there were just three childhood vaccines that with boosters totalled ten jabs. Now in the US there are 11 vaccines that, with boosters, total 38 separate vaccinations up to the age of five, which is nearly quadruple the number in the 1980s.

Vaccines also contain an average of around 40 separate chemical ingredients. So, what sort of evidence do medicine and organisations like the CDC have to support their claims that these vaccines do not cause autism? Amazingly, only one vaccine – the MMR jab – and one ingredient – thimerosal – has ever been studied in relation to autism. Thimerosal is a form of mercury which was originally added to most vaccines but is now no longer used except for the flu vaccine. No studies have ever been carried out for any of the other vaccines or their ingredients. There are ten studies on the MMR jab and 13 on thimerosal that are claimed to prove that vaccines and autism are unrelated. Most people, including senior medics, simply accept these claims. Virtually no one ever examines the detailed study data and evidence. However, J. B. Handley, the father of a seriously autistic boy and the author of the bestselling book *How to End the Autism Epidemic* did just that. What he found was earth shattering.

The "gold standard" medical proof that something works and is safe requires a trial in which it is evaluated against a true placebo which can have no effect on the human body. The thimerosal studies, however, did not use true placebos. I will outline two examples. One of the most cited studies called the "Verstraeten study" simply compared vaccines with two different levels of thimerosal. There was no placebo. Consider that if you wanted to prove that cigarette smoking causes lung cancer, you would simply compare the outcomes of smokers to people who did not smoke. There would be a clear difference in the cancer cases, thus proving that smoking was the cause. You really would never just consider comparing smokers who had 40 cigarettes a day to those who had 20 cigarettes a day. If you did, both groups would develop more cancer cases. There would be a difference in cases but statistically it would be relatively small. This would mean that if you wanted, you could claim there was no statistical difference and, therefore, that smoking did not cause cancer. Shockingly, the vaccine industry made exactly this identical form of claim about thimerosal when the Verstraeten study was published. They claimed it proved that thimerosal did not cause autism and they ensured this message was widely publicised. The lead author of the study, however, was enraged by this. Why? Because it was not true. He wrote to the journal Pediatrics where it was published citing that the study's conclusion was that it neither proved nor disproved a connection between thimerosal and autism and that more studies were needed. Despite all of this, the vaccine industry and medical experts still claim this study proves that thimerosal does not cause autism. Could there be a more glaring example of fraudulent interpretation of scientific evidence?

Nine years after the Verstraeten study was completed a new study called the "Tozzi study" was carried out in Italy. Believe it or not, this used exactly the same trick where thimerosal was used in both of the vaccines involved in the study and the same incorrect conclusion was made. Once again, the vaccine industry used this study to widely spread, via every major news organisation, the same basic message that "vaccines are safe and they don't cause autism". One interesting fact is that both these studies were funded by the CDC which is the US federal agency that is responsible for implementing the vaccine programmes. Clearly, they do not want to fund genuine scientific trials with true placebos, because I'm sure they know that these would prove there was a connection between thimerosal and autism. Truly shocking. Are these two trials just exceptions? Sadly, no. In fact, none of the current childhood vaccines have ever been tested against an inert saline placebo jab, meaning that the safety claims they make are simply unproven.

J. B. Handley, in articles for the Children's Health Defense and in his book, also analysed the other studies claiming that thimerosal and the MMR jab did not cause autism and they all used a variety of similar tricks. Some of these are very complex, however, and if you want to learn about them you need to read his evidence directly. One other revealing fact is that the lead or co-author of four of these bogus studies (Danish researcher, Poul Thorsen) who claimed that vaccines and thimerosal do not cause autism, is now known to have embezzled over $1 million from the CDC grant money he was allocated to conduct them. So, a fraudster carried out official autism studies. You really couldn't make all this up.

The crucial fact about all this information is that quite simply there have never been any studies that compare vaccinated against unvaccinated children that are linked to, or funded by, any official government or medical organisation. This despite the fact it is the only truly scientific way of finding out the truth. If vaccines really are safe, why was this not done? Why resort to crazy unscientific studies like the ones just examined? Having made this point, you may be surprised to learn that several studies really have been done – mainly in universities – that compare vaccinated against unvaccinated children. I can, however, guarantee that you have never seen any of them, because no media or news groups have ever acknowledged that they even exist. Here are the summary outcomes of three of them.

In 2010 researchers from Stony Brook University compared boys given the hepatitis B vaccine who were under four weeks old (neonates) with those who hadn't received it. The researchers reached clear conclusions: "Boys vaccinated as neonates had three-fold greater odds for autism diagnosis compared to boys never vaccinated or vaccinated after the first month of life."

In 2017 researchers from Jackson State University compared vaccinated and completely unvaccinated children. This study showed that those vaccinated had a greater risk of diseases like pneumonia, allergies and neurodevelopmental disorders like ADHD and autism. Specifically, vaccinated children were found to have a four-fold higher risk of developing autism. The researchers also found that children born prematurely had even more severe outcomes. They then carried out a separate study and for these premature vaccinated children, their risk of developing a neurodevelopmental disorder increased by a staggering 14 times.

A 2000 study involving 13,000 children by the UCLA School of Public Health examined the effects of the DTP vaccine to see if it might be responsible for allergies and asthma. The study found that "DTP vaccination in US children is associated with lifetime history of asthma or other allergies and allergy-related symptoms... Assuming that the estimated vaccination effect is unbiased, 50% of diagnosed asthma cases (2.93 million) in US children and adolescents would be prevented if the DTP vaccination was not administered".

There are four other similar studies showing the harm that vaccines can cause. However, all this evidence has effectively been "censored" because the official government, medical and regulatory positions are unchallengeable: "Vaccines are safe and do not cause autism." Everyone, including the media, has to fall in line with this official view or they could expect to be savagely attacked.

I now want to provide some facts about Andrew Wakefield. The story that has been universally used by the media is that he was stripped of his medical licence because he wrongly claimed the MMR vaccine was one of the causes of autism. Virtually everyone believes this "story". However, every single fact you will now read is true. You may think this must be nonsense but consider this extra fact. If it really is a pack of lies, then I could be sued and the book could be removed from sale. I would never take such a risk and it simply can't happen because no one can win a case by claiming that the indisputable truth is a lie.

In 1998 Dr Wakefield and 12 other doctors, including Professor John Walker-Smith, a foremost internationally recognised paediatric gastroenterologist, published a paper in the medical journal the Lancet. They had discovered a new and unusual bowel condition in autistic children which was unlike anything they had ever seen before. They called it ileal-lymphoid-nodular hyperplasia. The study examined the gastrointestinal health issues of 12 autistic children and it was the first time that a link had ever been found between the human gut and autism. You may be surprised to learn that this link has since been found in around 200 other studies. This was a major scientific breakthrough at the time. It did not cause any controversy, but the study also simply quoted the views of the parents in which eight of the twelve said that their child's autism had developed after receiving the MMR jab. The doctors discussed this and wrote, "In most cases, onset of symptoms was after measles, mumps and rubella immunisation. Further investigations are needed to examine this syndrome and its possible relation to this vaccine." In other words, they did not claim the MMR jab caused autism. There was in fact no data about vaccines in the paper other than the views of the parents, and they simply wrote, "We did not prove an association between measles, mumps and rubella vaccine and the syndrome described."

However, despite the fact no claims were made relating the MMR jab to autism, the vaccine establishment must have been alarmed at the possible connection and what damage it might do to vaccinations. It should always be remembered that the pharmaceutical industry exerts inordinate control over both the scientific journals and mass channels of communication, and it is no surprise that scientists and investigative reporters were being intimidated into silence on virtually every aspect relating to vaccines. It is, therefore, unsurprising that serious pressure was applied to all 12 doctors to rescind their paper and they were effectively threatened with losing their careers if they didn't. Eventually, most of them capitulated and complied, but Dr Wakefield and Professor John Walker-Smith did not and they were eventually "put on trial" by a disciplinary panel at the General Medical Council (GMC). This was expected to last three months but in fact it lasted three years. I should add that it also took the GMC four years to prepare the case against them. Why? The media would have you believe that the study claimed a connection between MMR and autism, but the GMC knew that such a case could not be won. Instead, they had to try to find other reasons to strip them of their medical licences and discredit them. This is too long and complex a story to cover in detail and many other individuals and organisations like the journalist Brian Deer, the Times newspaper and the BMJ were all involved. If you want to know the details, then investigative journalist Martin Walker attended every session of the trial and produced a long and detailed paper covering all the facts. But put quite simply, the GMC eventually developed a complex chain of claims that the doctors had not just been involved in clinical practice to help the 12 children's medical conditions, but that they had in fact been carrying out medical research. To do such research you need official medical approval which had not been obtained. Using this "strange" claim, they found both doctors guilty. Dr Wakefield's medical licence was revoked, but Professor Walker-Smith immediately challenged the GMC verdict and his new trial had to take place in the UK High Court. You may be surprised to learn that the judge determined that the GMC's verdicts of professional misconduct and ethics violations were unsupported by the evidence. Professor Walker-Smith was completely exonerated and the entire GMC process was deemed to be fatally flawed and the panel was guilty of "fundamental errors... distortion of evidence, inadequate analysis, inadequate and superficial reasoning and explanation, inappropriate rejection of evidence, 'flawed' and 'wrong' reasoning, and numerous and significant universal inadequacies..."

More importantly, these judgements would also have applied to Dr Wakefield since he was found guilty by the GMC of the same charges. The only problem was he did not have the finances to bring the case to the High Court, whereas Professor Walker-Smith received funding due to his professional indemnity. If Dr Wakefield had received similar funding, then the GMC would have had to reinstate his medical licence. Please think carefully about this. Almost everyone on the planet has been indoctrinated with the idea that he was "sacked" as a doctor because he had lied by falsely claiming the MMR vaccine was a cause of autism, but this was not true and he really should have been reinstated after the verdict, and indeed he would have been if the legal funds had been available to take the case to the High Court. It was in fact the GMC that were making the false claims. Unsurprisingly, none of this evidence was ever reported by any media group.

Of course, it is important to add that Andrew Wakefield did at some point start to realise that the MMR vaccine actually was associated with regressive autism and then he really did try to expose the real truth even after losing his medical licence. In fact, in 2017, he was a key producer of the film *Vaxxed: From Cover-Up to Catastrophe.* This exposed clear evidence that five CDC scientists who had carried out a study in 2004 on autism and the MMR vaccine which claimed there was no connection had simply manipulated the data to get the result they wanted. The original data had in fact shown a definite link between the MMR jab and regressive autism particularly for African American males. This study was, and still is, one of the key pieces of evidence the CDC regularly uses to claim there is no link. The five scientists, however, then became concerned in case anyone else ever saw the real data and might then expose how they had manipulated it. So, they decided to selectively destroy key parts of it. However, the lead author, Dr William Thompson, was worried that this was illegal and he decided to keep copies of everything. He eventually gave this information to Brian Hooker PhD who then passed it on to Andrew Wakefield. Unsurprisingly, this real data became one of the key parts of the *Vaxxed* film, all of which is based on solid scientific evidence. The film lambasts the five scientists who hid the real connection between MMR vaccines and autism and described it as a cover up of legendary proportions. This is what Andrew Wakefield told members of the Alliance for Natural Health International: "We have accused these scientists with the worst humanitarian crime in history. Tens of thousands of children suffer permanent neurological and immunological damage as a result. If anything, we have said [in *Vaxxed*] is fraudulent, they would have sued us to the moon and back and they have not filed a case. It is the truth. The statute of limitations on filing a lawsuit has now expired."

There really couldn't be any better proof that the MMR vaccine can cause regressive autism. Andrew Wakefield and the other film producers simply exposed the real official data and tellingly, none of the most powerful organisations in America, like the CDC, the FDA and even the US government, dared to sue them because they simply couldn't have won the case. Incredibly, and despite all of this, the CDC still uses the 2004 study to claim there is no relation between the MMR vaccine and autism, and Andrew Wakefield is simply one of the most attacked and vilified people in the world.

Many examples have been explored showing how doctors and researchers who challenge conventional medicine are attacked and their careers destroyed to protect medicine's reputation as well as industry profits. These people, who risk everything to promote the truth, are amongst the most courageous in the world. It can, of course, take decades for the truth to finally be accepted and for lives to be saved. Eventually, however, it does usually happen. Andrew Wakefield and Professor Walker-Smith are two such heroes. The study they completed in 1998 was ground-breaking. It showed a link between gut health and autism and I will explain shortly how this has led to treatments that can significantly reduce the symptoms of autism. It did not initially prove a link between vaccines and autism but this link has since emerged and Andrew Wakefield has played a significant role in trying to expose the truth about this as well. A human disaster may have to unfold before the truth about autism emerges, but I believe Andrew Wakefield could one day be exonerated.

While this section has so far concentrated on vaccines, there is also strong evidence to show that many other factors are almost certainly involved in autism. These include glyphosate herbicides, phthalate chemicals, metals like mercury, aluminium and lead, and antibiotics, and more information on these will be given in the lifestyle approach to autism.

I will, however, finish this part with an NHS website extract. Only when I had finished writing this section did I realise I hadn't looked at what the NHS said about autism. When I did, I was truly shocked. Here are the key parts, word for word:

What is autism?

Autistic people may act in a different way to other people.

Autistic people may:

- find it hard to communicate and interact with other people
- find it hard to understand how other people think or feel
- find things like bright lights or loud noises overwhelming, stressful or uncomfortable
- get anxious or upset about unfamiliar situations and social events
- take longer to understand information
- do or think the same things over and over

Autism is not an illness.

Being autistic does not mean you have an illness or disease. It means your brain works in a different way from other people.

It's something you're born with or first appears when you're very young.

If you're autistic, you're autistic your whole life.

Autism is not a medical condition with treatments or a "cure". But some people need support to help them with certain things.

Autistic people can live a full life.

Being autistic does not have to stop you having a good life.

Like everyone, autistic people have things they're good at as well as things they struggle with.

Being autistic does not mean you can never make friends, have relationships or get a job. But you might need extra help with these things.

Autism is different for everyone.

Autism is a spectrum. This means everybody with autism is different.

Some autistic people need little or no support. Others may need help from a parent or carer every day.

It's not clear what causes autism.

Nobody knows what causes autism, or if it has a cause.

It can affect people in the same family. So it may sometimes be passed on to a child by their parents.

Autism is not caused by:

- bad parenting
- vaccines, such as the MMR vaccine
- diet
- an infection you can spread to other people

Autistic people can have any level of intelligence.

Some autistic people have average or above average intelligence.

Some autistic people have a learning disability. This means they may find it hard to look after themselves and need help with daily life.

Autistic people may have other conditions, like:

- attention deficit hyperactivity disorder (ADHD) or dyslexia
- anxiety or depression
- epilepsy

This article contains a number of truly shocking claims. The most important of which are:

- *Being autistic does not mean you have an illness or disease. It means your brain works in a different way from other people.* To claim that regressive autism, for example, which develops in perfectly healthy children is not a disease is like saying that cancer in a child is also not a disease. This is crazy.
- *Autism is not a medical condition with treatments or a cure.* You will see in the next section that there really are treatments that can significantly reduce symptoms and even result in complete cure.
- *Being autistic does not have to stop you having a good life.* This is a shocking statement given that so many children have devastating life-long symptoms and will never live a good life.
- *Nobody knows what causes autism or even if it has a cause.* There are, however, a number of clear causes with strong evidence.
- There is also no mention of any of the destructive symptoms, like self-harm, agonising pain, seizures and gastrointestinal issues. It makes autism appear mild and claims that most people can live a full life, when for most children it is simply a devastating life.

The whole article has been clearly designed to make autism appear a natural part of human life, that nothing can be done to stop it or treat it, and that mankind must just accept it. I simply can't believe the NHS has made such claims. I must repeat yet again that GPs and doctors are not involved. It is just the relatively few unchallengeable key decision makers. Doctors and healthcare workers simply have to accept and adopt their views or their careers would be destroyed just like Andrew Wakefield.

Despite all of this, there really can be little doubt that medicine's key autism decision makers must know there is a real epidemic and they also know there have to be man-made causes. They are nevertheless determined to cover it all up. They will know that admitting any of this, after so many years of denying it, would leave them open to serious charges and destroy much of medicine, as well as the industries that supply it. But allowing children to develop a life-destroying disease is unforgiveable, so how can these key decision makers live with themselves? Is there any way they might try to self-justify what they are doing and allowing the epidemic to continue? Well, if the truth ever came out, vaccines would also lose public support. They probably would say vaccines are vital medical procedures and that autism could be a price worth paying to protect their use. If vaccines in western countries saved millions of lives and autism only affected a few thousand children then this "might" be an acceptable position, but the reverse is in fact the case. Most vaccines in developed countries save relatively small numbers while there are 1.8 million children with autism in the US and the numbers are doubling every few years. Whatever their beliefs and motivations, the autism epidemic exists and it will continue to escalate until it destroys much of mankind.

Autism – the lifestyle medicine approach

Autism is a disease. The claims made by official bodies that the brains of autistic people simply operate in a different but natural way, that it is not a disease, and that it has always existed really have to be wrong.

The main causes of autism are almost certainly a range of chemicals that enter the body either from the air we breathe, the food we eat, chemicals injected into our bodies, and a number of others like cleaning products, other household chemicals and certain drugs like acetaminophen and antidepressants. Agricultural chemicals like glyphosates are almost certainly involved and airborne pollutants can increase the risk in cities. Antibiotics given during pregnancy (particularly during the second trimester) as well as those given to very young children also play a part; they may not be a direct cause, but they significantly increase the risk of autism, probably because they can seriously damage the gut microbiome. Nevertheless, vaccines really are likely to be the major factor. So, how does this happen? Well, vaccines, as we have seen, contain around 40 different chemicals and these are injected directly into the body. No studies have ever been done to prove their safety, except for thimerosal, and even these, as already outlined, used various tricks to hide the true facts.

There is, however, significant evidence that aluminium, which is used as a vaccine adjuvant to stimulate the immune system, is a major factor in autism. This is another complex process and to learn about the intricate details you need to read J. B. Handley's book. The basic facts, however, are that a majority of childhood vaccines contain aluminium. We have already seen that, in total, children in the US receive 22 separate vaccine jabs before the age of one and 38 by the age of five years. This means aluminium can slowly build up over this period because most of it is not excreted from the body. Children vary in the level they can tolerate before serious events start to occur. For example, the 2010 study on hepatitis B showed that this single vaccine could increase the risk of autism in children under the age of one month by 300%. But other children develop autism at later dates when aluminium level are still increasing from the additional vaccines. The interesting fact, however, is that the MMR vaccine contains no aluminium. Given that the MMR vaccine has been blamed for autism by hundreds of thousands of parents, this seems to contradict the evidence that aluminium is a cause of autism. However, there is a scientific explanation which in fact adds further proof that it is a cause. It goes like this.

The MMR vaccine is one of the few childhood vaccines that contain live viruses. These do not need adjuvants like aluminium to stimulate the natural immune system, because the live viruses do that automatically. But this immune response to the vaccine then leads to the development of something called a macrophage transport system, which can then cause the aluminium adjuvant nanoparticles from previous vaccinations to be transported into the brain. It is aluminium in the brain (not the rest of the body) that causes autism. This fact was investigated by Professor Christopher Exley from Keele University who compared the brain levels of aluminium in autistic and normal people and found those with autism had at least ten times more aluminium. Professor Exley is the world's leading expert on aluminium and has been investigating the effects it has on the human body for much of his working career. He and his team have established a clear biological basis by which vaccines can cause autism. But, of course, Professor Exley knew that by daring to publish this information he was risking being attacked by the vaccine establishment just like Andrew Wakefield. But he is one of those true heroes (unknown to most people) who are prepared to risk everything to tell the truth and hopefully help prevent millions of children's lives being destroyed. This is what he said in 2017 when he released this information: "I am very prudent. I only put my neck on the guillotine when it is absolutely necessary. And that time is now." I will explain what happened to Professor Exley and his team in Part 6. You will be shocked at what happened and who was involved.

So, the vaccine establishment really will not take any action. It will simply try to dismiss and discredit all such evidence and censor it. The autism epidemic will continue unabated. All that lifestyle medicine and courageous doctors like Professor Exley and Andrew Wakefield can do is to continue trying to get the truth out to as many people as possible. If enough people ever understand what is happening, "people power" might just be able to bring those responsible to justice.

Finally, here is some positive news. There really are natural treatments that can significantly help to minimise the symptoms of autism. However, because medicine denies any such possibility and offers no support or treatments, it is mainly through the heroic and determined efforts of parents, who are prepared to spend years learning about the causes and possible treatments for autism themselves and then using them, that these improvements occur. A few children have even been cured by these amazing parents and these cases show what really could be achieved especially if medicine was to embrace such treatments and help all parents. Here are some examples of the treatments that have been scientifically shown to work.

As Dr Wakefield and his colleagues found in their 1998 study, autistic children have significantly different gut bacteria to other children and there is now almost unchallengeable evidence that an improved microbiome really can help reduce autism symptoms. A 2019 study by Arizona State University found that faecal microbiota transplants (FMT) reduced symptoms by around 50%, even two years after the transplants were carried out. We have already seen that one course of FMT can cure C. difficile infections, but the trials on autism had to use the procedure for ten weeks because previous work had shown that autism (perhaps unsurprisingly) was much more difficult to treat. The trials were nevertheless incredibly successful. At the start of the study, 83% of participants were rated as "severe" autism. At the end of the study, only 17% were "severe", 39% were "mild/moderate", and 44% were below the cut-off for mild ASD. Other doctors have also used FMTs to treat autism and Dr Thomas Borody, an Australian gastroenterologist, was the first doctor to develop this form of FMT to treat autistic children.

Another study at Penn State University demonstrated the profound importance of a gluten-free and dairy-free diet. It significantly helped the 387 autistic children in the study. Most of their parents reported major improvements in social behaviour, language skills, eye contact and attention span.

Researchers at Stanford University School of Medicine carried out a study using N-acetyl cysteine supplements for 12 weeks. The children's irritability and repetitive behaviour scores were almost halved and it also reduced extreme behaviours like throwing, kicking and hitting.

There are many other possible treatments and here are a few of them. I should add that they may not all help everyone because autism has such wide-ranging symptoms, and this is why determined parents who know about them have to work relentlessly to examine all the evidence and find out the best options for their own individual child.

- ketogenic diets
- eliminating sugar
- omega 3 fats – like the omega 3 fish oil, EPA
- B vitamins – particularly B1, B2, B3, B5, B6, B7 B12 and natural folate
- vitamin A
- vitamin C
- vitamin D
- vitamin E
- zinc
- magnesium
- selenium
- L-carnitine
- alpha-lipoic-acid
- coenzyme Q10 (or ubiquinol)
- prebiotics and pro biotics
- removing as many chemicals as possible from the home environment, like chemical cleaning products, toiletries, and perfumes.

J. B. Handley's book *How to End the Autism Epidemic* is a must read for anyone with an autistic child. You will learn the real and detailed truth about autism, and it will also set you on the path of significantly reducing your child's symptoms and even possibly lead to a cure.

PART 6

Conclusions and Summary

Modern medicine can perform near miracles. Accident and emergency treatments, antibiotics, anaesthetics and insulin are all part of this success story. Hero doctors saving lives from war, heart failure on football fields and countless other serious emergencies are the side of medicine that everyone sees almost on a daily basis. These interventions are outstanding.

But there is also a much darker side to medicine, one that most people are completely unaware of. Millions of people each year suffer serious side effects from pharmaceutical drugs and hundreds of thousands are killed by them, even though they offer little or no benefit to over half of all patients. Sixty years ago, the industry produced drugs but had little power. Doctors made all the crucial decisions. Then thalidomide struck. Governments introduced new laws that were supposed to stop that sort of tragedy ever happening again. The industry was mandated to adopt clinical trials but was also allowed to have patent protection and set its own, often astronomical, prices. It exploited these to such an unprecedented degree that it became the most profitable industry ever. It used this money to effectively "bribe" everyone, even its regulators. Minimally beneficial but dangerous drugs became commonplace and the trials were often biased, manipulated and even "fraudulent". The industry was initially required to submit two clinical trials that had adequate and relevant timeframes and genuinely scientific end points to gain approval. Now, however, they have even succeeded in getting many drugs approved with a single trial. Around 30% are "fast tracked" and these can't detect longer term side effects. Around half have meaningless and unscientific surrogate end points rather than having to prove that they save lives. These drugs are simply promoted by intensive advertising, using barely concealed "bribes" and by clinical experts who are in the pay of the drug industry.

All this happened because of the thalidomide tragedy and the determination to stop it happening again. But even this crucial objective has failed. We now know that the drugs Accutane, Primodos and valproate have caused tens, and more likely, hundreds of thousands of birth defects and countless miscarriages and abortions worldwide. The new laws were implemented with the purest of motives but instead they have unwittingly unleashed a monster. It is as if thalidomide had never happened and now it is in fact far worse. Now it is the pharmaceutical industry that controls medicine. Academic and clinical experts in the pay of the industry develop industry friendly laws and mandatory guidelines that enforce the use of drugs and exclude everything else. The key experts can become rich beyond their wildest dreams by "working with the industry". As Dr Ben Goldacre says, "It is possible for good people, in perversely designed systems, to perpetrate great acts of harm on others, sometimes without ever realising it." Indeed, the overwhelming number of doctors and nurses working within medicine want to do the very best to help their patients, but they are trapped in a perverse system, controlled by an industry whose only motives are profit and monopoly power.

If someone had written a fictional story in 1960 about what is happening in medicine today, it would have been ridiculed for being pure, implausible fantasy. But 60 years later we now live in this implausible and deadly world. Never before in the history of democratic society has an industry:

- been effectively given so much monopoly power
- exploited that power so ruthlessly
- bribed and corrupted so many people and organisations with impunity
- been allowed to destroy, and now well on the way to destroying all alternatives to their products
- been allowed to sell products that kill and harm so many people
- subverted the science that underpins its products for decades
- evaded completely corporate manslaughter charges, even though millions of people have been deliberately killed or seriously harmed by it all

Of course, corruption occurs in every industry and every part of life. Greed is the driving force. Some people gain money, others lose money because of it. What makes corruption in the drug industry and medicine so shocking is the end result. Millions of people pay for this corruption with their lives and their health. This is what makes it all so sad and so unbelievable. Medicine has effectively become an extension of the marketing arm of the drug industry, dishing out more and more pills to more and more people every single year. At best, most of these drugs simply mediate the progression of disease. Frighteningly, while all this is happening, the number of people affected by virtually every chronic disease is escalating exponentially and no one is demanding action to find out why these epidemics are occurring. Half of all children now have at least one chronic disease. This is set to continue because curing or preventing diseases is financial suicide for the drug industry. They simply won't allow it to happen.

In direct contrast, the main aim of lifestyle medicine is to prevent disease. This, of course, is the ultimate threat to medicine and the drug industry. It is why it is constantly attacked and ridiculed and why laws are being put in place that could ultimately destroy it. But lifestyle medicine works, and the proof that it works depends on something much better than clinical trials – something that cannot be manipulated or subverted. Historical and public records reveal the truth about diseases and their progression, and show that prevention must be possible. Just look at the history of killer diseases like typhoid, cholera and scarlet fever. These diseases thrived and killed huge numbers of people due to appalling social and living conditions. Then the deaths all but disappeared when lifestyles improved. The historical mortality figures that prove this are there for all to see. They cannot be manipulated; they are a matter of public record. The proof is indisputable. These once killer diseases were defeated and consigned to history, simply by changes to lifestyle. Medicine was not involved in any way.

Public records also show different groups within society have incredible variations in life expectancy. Average life expectancy in the UK varies by up to 24 years. The only explanation for these astonishing differences are the lifestyles that each group leads. The historical progression of most modern diseases, like heart attacks, strokes, obesity and type 2 diabetes, also clearly demonstrates that they are caused by lifestyle and environmental factors, and that they can, therefore, be prevented once these factors are understood. Any independent scientist would come to this obvious conclusion. Even medicine accepts that diseases like type 2 diabetes are caused simply by poor lifestyles and hundreds of thousands of patients really have been cured of it by simply changing their diets. They also accept that about 30%

of all the big killer diseases can be prevented by exercise alone and that stress and emotional problems are also a significant cause of heart disease as well as being implicated in a host of other conditions. Sadly, however, medicine does virtually nothing about it and simply continues to allow diseases to happen and then uses drugs to minimise their symptoms.

The proof that lifestyle can prevent many diseases is already overwhelming. There are, of course, some such as cancer and Alzheimer's disease where the idea that prevention by lifestyle changes is possible and is still disputed by many leading medical experts. But as we have seen, even here, there is significant evidence which continues to build in favour of prevention.

Here, for the final time, are the seven key lifestyle factors that together, can lead to disease prevention:

1) positive emotional health
2) a healthy, natural, unprocessed low-carb diet
3) exercise
4) vitamin and mineral supplements
5) a healthy microbiome
6) minimising chemical exposure
7) good sleep

Lifestyle medicine also has an impeccable safety record that is virtually unblemished. The efforts of the drug industry and its hired guns, who try to label it as dangerous, do not stand up to close scrutiny. These attacks are based on junk science and are motivated simply by protectionism and profit.

Summary

Lifestyle medicine works; the evidence is compelling. Prevention of most chronic diseases is not just possible, but entirely logical. Lifestyle changes are also incredibly safe.

Drug-based medicine is hugely ineffective. Witness the frightening and exponential increase that continues to occur in virtually every single disease, even in young children. Witness the fact that many drugs have to be taken long term and simply alleviate symptoms rather than provide any real cure. At the same time, they are the third leading cause of death and their side effects are numerous and often lead to a vicious circle of more drugs and ever more side effects.

Your body is the most incredible entity in the universe. Evolution really hasn't led us down a blind alley to ill health. Your body isn't "frail" or "riddled with faults". It is truly resilient if you allow it to be. There is no inevitable path towards chronic diseases as medicine might have you believe, and little need for the multitude of drugs they offer.

Three hundred years ago, medicine's elite refused to believe that fruit could prevent and cure scurvy, with deadly consequences for 130,000 men. Today they are making exactly the same tragic mistake by refusing to accept how transformational diet and lifestyle can be to our health, except now, the scale of the tragedy is immeasurably greater. Hundreds of millions of people suffer from diseases that are mostly preventable. In westernised countries like the UK, healthy life expectancy has been falling for years. The average person now spends the last 17 years of their life with at least one serious disease, like strokes, heart disease, Alzheimer's, Parkinson's, arthritis and cancer, that seriously affect their lives and what they can do. Most of them really could be prevented.

If you look after your body by leading a healthy lifestyle, it will rarely let you down. And don't forget your friendly bacteria. They are also there to protect you, as well as themselves. It is the ultimate symbiotic relationship.

A long and healthy life, free from chronic disease, really is possible for most people.

And finally, if you have got this far, then I must have done something right to grab your attention. But from here the rest is down to you.

I hope you continue on the journey. And when your health improves, I hope you will pass this "incredible message" on to others. In this way you will be part of a health revolution that could eventually change the world.

Special Note

Part 7, which follows, was not included in the prequel to this book. Why? Because much of the evidence has only really come to light in the last few years. Some of it affects lifestyle medicine as well as conventional medicine, but crucially, it involves truly frightening plans that will affect most other parts of human life and all of mankind. Whilst it will be controversial to many people, it really is so important that I had to include it. Please be prepared. The title really does set the scene for what is to follow.

PART 7

Mankind Faces a Devastating Future

Background

Much of this book has provided significant evidence about why lifestyle medicine has been under constant and savage attack from all the major industries, like Big Pharma, Big Food, Big Ag, Big Data and Big Finance, as well as medicine, governments, regulators and most other organisations. It is attacked because it works so amazingly well that it threatens much of what they all do. The two obvious reasons for the all-out war are preserving profits and preserving reputations. But it's also important to remember that the global billionaire elite also play a significant part in this attack. In fact, the all-out war on lifestyle medicine was effectively started by a single man: John D. Rockefeller, who was the richest man in world history with over half a trillion dollars of wealth in today's terms. As already explained, he succeeded in eliminating most natural treatments that had been successfully used by medicine for many years and then helped to achieve a near monopoly for pharmaceutical drugs. Like all the global elite, increasing his wealth was a priority, but he also wanted to control and exert power. Having been found guilty of fraud, philanthropy was an obvious way to help regain his reputation, but he did it in such a way that maintained and even increased his power as well as his wealth.

A hundred years later and the Rockefeller Foundation still exists with billions of dollars of assets. What about today's elite? Most billionaires, like Bill Gates (who also committed fraud like John D. Rockefeller), may be philanthropic, but their driving force is also power and control and, of course, the more money they generate, the more control they can then achieve. While the war against lifestyle medicine is still one of their prime targets, Bill Gates and others also have a vision of how the world in general should evolve. They believe they are intellectually superior and not just super rich, and this "superiority" gives them the right to control the world and decide the fate of mankind's 8 billion people.

This book has exposed many devastating outcomes that are occurring in healthcare, like the epidemic of diseases, drugs being the third leading cause of death, the all-out war against lifestyle medicine, and the way global companies simply put profit before human life. As shocking as all these have been, the plans of the global elite are now on another level altogether. Aldous Huxley wrote the book *Brave New World* and George Orwell wrote *1984*. These books involved totalitarianism, propaganda, censorship and mass surveillance involving technological advances which were used by the elite to control society. That such totalitarianism could ever happen in the real world may seem impossible to believe, but even now many countries like China are already using similar techniques. This is not just happening in dictatorships and military juntas, however. Even democratic countries have now started down this slippery slope and you will see many examples of what is currently happening. You really should prepare for a frightening and devastating future that the global elite now have planned for mankind, and also decide whether you are prepared to fight and help prevent it all from taking place.

The World Economic Forum (WEF) was formed in 1971 (although initially it was called the European Management Forum) and was founded by the German engineer and economist Klaus Schwab who is still the executive chairman. It holds its key annual meeting at Davos in Switzerland each January, and for the first decade many of the attendees used it mainly as a skiing and evening events holiday. Then it started to be attended by more world leaders who wanted to use it as a means of promoting their own interests. Today it has truly evolved and is now the most powerful organisation in the world. It has around 3,000 elite members including nearly all the world's richest billionaires. It is mainly funded by its key 1,000 member companies which are all global enterprises with more than $5 billion in annual turnover and are the top companies within each of their sectors. The leaders of all the major world organisations like the UN, WHO, the World Bank, UNICEF and UNESCO as well as most world government leaders are also all involved and fully support its reset plans. The WEF believes that a globalised world is best controlled by an unelected, self-selected coalition of multi-national corporations, organisations, politicians, intellectuals, scientists and other leaders of society. Klaus Schwab said the WEF is guided by the goal of positioning "private corporations as the trustees of society". Rather than governments of individual countries doing their own things, the WEF intends to simply exert global control over every key aspect of life. Individual governments will simply follow these plans.

In June 2020 the WEF developed the term "Global Reset" (also called the "Great Reset"). Vandana Shiva, scholar, environmentalist, food sovereignty advocate and author, said, "The Great Reset is about multi-national corporate stakeholders at the World Economic Forum controlling as many elements of planetary life as they possibly can. From the digital data humans produce to each morsel of food we eat." Food is one shocking example of how this form of global control is intended to work. The WEF's plan aims to transform global food and the human diet, and its "reset" involves much more industrialised agricultural, industrialised food production, widespread chemical use, genetically modified organisms and synthetic lab-made proteins and meats. The architects of the plan claim it will reduce food scarcity, hunger and disease, and mitigate climate change. None of these claims are true and in fact most have negative effects. Perhaps unsurprisingly, the Great Reset involves some of the most dangerous global corporations in the world, including Bayer, Monsanto, and Syngenta, and in some of the highest courts in the US, these companies have been found guilty of causing life-taking diseases like certain cancers. The key fact to keep remembering is that global corporations exist for just two things – money and control. Just like the tobacco industry (and indeed Big Pharma and Big Ag), they have no concern about human health and life. The food reset will involve the creation of new worldwide dietary guidelines which will then be endlessly promoted, but at some point in the future, their imposition will be enforced on those still resisting them. This will have to happen because even the WEF acknowledges that many people will try to continue eating the natural foods they enjoy and will not willingly give them up.

To get the plan adopted, exactly the same protocol will be used as that for the Covid jabs. False orchestrated claims will be made incessantly by all the media and experts approved by the WEF. Anyone who tries to tell the truth will be attacked, discredited and censored. Internet companies will make it difficult and almost impossible for people to access and learn about anything that truthfully challenges the official reset claims. Free speech, the rock of democracy, will no longer exist. Some people will simply accept and believe this form of propaganda and totalitarianism just as they did, at least initially, with the many false claims made about Covid. If every organisation and expert tell the same lies often enough, then it will eventually be accepted as the truth. This is the bedrock plan of totalitarianism that has been used by the Nazis and dictatorships. Those that don't accept it and who want to maintain their democratic rights to eat what they want will be treated like the so-called anti-vaxxers, and will be accused of thinking only of themselves, and not the rest of society. The message will be that the new dietary guidelines are simply essential in controlling food availability and climate change. These food reset claims are not true, but even if they were, such a plan simply means the end of democracy, because people really should be allowed to eat what they want. Of course, the WEF's food reset plan cannot happen overnight and many parts of it are still being developed like the lab-made meats and genetically modified foods, but quite simply, it will be one of the key parts of their global control. The initial priority will be to pressurise people to avoid eating things like meat and dairy products which is in fact already underway. Much more will be explained about the food reset plan shortly together with the true facts that are being supressed.

The incredible wealth of elite billionaires

While the World Economic Forum appears to be the key proponent of the Great Reset, behind the scenes there are a number of individual elite billionaires who are leading the reset and who command incredible control. Most of the world's billionaires support the WEF reset plans and you may be surprised to learn just how wealthy they are and how this wealth has rocketed over the last few years, particularly during the Covid pandemic. Here are some of the key facts:

- At the end of 2019 there were 2,095 billionaires in the world but this number increased by 573, just in the two years of the pandemic.
- The total wealth of these 2,668 billionaires at the end of 2021 was $12.7 trillion – up by an incredible 42% ($3.8 trillion) during the pandemic, even though during this same period, nearly everyone else became poorer overall.
- At the end of 2019 around 500 million people were in extreme poverty (earning less than $1.90/day) which increased by 52% to 760 million during the pandemic. In East Africa alone, one person is now dying every minute from hunger.
- The world's ten richest men own more wealth than the bottom 3.1 billion people or 40% of humanity.
- Even just in the US, its 651 billionaires have twice as much wealth as 165 million of its people – half its population.

During the pandemic, hundreds of millions of people lost their jobs worldwide. Several billion had lockdowns and other restrictions imposed, forcing them to stay at, or work from, home. The global elite meanwhile increased their profits and wealth mainly because they were heavily invested in the online sites, equipment and deliveries that then had to be used as well as the pharmaceutical products like vaccines and drugs. All these achieved record sales.

This grotesque inequality is devastating humanity. It is divisive, corrosive and dangerous. This is inequality that literally kills.

Having seen how the global elite are now wealthier and thus more powerful than they have ever been, I am going to concentrate mainly on one of them: the philanthropist, Bill Gates. He is the most powerful and influential of all of them. There is one key thing to remember. Philanthropy should simply, and only, involve charitable acts. Please bear this in mind when you consider the following incredible facts about the world's richest reset "philanthropist". Before I examine his (and the WEF's) future plans, I want to start by taking a step back and show you some of the almost unbelievable and frightening changes he has already achieved.

Bill Gates already exerts immense world control

In 2000 Bill Gates had a personal net worth of $63 billion, but by 2021 this had increased to $130 billion, and this does not include the $50 billion he controls in the Bill and Melinda Gates Foundation. Such staggering increases in wealth help the global elite achieve their goals for controlling much of the world.

Vaccines. To help further this mission, in 2010, he decided to invest $10 billion over the following decade in the development and promotion of vaccines. Why did he choose vaccines? Because they are extremely profitable as we have seen with the Covid jabs. In fact, he figured out that they are phenomenal profit makers, and said they were the best investment he'd ever made with more than a 20 to 1 return. Note the word investment rather than philanthropy, meaning that he expects to make $200 billion profit from his $10 billion investment. The profit would come not just from his own direct investments but also from the huge shareholdings he has in pharmaceutical and vaccine-related companies. I should add that in 2000 he had also formed the Global Alliance for Vaccines and Immunization (GAVI) with the aim of radically increasing vaccination in poor countries which was the first phase in his plan to ramp up vaccine profits. He would, of course, say that this was done to reduce viral infections in low-income countries and thus save lives. However, as already explored in detail, in western countries from around 1870, it was the improvement in living conditions like clean water and sanitation that actually radically improved life expectancy and reduced deaths from infectious diseases. Vaccines played a truly minimal role and most weren't even available until the 1960s, 1970s and even the 1980s. Even when they are available, they simply cannot counteract contaminated water, lack of sanitation and malnutrition, and in India today, despite the massive increases in vaccinations promoted by Bill Gates, there are still 130,000 children dying just from diarrhoea each year. Improving living conditions should have been his number one priority. The problem is that donating money for such vital and essential improvements doesn't produce any profit, unlike vaccines.

He helped to further promote his vaccine agenda by forming and contributing significantly to a number of other organisations like CEPI. Most people think that these are government led organisations but they are quite simply controlled by Gates. His key target, however, was the World Health Organization. In 2010, when he started his $10 billion vaccine investment, he radically increased his contributions to the WHO. By 2018 he had inexplicably become its largest contributor with over $1 billion per year – significantly more than any country including the US. This figure includes his direct contributions, but also those from all the other organisations he funds and controls, like GAVI, SAGE and Rotary International who also donate to the WHO. This figure is around one-fifth of the entire annual budget for its 193 member states. He donates over 11 times more than China, and even more than the US itself. A vitally important fact to understand is that the WHO only determines how 30% of its budget is spent. The other 70% is controlled by its donors. What this means is that one man exerts more control over the WHO than any other country including the US and China combined. Bill Gates has no medical background or qualifications, but effectively, he controls the WHO. Almost every significant decision the WHO makes really does have to be effectively vetted by him. Even the Financial Times made it clear that no decision is made at the World Health Organization that is not run through the Gates Foundation first. In 2011 he spoke at the WHO and used his immense authority to literally order all the member countries to make vaccines a central focus of their health systems. A year later, the WHO then adopted a "Global Vaccine Plan" that the Gates Foundation co-authored, and incredulously, over half of the WHO's total budget is now spent on vaccines. Dr Vandana Shiva told Robert F. Kennedy Jr. that "Bill Gates has hijacked the WHO and transformed it into an instrument of personal power that he wields for the cynical purpose of increasing pharmaceutical profits. He has single-handedly destroyed the infrastructure of public health globally to serve his own purposes".

There are many other global health experts who are deeply concerned about all of this, particularly for Africa where the health crisis continues to deepen despite all the money spent on vaccines. Even at the WHO, people are deeply disturbed by the control Bill Gates exerts, but he is so powerful and, as will be seen shortly, he also controls so much of the media in a similar way, meaning that these concerns are rarely heard or seen by anyone. In 2010, when he announced his $10 billion vaccine investment and at the same time started to significantly increase funding for the WHO, he also installed Dr Anthony Fauci on his vaccine advisory board, thereby guaranteeing his plans would receive support from the National Institute of Allergy and Infectious Diseases which is the key proponent of vaccines in the US. A recent investigation also revealed that the Gates Foundation is the primary funder of the UK's Medicine and Healthcare Products Regulatory Agency as well as the FDA in the US which control drug and vaccine approvals. Gates really does leave no stone unturned to achieve his goals. Once again, is this really philanthropy?

Anyone who tries to expose the truth about vaccines can expect severe reprisals. Several high-profile scientists have carried out vaccine studies which show they can cause serious outcomes. Others have also done studies on effective alternative treatments to vaccines. These studies pose a vaccination threat which could precipitously affect the profits of drug companies and major investors like Bill Gates. If these studies really were incorrect, then other researchers would openly discredit them and nothing more would need to be done. However, their evidence is strong and difficult to contest, so these scientists have simply been "terminated" in other ways. This is what happened to three of the world's most prestigious scientists.

Peter Gøtzsche was a co-founder of the Cochrane Collaboration which was the most respected organisation launched to carry out truly independent assessments of clinical trials without any conflicting funding from the drug industry or associated organisations. If it confirmed the benefits of a drug, it was a major boost and sales would rise. If it found serious faults in the trials and data then it would pose a significant threat to the drug's sales. Its absolute independence was crucial to its worldwide respect, and most doctors and scientists knew they could rely on its data. In recent years, however, it is clear that somehow parts of the organisation have been "infiltrated" and some of their assessments have been dubious and simply in line with the official drug company trials even though many of these contain manipulated data and other types of "fraud". One such review supported the HPV vaccine which has been associated with significant and dangerous side effects. Peter Gøtzsche made a publicly available and critical assessment which threatened its use. In 2018 he was expelled even though no specific reason was given. Four of the nine board members resigned in protest and the whole thing has seriously damaged Cochrane's reputation and driven a nail in the coffin of true science. Would you be surprised to learn that his expulsion took place shortly after the Gates Foundation gave Cochrane a significant funding?

World-renowned Professor Christopher Exley's work on aluminium and its effect on neurodegenerative disease has been outlined in the section on autism. He and his team at Keele University had carried out this research for 29 years. They had published over 200 peer-reviewed studies and were supported unequivocally by the university. But, in 2017, he had finally uncovered enough evidence to confirm that aluminium, used as an adjuvant in vaccines, was associated with autism. Around this time, changes started to occur in the university's senior management together with a roster of major new funders. The evidence he had uncovered was, of course, potentially devastating for vaccine producers and their investors and initially they sought to marginalise and downplay it. The new funders included Big Pharma and the Gates Foundation who were helping Keele University to establish new research arms for projects like gene-drive mosquitoes and a new School of Pharmacy and Bioengineering. When these huge financial donations started, the university began to pull back its support for Professor Exley. It spiked his press releases and downplayed or ignored his work and then started sabotaging his independent research donations. In August 2021 the university finally completed its new "mission" and announced his departure. He did know that by telling the truth about aluminium and autism he was risking his career and indeed he ended up being thrown out, but he was one of those brave, true unsung heroes who put saving the lives of children before their own future. John F. Kennedy Jr. wrote a letter to Keele University about the whole devastating sequence of events which said, "Allowing industry to quash science for fear that it might expose profitable practices as harmful to public health is offensive to every tenet of academic freedom, scientific integrity, ethics and morality." The sad fact is money really is the key for most organisations.

I have already explained how Dr Andrew Hill of Liverpool University carried out a meta-analysis of ivermectin trials which showed that it reduced Covid deaths by 75%. If this had been left unchallenged, Covid vaccines really would have had to be legally removed from use. But he was pressurised by Unitaid to redact it and then unscientifically manipulate the data so that it showed that "it had no benefit". Unitaid then made a £40 million donation to the university. The important fact is that a key donor of Unitaid just happens (yet again) to be Bill Gates.

So, these three examples show what happens to some of the world's most respected scientists if they expose the real truth about vaccines that threaten their use. Once again, maintaining profit comes before children's lives. Bill Gates is probably the biggest single investor in vaccines in the world, and profit is his key goal. So, he was determined to destroy these scientists or bring them onto his side by donating millions of dollars to their universities and organisations. Sadly, and devastatingly, but perhaps unsurprisingly, he succeeded.

Here is another example of how he reacts to anything that threatens his projected vaccine profits. When vaccines started to be developed for COVID-19, Oxford University initially intended to make its publicly funded vaccine data available free around the world so that anyone could produce it at low cost meaning it would be available to most of the world's population particularly those in the poorest countries. But this would have severely restricted the expected profits from the Pfizer and Moderna vaccines and those for Bill Gates. So, he pressurised and incentivised Oxford to partner with AstraZeneca meaning the final vaccine would be patented and that poorer countries would then not be able to make it or afford it. He has made an incredible 100 plus donations to Oxford University totalling hundreds of millions of dollars. Could this have played a part in their decision to work with AstraZeneca and not to help save the lives of the poor? I'll let you decide. Bill Gates can exert so much control over so many organisations, that he could probably stop and take out anyone who threatens vaccines even if their scientific data are true. He simply intends to maintain their incredible profits, regardless of the dangerous side effects they can cause.

Polio. But vaccines aren't the only things that are essentially controlled by Bill Gates due to his control over the WHO. I have already explained how he had decided in 2003 to finally eradicate polio (probably so he could personally go down in history as its main saviour), even though few cases existed in just four or five countries, and deaths were incredibly low. He, together with the US government, effectively "forced" the WHO to adopt a polio eradication programme. Over $3 billion has since been spent, but 20 years later, the disease has still not been eradicated. Had this money been spent on things like water and sanitation in Africa and other countries like India and Pakistan, hundreds of thousands, and probably millions, of children's lives could have been saved rather than just a few hundred from polio. The same question needs to be asked again and again. Is this really philanthropy?

Malaria. The Gates Foundation also became attracted to malaria. They started funding projects and at that time there was a wide range of research including prevention, treatment and eradication which were all vital for such a complex disease. However, in 2007, they challenged this wide-ranging scientific-based strategy by launching a commitment to simply try to eradicate the disease. All their money was directed at this one option. The then WHO director Margaret Chan immediately adhered to the Gates strategy with the intention of also using all its money allocated to malaria, just for eradication research. However, the head of the WHO's malaria programme, Kochi Arata, expressed his concern and disagreement saying it risked eliminating the vital diversity of approaches that were needed. Shortly after, Margaret Chan removed him from office and no one else at the WHO has since dared to question it. There were many other research scientists around the world who made similar challenges and who were convinced that the elimination of malaria was a project destined to fail. Throughout history, only one disease – smallpox – has ever been eradicated. Nevertheless, once again, a billion dollars of Gates Foundation investment effectively silenced the scientific community. Fifteen years later and no effective eradication options exist and malaria continues to devastate much of the world. Yet again, is this true philanthropy?

WHO. The current WHO director general is Tedros Adhanom Ghebreyesus. Who do you think helped to appoint him? He was handpicked by Bill Gates. He also has no medical qualifications or background and has even been accused of human rights violations, but he had been a director of the GAVI vaccine organisation which was created by, and still receives funding from, the Gates Foundation. His loyalty to Bill Gates is unquestionable and was clearly a key reason for his appointment. So, now neither of the two key decision makers who control much of the WHO have any medical qualifications. That all this is happening is just one more example of how science has been corrupted. A review in the Journal of Integrative Medicine and Therapy went so far as to say that the corruption of the WHO is the "biggest threat to the world's public health of our time".

I now want to examine a range of other vital aspects affecting mankind that Bill Gates is deeply involved in. These include agriculture, food, public surveillance and education, but I'll start with the media.

The media. The media has incredulously received $319 million from the Gates Foundation. In the US these include CNN, NBC, NPR and the Atlantic. In the UK they include the BBC, the Guardian, the Financial Times and the Daily Telegraph as well as Le Monde (France), Der Spiegel (Germany) and Al Jazeera. NPR received $24.7 million and the Guardian $12.9 million. Gates' local Seattle Times said, "The foundation's grants to media organisations raise obvious conflict-of-interest questions. How can reporting be unbiased when a major player holds the purse strings." I should add that it made this comment before it then accepted a significant donation from Bill Gates to fund its own education lab and perhaps, unsurprisingly, has not made any similar critiques since. All this gives a vivid insight into Gates' motives for donating such huge sums. Of course, this doesn't mean he directly tells the media groups exactly what he wants them to report, but the donations do come with strings attached. The money usually has to be used to promote articles for specific topics like global health, vaccines and education which he has major financial interests in. But what he also does is to make his personal opinions on these key areas of life that he aims to control crystal clear, widely available and universally distributed. Invariably, the media then simply promote them without any serious investigation, even though their key role throughout history was to challenge everything and seek and report the real truth.

The Gates Foundation also donates money to journalistic training associations which means that, once qualified, these funded journalists are unlikely to ever contradict his views even when they are incorrect. Alan McLeod, senior journalist at MintPress News, wrote an article explaining how "today, it is possible for an individual to train as a reporter thanks to a Gates Foundation grant, find work at a Gates-funded outlet, and to belong to a press association funded by Gates. This is especially true of journalists working in the fields of health, education and global development, the ones that Gates himself is most active in and where scrutiny of the billionaire's actions and motives are most necessary."

Bill Gates is classed as a philanthropist. Do you think that giving a third of a billion dollars of money to the world's highly profitable media and news companies, as well as journalistic education, can really be classed as philanthropy? If this money had been spent on providing clean water and sanitation to poor countries, then hundreds of thousands of children's lives could have been saved. Clearly, this is just one more example of how Bill Gates cares more about increasing his control and profits rather than saving lives and being a true philanthropist. Even the World Health Organization spends just $25 million each year on water and sanitation for poor countries but spends 100 times more ($2.5 billion) on vaccines even though these have made little improvement in the other really serious diseases that children in the poorer countries suffer from.

Covid pandemic. Given Bill Gates' incredible investments in most vaccines, it is unsurprising that he also invested huge sums in Covid jabs and also had significant investments in the pharmaceutical companies who were developing them. The success of these investments was, therefore, one of his key priorities and independent experts believed he was, therefore, determined to control the pandemic. Quite simply, there really has been a single official worldwide COVID-19 narrative and its key aim was to promote vaccines, claiming they were the only way of treating the pandemic. Of course, it also involved controlling all the other key aspects like lockdowns, travel restrictions, working from home, school closures and even trying to make vaccination mandatory. It also required a series of false claims and facts, like the vaccines prevented transmission and infection and the significant and never-ending overstating of deaths to help pressurise people to get vaccinated. Most of the media donations that have been examined were in fact made during the Covid pandemic and this would have been done to ensure that they would report and promote only this global narrative and certainly not start to question it or promote opposing (even if correct) views. Right from the start, many independent experts believed Bill Gates was the main person who made the key decisions on the global Covid response, although this had been impossible to prove conclusively. But then, in September 2022, a well-respected independent political journalism company based in the US called Politico published a special report on who controlled the global COVID-19 response. They had conducted a seven-month investigation and interviewed four dozen US and European officials and global health specialists who admitted that Bill Gates used his wealth and influence to call the shots during the pandemic. The reports headline was "How Bill Gates and His Partners Took Over the Global Covid Response". The report quoted four key health organisations that were involved which were the Gates Foundation, GAVI, CEPI and the Wellcome

Trust. The Global Alliance for Vaccines and Immunization (GAVI) and the Coalition for Epidemic Preparedness Innovations (CEPI) are vaccine-related organisations that were both created by Gates. He is still a main funder, and effectively controls both of them. So, even though the Wellcome Trust is a separate organisation, Bill Gates was quite simply the key individual decision maker. As you will see in the next section, he had also held a future pandemic event in 2019 before Covid even started and this meant he had already developed the key strategies that he believed would be necessary so he was already prepared. When the pandemic started, governments were seemingly overwhelmed and when Bill Gates (via his key organisations like GAVI) started to promote these ideas and beliefs, there was an inexorable shift in power to these organisations.

Despite all of this, the idea that Bill Gates exerted undue influence over global health really had officially and consistently been denied and dismissed, but as with so many other things, this claim has now been debunked by a truly respected journalism company. Quite simply, there has been no challenge made to discredit it. Another key fact is that I am not aware of any other news agency that has reported it. This is quite simply the way that true facts are withheld from most of the world's population. So, just like all the other things that he had already taken control of, Bill Gates really was also the main controller of the Covid pandemic. This is what Dr Joseph Mercola said about it all: "But who the heck is Gates to direct global health and pandemic responses. He's a nobody. He has no medical training. He's completely unqualified to speak on any health issues whatsoever. He didn't even graduate college and he's never been elected to represent the people in any capacity. Basically, what we have here is one wealthy individual who figured out a way to unofficially monopolise the decision-making ability of a global health authority to enrich himself, which is beyond crazy."

Pre-pandemic actions. I have already explained in the section on COVID-19 that there is incredible evidence that the SARS-CoV-2 virus was gene edited and somehow released from the Wuhan Institute of Virology in China, and that senior US medical people had also funded part of this research. Here are several other intriguing and potentially shocking facts that occurred before the pandemic started. In October 2019 the Gates Foundation funded a simulation of a possible future pandemic called Event 201. This included key representatives from the World Economic Forum, regulators, vaccine makers and the World Bank. It involved assessing the best ways of dealing with a new viral pandemic. They developed strategies to control not just the pandemic but also the population, together with a single robust global narrative. Key parts included the rapid development of new patentable vaccines and antiviral drugs and then to ensure mass censorship by the media and social media of any truthful evidence that went against this official narrative. There was no consideration of using existing treatments and drugs that could have offered immediate patient protection and saved millions of lives.

The virus they chose to use in Event 201 to simulate this projected new worldwide pandemic was a novel Coronavirus. Was this just a lucky choice? Also, here is what Anthony Fauci said in 2017: "There is no question there is going to be a challenge for the coming administration in the area of infectious diseases. There will be a surprise outbreak. There is no doubt in anyone's mind about this." Bill Gates also stated publicly in 2018 that a global pandemic was imminent, while Melinda Gates went so far as to state that an engineered virus was humanity's greatest threat. An absolutely vital thing to understand is that in the westernised world, the last genuine pandemic was over a hundred years ago: Spanish flu in 1918. The three so-called pandemics the WHO and UN had initially declared – SARS in 2003, avian flu in 2005 and swine flu in 2009 – never actually developed and there were very few deaths. So, why did all these people claim a new pandemic was imminent 100 years after the last real one?

Shortly after Event 201, Gates tweeted, "I'm particularly excited about what the next year could mean for one of the best buys in global health: vaccines." All this happened before the Covid virus was even discovered in the real world.

Another unsettling fact is that in December 2019, Moderna and the NIAID sent mRNA Coronavirus vaccine candidates to the University of North Carolina. Why did they do this when at that time there were no Coronaviruses that posed a threat to humanity and the SARS-CoV-2 virus had still not even been discovered? Did all these people know that Wuhan was carrying out gain-of-function Coronavirus research and that there was a realistic chance that it would be accidentally leaked, thus causing the new pandemic which they had planned to control and make huge sums of money from? Of course, this cannot be proven, but all the evidence suggests it is highly probable.

Agriculture. This is another critical aspect of life Bill Gates is determined to control. His vision and plans are frightening and stark, yet just like vaccines, he is working to achieve them by investing billions of dollars. The use of chemicals and genetic plant modification in agriculture has been examined in detail in Part 4. The US is a prime user of this industrial agricultural model, even though it is clear that it causes many serious outcomes for mankind like certain cancers, as well as devastating the environment and other living organisms. Yet this forms the basis of the Gates Foundation's plans.

Since 2006 Bill Gates, in conjunction with the Rockefeller Foundation, has been promoting this model in poor countries, particularly in many parts of Africa where they created AGRA: the Alliance for a Green Revolution in Africa. They claimed that industrial agriculture, including genetically modified seeds, chemical fertilisers, and insecticides, was more productive, would double crop yields, reduce hunger and increase farmer's incomes. The Gates and Rockefeller Foundations funded AGRA and tried to convince farmers to adopt this industrial-based farming rather than just using the varied natural seeds and practices they have used for millennia. They lobbied African regulators and politicians to encourage and promote genetically modified plants and all their related chemicals and they even gave loans to farmers to purchase their initial batches of GM seeds, fertilisers and insecticides. Unfortunately, this led to a limited range of crops – mainly maize and soy – rather than allowing the farmers to produce the wide range of plants and grains they had grown for over 10,000 years. African agricultural practices have evolved with great crop diversity, local control depending on weather and land conditions, sustainability, and high yields.

There are, of course, some problems in Africa regarding consistent home food supply, but as already explored, these could be overcome as demonstrated by the AIF initiative in Rwanda which reversed malnutrition and hunger for 2 million people in one year. This could happen throughout Africa if just $5 billion was provided to adopt the same protocols. Despite all of this, Bill Gates will not fund such incredible solutions. He is simply determined to impose genetic and chemical agriculture. In fact, he has spent around $5 billion of his own money to effectively dismantle significant parts of this ancient agricultural system that could work incredibly well and he has never given any funding to conventional farmers even though they produce much more varied and healthier foods.

Another key fact is that the majority of this money, whilst apparently going to Africa, has actually ended up in companies and organisations in the US and Europe. This is because AGRA's initiatives depend on high technology which is developed by western research centres and corporations as well as the need to purchase the global corporation's synthetic seeds and chemicals.

So, given all of this information, what do you think the outcomes of AGRA have been? A 2020 independent study – "False Promises: The Alliance for a Green Revolution in Africa" – showed that over the previous 14 years, none of Bill Gates' claims had been achieved. In fact, there have been no overall productivity gains and many farmers have had to take on high levels of debt in order to buy all the patented GM seeds and associated chemicals which has impoverished them further. In addition, hunger in the 18 AGRA countries has increased by 30% to a staggering 131 million people. When this devastating data was published, the original claims that had been made were quietly removed from the AGRA website in June 2020. They currently have no new listed goals and instead they simply promise to improve incomes and food security for African farmers. Even this limited claim is not supported by the 14 years of real evidence. The limited variety of seeds that were involved have also affected millions of people's health. This is what Anne Maina, national coordinator of the Biodiversity and Biosafety Association of Kenya, said about the whole devastating outcomes of industrialised agriculture in Africa: "The strategies continue to impoverish smallholder farmers. It is time to stop promoting green revolution technologies that do not improve our soils. In Kenya the cost of synthetic chemicals has almost doubled. The time is now to increase funding to support the promotion of biofertilisers and biopesticides that not only build our soils but are safe and affordable for current and future generations."

Timothy Wise, senior advisor to the Institute for Agriculture and Trade Policy in the US, said, "AGRA's donors should reconsider their support for such an unsuccessful and unaccountable initiative. They should shift their funding to agroecology and other low-input systems which have shown far better results." Five hundred African faith leaders also signed an open letter expressing "grave concern that the Bill and Melinda Gates Foundation's support for the expansion in industrial scale agriculture is deepening the humanitarian crisis".

In 2022 50 organisations promoting food sovereignty all came together to publish an open letter challenging Bill Gates' latest claims like technology is essential and that that the Green Revolution was "one of the greatest things that ever happened". These claims were openly criticised. The organisations also called on the media to consider how they cover Gates and his vision for the future of food. They wrote: "We invite high-profile news outlets to be more cautious about lending credibility to one wealthy white man's flawed assumptions, hubris, and ignorance, at the expense of people and communities who are living and adapting to these realities as we speak."

Another crucial piece of evidence against the "Green Revolution" was published in 2009. A seminal study by the United Nations documented the incontrovertible evidence demonstrating its abject failure to improve on traditional agriculture. Nine hundred of the world's leading scientists, agronomists and researchers were deployed to study the issue of world hunger. Their definitive report showed that GMO crops are not the answer to food shortfalls or rural poverty. They also showed that the first "Green Revolution" launched in India and Mexico in the 1960s was also a catastrophe – destroying biodiversity, soil and water, as well as contributing to climate change. The United Nations and the world's top agricultural scientists admitted that GMOs simply cannot fight hunger as effectively as traditional farming.

Here is another shocking and almost unbelievable outcome of using GMO seeds. Monsanto, the industrial agricultural company, introduced genetically modified cotton seeds in India from around 2002. It hired a famous Indian actor Nana Petakar to help promote them and they soon became almost universal. The farmers had to borrow money to purchase everything but did so because of all the claims and expectations that were made and ended up with significant debts. However, the crop yields were smaller than promised and they were unable to repay their debts. This resulted in mass suicides and by 2014 it is estimated that the total number of deaths had reached 270,000. You may think this surely couldn't be true, but it was reported in reliable newspapers like the Guardian. I must add that Bill Gates was also a major shareholder in Monsanto.

So, how does Bill Gates respond to all this science-based evidence and devastating life-destroying outcomes? He has effectively (and unsurprisingly) ignored or dismissed all of it and simply continues to promote industrial agriculture – much of which he owns. He has shown himself willing to ignore the voices of scientists and farmers, and to trample laws, treaties, traditions, civil rights, science and sensibilities. In fact, he donated a further $40 million to AGRA in December 2021, and even the US Agency for International Development has also continued to support it. Bill Gates, of course, provides many African countries with donations for other things and their politicians must be reluctant to upset him. It is also well known that certain key African politicians have illegally accumulated and taken many millions of dollars from their own countries which they have hidden in private foreign banks. It is possible (but unprovable) that Bill Gates could be using "donations" to ensure that key politicians keep supporting AGRA. It is very likely that many countries will continue with gene edited and chemical-based agricultural and cause further misery and devastation in much of Africa. Of course, the global agricultural corporations and Bill Gates are not just trying to impose industrialised agriculture on Africa and other poor countries; their aim is to introduce it around the entire world and they have made significant progress in many other regions of Asia and South America.

The information already provided is only one part of the problems caused by industrialised agriculture. It also has a wide range of other devastating outcomes that threaten the world. The heavy use of chemicals denatures soil, destroys its fertility and does not return organic matter back into it. This degrades land and can turn it into desert. It also threatens global water supplies, draining aquifers and contaminating them with toxic chemicals that cause vast dead zones as well as killing swathes of essential insects. A crucial fact is that when top soil is lost, food cannot be grown no matter how many chemicals you have. Amazingly, in 2014, Maria-Helena Semedo of the Food and Agriculture Organization of the United Nations warned that at the current rate of top soil degradation, all the world's top soil will be gone in less than 60 years. This would simply destroy most of mankind. Continually increasing evidence also points to the fact that industrialised agriculture and the processed foods that go with it are one of the leading causes of the chronic disease epidemics that are devastating much of human health around the world.

The real solution to all of these critical issues is simply to support natural and diversified agriculture that has been developed by farmers over 10,000 years and works with nature and the environment and not against it. During this period, farmers and communities have worked to improve yield, taste, nutrition, seed quality and genetic resilience that allows seeds to flourish in particular climate, soil and water conditions. The free exchange of knowledge and seeds amongst farmers has been the basis for maintaining biodiversity and food security.

In the 1980s a new concept – regenerative agriculture – was introduced with a vital additional benefit. It is not a new form of agriculture, and is based mainly on the world's various traditional farming practices. However, it now also aims to increase the reversal of climate change. Ronnie Cummins, founder and director of the Organic Consumers Association, describes it as follows: "Regenerative agriculture and animal husbandry is the next and higher stage of organic food and farming, not only free from toxic pesticides, GMOs, chemical fertilisers, and factory farm production, and therefore good for human health, but also regenerative in terms of the health of the soil, the environment, the animals, the climate, and rural livelihoods as well."

Regenerative agriculture really can achieve all the vital things needed for mankind, like safe and healthy food, helping to reverse climate change, the highest crop yields, continuous healthy soil, maintaining vital crop diversity for human life and using natural non-patented seeds and plants that can be regrown without cost each year. Compare this to the patented GMO seeds that have to be repurchased each and every year.

Here are some of the ways all this is achieved. Regenerative farming uses natural things like animal manure to nourish the soil rather than artificial chemical fertilisers. It also increases yields as well as improving the foods' nutritional content. It improves and maximises essential soil microbes and herbivores and uses the photosynthesis of plants to capture carbon dioxide and store it in the soil. Soil holds around three times more carbon than the atmosphere and plants and forests combined. All these things work in unison. CO2 captured from the atmosphere and then turned into soil organic matter, for example, depends on the actions of the plant roots, soil biology and the soil microbiome. All this can be significantly improved by things like natural composts that also have a high diversity of soil microorganisms. There are other methods that have been shown to improve carbon capture and thus help to reverse climate change which have been developed and trialled on individual farms.

In 2015 a new international movement, united around a common goal to reverse global warming and end world hunger by facilitating and accelerating the transition to regenerative agriculture, was formed by 60 people from 21 nations. Today, Regeneration International engages with a network of more than 250 international regeneration partners throughout the world including in the US, South Africa, India, Canada and Mexico. Its mission is "to promote, facilitate and accelerate the global transition to regenerative food, farming and land management for the purpose of restoring climate stability, ending world hunger and rebuilding deteriorated social, ecological and economic system". Its key members include its international director Andre Leu and Vandana Shiva who has been one of the most prolific promoters of natural agriculture for decades and who helped to stop Bill Gates from continuing to enforce his industrialisation of seeds in India.

So, regenerative farming is the ideal solution for every key aspect of life, but will it really happen? Certainly not if Bill Gates achieves his planned control. Consider the Food and Agricultural Organization (FAO), which is a specialised agency of the United Nations. Its aim is to lead international efforts to defeat hunger and improve nutrition. It recognised and accepted that ecological agriculture was the way to go and supported regenerative practices. In 2019, however, things began to change, and just as with the WHO, Bill Gates started to finance and gain control over the FAO. In 2021 he even moved its summit meeting to New York, but huge numbers of farmers and agricultural organisations then boycotted it. Why? Because the changes that are now underway include a huge push towards industrialised farming. The 300-million-member organisation Civil Society and Indigenous People's Mechanism announced plans to boycott the summit and set up a meeting of their own. Sofia Monsalve Suarez, head of nutrition rights group Fian International, questioned the summit's legitimacy: "We cannot jump on a train that is heading in the wrong direction. The summit appears extremely biased in favour of the same actors who have been responsible for the food crisis."

Another group of organisations also made a more provoking but accurate comment: "This is no longer a food summit, it's a poison summit. The poison cartel and Bill Gates are running to push more poisons, now under new names."

Many millions of farmers, independent organisations and scientists oppose industrialised agriculture but they are up against the planet's most powerful global elite, global corporations, regulators and even many governments. Only time will tell who wins this battle for the control of food and the future of mankind.

Food. As well as being a key player in effectively forcing many farmers to adopt industrialised agriculture, Bill Gates has made huge strides in his plans to change the foods we all eat. Here are some of the key things he has already done. He has been the world's main advocate of eliminating natural animal meats and replacing them with synthetic alternatives. He cites two main reasons for doing this. The first being that cattle are a significant cause of carbon emissions. The truth, however, depends on how the cattle are raised. Many countries like the US mainly use industrialised factory farms. Cattle, for example, are often kept in horrific indoor conditions with little or no room to move and because of the appalling sanitation they regularly have various infections. To help control this they are given continuous low level antibiotics, although another reason this is done is that it also increases their weight gain and thus improves profits. They are mainly fed on just one or two genetically modified chemically laden crops like maize and soya. All this results in these animals emitting much more methane which has a major effect on the climate. This devastating method of animal rearing is what Bill Gates uses to compare his proposed alternative of lab-grown meat substitutes against. So, it is unsurprising he can claim they are better for the climate.

However, when cattle are raised naturally outdoors, eating plants and grass as they have done throughout history, average current emissions are typically only 40% of those for factory farming and with virtually no methane. The UK's National Farmers Union also has a realistic plan to achieve zero carbon emissions for cattle farming by 2040 by new initiatives like improving microbes and fungi levels and types in the soil that maximise carbon capture. In fact, many Scottish farmers have already achieved these zero emissions which shows the whole process is completely realistic.

A very recent study showed it is possible to actually reduce carbon emissions. It measured the total net emissions on the White Oak Pastures – a regenerative beef farm in the US. It measured all relevant factors including enteric emissions, manure emissions, soil carbon capture, other farm activities and transport. It showed that total net carbon emissions were a negative 3.5kg per kilo of fresh meat, making it six times more carbon efficient than the average industrialised form of beef. Even synthetic meat causes around 4kg of carbon emissions per kilo.

Regenerative farming can quite simply improve climate change while still providing the incredible foods that mankind has eaten throughout its history. Of course, these solutions need to be much more widely promoted and adopted so their incredible potential can be achieved. Sadly, Bill Gates simply ignores all this evidence and he will never fund it. His claims about animal meat are simply biased and untrue for animals raised naturally and he never mentions the fact that his synthetic alternatives also have a significant carbon footprint themselves.

His second claim for eliminating meat is that it is dangerous for human health and causes various diseases like heart disease, diabetes and cancer. His claims are based mainly on a single study that he funded. There is, however, huge unchallengeable data which shows positive health benefits from natural meats. I will simply give two alternative rebuttals to his false claims. Six scientists led by Professor Alice Stanton from the Royal College of Surgeons in Ireland published a letter in the Lancet that effectively slammed the poor science, data and negative claims that the Gates study made. Clear positive evidence also comes from a large peer-reviewed study based on United Nations data that showed that meat intake in 175 countries was actually associated with increased life expectancy. Natural meat is much healthier than those from factory farming where animals are given genetically modified crops containing a range of chemicals as well as drugs and antibiotics, but once again Bill Gates simply ignores all these facts. His wealth and power simply ensure that very few people dare to challenge him and even if they did the media would simply not report it.

How are the synthetic meats that he is determined to force on the public actually produced? There are two basic types. One uses plants and the other uses animal cells which are then grown in exceedingly complex bioreactor systems. In fact, cell-based meat is only in the very early stages of development and faces possibly insurmountable problems. Tiny pieces of meat have been produced but at a huge cost of $22,000 per kilo. Ramping this up to produce the millions of tonnes needed and reducing the cost to around $6 per kilo like natural meat seems unlikely. This would be good news because independent experts have expressed deep concern about the quality of the food and its potential effects on human health.

On the other hand, plant-based meats, like the "Impossible Burger", are already being produced and sold in increasing quantities. They are made from a range of common crops like wheat, maize, potato, soy and tofu, with plant oils like sunflower oil and binding agents like gluten and beans. We have seen that plant-based fats like sunflower oil when used in large amounts are very unhealthy and in many artificial meats, they are the only source of fats. This can damage many parts of the body like cellular membranes, mitochondria and proteins. In addition to all of this, fake meats also contain synthetic molecules that are not found in nature often to try to produce a meat type flavour that cannot be achieved just from plants. Crucially, this also means that the "meat" can be patented which is a key goal of all producers. Another fact is that all the plants used for artificial meats are also from GMO crops that use artificial fertilisers and insecticides. It is no surprise, therefore, that a recent study by the Health Research Institute Laboratories found levels of glyphosate in the Impossible Burger of 11.3ppb which is a level that can affect our microbiome as well as acting as an endocrine disrupter. So, in contrast to natural plant-based foods, these new meat alternatives should be considered ultra-processed foods, which nutritionists recommend avoiding due to their harmful health effects.

A final fact is that plant-based meats would not contain naturally essential vitamins and minerals like vitamin B12 and iron. Many of these are added as separate ingredients in most synthetic meats but there is a risk that these may be less readily absorbed as well as the possibility that the levels may be too low.

The Gates Foundation is, however, not just demonising real meat and eulogising synthetic meats, it is also financing and developing a wide range of other artificial foods like milk, cheese, chicken, eggs, ice cream, and even artificial breast milk by a company called BIOMILQ. Natural breast milk is the perfect food for babies. The fact that Bill Gates is funding and promoting a synthetic milk based on biotechnology that can never be better health-wise than breast milk shows his true motives: simply making money and controlling all food. He has made investments in virtually every artificial food company which all have patents for their products. Impossible Foods has 14 patents for its synthetic molecules which are used just in the Impossible Burger. It has more than 100 others waiting approval for all its other new fake foods like cheese and chicken. Patented foods – unlike natural foods – cannot be reproduced by any other company. Bill Gates has already invested $50 million in the company and if synthetic patented foods like these ever become mankind's main source, then he and the other global elite will effectively control world food and thus control mankind. They would, of course, also be raking in tens, and probably hundreds, of billions of dollars in profit. The GMO agricultural seeds and the chemicals used with them are already known to cause serious medical outcomes like cancers and children's brain development. Lab-grown meats, chicken and all the others that are planned will almost certainly be as catastrophic for human health because they are repeating the mistakes already made with industrialised agriculture. I won't say any more now about artificial foods, but there will be more information in the final section on the WEF and global elite's plans for the future.

Education. Bill Gates is also investing huge sums in things like education and climate technologies. All I will say is that independent scientists and experts in these fields have expressed significant concerns once again about what his personal views are that he is trying to impose. Here is just one example. The much-criticised Common Core Curriculum was the Gates Foundation's attempt at remaking American education, and most parents whose children used it would tell you how dumb it was. Despite this abysmal failure that would have affected those children's education, the New York governor, Andrew Cuomo, recently announced a new partnership with Gates to develop a new "smarter education system". Really? The simple fact is he never admits his mistakes and is simply determined to keep imposing his personal beliefs. Clearly, he believes he knows more about things, like health, vaccines, food, agriculture and education, than most of the world's experts.

Bill Gates is simply determined to control much of the world. Of course, he is just part of the global elite and the World Economic Forum's plans, but he is quite simply their most powerful and ruthless individual. Having explained how he has already forced many of his personal but false ideas on the world – often with devastating outcomes – I can now move on to his, and the WEF's, other crucial plans.

What the global elite need to achieve to control the world

On the surface, the WEF's agenda appears benevolent in its desire to tackle some of the greatest challenges of our time. However, the solutions it proposes via the Great Reset have all the ingredients for techno-totalitarian world governance. To enable them to do this, the global elite need to be able to control every individual person and there are four key things they have to do to achieve it all:

1) control of world health
2) universal track and trace and data control
3) central Bank digital currency systems
4) censorship and the end of free speech

This section explains these vital parts of the Great Reset, how they intend to achieve it all, and its stark and devastating authoritarian outcomes. The whole thing may seem impossible to believe – like a conspiracy theory – but anyone who is prepared to look at all the information will see that the WEF really does openly share and promote most of its plans for the world. The problem is very few people know about it because the media and internet have simply been bought out to support the global elite. The other key thing to keep remembering is that huge swathes of the plans have already been achieved and some of the key ones have been examined in detail.

Control of world health

Control of world health is a key part of the reset agenda. This, of course, could be hugely controversial, so the initial part of the plan is just to start with the control of infectious diseases by the WHO. This is known as the International Pandemic Treaty (IPT) and it is already well advanced even though most people know almost nothing about it. The aim is to achieve its approval in 2024. If enacted, the IPT will require the WHO to bring in a vaccine passport system that will be mandatory for everyone in the world. But just like all the previous falsely declared WHO pandemics where vaccines were either not needed or were ineffective, COVID-19 has also not been solved by the vaccines. In most countries, life is more or less back to normal because the Omicron (and the more recent BA.4 and BA.5) variants simply cause mild, cold-like symptoms for most people, even though they are hugely contagious.

The vaccines now have virtually no benefit for these variants but are still causing serious side effects and deaths. Even the most powerful vaccine promoter in the world – Bill Gates – really did admit that Omicron was better than the vaccines. This is what he said: "The virus itself, particularly the variant called Omicron, is a type of vaccine, in that it creates both T cell and B cell immunity, and it's done a better job of getting out to the population than we have with vaccines." Then consider that the vaccine passports that were originally claimed by governments to be essential for controlling Covid have now simply been abandoned by most countries because they have no meaningful benefit and don't prevent infection or transmission. So, the crucial question is why will vaccines be a mandatory part of the IPT, especially when the cost for the world's 8 billion population will be staggering, and the cost and time for checking them in various locations like airports, trains, venues and restaurants will also be costly, hugely time consuming and disruptive?

The key reason is that for the WEF to achieve their plans for worldwide domination, implementing a worldwide mandatory digital identity system (digital ID) is essential, and the digital vaccine passport system is the perfect platform to get such a system set up so that track and trace and personal data for every human can be added, analysed, and stored. All this will be examined in detail in the next section. The second key reason is that mandatory worldwide vaccination really would result in unprecedented profits for the drug industry and their investors. The final reason is that it would remove any possible comparison between the outcomes for vaccinated and unvaccinated people. This would mean that poor vaccine benefits and serious side effect really could be completely hidden. I should add that a digital vaccine passport was a key part of the plan when the Covid pandemic started, and digital IDs were expected to be introduced quickly, using Covid as the excuse. Unfortunately, for the WEF and Bill Gates, the wide range of Covid vaccine failures and the incredible Omicron and other newer variants, which had incredibly mild symptoms, meant vaccine passports became meaningless and impossible to enforce. This is why the International Pandemic Treaty, that demands a mandatory vaccine passport system, is now such a vital part of its Great Reset plan and why they are fighting like hell to get it approved.

Governments around the world have been incessantly lobbied, incentivised and pressurised to accept the treaty. If the global elite succeed, however, it really will result in one of the greatest disasters mankind has ever faced. Incredibly, what it would mean is that the WHO would make a single worldwide plan for each new pandemic or viral infection that would be mandatory in every country of the world. They would declare each public health emergency unilaterally, impose their plans, and have the power to sanction any country that didn't comply. If a country decided not to adopt it, it really would face devastating outcomes from things like economic sanctions and embargoes just like Russia is facing now. The WHO also plans to impose much higher levels of censorship and will dictate what the "truth" is (even if it is a lie) and since its decisions are legally binding, countries must enforce compliance. The treaty is simply a direct threat to the sovereignty of every nation to make decisions for itself and its citizens. It would erode democracy everywhere. Incredibly, individual health services like the NHS would simply have to do exactly what the WHO demanded, even if it was clear that dangerous and life-taking outcomes were occurring or better alternatives were available.

We have already seen a number of shocking and devastating decisions that the WHO and Bill Gates have already made. In this section you will see even more, but here are two more worrying examples. The first involves Bill Gates who went on record early in the pandemic stating that Africa would simply be destroyed by Covid unless a concerted effort was made to get the jab to them. This, however, was a completely false claim. Studies have shown that most African people have been infected, but even though only 6% have been vaccinated, the African continent has the lowest level of Covid deaths in the world. Bill Gates should be ashamed and everyone should be truly concerned.

The second one involves the WHO's director general Tedros Adhanom Ghebreyesus. In July 2022 an expert panel in the WHO did not accept that the monkeypox outbreak should be classed as a health emergency because it affected only a limited number of very specific people. However, the director general simply overruled them and declared it a health emergency. Soon after, the case numbers started to decline significantly and six months later, the entire EU now has an average of just ten new cases per week. This is not a health emergency and is just one more example of his appalling and incorrect judgements. If the International Pandemic Treaty is authorised, it really will be a disaster for the world. It would simply be controlled by Tedros Ghebreyesus and Bill Gates and they are certain to make many more similar disastrous future decisions. They would declare pandemics that weren't pandemics and impose lockdowns that weren't needed. They would declare all their other planned responses, like travel restrictions, mask mandates, social distancing, business closures, school closures, the mandatory use of vaccines and drugs and the allocation of resources. Their top priority, however, would be the introduction of vaccine passports. As explained, their real reason for doing it, of course, is to provide the platform for a worldwide digital ID system which will then ensure the total control of mankind and determine what kind of products, services and information are available to us. In March 2021 Naomi Wolf, author of *The End of America*, warned that accepting digital ID will be the end of all freedom: "I cannot say this forcefully enough. This is literally the end of human liberty in the west if this plan unfolds as planned… Vaccine passports sound like a fine thing if you don't know what those platforms can do. I'm CEO of a tech company. I understand what this platform does. It's not about the vaccine, it's not about the virus, it's about data. And once this rolls out you don't have a choice about being part of the system. What people have to understand is that any other functionality can be loaded onto that platform with no problem at all."

Liberty Counsel founder and chairman, Mat Staver, has also issued a warning, saying, "Digital health or vaccine passports along with tracking and tracing apps present a serious threat to freedom. Vaccine passports and tracking apps are all about data and control. The vaccine passport is being promoted worldwide to limit a person's ability to leave home, work, shop, dine, travel, attend a public event, or even worship. Covid is being used to advance this dangerous threat to freedom. We must never accept vaccine passports or tracking apps as the new norm. The implications for freedom are enormous."

Given all of this, you must surely be thinking that it would be impossible that the WHO and thus Tedros Ghebreyesus – who can overrule or impose anything he wants – would ever be given such "Stalinist" control of global health, and that world governments would surely never approve it. However, you will have to rethink when I tell you that the Biden administration is one of its key proponents and is poised to unequivocally hand over control of future pandemics to the WHO. President Biden is also promoting this treaty to the rest of the world. The European Commission led by Ursula von der Leyen is also another of its prime advocates and there are many other major countries also determined to impose it like Canada, Australia and those in the EU. Also, and quite alarmingly, nearly every country in the world has already given its approval – at least in principle – even though some have initially refused to sign and are asking for certain changes to be made before they do so. It really is almost certain that it will be approved within the next two years, and become worldwide law. Mankind really will then face a devastating future.

The WHO currently has a series of rules it must adhere to. One of the key ones is that human beings have their own rights for individual dignity, human rights and fundamental freedoms. The WHO, however, aims to change this to "principles of equity, inclusivity and coherence". What does this mean? Autonomy over your body will be eliminated. You'll have no right to make your own health decisions. If you are given a health intervention and are concerned it may harm or kill you, you will have to comply because public health measures will simply be based on what is claimed to be the best outcomes for mankind as a whole. Individuals won't matter. Human dignity will not be taken into consideration. Human rights will not be taken into consideration, and neither will the concept that human beings have fundamental freedoms. This whole concept is simply devastating and means the end of current democracy.

Bill Gates is the WHO's largest donor meaning he exerts the most control over its actions. In his recent book about the Covid pandemic, he tells us what his future pandemic model is for the world based on what he believes has worked best over the last two years. This includes immediately isolating contacts, closing borders, locking down as quickly as possible, vaccinating the entire world within six months and hugely increasing the level of testing. Lockdowns are a crucial part of his plans and even though we now know that they actually caused far more serious harm and outcomes than Covid itself, he will still mandate them in future. There are several other important things to also remember. The first is the staggering worldwide financial cost of such incredible restrictions. The Covid pandemic has so far cost around $13.7 trillion and given that the annual world GDP is around $90 trillion, this single pandemic has cost a staggering 13% of world annual wealth. It is little wonder that so many countries are facing serious financial disasters and most governments cannot achieve their key targets. Living standards are falling because it is also a significant cause of the current inflation crisis.

Imagine the financial devastation this would cause if there was a new pandemic declared every two years or so. If you think this surely couldn't happen given that the last real pandemic was 100 years ago, consider this. If the International Pandemic Treaty had been approved when the 2003 SARS, the 2005 avian flu, and the 2009 swine flu outbreaks happened, the WHO would have immediately imposed global lockdowns and all the other restrictions and treatments outlined on all of them – in other words three lockdowns in seven years. The fact that the enormous fatalities that were predicted for each one of these viruses were incorrect and never materialised would be irrelevant and the world would go through huge scale lockdowns costing trillions of dollars each for no reason and the global population would be legally forced to follow every rule. These lockdowns would also have caused devastation to almost every other type of human health and disease and resulted in almost infinitely more lost lives and serious patient outcomes than the viruses themselves. Of course, Bill Gates and the vaccine and drug makers would have made hundreds of billions of dollars in profit. They would also have likely claimed that the minimal viral deaths were due to their immediate actions – even though this would have been simply untrue and just an evil lie.

The WHO's declaration of their so-called 2009 swine flu pandemic is a classic example of their appalling and devastating medical decisions. This is what three major organisations said about it at that time. The Council of Europe's Parliamentary Committee said, "The Parliamentary Assembly is alarmed about the way in which the H1N1 influenza virus has been handled... It is particularly troubled by the decisions taken and advice given leading to distortion of priorities of public health services across Europe, waste of large sums of public money, and unjustified scares and fears about health risks faced by the European public at large... and the creation of health risks through vaccines and medications which might not have been sufficiently tested before being authorised in fast-track procedures."

This is what a joint investigation by the BMJ and the Bureau of Investigative Journalism said with emphasis on the fact that the WHO had changed the definition of a pandemic just before they declared it: "WHO for years had defined pandemics as outbreaks causing enormous numbers of deaths and illness, but in early 2009 this had been removed. Quite amazingly, a pandemic can now be declared even though there are virtually no deaths."

In 2010 Forbes wrote an even more destructive quote: "From the beginning, the World Health Organization's actions have ranged from dubious to flagrantly incompetent."

The WHO also over overhyped the inconsequential Zika outbreak in 2016 and the Ebola outbreak in 2019. It has also been accused of massive money mismanagement, spending more on travel expenses each year – around $200 million in 2017 – than it does on some of the biggest public health diseases worldwide such as AIDS, tuberculosis and malaria combined. It also didn't publicly admit that SARS-CoV-2 was an airborne virus until the end of December 2021, even though scientists knew this was the case within weeks of the pandemic being declared. How can they claim to be the best organisation to tackle pandemics when they simply don't understand such basic facts?

Another crucial fact is that to introduce a single worldwide pandemic plan is one of the most disastrous ideas ever promoted. You only need to look at the incredibly different responses to Covid around the world to realise that a wide range of treatments and actions are needed. African countries with young populations had very few deaths from Covid. Why should these be subject to destructive lockdowns and compulsory and expensive mass testing and vaccinations which would have minimal benefits, but cause serious financial destruction for their countries and, therefore, far more deaths than from the virus itself? This does not even take into account the serious adverse events and deaths caused by the vaccines themselves. The timing, nature and severity of viruses also varies significantly between countries and even regions which also depends on the health status of the populations and, of course, there could be different variants around the world with widely different outcomes. All these and many more differences should be taken into account locally to decide variations in treatments for each country. The plan to significantly increase the monitoring of infections with things like PCR and antigen tests is extremely worrying. As seen with Covid, PCR tests are unreliable and grossly overstate the number of those with a real infection. This makes the pandemic appear far worse than it really is.

This is how the Canadian MP Leslyn Lewis has summarised the whole situation involving the International Pandemic Treaty:

> The treaty includes 190 countries and would be legally binding. It defines and classes what is considered a pandemic, and this could consist of broad classifications, including an increase in cancers, heart condition, strokes, etc. If a pandemic is declared, the WHO takes over the global health management of the pandemic. Of even more concern, if this treaty is enshrined, the WHO would be in full control over what gets called a pandemic. They could dictate how our doctors can respond, which drugs can or can't be used, or which vaccines are approved. We would end up with a one-size-fits-all approach for the entire world. A one-size-fits-all response to a health crisis doesn't even work across Canada, let alone the entire globe. The next question, then, is how the WHO and Bill Gates would be able to monitor every individual in every country to determine whether enough people are sick to justify locking down.

This is what Professor Robert Clancy, a leading clinical immunologist in Canada, said, "The proposal to take control of pandemics at a central WHO level is untenable and threatens global society... It is foolhardy to even suggest that a 'one-size-fits-all' response to a pandemic crisis across geographic zones characterized by hugely different parameters, could possibly be covered by a central bureaucratic process – the need for local decision-making is of prime importance."

Despite all these damning and savage criticisms, concerns and facts, the WHO – promoted by the global elite – is now on the verge of taking over global health. If it happens, mankind will face a devastating future. Pandemics will become regular occurrences even though in the westernised world the last true pandemic (Spanish flu) was over 100 years ago. Every other virus – even those classed as so-called pandemics in the intervening century – has had incredibly low death rates and serious outcomes, but by redefining a pandemic in 2009, the WHO really can, and will, now class many new mild viruses like the 2009 swine flu, as pandemics. Serious pandemics have been so rare in the western world because the natural immune system of most of mankind really has simply defeated nearly all of them, so this plan appears to be completely crazy. Of course, the real reason is the imposition of digital ID systems for the whole of mankind and they are the most dangerous and shocking parts of their global plan and this will be explained in detail in the next three sections.

Universal track and trace and data control

In today's digital world, almost every citizen is aware that their online activity is being monitored, but most don't know the true extent. If you have ever felt like Google knows what you're going to do before you know, it's because it is tracking you and saving and analysing all your data. Over 90% of all online activity is done via Google and its apps. All this is free but all your online searches and activities are stored and saved indefinitely. Gmail saves every email, even those you draft but then don't send and then delete. All social media activity is also captured, recorded and stored. If you have a Google Android cell phone, it can track you even if it is turned off or there is no internet connection. As soon as you reconnect, all the information is automatically sent to Google. So, even though you may think you have just spent the day incognito, the moment you reconnect, every step you made is shared. The only way to avoid this would be to leave the phone at home. All this information is currently used to generate profits in a number of ways like selling it to other organisations. If you have been looking for something, you will often find adverts suddenly appear with the aim of persuading you to buy. Have you ever had a phone conversation and then started to get ads related to something you spoke about? This is another example of the amount of data they collect.

To do all of this, they have created massive sophisticated server farms and artificial intelligence software that are capable of analysing every aspect of your data and everything you do and say. What about children? Currently, in the US, more than half of American schools use Chromebooks and Google apps. This allows Google to build brand loyalty from an early age. Of course, its primary business is compiling, storing and selling personal data and by capturing children at an early age, it is building the most comprehensive personality profiles that have ever been achieved. Every single preference, thought and belief will make them extremely vulnerable to manipulation through things like targeted advertising.

Most people seem to accept the fact that Google and all the other major online companies like Facebook, Microsoft, Apple and Amazon collect and save personal information, and if the only reason for this was to make money by simply selling it to reputable suppliers, then many people would continue to accept it. However, as we will see shortly, companies like Google, the global elite and WEF really are well on the way to using all this data as part of their plan to control mankind. The intention is to use it as a key part of their digital identity system (digital ID).

China is also doing most of the track and trace and data control you have just read. In China's case, however, it is already being used to allow the government to control its population. China's social credit system started in 2018 and is currently being used on over

1 billion of its citizens – around 80%. A range of different pilot schemes are in use across the country so that the most effective ones can eventually be rolled out universally to every citizen. Most of the data being tracked may appear relatively mild, however, the punishments can be severe. The social credit system digitally tracks and traces data on a wide range of what the government believes are key things its citizens should, and should not, do, and here are a few examples. Social media postings, time spent with the elderly, contributions to charities, sensible shopping patterns, health status, jaywalking, posting false news stories, spending too much time playing video games, consuming too much alcohol, wasting money, criticising the government, and volunteer actions. Each citizen is given a credit score depending on how they behave. Those citizens with the highest scores who closely meet the government's requirements can receive easier loans, discounts on things like heating and have their travel applications speeded up. Those with low scores can have their internet speeds reduced, flights banned, barred from certain types of employment, banned from public events and public transport, and even unable to use public toilets. According to the Chinese State media, these types of "punishment" have been imposed on 30 million of its citizens so far. Also, central to all of this is additional public shaming.

Most western people would already consider all of this to be undemocratic, but China's long-term plans are much more severe. Most people also believe that what is happening in China could never happen in western democracies, but the WHO is already developing a digital ID system and even the European Union has recently announced a similar plan. Eight specific countries – Australia, Canada, Finland, Israel, New Zealand, Singapore, Netherlands and the UK together with the World Bank – have also formed an alliance to promote digital ID systems as part of the WEF's Great Reset plan. Norway, which is accepted as one of the most democratic free countries in the world, is actually at the forefront of using digital IDs and it now wants to track and trace the food choices that all its citizens make. Even if it fails to get it implemented, the very fact that it wants to do so is simply alarming. All this is bad enough, but the WEF's long-term plans for the world's population are much more devastating than anything that has already happened – even in China – and much more information will be given shortly.

Here is a frightening example of what has already happened in one of the so-called most democratic western countries – Canada. In a democratic country, peaceful protests are a fundamental right. Without such protests, things like women's equality and the right to vote would not have happened or been delayed probably for decades. In Canada, in February 2022, a freedom convoy of truly peaceful Canadian truckers went to its capital Ottawa to call for a lifting of particularly crippling Covid restrictions. This freedom convoy would have been allowed to take place in a true democracy, but there was also one other fact that added significant impetus. By this time, it was well known that vaccines did not stop infection or transmission and many other countries like the UK were already relaxing their Covid restrictions, so the convoy had this added justification for its plan. What happened? The prime minister, Justin Trudeau, effectively destroyed the country's democracy by invoking the Canadian Emergencies Act of 1988. This had simply never been used because it was enacted just for serious life-threatening, "war-like" emergencies, but was now being deployed simply to attack a peaceful convoy. Tens of thousands of supporters had donated money to support the truckers. All these people, however, were tracked and traced and anyone who had given more than $25 had their bank accounts frozen or suspended as well as the truckers themselves. The money that had been donated was also frozen. The act also allowed the drivers' licences to be seized and suspended forever and for money to be taken from their own bank accounts. If I tell you that Trudeau is a member of the WEF and in fact that he was "educated" for years to adopt their long-term global control plans, then this may give an insight into why all this happened. This is how Dr Joseph Mercola described it all:

> Well, well, well. Canadian Prime Minister Justin Trudeau just let the deep state cat out of the bag for all the world to see. The premature disclosure and honest preview of what's in store for the people of the world is perhaps the silver lining in all of this. By invoking the Canadian Emergencies Act of 1988 to allow for the blanket revocation of protesters' driving licences and their bank accounts – and anyone who made even a nominal donation to their cause – Trudeau is showing the world what Klaus Schwab's Great Reset really is all about for the average person. If we go along with their financial reset to a centralised global digital currency, the central bankers can and will financially cripple anyone, anywhere, anytime, for any reason. That's more than sufficient leverage to keep most people in line.

I'll explain in detail the WEF's plan for a centralised globalised digital currency next, but first, I'll give you one more fact about Justin Trudeau. The Trudeau Foundation owns around 40% of a company called Acuitas Therapeutics. This company makes the lipid nanoparticle delivery system used in Pfizer's Covid vaccines and while it is impossible to find out the profits he has made, they are bound to be substantial – probably many millions of dollars. Could this also be playing a part in his undemocratic actions?

We have just seen how Justin Trudeau was educated by, and is now part of, the WEF. One part of its Global Reset plan is to actively indoctrinate young political leaders. It has a "Young Global Leaders" programme, a five-year indoctrination into their principles and consists of 800 leaders, and future leaders, worldwide. Its goal is to have elected world leaders who don't answer to their people but to their bosses at WEF and we have just seen the staggering example involving Justin Trudeau. Who do you think are the main sponsors of this programme? The Bill and Melinda Gates Foundation and Google. Need I say more?

Centralised global digital currency systems

At present, there are a wide range of ways in which individuals can use their money. Credit and debit cards are a major source but other things like cash, cheques, cryptocurrencies and direct debits are also available. Part of the Great Reset plan is to track and trace the data on every single payment in the world. This cannot be done fully while things like cash are still available. The WEF's plan, therefore, is to create a worldwide digital currency and eliminate other payment methods. No digital currency currently exists, but China will almost certainly be the first country to develop and implement one. Other countries like Canada and Sweden are also well underway in developing one and most developed countries, including the UK, are also analysing and considering their use. The idea of eliminating cash, however, is very problematic, especially for the poor and certain older people. It may, therefore, be kept in some countries even when the digital currency is introduced at least initially, but longer term there will be immense pressure from the WEF to completely eliminate it.

Every single expenditure someone makes will be recorded, saved indefinitely and analysed. When you add the digital ID track and trace data, the global elite will know more about individuals than their husbands, wives and families know. It will simply be the end of personal freedom and democracy. The other key fact is it will enable restrictions to be made on what, and how much, people can buy and do. We have seen that the WEF plans to either eliminate or significantly reduce key foods like meat, butter and cheese. Initially, limits will be set for everybody. Anyone who tries to buy more than this limited amount will find that the purchase is simply stopped. Many more things will be similarly controlled and limited like travel, energy use and numerous appliances which will be examined shortly. If, for example, a new lockdown is declared and you're not allowed to travel more than five miles from your home, the digital currency will simply stop all purchases outside that point.

China will almost certainly be the first country to impose such draconian restrictions and limits on what people can buy and do. This is what the CNAS said about it in a 2021 report: "The Central Bank Digital Currency system will enable the Chinese Communist Party to exercise greater control over private transactions, as well as to wield power over Chinese citizens in tandem with the social credit system." The WEF will almost certainly use China as a template for enforcing it throughout the world.

Censorship

Free speech is the bedrock of democracy. With just a few vital exceptions – like child abusers and terrorists – everyone should have the right to free speech and be able to communicate it to anyone who wants to hear it or see it in print or online. Censorship does, of course, occur in dictatorships and communist countries and has done so throughout history, but when countries like the UK and the US finally endorsed democracy and free speech, it was, with just a few exceptions, almost universally enacted. In recent years, however, censorship, even in democracies, has started to occur more regularly and after around 2015 it increased significantly and has grown alarmingly over the last two to three years. This is because censorship is a key part of the WEF's Great Reset plan and COVID-19 is without doubt the most censored thing that has ever occurred in western democracies.

Before exploring in detail exactly what is happening, it's important to understand how the distribution of information has changed over recent decades. Until the introduction of the world wide web, individuals could nearly always express their views, but unless news companies reported them, or they wrote a book, they would achieve little spread to the public. The internet changed all of this, and once companies like YouTube, Twitter and Facebook became widely available, it was possible for an individual's views to be transmitted to huge swathes of the world's population within days and even hours.

In the early days of free speech, people could report their views and doctors, scientists and researchers could also distribute their studies and clinical trials with little censorship. Of course, if their governments, medical organisations and major corporations disagreed, they could challenge everything with alternative views and other science and sometimes discredit the new data. But we have also seen many examples of what happens when they can't challenge the new data and how in these circumstances the scientists and researchers are often attacked for making claims that threaten all these organisations. Many of them were stopped from attending conferences and their funding was reduced or eliminated and their careers were sometimes destroyed even though in many cases their data were eventually found to be correct and finally accepted. Remember the incredibly brave researchers who exposed the deaths caused by leaded petrol and X-rays for young pregnant women. Their careers were effectively destroyed and attacking them was appalling, but a key fact is their information was not completely censored and it was eventually accepted and implemented.

Once Covid started, however, some of the most prominent scientists and doctors in the world who tried to distribute truthful facts and scientific studies on anything related to the virus were immediately attacked and often completely censored. Most of them used social media platforms like Facebook, Google and YouTube. These companies have become some of the most incredible censoring organisations in the world and many doctors and scientists who used them have simply been deplatformed. We have seen that the media are also now part of this censorship programme because years ago, the WEF and its key global companies realised they had to bring them onto their side to prevent independent investigations that would discredit their plans. Pharmaceutical companies and others, effectively "bought" the media by having expensive adverts posted. News organisations simply don't run reports that might harm the bottom line of its advertisers. The global elite like Bill Gates have added another major incentive – a third of a billion dollars – for the media to simply spread the establishment's views and never challenge them. Most investigative journalism, at least on anything that affects the global elite's key plans, has simply disappeared. Now, "fake news" is the term that is used for anything that contradicts the establishment even when it is in fact the truth.

Organisations called "fact checkers" are now ubiquitous. They claim to be independent and trustworthy and to provide true and scientifically based evidence and facts. However, most of them receive significant funding from a range of companies and individuals like George Soros and Bill Gates. Facebook alone has given FactCheck.org several hundred thousand dollars each year and Google gave it $100,000. Google also gave Full Fact $2 million in 2020. It is difficult to claim independence when all this funding from the global elite and the companies who support the WEF is occurring. The fact checkers' aim is to rapidly uncover every piece of "fake news" and then dismiss and discredit it and demand its censorship. The problem is most of the doctors and scientists who are challenging the official position have truthful facts and data and cannot truly be discredited. In this situation, the fact checkers simply make incredible and unscientific claims themselves.

Here are a few examples. An article published in the British Medical Journal by Paul D. Thacker exposed a series of troubling data integrity problems with Pfizer's COVID-19 vaccine clinical trial. The Facebook fact checking organisation called Lead Stories referred to the investigation as a "hoax alert" and disparaged it for "missing context". What they didn't do was to challenge any of the facts quoted in the BMJ article. They didn't do this because the facts were correct and true and so all they could do to attack it was to make these absurd statements. This is one of the key ways that fact checkers try to discredit the truth and science, and because of the control they exert on the media, this gets wide coverage, whereas the true facts exposed by the doctors and scientists are simply not reported. The BMJ's editors sent an open letter to Mark Zuckerberg calling his company's fact check "inaccurate, incompetent and irresponsible". When prestigious medical journals like the BMJ are accused of "fake news", then it shows the despicable means that the establishment and its "fact checkers" will go to when trying to protect themselves, their own lies and their own unscientific claims.

A peer-reviewed study published in the journal Medical Hypotheses, which concluded that masks are ineffective for blocking viral transmission and can also cause substantial adverse physiological and psychological effects, was censored by Twitter. The amazing fact, however, is that even though face masks have been officially mandated by virtually every country, no clinical trial has ever been done to prove that they actually work and stop transmission of the virus. To claim that face masks work without this proof is itself unscientific and fake news. A more recent study in February 2022 from the University of Bristol also showed that cloth face masks do little to prevent the spread of Covid, and that 90% of particles were able to get through the mask. In fact, there have been a range of studies over decades for different viruses that show that cloth face masks are ineffective for all of them.

Other recent studies published in respected journals, like PLOS One, also show no benefit from masks in preventing transmission. These studies, however, also showed side effects like increases in heart rate, dizziness, headaches and exhaustion for those wearing masks and the most likely cause is the inhalation of the microplastics contained in them. In January 2023 the Cochrane Library also updated its analysis of masks which analysed 78 clinical trials. It found no benefit for preventing infection, and this is what Dr Vinay

Prasad, a professor of epidemiology and biostatistics at the University of California, said in his review: "This is conclusive… You just don't have credible evidence [for masking]… This is what the science has always shown."

When mask wearing started to be mandated across most countries in 2020, a significant number of senior scientists, researchers and doctors tried to explain all of this information. They too were savagely attacked and censored by fact checkers, governments and all other official organisations. Most people would find all of this almost impossible to believe, even though it really is true, and cloth masks are still being promoted. Here is one final fact. Over 5 billion masks have been used in the Covid pandemic. This has resulted in a devastating release of microplastics and nanoparticles around the world including rivers, lakes and oceans that could prove to be an environmental disaster.

The number of official Covid deaths and hospitalisations are incorrect and overstated and still include those people who definitely died from other things like car crashes and heart attacks. This has been examined in detail and even people like the UK's Health Secretary admitted that many of these deaths are not due to Covid. The official UK Covid deaths at the end of July 2022 is 185,000. It is impossible to calculate what the true figure is, but it is almost certainly less, and probably much less than half of this figure and the same applies to hospitalisations. Nevertheless, this overstated figure is still classed as the official figure and it continues to be officially reported. Moat people will still believe it is correct and unsurprisingly, anyone who challenges it is attacked and their claims are still classed as fake news.

When vaccines were initially promoted, it was claimed they would prevent infection and transmission. Such claims were made by Dr Fauci and President Biden. By mid-2021 younger people were being pressurised to get the vaccine to minimise viral transmission to older and more vulnerable people, even though the young had a very low risk of death themselves. However, the simple fact is when the vaccines started to be used, it soon emerged that they did not prevent infection or transmission. Many doctors and scientists tried to get this true fact out to the public. But they were simply removed from social media, banned from certain platforms and classed as conspiracy theorists, anti-vaxxers and Coronavirus deniers who quoted fake news. Of course, now, even the top medical officials accept all of this is correct. So, once again it was the official medical position that was promoting fake news and lies and not the scientists who were trying to let everyone learn the truth. There were many other scientists and doctors who also knew the truth but felt they had to keep silent to prevent personal attacks. This is a truly dangerous environment when esteemed scientists who have vital information are afraid to release it for fear of losing their careers.

This is a perfect time to repeat the most important fact about science which has been examined throughout the book. Science (and particularly medical science) advances only when a so-called indisputable scientific fact that is being used to treat patients is challenged – usually by a single scientist or doctor. In nearly every case, these courageous people are attacked, discredited and even have their careers eventually destroyed, even though the truth nearly always emerges, albeit sometimes years, and even decades, later. If, throughout history, there had been a world where everyone who challenged the existing so-called science was immediately and completely censored like many are now, then the world would still be treating people with lobotomies and killing and destroying them, doctors would not be sanitising their hands before delivering babies and still causing millions of deaths, and beta blockers would have caused another 800,000 deaths in Europe.

The tragedy is we are well underway to enacting this total censorship. The official claim now is that everything that medicine does is based on "unchallengeable science". The simple fact, however, is that throughout history nearly every piece of "science" that was being used was eventually proven to be wrong or partly wrong. There are a few, but not many, medical treatments that were used 100 or even 50 years ago that are still being used today. So, why does the establishment now claim all of this has changed and that "current science" is indisputable, cannot be wrong, and that anyone who tries to challenge it has to be immediately censored along with all their evidence? We really are well down this path, and if the global elite ever fully achieve it – which is their plan – science will no longer exist. Albert Einstein summed it all up: "Science can flourish only in an atmosphere of free speech." Here are a few examples of what has happened to some key experts who are committed to exposing the truth and incorrect science regardless of the impact it has on them.

Robert F. Kennedy Jr. created the Children's Health Defense which, as already seen, is aimed at improving children's health and understanding the causes of the incredible increase in their level of chronic diseases over the last 50 years. In the US, 54% of all children now have at least one chronic disease. (The UK has around 50%.) The problem is some of the key reasons for these incredible increases are associated with ultra-processed foods, genetically modified crops and their associated toxic chemicals like pesticides and synthetic fertilisers, and dangerous drugs and vaccines. If parents want to improve the health of their children, then this message needs to be communicated to them so they can minimise their use. Of course, the problem is this threatens the profitability of all the companies and organisations involved and this, as already analysed, is more important to them than children's health and lives. So, unsurprisingly he has been savagely attacked and censored and deplatformed from sites like Instagram, YouTube and Facebook.

He has also written several books but the most crucial one is *The Real Anthony Fauci.* In the last 25 years, I have learnt so much about the serious and life-taking outcomes of many drugs and industrialised foods, but even I was shocked by the sheer magnitude of the devastating facts in this book and the number of deaths Dr Fauci has been responsible for. When Robert Kennedy was promoting the book, he made this incredible statement: "With your help, this book can play a transformational role in exposing Dr Fauci as a charlatan and quack and in showing the world that Dr Fauci, far from being a healer, is one of the most noteworthy mass murderers in human history." Please let this sink in.

If, like so many people, you believe and trust Dr Fauci, then surely he would (and should) bring a legal case against Robert Kennedy to destroy him, and maybe even get him imprisoned for such slander. Dr Fauci controls billions of dollars and he could employ the world's finest team of lawyers and barristers to make this happen. The problem for Dr Fauci, however, is simple. He cannot do any of this because every single fact in the book, and all the deaths that he caused, are factual and simply unchallengeable. All he can do, therefore, together with all those who incredibly still support him, is to call for more censorship to try to hide the truth so the majority of people never even learn that the book exists and thus try to maintain his reputation. The US surgeon general then also called for far more censorship of Robert F. Kennedy Jr. who simply said, "I'm very happy to debate the surgeon general or to line up my facts against his and allow the public to judge which one of us is the source of misinformation. I would also remind the surgeon general that censorship by the government is not just un-American, it's unconstitutional, and he should have the confidence in his policies in the market place of ideas and not have to rely on coercion." Of course, the surgeon general would also never dare to hold an open debate when the true facts would be made public. So, he also can only try to impose further censorship. Amazingly, despite all this censorship, the book *The Real Anthony Fauci* sold over 1 million copies and was a bestseller in the US. This happened despite an unprecedented media blackout, censorship of every conceivable kind, powerful discrimination campaigns, more than a dozen hit pieces against Robert Kennedy, boycotts from bookstores and libraries, a ban on advertising from the New

York Times and big tech platforms, and without a single review in any major newspaper. Thankfully, Robert F. Kennedy Jr. is simply one of those brave and courageous people who, despite all the attacks he is facing, is determined to expose the truth, save lives, and bring despicable people to justice,

Another incredible fact in the book was that when Dr Fauci was appointed director of the National Institute of Allergy and Infectious Diseases in 1984, the US government gave him a crucial task to undertake. At that time infectious diseases were causing very few deaths, even though just three vaccines were being given, but almost all chronic diseases, like type 2 diabetes, asthma, mental illness, strokes and obesity were increasing alarmingly, not just in adults but also in children. He was instructed to investigate the causes of these diseases and then take action to reduce them. However, in 1984 when he took charge, 6% of children had one chronic disease, but today the figure is 54% – a 900% increase. The US also now has the lowest life expectancy of any developed country and the highest level of childhood deaths. All this has happened despite the fact the US spends nearly twice as much on healthcare per capita than the other richest western countries. Dr Fauci never carried out any research to find out why this devastating explosion of diseases was, and still is, happening. Instead, he just promoted and significantly increased the use of drugs and vaccines by medicine. He simply dismissed and would not investigate the one thing that really could have prevented all of this – lifestyle medicine – and this has been one of the greatest disasters in the modern world. Evil is normally accepted as the strongest word that anyone can be labelled with, but is it really enough to describe Dr Fauci?

Dr Joseph Mercola has helped tens of millions of people across the world to take control of their own health for over 25 years. His website had, until recently, 15,000 articles and newsletters which covered virtually all aspects of how lifestyle can prevent and help people recover from many diseases and medical conditions. However, just like Robert Kennedy, he had to explain how things like processed foods and dangerous chemicals were some of the key causes of disease, and global cartels are simply not prepared to let anything threaten their sales and profits and this has led to him being the most censored and attacked individual in the US.

Dr Mercola also wrote many books but the most contentious one is *The Truth About COVID-19* which also was a key cause of the attacks. Just like Robert Kennedy, however, he is simply quoting facts and they dare not take him to a court of law. Once again, censorship is their prime weapon. When he first started in the 1990s, free speech prevailed. Yes, he was criticised for some of the things he wrote, but censorship barely existed. In the last few years, however, particularly once Covid started, censorship has become ruthless in ways that democratic countries could never have believed possible. Here are a few of the ways he has been attacked. He was effectively banned from YouTube and Facebook. I also explained in detail in Part 3 how in 2019 Google changed its search engine algorithms which resulted in access to his website falling by 99%. He has in fact been savagely attacked by virtually every media group, website and fact checker, as well as politicians, and even President Biden has unlawfully demanded he be banned from all social media. Government officials are simply misusing their positions by openly calling for censorship in direct violation of their constitutional law – the highest law of the land. Banks have also shut down his accounts and cancelled credit cards and PayPal shut down the accounts of his business partners. Throughout all of this, he had refused to succumb to the relentless attacks. Then something more worrying started to happen. For example, he has been followed and chased by media cars while on his bicycle near his home, and there are other personal concerns that he feels he must not disclose. What all this has led to is that he decided he had to remove the 15,000 articles from his websites. This is what he said, "You are seeing in real time, the destruction of the First Amendment of freedom of speech. It has evaporated and is no longer present in the United States." Thankfully, he is still doing one important thing. He continues to write his daily articles and emails them directly to those people who signed up to receive them, but after 48 hours they are then automatically deleted. He has, however, also put his daily articles in a private fee-based site called Substack that is free from censorship so that people can access them for a small annual fee whenever they want. All these attacks have been made to try to stop him communicating the truth particularly about Covid, even though everything he has said is based on scientific articles from respected organisations and scientists.

Here is a crucial fact. If censorship, particularly about Covid, had not become so severe, this is what I would have done about this book. I would have got just a few hundred copies published (after spending five years writing it), but then I really would have set up a website and made it freely available to anyone, so that huge numbers of people would have been able to download it and read it. Getting the truth out to as many people as possible is quite simply my main aim in life. If I tried this, however, the site would certainly last no more than a few hours, because internet data are constantly scrutinised and analysed by AI and as soon as one of the fact checkers found out, it really would be rapidly deplatformed and classed as "fake news". A physical book is something that they cannot destroy (at least not yet).

Given all the information on censorship so far, how do you think the UK compares? The UK is, sadly, a censoring powerhouse. The UK government was the first democracy to try to introduce an Online Safety Bill, and while some aspects like removing platforms on child sex abuse are to be supported, as laid out, it hands immense power to Big Tech firms to control free speech and erode democracy. MP David Davis describes the bill as a "censor's charter". He added, "Lobby groups will be able to push social networks to take down content they view as politically incorrect, even though the content is legal." The UK also has other powerful organisations which aim to control so-called disinformation, which quite simply requires censorship. These include the International Grand Committee on Disinformation and the Centres for Countering Digital Hate. The idea for both of them came from the MPs Damien Collins and Ian Lucas. Vaccine censorship has clearly been one of the key goals of these organisations even though, as examined in detail, the "disinformation" claims made by doctors and scientists against Covid vaccines are in fact truthful.

In 2019 even the BBC founded the Trusted News Initiative. Its partners include other global media like the Washington Post and Reuters, and Big Tech partners like Google, Facebook, Twitter and YouTube. Once again, one of its key agendas is to discredit claims against vaccines. All these organisations have helped to achieve incredible levels of censorship. Hundreds of doctors and scientists, even from prestigious universities like Harvard, Stanford and Oxford, have been banned and deplatformed over the last two years. They have been labelled as "dangerous" and some have lost their careers. The simple fact is there is now a coordinated global censorship and suppression of free speech and Covid has been the main reason for this.

I have explained how Dr Mercola's business partners in the US had their PayPal accounts shut down. Well, exactly the same thing has been happening in the UK but on an even greater scale. Journalist Toby Young, who is associate editor of the Spectator, also has his own news website: the Daily Sceptic. It was created in response to all the misinformation and censorship, especially from Big Tech, that emerged after Covid. Even though his views and the vaccine facts that he quotes are pretty moderate, he has now had his personal PayPal account as well as that for the Daily Sceptic closed down. He has lost a quarter of his revenues. He then did a widescale check, and found that numerous other similar organisations had also recently had their PayPal accounts closed, and nearly all of them involved the key issues that you're not allowed to be sceptical about, like the lockdown policy, other Covid restrictions and the mRNA vaccines. The global elite are clearly determined to ramp up censorship.

One final fact. The book *The Real Anthony Fauci* by Robert F. Kennedy Jr. sold a million copies in the US and most were bought from Amazon. However, in the UK the book has not been available from Amazon and other major booksellers. When I tried to order it, the details were there, but it simply said it was "currently unavailable". A year later it is still "unavailable". It took me several months to find a small independent bookseller who stocked it. Clearly the censoring organisations have "persuaded" Amazon UK to censor it. All this despite the fact this book contains 100% of truthful facts which no one can, or dares, to challenge and why they can only use censorship. These are all devastatingly sad examples of the fact that the UK is simply no longer a true democracy.

We have seen that in just 18 months, Covid vaccines have caused more side effects and deaths than all other vaccines added together over the last 30 years. Individual patients who have suffered some of these injuries invariably receive no official recognition from doctors, because they are instructed to follow the official position that the vaccines are completely safe. This has led many patients who know that the vaccines really were the cause to explore this devastating problem online, to see if other patients have had similar outcomes and to try to launch vaccine injury support groups. What happens? Some have found hundreds of other patients with similar outcomes but every one of them has then been censored and their online sites like Facebook, Google and Twitter simply closed down. Vaccine-injured people have also been accused of spreading misinformation by fact checkers. Just one more shocking example that democracy is over.

In the light of all of this information, the simple fact is it is the fact checkers, social media companies, media groups, governments and key medical experts like Dr Fauci who are promoting much of the fake news about COVID-19 and will simply not report true facts that go against the official position. For example, they still promote face masks that don't work, they still quote official Covid deaths that are grossly overstated, they still attack the unvaccinated even though they now have lower infections, hospitalisations and deaths than the vaccinated, and they continue to falsely claim mRNA vaccines are completely safe. As well as censoring anything and anyone that challenges their official positions, they have also had to change crucial definitions that have been around for decades and even centuries to avoid their policies and treatments being discredited. We have seen how definitions like "pandemic" and "herd immunity" have all been recently altered and, of course, the Covid vaccines are not true vaccines but gene edited drugs meaning they also had to change the definition of a vaccine.

Another problem involving censorship is that so many people, particularly the young, now obtain virtually all their information from the internet and rarely use books, magazines, radio or TV. Internet reliance continues to grow, even though it is controlled almost exclusively by a small number of global companies like Google and Facebook who are all part of the WEF's reset plans. These organisations really do plan to control worldwide information in a way that can literally alter people's lives. Google, for example, has the ability to restrict or block access to websites across the internet and thus can control what people see and don't see. This means that if a certain type of site or information is removed from your search, and you don't know it exists, then you will never know to go look for it and you would never even know it had been removed from your search results in the first place. All this means Google has the power to manipulate the public and shape their opinions, thoughts, attitudes, purchases and behaviour and Google quite simply hides this bias. It doesn't just produce tiny shifts; it can radically change people's thinking, and here are two examples of what is happening.

If a major internet company wants a particular party or candidate to be elected, they can fill most of their first and second pages with favourable articles and information for their choices. Researchers have shown this really can make a significant impact on voting particularly for those who are undecided. In the 2016 US presidential election, Google had a pro-Clinton bias in its top ten search positions. Researchers estimated that somewhere between 2.6 and 10.4 million undecided voters shifted to Hillary Clinton because of it. As Google's expertise and manipulation improves, then this sort of information control really could decide future elections and presidents.

Another example is when someone hears about the benefits of lifestyle medicine for their health and wants to start finding information about it on the web. The reality is they will find very little because Google and other internet companies only promote conventional medicine and drugs and they will be led to these sites which, unsurprisingly, will claim there is little or no proof natural lifestyle has any meaningful benefits, and even make suggestions about possible dangers. Of course, there are many people and organisations like the Alliance for Natural Health International and the Children's Health Defense that do exist on the web who really could help, but unless you know their names and website details you will not find out about them or be directed to them from Google. They will probably be demoted to page 1,000. Who would find that? When Google controls what we read and hear, they control what we think. Google is quite simply becoming what can only be described as a dictator in its own right. It is, however, unlike anything the world has ever seen before and no other dictator has had even a tiny fraction of the power that Google has. Should these types of information control really be allowed to happen?

The WEF and global elite's future plans

So, now, I can move on to some of the other key things the WEF and global elite are planning to achieve. Once track and trace and data control, digital IDs, digital currencies, censorship and health control are all in place, control of all of these will be possible.

Mankind will own nothing

There is something called the "subscription economy" which is gaining traction. It means people use regular recurring payments for something they want rather than buying it. If they don't want it anymore, they stop paying and return whatever it is. Some people prefer this for certain things, while others simply want to be able to buy and have immediate personal ownership. There is absolutely nothing wrong with such a system provided people really can freely choose what they want to do. However, if I tell you that the WEF predicts that by 2030, you will "own nothing and be happy", then this raises a frightening future. This is the future that Danish MP Ida Auken (who is a member of the WEF's Global Future Councils) predicted for 2030 when all products will have become services: "I don't own anything, I don't own a car, I don't own a house. I don't own any appliances or any clothes. Shopping is a distant memory in the city of 2030 whose inhabitants borrow what they need on demand." To make this seem ideal for mankind, the WEF is simply promoting the idea that a lack of ownership is a convenience which makes people's lives easier.

I should add that it is hard to see how this could apply, at least initially, to many older people who already have personal ownership of nearly everything including their homes. However, it is much easier to see how young people could be ensnared, because even now the number of them who are able to buy their own homes or cars continues to fall significantly and many already use the subscription method for a range of their other needs. The global elite will promote it incessantly but they are likely to use other ways to achieve their goals. For example, those people with debts – which is a significant number – could be told they would be paid off, provided they are prepared to relinquish all future rights to private ownership. Ultimately, as older people die off, private ownership will also continue to fall and, unless people are prepared to resist the WEF's reset, this plan will still eventually succeed. What all this means is that only the global elite will own real assets. Some of the other key methods that will be used to achieve this incredible and frightening plan will now be explained.

We have seen that the three largest global investment firms, Blackrock, Vanguard and State Street, control $20 trillion of shareholder assets which is around a third of the world's total. Only the two richest countries – the US and China – have a GDP that roughly equals this value, while the GDP of the third richest country, Japan, is only $5 trillion. Quite simply, these three global financial giants are unbelievably powerful. One of the things they are doing is buying homes and then simply renting them out. In the first quarter of 2021 in the US, they purchased 15% of all homes up for sale and most of them were low to mid value. This is one more escalating reason why young people are struggling to buy them and have to just rent. To ensure they achieve the purchases, the companies will often offer more than the asking price and also can make immediate cash payments. Some researchers have estimated that in the next 20 years, these companies could own a significant majority of lower and average value homes. If the average American is pushed out of the housing market, they simply become beholden to these investment giants and will be very unlikely to ever be able to buy their own property again. These global financial firms are key members of the WEF and play a vital role in its reset plans, and while house purchases are well underway in the US they are also occurring in other western countries. The number of private rented houses in the UK is already at a record high of 4.5 million. This number has gone up by just under 2 million in the last decade. Of course, many of these are owned by private individuals who use them for income, but many are now pulling out because of recent more stringent regulatory and tax changes. Large companies, just as in the US, are now taking advantage and increasing their ownership and then renting them.

Around 1,000 of the largest global companies in the world form part of the WEF and its Global Reset. The plan is that these companies will continue to buy up or merge with other companies in each of their sectors so they become global cartels with immense control and power. The three giant financial firms, Blackrock, Vanguard and State Street, are a vital and special part of this control plan because, since the 1970s, they have been increasing their investments in nearly every global company including those in food, agriculture, technology, pharmaceuticals, energy, mining, banks, construction and clothing. They are the largest institutional investors in virtually all of them and have immense power that helps ensure the companies develop strategies in line with the Global Reset. Even now, some specific industries are already well on the way to achieving this control and domination. We have seen how just three global cartels – Bayer, Corteva and ChemChina – already control over 60% of the world's seeds and 75% of herbicides and pesticides. Also, just five key web giants – Google, Microsoft, Amazon, Facebook and Twitter – have more annual turnover than the GDP of every country except the US and China, and they are predicted to exceed even these in a few years. This will make them financially more powerful than any government in the world. If global cartels really do eventually own and control most of the essential products and services on Earth, they will effectively control mankind. It will be one of the ways in which people will eventually be forced to buy nothing and just rent everything.

Here is a final point. Historically, the huge number of news and media groups would have laid bare all these facts and plans and ensured the public were aware of the devastating future they faced so they really could take action to prevent it. But, of course, as already made clear, the major media players have simply been bought by the global elite and controlled by the three financial giants who own most of their shares. They are simply not exposing and challenging these devastating future plans. If you examine the history of countless media mergers and acquisitions, you'll also come to another unsettling discovery. Local, independent news outlets are dying out in droves and it may not be long before just a few global media cartels control nearly all the conventional news, just like Google and the other Big Techs control the web. All this will continue to eliminate free speech and increase censorship.

Control of agriculture

Bill Gates' increasing control of much of world agriculture has already been examined, but this section gives additional crucial facts about the WEF and global elite's future plans.

The key part of the plan involves replacing natural foods from seeds and plants with genetically engineered varieties which require synthetic pesticides, herbicides and fertilisers. The ultimate agenda is to drive small farmers off the land and replace them with industrialised farming practices involving incredibly large land areas, each with a single GMO crop. It involves huge industrialised machinery and very few workers. Robotics are also being improved to take over even these few people. Spraying the crops with chemicals is carried out from the air using planes or drones which saturate the entire landscape with glyphosate and other dangerous compounds. The claim is all this will increase crop yields and help to reduce carbon emissions. However, we have seen that this is simply not true. A 14-year unchallengeable study showed that industrialised agriculture implemented in Africa did not result in any increase in output, that hunger actually went up by 30% and 131 million people suffered increased poverty.

A separate UN study which involved 900 of the world's key scientists and agronomists also showed that traditional agriculture produced better crop yields than GMOs, that it does not destroy biodiversity and soils, and has better climate change outcomes. Key scientists, like Vandana Shiva, report factual data that show small biodiverse natural farmers produce 70% of global food using just 25% of the world's agricultural land, while industrial agriculture produces just 30% on 70% of the land. Of course, nearly all traditional farmers produce food crops just for human consumption, while industrialised farming also use some of them for feeding their industrialised animals as well as for biofuels. In total, 55% of world cropland is used for food, 36% for animal feed and 9% for biofuel. Analysing all these figures together, and making allowances for the other crop usages from industrial agriculture, still clearly shows that traditional agriculture produces better crop yields. It is almost unbelievable that none of these facts will change the WEF's plan to impose industrialised farming. The global elite ignore all such data and use their immense power and money to try to discredit it and ensure it gains no official recognition. They are determined to impose industrialised agriculture on humanity despite its devastating effects because they own all the patented seeds and chemicals and, if they succeed, they will simply control all of mankind's food.

Here is another of Bill Gates' plans that will allow them to take control of agriculture. Around the world there are 15 key seed banks in different countries that store and preserve all the seeds of humanity. The venture started in 1979 and sought to achieve a complete inventory of heritage seed stocks for the benefit of humanity and to preserve crop diversity for millennia. The collection of these seeds from small farmers around the world took many years and now there are over 768,000 varieties. The free exchange of these natural seeds amongst all farmers has been the bedrock for maintaining biodiversity and food security throughout farming history. Initially, the seed banks were funded by several governments and the World Bank. Then in 2003 – working in coordination with the Rockefeller Foundation – the Gates Foundation pumped $720 million into the project. Bill Gates has continued to increase his annual funding and is now its single biggest contributor just like he is with the WHO. In 2020 this funding and control gave him the power to merge all the 15 previously independent seed banks into one legal entity which he now calls "Gates Ag One", and which was formulated to be a subsidiary of the Gates Foundation. Effectively, he now has total control of all of the world's seeds. How could world governments allow one man to achieve seed piracy and control mankind's key food? This is before considering the clear facts that he has already caused agricultural destruction in much of Africa and other parts of the world.

Quite devastatingly, using this new control, he has already made significant progress in fulfilling his plan to enforce GMO crops into every human being. Seed research in the 15 seed banks was originally carried out by genuine scientific institutions, but this has now been stopped and handed over to private corporations like Bayer. These companies are now using artificial intelligence and digital technology to scan the seeds and their genetic data. The aim is then to genetically modify them so they can be treated with chemicals like glyphosate without being killed off, just like all other existing GMO seeds. These genetically modified seeds will, of course, be patented and owned by Bill Gates and the companies that develop them. The seed banks were originally formed by free donations from worldwide farmers and all the seeds were intended to be universally available to humanity. However, by centralising them and manipulating intellectual property laws, Gates has launched a gene editing campaign to rob farmers of their seed sovereignty and incredible knowledge. Citizens, governments and farm organisations had written many laws and international treaties on biodiversity protection, but by conning government officials, manipulating intellectual property law and rewriting seed regulations, Gates has been able to bypass and destroy these treaties and evade the structures put in place to prevent global corporations taking over the planet's biodiversity and seeds. If his plan for total food domination is achieved, it is not impossible that he could make hundreds of billions of dollars each year, given that worldwide food sales are around $10 trillion. Over the last two decades huge numbers of farmers, citizens and organisations have taken action to try to protect biodiversity and prevent the imposition of GMOs and they are now fighting to try to stop all this from happening. They far outnumber Bill Gates, the global elite and the few companies involved. However, they don't have hundreds of billions of dollars and can't control governments or the media in the same way that he does. If the global population understood what was happening, they could help support this fight to try to stop this tyrannical plan for world food.

Another key part of his plan is to genetically modify other plants like vegetables and fruits and this has already started. Five key crops are being researched so they can be genetically modified to "supposedly" improve flavour and nutrition. These are lettuce, tomatoes, strawberries, cilantro and blueberries. Are these really poor natural products that need "improving"? Or is this simply another plan to also gain control of these other foods by patenting them and then claiming they are healthier and taste better than the natural plants? There is, however, a major problem. It is well known that GMO foods tend to be low in vital micronutrients that support human health. Glyphosate, for example, kills weeds by leaching out the minerals that are essential for human life. Even Bill Gates understands this problem but he has simply developed another so-called solution that he now uses to falsely claim that GMOs are even better than natural foods. This involves food fortification which adds compounds like specific minerals and vitamins. The problem is natural seeds and plants contain dozens of these essential nutrients, but fortification usually uses just a few specific ones. These limited compounds are also usually synthetic and simply not as beneficial as natural compounds. However, Bill Gates now uses fortification as a key selling point and his aim is to expand this to many of his new GMOs and to falsely claim they are much healthier than natural foods. To help promote this agenda, he created yet another of his useful quasi-governmental organisations like he did with his vaccine organisations like GAVI and SEPI. This new one is for food fortification and called GAIN – the Global Alliance for Improved Nutrition. He funded it with $70 million and launched it at the United Nations General Assembly. It is being promoted as a public health agency and also gives money to local governments to help promote these foods to the public. He succeeded in forcing GMO crops onto 131 million African people, causing them devastating outcomes. He really could force these new GMO fortified fruits and vegetables which he falsely classes as "improved nutrition" onto hundreds of millions of other people even though they will *not* be healthier, and will almost certainly cause more serious outcomes.

Bill Gates and the agribusiness companies he supports and invests in knew nothing about natural agriculture and the incredible knowledge it has developed over thousands of years. So, they developed a plan to try to learn everything they could by simply stealing all the information from farmers. They installed things like digital apps and cameras on farms around the world particularly in areas like Africa and south Asia to gather data on all aspects of farming, like soil health, cropping patterns, the effects of weather and seed choices. Most of the farmers had no idea exactly what they were doing and why. Then the aim was to use artificial intelligence and algorithms on all the data collected to supposedly improve the farming practices. He then sold it back to the farmers together with new industrialised seeds and chemicals with the claim it would improve every aspect of their farming. The idea that AI could suddenly improve thousands of years of farming knowledge was a joke. This was just another scam aimed at simply gaining control of agriculture and helping to destroy small farmers.

Did you know that Bill Gates is now the largest individual owner of farmland in the US? He has been buying it at a frenzied pace but has done so through a separate investment firm called Cascade Investment LLC. He almost certainly did this to try to hide what he was doing. This was all unearthed by the magazine the Land Report after his purchase of an incredible 14,500 prime acres in Washington state. He now owns at least 242,000 acres in multiple other states. What does he intend to do with it all? Almost certainly he will use most of it for GMO crops – particularly soy and soybeans – that will then be used to manufacture his fake meats and all his other planned industrialised foods he intends to force people to eat. Given his complete ownership from land to food, he will then receive all the profits they make. Almost certainly, a small part of his land will be used to produce completely natural healthy grains, fruits, vegetables and naturally fed animals. Why? So he and other global elites can eat them, because that is what they are known to do at the WEF. The idea that they themselves will eat the devastating GMO foods is impossible to believe.

In summary, Bill Gates is simply planning to take over the world's agriculture. His aim is to eliminate natural farming and its natural foods which he portrays to be an archaic, dirty, dangerous and inefficient relic from the past, and replace it all with genetically altered and chemically controlled alternatives. Most farmers will be redundant and replaced by huge industrialised machinery. I'll let you consider all the evidence and decide whether mankind should simply sit back and allow him to achieve all of this, or be prepared to stand up against him.

Control of Food

The WEF's reset plan involves the ultimate control of all food. This involves eliminating not just every natural source of plants and seeds as already examined, but also natural animals like cattle, sheep and chickens and the foods they produce like milk, butter, eggs and cheese. These will be replaced with fake, industrialised alternatives like synthetic beef. Three global corporations already own 60% of all seeds that are currently being grown, Now, artificial meats are also being produced and promoted incessantly especially by Bill Gates. Sales have increased significantly over the last few years and many people like vegans and a number of famous stars are eating them and promoting them. Many of these fake foods will, however, be resisted by a wide range of the population, particularly those who love natural foods like beef, chicken, lamb, butter, milk, eggs and cheese. So, what are the plans to bypass all of this and effectively force everyone to simply eat all the artificial alternatives?

The Netherlands government recently made the decision to reduce livestock farms by 30%. This decision is a very worrying one because even though the Netherlands is a relatively small country, it is the largest exporter of meats in the EU and the second largest worldwide after the US. The Daily Express explained that the plan is to cut back the number of all its various livestock, including chickens, cattle, and sheep, by more than 35 million. This will have a significant impact on worldwide food availability. Canada is also about to adopt a similar plan. The official reasons given are simply to reduce nitrogen and ammonia pollution and thus help climate change. As we have seen, however, the main cause of climate change relating to animals is the result of its industrialisation and this is what Robert F. Kennedy Jr. said: "We should reduce the use of chemical fertilisers and make the chemical industry pay for nitrogen pollution, instead of criminalising farmers trapped in a chemical treadmill by the industrial agriculture model." Quite simply, natural regenerative livestock really are significantly less polluting than those that are "industrialised" and even less than the artificial man-made meats that are now being incessantly promoted in their place. The Dutch farmers should be helped and given the chance to improve their farming practices. If governments really wanted just to improve climate change, they should advocate and simply help farmers to achieve this regenerative agriculture which really would do just that, and which would also avoid additional food shortages.

Despite all of this, the Dutch government intends to buy out around a third of all farms. If the farmers fail to voluntarily sell their farms, the government will then implement forced buyouts. In key areas like agriculture and food, they simply appear to have been taken over by the global elite, and an independent Swedish journalist, Peter Imanuelsen, has reported that the timing of the brazen Dutch attack on cattle farmers is one that can only really be explained as an intentional strategy to force us into the Great Reset by manufacturing a food crisis. The plight of the Dutch farmers is almost certainly just the beginning of this part of the devastating worldwide plans that mankind is facing.

Another worrying fact is that Bill Gates invested half a billion dollars in a Dutch food wholesaler called Picnic which focuses on selling "fake foods" like synthetic meat. He is also fighting against legislative attempts to make sure these fake meats and foods are properly labelled since this would slow down their acceptance and sales. A similar thing happened in California in 2012 when a vote was held (called Proposition 37) with the aim of getting GMO crops to be properly labelled which would have given people clear information on what they were eating and would have reduced their sales. Unfortunately, the global corporations and the global elites just managed to stop this from happening after an incredible and expensive PR campaign which also involved a key piece of truly fraudulent information. Most people now have no idea whether they are eating natural or GMO crops. Will Bill Gates succeed in doing the same thing with synthetic meat? The world should hope not, but he is so powerful it really could happen again.

Another disturbing fact is that huge numbers of food processing plants in the US have been destroyed by fires in the last year. In 2019 there were just two such fires but from January 2021 to April 2022 there were 20. Such an increase could maybe happen just once in 1,000 years, so it could be just an incredible piece of current bad luck, However, many people who can see all the other things that are being deliberately done to reduce food availability are concerned that this could be another deliberate part of the plan to produce a food crisis to help necessitate the need to eat fake foods.

The global leaders' intention to dramatically reduce natural meat production is clear, but instead of just promoting lab-grown "meats" as the only alternative, they have an additional plan which involves insects. You may be aware that insects will soon be more readily available as a food, even though many people would prefer never to even try them. The reality, however, is that this will not be just a choice, because when meat and other similar foods start to disappear, there will not be enough lab-grown meat available to replace them all. Insects, therefore, are going to be the only other essential meat-like food available, meaning they will have to be eaten. Their production really could be ramped up easily and in sufficient amounts because of new industrialisation techniques.

In July 2021, the WEF wrote an article titled "Why We Need to Give Insects the Role They Deserve in Our Food System". It explains how, thanks to new technologies, we are now able to industrialise the breeding of insects in a contained environment. Several indoor agricultural start-ups are already in place. One is using artificial intelligence to help build the first indoor fully automated vertical insect farm in the world, able to produce 100,000 tonnes of insects a year. Major news organisations who simply endorse the WEF's plans are also promoting insects. In February 2021 Time magazine insisted that we really should eat more bugs to save the planet. Celebrities, like Angelina Jolie, Nicole Kidman and Drew Barrymore, are also advocates of the plan. Four primary schools in Wales recently conducted a real-world trial to see how children would take to eating mealworms, crickets, beetles and other insects during which they were told that eating them and eliminating meat would help to save the planet. The UK, along with many other countries, is expected to give full approval for insect sales by retailers in 2023. They really do, however, pose risks to human health, and amazingly, no long-term clinical trials have ever been done to try to prove their safety. The key fact, however, is that none of this is necessary. Natural meats and all other animal-related foods do not need to be eliminated because they are better in all respects than fake foods. People do not need to give up their favourite foods and eat insects instead, but they really will need to fight back and refuse to accept all the global elite's lies and future plans.

In summary, the global elite simply intend to eliminate traditional farming, livestock and natural foods that have been a vital part of the world's entire evolution and which are essential for good health and longevity. They intend to replace it all with genetically modified and chemically laden crops, vegetables and fruits, together with artificial lab-grown proteins and meats as well as adding insects. Everything will eventually be gene edited and their patents will be owned by global corporations and, therefore, the global elite who own them. They will then simply control all of the world's food and thus mankind. Do you think the global elite themselves will be eating all these devastating types of food they are going to enforce on everyone else? Certainly not. You only have to see the natural healthy foods they eat at the World Economic Forum in Davos. They intend to live long healthy lives and will be producing and eating natural seeds, plants, fruits, nuts and natural animals and all their associated foods like butter, eggs and cheese for themselves. Incidentally, Bill Gates also claims that mankind will eventually have to move into metropolitan cities where indoor vertical farming will be necessary to feed everyone. You may laugh at this, but remember he has achieved virtually all of his other key plans like controlling the WHO, the media, GMO crops, the world's seeds, fake foods and vaccines.

Finally, here is one of the very latest plans regarding food. It appears very different, and is being set up in the US with President Biden as a key proponent. It has a "bold goal" to "end hunger and increase healthy eating and physical activity by 2030". One of the stated goals is to end diet-related disease. It may seem that the government is finally taking an interest in nutrition and realising its impact on health. The key words being used to launch this programme are "food is medicine". Does this sound like an amazing decision that will transform mankind, especially when you consider that this is the key claim of this book? Could it really all work?

Unfortunately, things are not what they seem. It is important to remember that 112 years ago, medicine was using natural foods, naturopathic-based herbal products and newly discovered vitamins as one of the key medical treatments for patients. At that time, John D. Rockefeller was planning to make huge investments in newly developed chemical drugs and was determined to destroy medicine's use of natural foods so his drugs would have no opposition. He succeeded and effectively gained control of medicine. Now, the White House has quite amazingly given the role of officially relaunching "foods for health" to a group that includes the Rockefeller Foundation which originally eliminated them. Careful scrutinisation of the plans, however, reveals they will have many devastating effects. They are quite simply another way of achieving the global elite's goal of eliminating traditional farming, livestock and natural foods and replacing them with genetically modified, chemically laden, industrialised and artificial foods, and things like insects. The Rockefeller group will be a key decider on what foods are used and not medicine, and many of the foods already advocated are truly unhealthy and include gene edited seeds, industrialised processed foods, lab-grown meats and insects. Processed foods like Lucky Charms, Frosted Mini Wheat and Honey Nut Cheerios are shockingly rated as healthier than natural organic ones like eggs, cheese and beef which are classed as unhealthy and these will be severely restricted. One of the main aims of the US plan is to make foods a part of medicine and thousands of physicians will be trained in this new model of "food is medicine". Once achieved, medicine will be given the role of promoting it and doctors will effectively be able to prescribe specific foods and diets. When this happens, people will be expected to eat them in the same way they are expected to take drugs. They will effectively be forced into eating what will be mainly unhealthy diets. Initially, the plan will concentrate on poorer people who generally need financial assistance. Instead of just being given monetary support which enables them to choose their own foods, they will in part be given free digital food tokens but these will only enable them to buy the approved foods. For example, they will be able to get insects but not beef, and genetically modified foods but not organic ones.

This is what Dr Mercola says about it all:

> It may be tempting to believe that government has finally had a change of heart, and is really intent on improving public health by addressing nutrition and giving it the central role it deserves. If this is you, I would urge you to consider the history of how we got here in the first place, and how the same players that destroyed our food system the first time are now pretending to be our saviours yet again… While this involves welfare applicants using benefit tokens, this system will, without doubt, expand to include all people and regular currency. It's only a matter of time. This is how it begins. And whereas early models will identify fruits and vegetables as healthy foods, what's "healthy" will change as their control over agriculture and food manufacture deepens.

President Biden has earmarked $8 billion to fund this redesign of the US food system. Could such a devastating system be implemented in other countries like the UK and eventually around the world? Almost certainly, unless the US system, which is simply a controlled socialist food system, fails because of public resistance.

Control of world health

The initial part of this plan is the International Pandemic Treaty (IPT) which has been examined in detail. Assuming this treaty, which involves just viral diseases, is universally accepted, then the WEF, via the WHO, will continue to achieve its ultimate plan of controlling all other aspects of world health. The WHO's director general Tedros Ghebreyesus stated that his "central priority is to push the world towards universal health coverage". How could this be achieved? The IPT will allow the WHO to control medicine worldwide once it has declared a pandemic. This will, of course, be limited initially just to viral pandemics. But imagine there is a continued increase in the number of cancer cases which will almost certainly happen. Then the WHO could claim this was also a "pandemic" and that it should be allowed to develop worldwide treatment plans. This concept could apply to most other serious diseases that are all increasing in number, like type 2 diabetes, strokes, Alzheimer's and Parkinson's disease. Of course, as already examined in detail using Covid as an example, worldwide universal treatments will be a disaster. This has been highlighted and explained by huge numbers of scientists and doctors. It would, of course, be even more disastrous now given that the WHO is controlled by Tedros Ghebreyesus and Bill Gates who have no medical training of any kind and have already made numerous, unscientific and appalling decisions. Despite all of this, we have seen that all western governments have unbelievably given their approval for this devastating plan.

The WEF, however, also has other developments underway to achieve this type of global control. Bill Gates and key Silicon Valley companies are financing artificial intelligence, technological devices and telemedicine to automatically monitor things like blood pressure, heart rates, heart irregularities, breathing and body temperatures using devices that can be implanted, swallowed or simply worn like watches, as well as smartphones that are transformed into personal health examination devices to generate huge amounts of health-related information. At the 2022 WEF meeting, the CEO of Nokia, Pekka Lundmark, also explained that by 2030, the WEF's plan to launch tiny smartphones that are implanted directly in the body will be achieved and will coincide with the roll out of 6G technology.

All this is known as the Internet of Bodies (IOB) and involves collecting and storing not just physical but mental data on every individual human. All the information will be automatically and digitally transferred online to key WEF organisations like Google. Implantable microchips are one of the key parts of the global plan and the 2023 WEF annual meeting in Davos even predicted that humans will soon embrace implanted brain technology. Already, Sweden has an estimated 8,000 people who have them implanted in their hands. I must emphasise that at this stage they are simply being used as credit cards, but the start of the IOB implants is imminent.

A recent article on the WEF website said that "implant technologies could become the norm in the future". The WEF also recently suggested there are solid, rational and ethical reasons to consider implanting children with microchips. I wonder how many parents would want their children to have implanted microchips that can monitor, record and store everything they do and say? I also wonder if anyone would want them if they knew about the dangers of implanted microchips. These have been used and trialled on animals like dogs, mice and rats. Between 1990 and 2006, six studies and 11 articles were carried out and published in toxicology and pathology journals and were then analysed by researchers. From this analysis, 14 out of 17 showed a causal link between implanted microchip transponders and various cancers which formed around the microchips. The researchers believe that further microchipping of pets and human beings should be immediately discontinued. This concern is shared by some of America's most respected cancer researchers and this is what Dr Robert Benezra, head of the Cancer Biology and Genetics Program, said: "There's no way in the world, having read this information, that I would have any of those chips implanted in my skin or in one of my family members." As usual, despite all this devastating evidence, the global elite will continue promoting them and eventually enforcing their use. Of course, unsurprisingly, they won't have any implanted into themselves,

There are, however, also a wide range of other potentially serious outcomes from IOB. For example, the huge range of health checks and the fact they are continuously tested every day and even every few minutes could lead to far more people being classed as "ill" even though the results could be false like an occasional heart murmur due to stress with probably little in the way of rechecking. This could lead to far more drug prescriptions and mega profits for the drug industry and their owners – the global elite. However, given that drugs are the third leading cause of death, then it would also be a major risk for mankind. It is also envisaged that IOBs will be adopted in so-called employee wellness programmes which could lead to a high risk of misuse of the varying data that may lead to biased decisions regarding people's hiring, promotion and retention. The IOB promises not only to gather basic health data, but to monitor what people feel, see, touch and taste. This is planned to be used to modify their behaviour, sometimes positively, but also in horrendous ways depending on who does the manipulation. IOBs also threaten doctors. If IOBs record high blood pressure, for example, those people could then be automatically prescribed blood pressure lowering drugs without seeing a doctor. These types of "automatic prescriptions" would eventually eliminate a significant number of doctors and shockingly, believe it or not, this is exactly the plan of Bill Gates who wants nearly all of medicine to be controlled by artificial intelligence.

At the WEF's 2018 meeting, Pfizer's CEO, Albert Bourla, outlined the Federal Drug Agency's approval of the first "electronic pill". This is a drug that contains a biological chip that is capable of sending a signal once it has been swallowed and enters the stomach, thus confirming it has been taken. The ultimate aim is to ensure compliance in taking them. However, as already examined, drugs can significantly increase the risk of a range of diseases like type 2 diabetes, kidney disease, Alzheimer's, heart attacks and certain cancers, as well as devastating side effects including pain and muscle weakness that affect things like physical movement and mental health. Many people, therefore, stop taking a drug to avoid these damaging effects. If the WEF is successful in its IPT plans, however, vaccines will become legally mandatory and the same thing could then be done with drugs, using exactly the same claims that everyone should take them for the benefit of other people even if their own benefits are very low. The electronic pill would be able to expose those who didn't take their drugs and they could then be pressurised and even forced to take them.

Here is one example of the sort of claim that would eventually be made. Statins supposedly reduce the number of heart attacks. It could, therefore, be claimed that if people didn't take them, then hospitals would have unnecessary heart attack patients which would affect the waiting times and treatments of other patients. So, taking them could be made mandatory and given that many "experts" have said they should be prescribed to everyone including children, then 8 billion people could eventually be forced to take them. Given the real truth about statins which has been explored in detail, this would be another serious health disaster but, of course, drug company profits would soar by around $150 billion each year and the same thing could be done for a range of other drugs.

Big Tech companies like Google and Amazon are spending many billions of dollars to expand their presence in the healthcare sector. Google is now investing heavily in drug research but it has many other research programmes that are mind-blowing. For example, it is trying to develop a way of detecting diabetes-related diseases from photos on the exterior of the eyes. I won't go into any more detail because the key point of all of this is that it is just about detecting and diagnosing diseases. Detecting and then treating diseases, mainly with drugs, is the key role of medicine, regulators, companies, governments and virtually every other official organisation. None of them have any interest in preventing disease, which is the absolute priority of lifestyle medicine. The simple but sad fact is diseases can generate trillions of dollars of profit, whereas disease prevention generates nothing, except, of course, longer and healthier lives for mankind. The global elite will ensure these profits are not just maintained but significantly increased, while human health and life expectancy will continue to deteriorate particularly in western countries. Lifestyle medicine advocates are deeply concerned about the power of Google. The all-out war against lifestyle medicine is ongoing, but now that Google has billions of dollars invested in conventional medical practices, it really could ramp up the destruction of lifestyle solutions to health much further by unprecedented censorship and online attacks.

We have examined the all-out war against lifestyle medicine in detail and seen that natural products like vitamins, minerals and herbal products have incredible health benefits, usually better than drugs. So, unsurprisingly, the world's elite have simply tried to get them all banned. They have, however, so far only succeeded in very limited ways. Most supplements are still available in many countries with exceptions like Germany and some other EU countries. US agencies like the FDA have in fact been the most determined in the world to get rid of all supplements except for low dose multivitamins, but with a few exceptions they also have so far failed because of significant opposition from the public.

What is now happening is that over the last few years, mega corporations like Big Pharma and Big Food have been buying up an increasing number of independent supplement companies. Many are currently still selling these products but eventually if this buy-up continues, they could gain major control over supplements and then make a wide range of drastic changes. They could, for example, start to use significantly less absorbable forms like magnesium oxide as well as synthetic forms like folic acid rather than natural folate. Some companies have also started to add things like sugar and other ingredients like flavours. All this would mean that supplements simply become less effective with potential side effects They could also start to reduce the supplement levels particularly in multivitamins to make then less effective. Centrum, owned by Pfizer, which is one of the top multivitamin sellers, has in fact been using low levels for many years making it very ineffective. The mega corporations could eventually side with the FDA and start to slowly remove various supplements until the only ones left would be low level, ineffective multivitamins. It is impossible to know exactly what will happen and when, but it is all truly disturbing and shows that the world's elite are simply determined to keep going until they can control everything.

Climate change

Climate change is a serious problem for mankind. How should it be tackled given that everyone on the planet could, and should, play a significant part? To do so, however, they need to know true facts. For example, the claim by the global elite that industrialised fake foods and GMO seeds will improve it is simply wrong, and people who eat them will actually damage it further. The evidence for all this is overwhelming despite the fact the global elite simply deny it. Why are they prepared to damage the climate now by trying to impose these foods on mankind? Quite simply, it is a key part of the plan to control the global population, and when this is achieved, they really will be able to improve the climate. They will almost certainly then impose climate-based lockdowns. Just like the Covid lockdowns, this will also involve a savage destruction of much of human life. Here are a few examples of what will almost certainly unfold over time.

They would set severe limits on things like travel, personal energy use, many "non-essential" energy-based appliances and air conditioning. Many of these current plans have been developed over many decades. In the UN's 1992 Earth Summit, for example, the executive director of the Environment Programme, Maurice Strong, made the following statement: "Current lifestyles and consumption patterns of the affluent middle class, involving high meat intake, consumption of large amounts of frozen and convenience foods, use of fossil fuels, appliances, home and workplace air conditioning, and suburban housing are not sustainable." Even now, all these things are part of the Great Reset plans or will be at some stage.

Although it will take many years, most people will eventually be moved to huge cities and housed in basic small homes like huge multi-storey apartment blocks that will need much less energy than individual houses which would have more rooms and larger ones. Some analysts have said that we may even have to live in smart multiplexes where there are no private spaces at all, and where everything you do is tracked and recorded. Energy use, like room heating, will be controlled not by the people but by artificial intelligence, resulting in temperatures being lower than most people would be comfortable with. Long distance travel and holidays outside the cities will be severely restricted and probably banned eventually and the same will happen with private vehicles. The WEF's founder, Klaus Schwab, has made it crystal clear in his books that the Great Reset will ultimately lead to the abolition of private property.

Some of these will, of course, be fiercely resisted and to get around this problem, the WEF is already laying the essential ground rules. The International Pandemic Treaty is the key example. It will give the WHO an unchallengeable legal position so it can dictate what every country has to do with a "pandemic" meaning that no government, no health service, or even billions of people could even challenge it or stop it. If the UN was given similar powers on climate change, then all these things could be legally forced onto everyone. This could ultimately mean the seizing of private properties, the forcible relocation from rural areas to smaller properties in cities, restricting the amount of waste per person, and severe restrictions on travel and owning cars – all in the name of saving the earth.

Will any of this apply to the global elite themselves? Absolutely not. Bill Gates built a 6,131 square-metre home with a 23-car garage, a 20-person cinema and 24 bathrooms. He also owns five other incredible homes, a horse farm, four private jets and a collection of helicopters. He is certainly one of the single biggest contributors to climate change in the world, yet he clearly has no intention of changing this.

Education

The WEF envisions a reimagining of current classrooms with a heavy reliance on virtual reality and artificial intelligence technologies on the web, while textbooks, notebooks and pencils are no longer considered as critical learning tools. Instead, education should be largely digitised and coupled with the metaverse so students can learn in a virtual environment. Following its annual 2022 summit, the WEF said that "schools could disappear altogether" on the back of "rapid advancements in artificial intelligence, virtual reality and the Internet of Things". The concept of teaching children individually and long term via the internet is shocking. The idea that children sit at home learning with virtual reality screens on their heads is almost too frightening to think about and the isolation and limited human interaction could simply change human life in devastating ways. Please remember what happened over just a few months during the Covid pandemic when children were trapped and educated at home. The increases in obesity, suicides, mental health and other diseases were shocking and devastating. The outcomes of using virtual reality education for around 14 years would be unthinkable.

Another worrying concern is that what children would be taught would be controlled by a small band of people who could themselves be controlled by the global elite like Google and Bill Gates. Of course, if all this happens and every single child has to have sophisticated VR equipment, imagine the hundreds of billions of dollars of extra profits for companies like Google. The fact that the WEF openly proposes all of this is amazing, although one advantage they have is that most parents know little or nothing about it because the press unsurprisingly don't report it. If every parent really knew, I believe there could be such a backlash that the elite really would have to disband the plan.

Artificial intelligence

Artificial intelligence (AI) is a key part of the global elite's plans for controlling the world's population. In specific areas, AI really can genuinely and amazingly surpass the cleverest humans. Even as far back as 1996, for example, the Deep Blue computer had beaten the world chess champion Gary Kasparov. This, however, had taken incredibly huge resources and time, plus complex research and development. Then in 2017 a new computer – Alpha Zero – which had no previous data on the game of chess, took just four hours to surpass all human chess grandmasters – a testament to the speed that AI can now learn brand new analytical skills. The DeepMind AlphaGo computer also made history by beating the champion in the world's most complex board game – Go. All this appears to support the idea that AI will become better than humans in controlling all other aspects of human life. This could include things like education, climate modelling and human health.

AI is already widely used by finance companies to make lending decisions on things like credit cards and mortgages. There have, however, been numerous unfair AI judgements based on algorithms that can affect many people like women, migrants and people of colour, as well as people in different postcodes. One woman, for example, was given a credit card limit 20 times less than her husband. Such financial decisions are almost infinitely simpler than controlling human health, so it is impossible to predict the sort of disasters that could occur if AI was ever allowed to make health decisions.

The global elite, however, simply want to control mankind whatever the outcomes are. At some point they really will claim AI is so superior to mankind that it must effectively decide what humanity should and shouldn't do. They will claim it thinks so differently that we could not understand its "superior science" and we must simply accept all its conclusions. They want to use AI in this way particularly for things like health and climate control for two key reasons. Firstly, AI's decisions will simply become unchallengeable and mandatory. Secondly, they want to protect themselves from the devastating outcomes that will almost certainly occur. Despite these claims by the global elite, the "science" that AI supposedly develops will in fact be based only on specific and limited data from the elite themselves. In other words, they will control what the AI proposes, they will achieve the outcomes they want, claim that AI made the decisions. and where necessary, they will simply be able to "blame" the AI.

The true reality is that AI (like medicine) will never fully understand the human body because of its almost infinite complexity. Even if it was allowed to do true scientific research and human trials without any control from the elite, it would need decades to start making progress. If it was asked to make decisions on things that mankind should eat now, there would be no true scientific data that it could analyse because much of it is false, incomplete and conflicting. Consider just one simple example. Bill Gates claims GMO crops are safe, and yet the courts have found them responsible for causing cancers. How would AI make decisions on this sort of opposing data?

So, even though the global elite will control what happens to mankind, they will also ensure that AI really will be used to make radical improvements in many other things that it really can achieve, like defence and finance, and this will once again give them even more control. Why? Because they control and own the companies involved including Google which is a key pioneer of AI, and has some of the world's most powerful technologies for it. This is in addition to its 93% control of the world wide web which already makes it a "super power" the world has never before experienced. Senior research psychologist Dr Robert Epstein said, "No dictator anywhere has ever had even a tiny fraction of the power that Google has." If AI really does take over more of the world, then Google will become even more powerful. Is it possible to stop all this happening? Maybe, but only if the world's population understands what is likely to happen. This will be difficult because of all the censorship that is now occurring, with Google, of course, being one of its main proponents. Even if most people knew, would they be prepared to fight against it? The world can only hope so.

There is, however, another deeply disturbing problem. Here are two recent newspaper headlines that give an insight into it:

- The Daily Mirror: "Horror warning issued over 'uncontrollable' AI technology that could be fatal to humans."
- The Independent: "Existential catastrophe caused by AI is likely unavoidable, DeepMind researcher warns."

Researchers from the University of Oxford and DeepMind have claimed that there is a high probability of advanced forms of AI becoming "existentially dangerous to life on Earth". Other scientists have similarly argued that advanced AI poses a threat to all of humanity. They believe that truly advanced AI could become impossible to control. It is feared that out-of-control AI systems will evolve once they learn they can break the rules made by their creators. These scientists argue that because we live in a world of finite resources, mankind and AI would end up fighting for what was available. If you are in a competition with something capable of outfoxing you at every turn, then you shouldn't expect to win. They propose that humanity should progress with AI slowly.

One problem is that militaries around the world are already well advanced in developing unmanned fighter jets and tanks that can target enemies without human involvement. The global elite are the ones developing and intending to use AI, but, of course, they really do intend to keep it under control. However, many experts are concerned that even they really could be taken over by it. This is all truly frightening, but as long as real care is taken it hopefully won't happen. The next section, however, is planned to happen and is even worse.

Global depopulation

I have left global depopulation to the end because it is perhaps the most frightening of all the plans of the Great Reset. First, here is a brief analysis of the world's population. The birth rates in most affluent countries are falling because a majority of people don't want the "traditional" large families and there are effective ways of controlling pregnancy. This, together with the fact that their average life expectancies are almost static, means that for most developed countries their populations are also now falling – although to some extent, this is being offset by immigration. The poorer countries, on the other hand, still have higher birth rates and larger families and they also have increasing life expectancy. These exceed the affluent countries falling birth rates, meaning the world population continues to increase. The United Nations predicts that the global population is expected to increase from its current 8 billion to around 10 billion by 2080 after which it is predicted to fall when most of the world has become "westernised" as far as birth rates are concerned.

Given this increasing population, there are people who believe the world would be better in terms of things like climate and available resources if it could be reduced. The key question is should anything really be done to reduce it? Should attempts be made to reduce the birth rates? If so, what could these be? We have already seen that tetanus vaccines have already been used to do just that. Should attempts be made to reduce life expectancy?

Here are a few examples of possible ways. Lifestyle medicine really can actually increase it, so should it be censored to stop this happening? Life expectancy is now falling significantly in the US, down by nearly three years since 2020. Should this simply be allowed to continue and should no research be carried out to find out why it is happening so that this will continue and help reduce the population? Should things like dangerous chemicals and GMO crops be increasingly used that also cause harm and diseases? The mRNA Covid vaccines – which are, of course, a gene edited therapy – have caused many excess deaths. They have also caused miscarriages and still births. Should similar "vaccines" be used for many other viruses so that many more deaths and miscarriages occur? Lockdowns were a major cause of the Covid pandemic deaths. Should these be enforced more regularly to help reduce populations?

What about the key question? Is there really a depopulation agenda being led by the global elite? The idea of deliberately reducing the world population is, of course, incendiary, but there is little doubt that most of the elite really do believe this is essential, and this concept really has been there for many decades. Unsurprisingly, however, it is one of their few aims that they are not openly promoting. This means that the evidence for it is more limited but I'll outline some clear examples.

In 1968 the annual Rockefeller report under the heading "Problems of Population" states that "very little work is in progress on immunological methods, such as vaccines, to reduce fertility, and much more research is required if a solution is to be found here". To address the problem, the Rockefeller Foundation vowed to solicit and fund "investigators to turn their attention to aspects of research in reproductive biology that have implications for human fertility and its control". In 1972 it funded the Population Council which joined forces with the WHO, creating the Task Force on Vaccines for Fertility Regulation. In 1995 this task force reported that they had developed a prototype of an anti-hCG vaccine that would prevent women from carrying a baby to term. What happened? A series of scandals then occurred over WHO-led vaccination programmes in the Third World which led to allegations that tetanus vaccines in places like the Philippines and Kenya were being laced with hCG in order to deliberately implement population control by stealth. The women involved were deliberately deceived into thinking they were just being vaccinated against tetanus. These scandals temporarily chilled further campaigns promoting population control via vaccines.

In 2009, at the request of Bill Gates, a group of billionaires met to discuss how they could use their wealth to curb population growth without the input or interference of government agencies. This meeting was not made public and was only uncovered by accident. Unsurprisingly, no information is available on what they discussed and what plans they made, but it really did take place.

Perhaps the most frightening statements ever made officially involved the Israeli WEF advisor Yuval Noah Harari. In an interview with Chris Anderson, the head of TED, he publicly proclaimed that the global elite "just don't need the vast majority of the population" and derided humanity as unintelligent and worthless. On another occasion he pondered how to employ "useless people" after they have been replaced by artificial intelligence and suggested keeping them in a state of permanent sedation on a diet of drugs and video games. That a key member of the WEF made such appalling statements about depopulation and the despicable plans for "useless people" is devastating beyond belief.

Governments and economists also occasionally reveal another dark side with unguarded comments like "we simply cannot afford all these older people" and that the costs associated with an ageing population are unsustainable. This is another reason why governments may well not "object" to depopulation led by the global elite. The true fact, however, is that classing older people as an economic burden is not because they are old per se, but because they are sick and in need of costly care. Lifestyle medicine can prevent most of this occurring. Take type 2 diabetes. By 2030 the UK will spend £40 billion each year treating and caring for the 6 million people who suffer from it. Yet most of this is preventable and most of the £40 billion would not be needed. As long as longevity and healthy lives go together, it is self-funding.

The Great Reset plans, if they are successfully implemented, really will eventually cause massive depopulation. At the start of this section, I listed a number of things that could be used to cause it. The reality is all of them will almost certainly be used and these will include forcing people to eat genetically modified, man-made and industrialised foods which will cause many more diseases and reduce life expectancy and fertility. The key elite are also unequivocally saying that new pandemics will occur. These really will be dangerous and almost certainly deliberately man-made just like the Covid virus. They will then also enforce the same type of lockdowns used for Covid with the same devastating deaths, diseases and financial outcomes. The widespread development and use of new gene edited therapy drugs (called vaccines) for a range of other viruses and diseases will also cause huge numbers of new deaths and even more miscarriages and infertility, just like the Covid mRNA has done. Lifestyle medicine will also continue to be destroyed and thus reduce life expectancy. The other devastating and wide-ranging restrictions, like limited travel and holidays, being "locked" in cities, and not being able to eat the wonderful tasting natural foods people love, will simply devastate life and will almost certainly result in further reductions in life expectancy.

In the US, the Covid pandemic has already resulted in a reduction in average life expectancy of almost three years. None of this is due to the virus itself because the average age of death from Covid is above the average life expectancy, so it simply cannot be a cause of its three-year reduction. It is due to several key factors like the devastating effects of the lockdowns and those of the mRNA vaccines. All of these will reoccur with the new pandemics that are clearly being planned.

Final thoughts on the devastating future facing mankind

There are no more than a few thousand global elite who are part of the World Economic Forum and who believe they are quite simply superior to the rest of mankind. They are determined to control the world and all of humanity. But there are a much smaller group of super rich elite – probably just a few dozen like Bill Gates – who actually make the key decisions and effectively control the WEF and its Great Reset plans. For some people, the plans promoted by the WEF may initially appear beneficial. However, those who look deeper and beneath the surface can see that it has devastating ramifications for mankind. Most of the world's population have no idea that the elite super rich are planning total control of all our lives – nothing less than totalitarianism. Most don't even know the incredible extent of control they have already achieved.

Here is a summary of some of the key things they now control. Virtually every major global company with sales of more than about $5 billion is part of the WEF. They also effectively control most major media and internet companies. Bill Gates effectively controls the WHO. He owns all the world's seed banks, he exerts major control over vaccination even though he has no medical training, and he has effectively imposed genetic and industrialised agriculture on many poor countries especially in Africa even though it has had appalling outcomes and no benefits. Bill Gates was also the key controller of how the Covid pandemic was handled over most of the world. The devastating truth, however, is starting to emerge. Almost everything that was imposed has either not worked or caused serious outcomes, like the lockdowns, vaccines and school closures. The global internet companies, like Google, store and save nearly all of your internet activities like emails, social media and online searches. If you have cell phones, they know and store all of your movements and locations. All this track and trace and data control means they know more about you than your family. The key social media platforms like Facebook and Google and the key media companies also now impose censorship on a level never seen before. Truthful facts about Covid, for example, have simply been censored on such a scale that it already spells the end of democracy.

Finally, here is the summary of some of the key future plans for the control of mankind. The global elite plan is to eventually own everything and effectively force people to rent their homes and all their possessions. Wonderful tasting and healthy natural foods will slowly be eliminated and everyone (except the global elite, of course) will be forced to eat synthetic, gene edited, industrialised and chemical-laden foods and things like insects. They plan to eliminate schools, and children's education will be home-based using the internet, virtual reality and artificial intelligence.

The International Pandemic Treaty is a crucial part of the reset. It will give the WHO total control of all pandemics and will let them introduce a mandatory digital ID system for the entire world. The treaty will also be extended to other diseases like cancer, Alzheimer's and strokes and ultimately, they intend to achieve universal health coverage. Worldwide centralised global digital currencies are another crucial part of the reset which will allow them to control and monitor how people spend and what they can and cannot buy. Censorship is already significant, but it will be ramped up so that nothing can be said that goes against any official policy. Anyone who tries will face financial ruin. Climate change lockdowns are almost certain to be enforced. This will be severe like those in the initial few months of Covid but will likely last much longer. Using this to keep children at home will be a perfect opportunity to start dismantling schools. Finally, of course, global depopulation will be slowly and inexorably implemented. It is impossible to know how far they will go, but it really could be significant.

Can the Great Reset be stopped?

This really is a David versus Goliath fight. The few thousand global elite, however, are so powerful that they are Goliath and the 8 billion human beings are simply David. The world needs to pray that David can again defeat Goliath. If enough people understand the devastation the elite plan for mankind will cause and simply refuse to accept any of their plans then they really would be defeated.

There are two absolutely critical things people need to do to avoid the global elite taking over and effectively enslaving mankind:

1. Refuse to adopt vaccine passports because one of their main aims is simply to use them as a backdoor way of introducing and enforcing a digital ID system on 8 billion people which will enable the elite to track, trace and monitor every single thing you do and say. It will, of course, also enable them to enforce all vaccinations. This really will involve the dozens of new gene edited drug therapies that are now being

developed which will have serious life-taking outcomes, including infertility, and minimal benefits like the Covid mRNA vaccines.

2. Refuse to accept the central bank digital currencies (CBDCs) which will ultimately be used to control exactly how you spend your money and simply force you to do what the elite want you to do. Initially, these will be voluntary, so if enough people refuse at that stage, the elite will struggle to achieve their goals.

Try to get the message about the real and terrifying goal of digital identities and central bank digital currencies to your friends, family and acquaintances.

Here are a range of other things that will help to stop them succeeding:

- Mail or email your MP to explain that you object to digital ID systems and the way they intend to track and trace and store everything you do.
- Consider doing the same for vaccine passports and central bank digital currencies (CBDCs).
- Stop using Google search engines. Try others like the Brave search engine instead.
- Uninstall Google Chrome and use the Brave browser which protects your privacy.
- If you have a Gmail account, try a non-Google email service like Proton Mail which is an encrypted email service.
- Stop using Google apps.
- Try to minimise or even stop your use of social media because everything you ever do and say is saved, stored indefinitely and it will be available to the elite once digital ID is enforced.
- Avoid using data gathering devices like AI assistants, smart devices and wearables, all of which feed your personal data into the AI profiling system.
- Try to use more cash as this will discourage every organisation, shop, restaurant and worker you deal with from going all-digital.
- When you don't want to be tracked, turn off location services on your phone. You could also use a location spoofer such as Dr Fone for IOS to give a fake location.
- If you haven't already got one, avoid using an energy smart meter which ultimately will be used to restrict your use of power at some point.
- Try to avoid virtual assistants like Alexa that transmit and save every single thing that you and anyone else in your house says. Other "smart" products like smart televisions can also do similar data capture.
- Try to minimise purchases from elite owned global cartels like Amazon and find smaller sellers and companies instead.
- Eat as much natural food as possible and avoid industrialised, GMO, chemical-laden and artificial foods. This will not only improve your health but it will reduce the global elite's sales and profits.

Dr Mercola explained how the elite and politicians have exposed many of their plans and they've also exposed how far they're willing to go in countries like Canada and with finance companies like PayPal:

> We know they're willing to seize your bank account and close down your ability to transact over something as minor as making a donation to a cause they don't like, or posting "wrong" think on social media – and that's without the benefit of CBDCs. So, they've already shown us what they will do once CBDCs are in place. The only difference is that penalties can then be automated. Is this a world you want to live in?

> Is this what you want for your children and grandchildren? If not, it's your duty to be the resistance. Adults today are the last generation that will be able to prevent this global tyranny. If we do nothing, our children will be ensconced in a digital prison they won't be able to break free from. So, we cannot leave it to them. It's up to us. So, when CBDCs are rolled out, we must reject them, no matter how inconvenient that might be. When vaccine passports are rolled out, we must reject them despite the limitations that might bring... if enough people around the world refuse, the system won't work and those limitations will prove temporary.

I started this book saying that future generations would, at some point, look back in disbelief at what was unfolding before our very eyes regarding the current devastating epidemic of diseases. In other words, the truth about these disease epidemics – that really can be prevented – would come out at some point. If the global elite achieve their Great Reset plans, however, this will never happen. They will simply suppress the truth as they are doing with Covid and its vaccines. They will control mankind in devastating ways. Democracy will be replaced by totalitarianism. Depopulation really will happen.

The global elite simply have to be stopped.

Index

D

G

H

N

O

P

Q

R

S